Perinatal Psychopharmacology

Faruk Uguz • Laura Orsolini
Editors

Perinatal Psychopharmacology

Second Edition

Springer

Editors
Faruk Uguz
Department of Psychiatry, Medova Hospital
Faculty of Medicine, KTO Karatay
University
Konya, Türkiye

Laura Orsolini
Unit of Clinical Psychiatry, Department
of Experimental and Clinical Medicine
(DIMSC) Faculty of Medicine and Surgery
Polytechnic University of Marche
Ancona, Italy

ISBN 978-3-031-99719-8 ISBN 978-3-031-99720-4 (eBook)
https://doi.org/10.1007/978-3-031-99720-4

This Springer imprint is published by the registered company Springer Nature Switzerland AG
The registered company address is: Gewerbestrasse 11, 6330 Cham, Switzerland

Contents

Part I Introduction to Perinatal Psychopharmacology

1 Epidemiology of Use of Psychotropic Drugs in Pregnant and Nursing Women 3
Sura Alwan and Anick Berard

2 Maternal and Infant Pharmacokinetics of Psychotropic Medications During Pregnancy and Lactation 21
Nikolaos Kokras, Eleni Poulogiannopoulou, Marinos G. Sotiropoulos, and Christina Dalla

3 Safety Parameters and Risk Categories Used for Psychotropic Drugs in Pregnancy and Lactation 45
Yusuf Cem Kaplan, Hilal Erol, and Elif Keskin-Arslan

4 General Approach to Psychopharmacological Treatment During the Perinatal Period 65
Cesario Bellantuono

5 The Role of Paternal Mental Health During the Perinatal Period: From Preconception to Postpartum 79
Giulia Francesconi, Rosa Volgare, Umberto Volpe, and Laura Orsolini

Part II Safety of Psychotropic Drugs During Pregnancy and Lactation

6 Antidepressants in Pregnancy 101
Esra Yazıcı and Özlem Akçay Ciner

7 Antidepressants During Lactation 139
Pierre Desaunay, Camille Blouet, Mélanie Alexandre, and Fabian Guénolé

8 Antipsychotics in Pregnancy 167
Carolyn Breadon and Jayashri Kulkarni

9 Antipsychotics During Lactation 237
Adele C. Viguera, Alexia M. Jones, Joshua Niforatos, and Carrie Swetlik

10 Mood Stabilizers in Pregnancy 261
Anne-Laure Sutter-Dallay and Florence Gressier

11 Mood Stabilizers During Lactation 275
Sandeep Grover, Devakshi Dua, and Nidhi Yadav

12 Benzodiazepines and Z-Drugs in Pregnancy 289
Cesario Bellantuono

13 Benzodiazepines and Z-Drugs During Lactation 303
Betül Bakay and Faruk Uguz

14 Miscellaneous Drugs During Pregnancy and Lactation 311
Hasan Bakay

Part III Pharmacological Management of Psychiatric Disorders During the Perinatal Period

15 Major Depression 331
Sonya Rasminsky and Vivien K. Burt

16 Bipolar Disorder 349
Michael Thomson and Verinder Sharma

17 Schizophrenia and Related Psychoses 371
Selma Bozkurt

18 Obsessive-Compulsive Disorder 383
Faruk Uguz

19 Anxiety Disorders 401
Benyamin Daniel Daniel, Caterina Dell'Anna, and Carlo Marchesi

20 Posttraumatic Stress Disorder 427
Mine Sahingoz and Serap Sari

21 RETRACTED CHAPTER: Alcohol Use Disorders 447
Laura Orsolini, Rosa Volgare, Giulia Francesconi, Giovanni Martinotti, and Umberto Volpe

22 Substance Use Disorders 467
Laura Orsolini, Giulia Francesconi, Rosa Volgare, Fabrizio Schifano, and Umberto Volpe

23 Pharmacological Approaches to Managing Common Sleep Disorders 495
Laura Palagini

24 Psychiatric Aspect and Psychopharmacologic Treatment of Hyperemesis Gravidarum 535
Goksen Yuksel

Retraction Note to: Alcohol Use Disorders C1
Laura Orsolini, Rosa Volgare, Giulia Francesconi, Giovanni Martinotti, and Umberto Volpe

Part I

Introduction to Perinatal Psychopharmacology

Epidemiology of Use of Psychotropic Drugs in Pregnant and Nursing Women

1

Sura Alwan and Anick Berard

1.1 Introduction

Psychiatric disorders include a wide range of illnesses that are usually chronic and relapsing during an individual's lifespan. The most commonly encountered psychiatric disorders include depression, bipolar affective disorder, schizophrenia, obsessive-compulsive disorder, and anxiety disorders. Women of reproductive age are more likely to develop some of these common conditions (Deierlein et al. 2024) and can be specifically vulnerable when they are affected in the perinatal period, defined as "including the entire period of pregnancy, the periconception period and up to 12 months postpartum" (Koukopoulos et al. 2020). In the United Kingdom (UK), it is estimated that about 25% of women aged 20–35 years who commit suicide do so in the perinatal period, and that these women were twice as likely to have been receiving mental healthcare mostly with regard to anxiety and depression illnesses (Kim and Silver 2016). Another study that reviewed pregnancy-related mental health deaths, including suicides and accidental overdoses, in the United States (US) indicated 11% of pregnancy-related deaths to be due to mental health conditions and that three-quarters of people with a pregnancy-related mental health cause of death had a history of depression; more than two-thirds had past or current substance use (Trost et al. 2021).

Pregnancy is believed to be neither protective against mental illness nor a specifically high-risk period. There appears to be no significant differences in the prevalence of psychiatric and mood disorders between pregnant and non-pregnant women

S. Alwan (✉)
Department of Medical Genetics, University of British Columbia, Vancouver, BC, Canada
e-mail: alwans@bcchr.ca

A. Berard
Faculty of Pharmacy, University of Montreal, and Research Center, CHU Sainte-Justine, Montreal, QC, Canada

F. Uguz, L. Orsolini (eds.), *Perinatal Psychopharmacology*,
https://doi.org/10.1007/978-3-031-99720-4_1

of reproductive age (Mota et al. 2019). Few studies, however, report on the impact of pregnancy on severe mental and psychiatric conditions (Vigod et al. 2014; Molenaar et al. 2023). Bipolar disorder has been most studied in this regard, and it appears that its overall recurrence risk in the perinatal period may exceed 70% (Alcantarilla et al. 2023; Perry et al. 2021). Furthermore, untreated maternal mental and psychiatric illness in pregnancy can have negative impacts on both the mother and the baby by increasing the risk of developing postpartum depression and maternal suicidal thoughts (Hagatulah et al. 2024). When left untreated, these conditions can also lead to unhealthy lifestyle habits adversely affecting pregnancy outcome, such as poor nutrition, smoking, alcohol drinking, and substance use (Wohrer et al. 2024), and developing certain conditions, including diabetes and other pregnancy complications, such as pre-eclampsia (Kozhimannil et al. 2009; Bergink et al. 2015). There is also evidence in the literature that untreated maternal mental illness itself, including stress and other psychiatric conditions, is associated with various adverse pregnancy outcomes including spontaneous abortions (Nikfar et al. 2012), preterm birth, low birth weight, intrauterine growth restriction, and operative delivery (Mohamed et al. 2023; Walsh et al. 2019), as well as long-term neurodevelopmental and health outcomes (Caparros-Gonzalez et al. 2021).

Besides risk of the untreated illnesses, pharmacotherapy of these disorders is further complicated by concerns over potential risks to the pregnant woman and her prenatally exposed or breastfeeding infant, including structural and behavioral teratogenicity, neonatal toxicity, and other adverse reproductive outcomes. The absence of randomized control trials (RCTs) in this field due to the difficulty and ethical concerns of conducting them during pregnancy results in most safety and/or risk data being extrapolated from observational studies, which need to be interpreted carefully because of their specific potential biases. Several qualitative studies across different geographical regions found that many women were concerned about the potential adverse effects of psychotropic medications during pregnancy and the nursing period, often reporting that professional advice was lacking in detail which affected their decisions (Stevenson et al. 2016; FrayNE et al. 2023; James et al. 2024). Thus, it is essential to maintain clear communication and collaboration between healthcare providers and patients to facilitate informed decision-making regarding medication use during the perinatal period.

Fortunately, the availability of online clinical teratology knowledge databases, such as *TERIS* (https://terisweb.deohs.washington.edu) and *REPROTOX* (https://reprotox.org), has greatly simplified the process of collecting and analyzing the data from the published literature and translation into proper clinical assessment of human teratogenic risk. In addition, pharmaceutical labels are now developed in accordance with the revised US Food and Drug Administration (FDA) Pregnancy and Lactation Labeling Rule and the European Medicines Agency (EMA), along with an opportunity for alignment across regions being actively discussed (Kappel et al. 2023). Furthermore, access to information on the effects of drugs and other exposures in the perinatal period, via phone, text or online chat, is also provided to the public through Teratology Information Services (TIS) in the United States (https://mothertobaby.org), in collaboration with a Canadian platform (https://www.

healthypregnancy hub.ca), and in Europe and other parts of the world (https://www.entis-org.eu/). TIS centers continue to combine multidisciplinary expertise and consolidate knowledge from the fields of teratology, dysmorphology, toxicology, pharmacology, epidemiology, clinical genetics, obstetric medicine, infectious disease, and occupational health. Such a collaborative approach enables these services to provide timely, evidence-based information to patients and healthcare providers regarding exposures during pregnancy and breastfeeding (Alwan and Grant 2024).

1.2 Psychopharmacology in Pregnant and Nursing Women

Management of mental and psychiatric illnesses in the perinatal period is challenging and becomes more difficult when the pregnancy is unplanned, which is the case in nearly half of pregnancies (UNFPA 2022). Therefore, it is important that healthcare providers discuss pharmacological risks of pregnancy at the time of administration for all women of reproductive age as well as alternative treatment options such as psychotherapy. Psychotropic medications in the perinatal period are prescribed for women experiencing moderate to severe psychiatric conditions, whether newly developed during pregnancy or as a relapse of pre-existing disorders (Payne 2021). It is estimated that at least 10% of women are prescribed a psychotropic medication in the perinatal period (Hanley et al. 2020; Robiyanto et al. 2023; Leong et al. 2017; Bérard et al. 2019), with usage varying by geographical region, over time, and over the course of a pregnancy, underscoring the importance of continuous monitoring and evaluation of these agents in the perinatal period to inform guidelines and ensuring safety of both maternal and fetal health. Prescribed psychotropics can generally fall into five main classes of medications: antidepressants, anxiolytics, antipsychotics, mood stabilizers, and stimulants. An update on the epidemiology and patterns of use of these drug classes (and subclasses) will be discussed below.

1.2.1 Antidepressants

Depression affects about 1 in 10 women of childbearing age (Guo et al. 2018). The increasing use of antidepressants over the past two decades, specifically with regard to the selective serotonin reuptake inhibitors (SSRIs), has put these medications among the most common therapeutic prescriptions worldwide. In the United States, for example, the National Center for Health Statistics reports that between 2015 and 2018, antidepressants were the first most commonly prescribed class of medications among females (17.7%) (Brody and Gu 2020), with the rate continuing to increase significantly over the years.

Prevalence of exposure to an antidepressant at some point during pregnancy has ranged between 2% and 10% (Alwan et al. 2011; Huybrechts et al. 2013; Jimenez-Solem et al. 2013; Bénard-Laribière et al. 2018; Molenaar et al. 2020; Donald et al. 2021; Bérard et al. 2017b), with the lowest rates being reported in Scandinavian populations, while the highest observed in the United States. The increase in antidepressant use in the perinatal period over time has also been established worldwide. In Denmark, studies reported a six-fold increase in the use of an antidepressant at some point during pregnancy, where the exposure rate increased from 0.4% in 1997 to 3.1% in 2016 (Jimenez-Solem et al. 2013; Sun et al. 2019). In a study utilizing the UK Clinical Practice Research Datalink (CPRD) Pregnancy Register, antidepressant prescribing during pregnancy increased from 3.2% in 1996 to 13.4% in 2018 (Martin et al. 2024). Notably, most women discontinued antidepressant use at some point before the end of pregnancy, but post-pregnancy resumption was common. Similarly in the United States, reports of antidepressant use in pregnancy have shown increases from around 1.5% in 1996 to 8.1% in 2005 (Cooper et al. 2007; Alwan et al. 2011; Andrade et al. 2008; Huybrechts et al. 2013). A study published in 2023 analyzed data from privately insured individuals in the United States diagnosed with perinatal mood and anxiety disorders (PMAD) between 2008 and 2020 (Hall et al. 2024). The findings revealed that antidepressant prescriptions increased significantly during this period, particularly after the issuance of clinical practice recommendations in 2015–2016 regarding PMAD screening and treatment. This suggests that updated clinical guidelines may have contributed to increased access to antidepressant treatment for pregnant and postpartum individuals.

Dispensing of an antidepressant medication during pregnancy is more common among older women, non-Hispanic White race, women living in the Midwest, and those with higher education (>12 years) (Huybrechts et al. 2013; Molenaar et al. 2020). Other commonly reported predictors of antidepressant use in the perinatal period are periconceptional smoking or alcohol use and having comorbid disorders, such as pre-pregnancy type 1 or 2 diabetes and hypertension (Bakker et al. 2008; Jimenez-Solem et al. 2013; Bénard-Laribière et al. 2018).

During the course of a pregnancy, a sudden decrease in use of an antidepressant, regardless of the type, was observed in many studies around the third month of conception, which appears to be related to the time at which pregnancy was recognized and may indicate the possibility of healthcare providers being reluctant to continue treatment after the occurrence of pregnancy (Noh et al. 2022; Liu et al. 2022). However, the attempt to decrease the fetal risk of antidepressant use during pregnancy by discontinuing treatment in women with severe depression has been associated with increased risk of relapse of the depression with its associated adverse pregnancy outcomes (Bayrampour et al. 2020).

1.2.1.1 Selective Serotonin Reuptake Inhibitors

SSRIs account for about 80% of all antidepressant prescriptions and are being prescribed for a variety of conditions, other than depression (Harman et al. 2009). Fluoxetine was the first introduced SSRI in 1988 and became the most frequently prescribed antidepressant worldwide (Morrison et al. 2005). Other SSRIs currently available on the market include citalopram, and its pharmacologically active s-enantiomer, escitalopram, fluvoxamine, paroxetine, and sertraline. SSRIs share a similar mechanism of action by blocking the reuptake of serotonin (5-HT) via the serotonin transporter (SERT). However, each SSRI differs from another with regard to its chemical structure and pharmacokinetic properties (Hiemke and Hartter 2000), and therefore has the potential to affect the developing fetus in various ways.

Maternal use of SSRI medications in pregnancy has gained considerable clinical attention over the past two decades. Evidence from the literature include slightly elevated risks for organ-specific birth defects, heart defects in specific, with first-trimester exposure to certain SSRIs (De Vries et al. 2021) and risks of neonatal withdrawal syndrome and behavioral alterations (Forsberg et al. 2014), persistent pulmonary hypertension of the newborn (PPHN) (Huybrechts et al. 2015; Alwan et al. 2016; Bérard et al. 2017a), preterm birth, low birth weight and small for gestational age birth associated with late intrauterine exposure to any SSRI (Hogue et al. 2017). Although concerns have been raised with regard to elevated rates of autism spectrum disorder diagnoses in children born to mothers who were treated an SSRI in pregnancy (Kaplan et al. 2017), several large record-linkage studies suggested that such associations may not actually be causal, but instead reflect genetic and shared familial environmental factors (Brown et al. 2017; Sujan et al. 2017).

The US FDA has initially issued two public health advisories in 2005 and 2006 regarding the potential risk for cardiac defects with maternal paroxetine use, and later of PPHN in relation to any SSRI use in pregnancy, which ultimately affected the pattern of use of SSRIs among pregnant women at the time. A later advisory from the FDA in 2011 was issued, based on the results of subsequent studies, recommending healthcare providers to treat depression during pregnancy as clinically appropriate (U.S. Food and Drug Administration 2011). Additionally, in 2011, the UK's Medicines and Health Care products Regulatory Agency (MHRA) warned that first-trimester exposure to fluoxetine might slightly increase the risk of congenital cardiac malformations in newborns and also highlighted a small increased risk of postpartum hemorrhage associated with the use of SSRIs in the month before delivery. The MHRA reminded healthcare professionals of the potential risks of PPHN and neonatal withdrawal or toxicity reactions linked to these medications, emphasizing the importance of balancing these risks against the consequences of untreated depression during pregnancy.

Sertraline remains to be reported the most frequently prescribed SSRI during pregnancy in the United States and France (Bénard-Laribière et al. 2018; Andrade et al. 2016), while in other European countries, citalopram in Scandinavian countries (Jimenez-Solem et al. 2013; Kallen et al. 2013) and fluoxetine in the UK (Ban et al. 2014) have been reported to be the most commonly used SSRIs in the perinatal period. Despite the fact that paroxetine use during pregnancy has been initially contraindicated, it has been reported to be the most frequently dispensed SSRI to women in the perinatal period in Italy and the Netherlands, with no reduction in its use following the US FDA warnings (Charlton et al. 2015). In Canada, a decrease in the use of paroxetine during pregnancy has been noted (Bérard et al. 2017b), while rates for sertraline and citalopram remain to be the highest in this population.

Within the perinatal period, patterns of maternal SSRI continuation versus discontinuation also differ by geographical region. For example, in a European pharmacoepidemiologic study based on six electronic healthcare databases (Charlton et al. 2015), at least 40% of women with a prescription to an SSRI during the year before pregnancy discontinued use before pregnancy and did not restart the medication during the year following delivery. Continuing treatment with an SSRI throughout pregnancy and following delivery was more common among women in Denmark and the Netherlands compared to those living in Italy, with the lowest rates.

In terms of breastfeeding, SSRIs vary in the degree to how much they cross into breast milk, but sertraline and paroxetine appear to be more tolerated by nursing babies than other SSRIs (Uguz 2021). However, most studies regarding the safety of antidepressants among nursing women are confounded by prenatal exposure to the same drug, which may increase the risk of early adverse effects, as well as other lifestyle risk factors, including smoking and alcohol and substance abuse, and no studies exist on the long-term cognitive and behavioral development on the breastfed children.

1.2.1.2 Bupropion

Bupropion is an aminoketone that is structurally and chemically different from other antidepressants on the market. It is a weak inhibitor of neuronal uptake of dopamine, norepinephrine, and serotonin and does not inhibit monoamine oxidase (Ascher et al. 1995). It was first marketed as an oral antidepressant (Wellbutrin®) and was subsequently developed as a non-nicotine aid to smoking cessation (Zyban®). Because women who smoke are encouraged to stop doing so when they become pregnant (Tong et al. 2008), it is therefore not surprising that many women are treated with bupropion in early pregnancy (Berard et al. 2016). Regardless of the indication for use, bupropion is the second most commonly used non-SSRI antidepressant in the perinatal period, with a reported frequency of 0.7–1.0% among pregnant women in the United States (Alwan et al. 2011; Hanley and Mintzes 2014). Maternal treatment with bupropion during pregnancy appears to be relatively uncommon in Europe, though specific prevalence rates are not extensively documented.

Available data on the safety of bupropion in human pregnancy is also limited. Some studies have reported a slight increase in the rate of congenital heart defects, in particular, left ventricular outflow obstruction defects following bupropion use in early pregnancy (Alwan et al. 2010; Louik et al. 2014; Thyagarajan et al. 2012; De Vries et al. 2021), but the absolute risk was estimated at 2.1–2.8 per 1000 births.

1.2.1.3 Other Less Commonly Used Antidepressants

Tricyclic antidepressants (TCAs) were once the treatment of choice for depression and panic disorder before the introduction of SSRIs. They remain commonly used for comorbid conditions and when treatment with an SSRI has failed. About 0.2% of women are exposed to a TCA sometime during their pregnancy (Alwan et al. 2011, Hanley and Mintzes 2014), and some neonatal withdrawal symptoms have been reported with their use in late pregnancy (Ter Horst et al. 2012). The most commonly used TCA is amitriptyline, which has a mechanism of action similar to SSRIs with regard to the blocking of SERT. Some reports have shown that amitriptyline use during gestation was associated with an increased risk of birth defects and other long-term neurodevelopmental outcomes (Bérard et al. 2017b; Boukhris et al. 2017).

Selective norepinephrine reuptake inhibitors (SNRIs) work in a similar mechanism to SSRIs, but they also block the reuptake of the neurotransmitter norepinephrine along with serotonin in the brain to help relieve depression, and are also commonly prescribed for other conditions, including anxiety disorders and long-term chronic pain. SNRIs are increasingly being used in pregnancy with an overall reported frequency of up to 0.8% based on a US population (Hanley and Mintzes 2014). In a Scandinavian population-based study encompassing Denmark, Iceland, Norway, and Sweden, 0.5% of pregnant women were exposed to SNRIs (Zoega et al. 2015). Notably, SNRI use varied by country, ranging from 0.3% in Norway to 0.9% in Iceland. Additionally, the study observed a decrease in SNRI use as pregnancy progressed: 0.5% at conception, 0.4% in the first trimester, 0.3% in the second trimester, and 0.2% in the third trimester. Venlafaxine has been the most frequently used SNRI in pregnancy and lactation, with the majority of studies reporting on its safety when taken in early pregnancy (Richardson et al. 2019; Furu et al. 2015). However, some studies have indicated slightly elevated risks of cardiac defects and spontaneous abortion with early pregnancy exposure (Bérard et al. 2017b; Anderson et al. 2020; Kolding et al. 2021).

1.2.2 Anxiolytics

Anxiety constitutes the most common mental disorder among women of reproductive age, and specifically women in the perinatal period. In fact, it appears to be that among women taking antidepressant medications in pregnancy, anxiety diagnoses are nearly as common as depressive diagnoses, and antidepressant users with an anxiety disorder are twice as many as antidepressant users with a depression disorder (Hanley and Mintzes 2014). Even though there is evidence in the literature that maternal stress and anxiety in the perinatal period can negatively affect both mother and baby (Monk et al. 2020), women's perceived concerns of the teratogenic risk of medications may lead to low adherence and discontinuation of needed therapy upon recognition of pregnancy (Denton et al. 2020). Nevertheless, antianxiety medications, or anxiolytics, are the second most commonly used medications in the perinatal period after antidepressants. Anxiolytics include benzodiazepine and benzodiazepine-like medications. Most women often use benzodiazepines to manage anxiety as needed more than regularly. A few studies have looked into patterns of use of anxiolytics in the perinatal period, and in one US study, the rate of use of benzodiazepines and benzodiazepine-like medications was estimated at 3.9% in pregnancy, with zolpidem being the most common one dispensed among pregnant women (2.4%) followed by alprazolam (0.8%) (Hanley and Mintzes 2014). Diazepine use in pregnancy was much lower at 0.6% and only 0.05% refilled more than one prescription for it in pregnancy, which is probably related to its association with cleft lip and palate in the infant in earlier reports that have not been confirmed in several later studies and reviews (Iqbal et al. 2002). Notably, anxiolytic use was more frequently initiated during pregnancy (2.7% incident users) than continued from preconception (1.2% prevalent users), suggesting that some women may begin anxiolytic treatment after becoming pregnant (Hanley and Mintzes 2014). Another study focusing on benzodiazepine dispensing patterns among commercially insured pregnant women in the United States from 2007 to 2015 highlighted a significantly increased shift of prescribing these medications in recent years (Qato and Gandhi 2021). In this study, benzodiazepine dispensing increased in the pre-conception period from 2.3% to 3.8%, first trimester from 1.1% to 2.1%, and second trimester from 0.3% to 0.5%; however, it decreased post-delivery from 2.4% to 2.1%. However, it is important to note that maternal use of benzodiazepines during pregnancy has been associated with certain risks, including an increased likelihood of spontaneous abortions (Sheehy et al. 2019) and potential congenital anomalies (Grigoriadis et al. 2019). Therefore, short acting prescription should be prioritized during this period.

1.2.3 Antipsychotics

Use of antipsychotic medications is indicated for a number of conditions, including psychosis, schizophrenia, and bipolar disorder. However, use of antipsychotics has increased over the past two decades, partly because the approved indications for these agents have expanded beyond these conditions to also include depression, obsessive-compulsive disorder, anxiety disorders, and autism spectrum disorders (Olfson et al. 2012; Alexander et al. 2011). Apparently, as many as 25% of patients with depression and up to 50% of patients with bipolar disorder also have psychotic symptoms (Smith and Dubovsky 2017). The rate of antipsychotic medication use during pregnancy has also increased over time (Toh et al. 2013; Robiyanto et al. 2023), and their use in pregnancy constitutes an important clinical challenge because of concern over their risk to the fetus. Reported adverse outcomes of prenatal antipsychotic use include congenital malformations, preterm birth, small for gestational age (Terrana et al. 2015; Coughlin et al. 2015), as well as short-term delay in development and lower neuromotor performance (Peng et al. 2013; Johnson et al. 2012).

Confounding by indication could not be ruled out in the observed increased prevalences of adverse outcomes. Schizophrenia is the best studied in pregnancy, and the untreated condition appears to be associated with low birth weight, small for gestational age infants, and preterm delivery (Lin et al. 2010). It is important to note that schizophrenia patients are more likely to have unplanned pregnancies along with lower educational levels and higher body mass indices (BMI), as well as adverse lifestyles, including smoking and alcohol use and lower adherence to multivitamin (Habermann et al. 2013), all of which may contribute to an increased risk of adverse pregnancy outcomes. Furthermore, since psychosis interferes with commitment with prenatal care and parenting, it is believed that risks of not managing schizophrenia outweigh risks of managing it therapeutically (Edinoff et al. 2022). However, indications for use of both first-generation and second-generation antipsychotics include depression in more than 50% of cases, followed by bipolar disorder and schizophrenia (Toh et al. 2013).

1.2.3.1 First Generation Antipsychotics (FGAs)

The neuroleptic FGAs, also known as the typical antipsychotics, were the first antipsychotic treatment of choice for psychiatric disorders. These medications act through blocking dopamine receptors in the dopaminergic pathways of the brain, as excessive dopamine release is associated with psychotic experiences. The most commonly used agents of this class in the general population and among women in the perinatal period are chlorpromazine and haloperidol. Because they have been available longer on the market, they have an established safety record as monotherapy, specifically with regard to haloperidol (Patton et al. 2002; Straub et al. 2022). However, over a ten-year period between 2001 and 2010, the rate of use of FGA drugs during pregnancy in the US population has remained constant at 0.1% (Park et al. 2017), which is probably due to the recently introduced atypical antipsychotics among women of reproductive age (Robiyanto et al. 2023). Over the course of a pregnancy, the prevalence of FGA use is reported highest in the first trimester then drops by the second and third trimesters (Toh et al. 2013), indicative of inadvertent exposures before the pregnancy is diagnosed.

1.2.3.2 Second-Generation Antipsychotics (SGAs)

The first atypical antipsychotic, clozapine, was introduced in the 1960s and has been widely used since then. Subsequently, several SGA agents became available in the market in the past three decades and have received approval for various indications, including irritability in autism spectrum disorders, mood stabilization in bipolar disorder, and additional therapy for major depression. The diagnoses of these conditions have notably increased, leading to a significant rise in SGA use among the general population, which also translated during the perinatal period. For example, a threefold increase in the prevalence of use of SGA among pregnant women in the United States, from 0.4% to 1.3% over a ten-year period, has been reported (Park et al. 2017), with the most frequently reported SGA used being quetiapine and aripiprazole. In the same study, polytherapy with other antipsychotics and antidepressants is reported in more than half of pregnant women on an SGA, and about 25% of them also take a mood stabilizer or a benzodiazepine simultaneously.

In Europe, the prevalence of women on antipsychotic medications in general is lower than in the United States, and ranges between 0.1% and 0.3% (Margulis et al. 2014). About 50% of women discontinue therapy with an SGA upon recognition of pregnancy, while 60–70% stop taking an SGA by the third trimester of pregnancy (Park et al. 2017). Furthermore, among those who switch at the beginning of pregnancy, the majority are reported to switch to quetiapine (Park et al. 2017). The overall prevalence of antipsychotic use in pregnancy in the Netherlands doubled due to increased use (in terms of both continuation and initiation of SGAs), which escalated from 0.3 in 1994 to 2.6 per 1000 in 2011 (Robiyanto et al. 2023).

It is not surprising that quetiapine is most reported among women in the perinatal period as it has a wide range of off-label indications such as generalized anxiety disorder, insomnia, and post-traumatic stress disorder (PTSD) in addition to its approved uses for bipolar disorder and schizophrenia (Maan et al. 2025). Quetiapine also has an established safety profile including a lower placental transfer compared to other antipsychotics (Creeley and Denton 2019), and is recommended for nursing women with low concentrations of the drug passed into breastmilk (Van Boekholt et al. 2015).

1.2.4 Mood Stabilizers

Due to the chronic nature of bipolar disorder with a relapsing-remitting course, most patients require long-term treatment with several psychotropics, particularly with mood stabilizers. There has been an increase in bipolar disorder diagnoses among women in the perinatal period, which is consistent with the increase observed in the general population, possibly due to improved classification of people who were previously misdiagnosed as having unipolar depression or overdiagnosis of this condition (Masters et al. 2022). Evidence also shows increased recurrence of the condition during the perinatal and postpartum periods, especially after abrupt discontinuation of mood stabilizers (Wesseloo et al. 2016). Whether treated or untreated, bipolar disorder may increase the risk of various adverse pregnancy, obstetric, and neonatal outcomes which may be worse in untreated cases (Rusner et al. 2016; Boden et al. 2012).

Mood stabilizers that are used to treat bipolar disorder include lithium and anti-epileptic drugs, most commonly, carbamazepine and valproate. Lithium is the only medication consistently shown to be effective for acute mania, bipolar depression, and long-term relapse prevention (Smith and Dubovsky 2017). Lithium use in early pregnancy has been associated with an increased risk of congenital heart defects (Patorno et al. 2017; Hastie et al. 2021). Prenatal diagnosis by fetal echocardiography should be offered to women who have been treated with lithium in early pregnancy. Both valproic acid and carbamazepine are contraindicated in pregnancy because of their association with high prevalences of malformations and other adverse outcomes, including long-term neurodevelopmental disorders (Blotière et al. 2020). On the contrary, both medications are considered for nursing because of their low serum levels in breast milk, but close monitoring is still recommended (Wisner and Perel 1998; Kacirova et al. 2019). As per the product labelling, lithium is not recommended for nursing mothers because of the risk of accumulation while the neonatal kidney is still immature. However, a recent study suggests that with careful monitoring, lithium use among nursing women might be feasible (Viguera et al. 2007; Heinonen et al. 2022).

The use of lithium during pregnancy and breastfeeding varies significantly across different regions and clinical practices, influenced by concerns about potential risks to both mother and infant, even though it has been recommended as the first-line mood-stabilizing treatment during pregnancy (Poels et al. 2018). In Denmark, a study revealed that only 16% of pregnant women with bipolar disorder continued lithium therapy, with just 6.3% maintaining usage into the third trimester (Broeks et al. 2017). Similarly, in the UK, high discontinuation rates were observed, with only 17 out of 52 pregnant women persisting with lithium treatment (McCrea et al. 2015). In terms of breastfeeding, a retrospective review at a single academic medical center from 2013 to 2023 found that 39% of postpartum patients on lithium chose to nurse their babies (Kummerlowe et al. 2024). Most of these patients had been on long-term lithium therapy, initiating treatment prior to pregnancy.

These patterns underscore the need for individualized risk-benefit assessments and multidisciplinary collaboration when considering lithium therapy during pregnancy and breastfeeding. Ongoing research and education are essential to support informed decision-making and ensure the safety and well-being of both mother and child.

1.2.5 Stimulants

Prescription stimulants, including amphetamines and methylphenidate, are a group of psychoactive drugs that affect the central nervous system and the autonomic nervous system, and used to treat attention-deficit hyperactivity disorder (ADHD) and narcolepsy. A significant increase in the use of stimulants among women of reproductive age has been observed in the past decade in different parts of the world. The percentage of females aged 15–44 years with prescription stimulant fillings increased from 3.6% in 2016 to 4.1% in 2021 in the United States (Danielson et al. 2023). In Norway, the prevalence of ADHD medication use among females aged 18–64 years increased nearly sixfold, from 3.0 per 1000 in 2006 to 18.1 per 1000 in 2022 (Hartz et al. 2024). In a Canadian study, a rising 14-fold from 0.08% in 1998 to 1.2% in 2015 was reported, with methylphenidate use being the most common (Lemelin et al. 2021). Many women opt for discontinuation of stimulants upon recognition of pregnancy because of lack of knowledge on their safety. Another US study utilizing data from 2013 to 2018 found that among 15,413 pregnancies with pre-pregnancy stimulant use, 42% discontinued treatment before conception, 39% during the first trimester, and only 19% continued into later trimesters (Murugappan et al. 2022). A Danish cohort study reported nearly 60% of women discontinued ADHD medication during pregnancy, whereas 17.2% halted medication during pregnancy but resumed after delivery (Bang Madsen et al. 2024). These findings underscore the prevalent pattern of discontinuing stimulant medications during pregnancy, primarily due to uncertainties regarding their safety.

1.3 Conclusion

In balancing the necessity of pharmacotherapy for pregnant or nursing women with psychiatric conditions, it is imperative to evaluate the risks posed by medication exposure to the unborn child against the dangers of untreated maternal illness. Although confounding by indication has been a common limitation in earlier studies affecting both treatment decisions and outcomes, recent observational studies have significantly improved methodologically, particularly in their ability to adjust for indication. This improved understanding aids decision-makers to better inform their patients with effective and safe therapy choices. However, pregnant women are often affected by more than one mental health disorder and may require combination therapy with various psychotropic drugs, which can complicate treatment decisions. Consequently, given the high prescription rates and expanding indications for these drugs among women of reproductive age, it is essential to have a comprehensive risk assessment understanding of pharmacotherapy options. This ensures that treatment decisions and preconception planning are based on the best available evidence, optimizing outcomes for both mother and child.

References

Alcantarilla L, López-Castro M, Betriu M, Torres A, Garcia C, Solé E, Gelabert E, Roca-Lecumberri A. Risk factors for relapse or recurrence in women with bipolar disorder and recurrent major depressive disorder in the perinatal period: a systematic review. Arch Womens Ment Health. 2023;26:737–54.

Alexander GC, Gallagher SA, Mascola A, Moloney RM, Stafford RS. Increasing off-label use of antipsychotic medications in the United States, 1995-2008. Pharmacoepidemiol Drug Saf. 2011;20:177–84.

Alwan S, Grant KS. Maternal medication use in pregnancy: a narrative review on assessing and communicating the "risk" of birth defects to the patient. Pharmacoepidemiology. 2024;3:336–49.

Alwan S, Reefhuis J, Botto LD, Rasmussen SA, Correa A, Friedman JM. Maternal use of bupropion and risk for congenital heart defects. Am J Obstet Gynecol. 2010;203(52):e1–6.

Alwan S, Reefhuis J, Rasmussen SA, Friedman JM. Patterns of antidepressant medication use among pregnant women in a United States population. J Clin Pharmacol. 2011;51:264–70.

Alwan S, Bandoli G, Chambers CD. Maternal use of selective serotonin-reuptake inhibitors and risk of persistent pulmonary hypertension of the newborn. Clin Pharmacol Ther. 2016;100:34–41.

Anderson KN, Lind JN, Simeone RM, Bobo WV, Mitchell AA, Riehle-Colarusso T, Polen KN, Reefhuis J. Maternal use of specific antidepressant medications during early pregnancy and the risk of selected birth defects. JAMA Psychiatry. 2020;77:1246–55.

Andrade SE, et al. Use of antidepressant medications during pregnancy: a multisite study. Am J Obstet Gynecol. 2008;198:194–5.

Andrade SE, Reichman ME, Mott K, Pitts M, Kieswetter C, Dinatale M, Stone MB, Popovic J, Haffenreffer K, Toh S. Use of selective serotonin reuptake inhibitors (SSRIs) in women delivering liveborn infants and other women of child-bearing age within the U.S. Food and Drug Administration's mini-sentinel program. Arch Womens Ment Health. 2016;19:969–77.

Ascher JA, Jo C, Colin JN, Feighner JP, Ferris RM, Fibiger HC, Golden RN, Martin P, Potter WZ, Richelson E, et al. Bupropion: a review of its mechanism of antidepressant activity. J Clin Psychiatry. 1995;56:395–401.

Bakker MK, Kölling P, et al. Increase in use of selective serotonin reuptake inhibitors in pregnancy during the last decade, a population-based cohort study from The Netherlands. Br J Clin Pharmacol. 2008;65:600–6.

Ban L, Gibson JE, West J, Fiaschi L, Sokal R, Smeeth L, Doyle P, Hubbard RB, Tata LJ. Maternal depression, antidepressant prescriptions, and congenital anomaly risk in offspring: a population-based cohort study. BJOG. 2014;121:1471–81.

Bang Madsen K, Bliddal M, Skoglund CB, Larsson H, Munk-Olsen T, Madsen MG, Hove Thomsen P, Bergink V, Srinivas C, Cohen JM, Brikell I, Liu X. Attention-deficit hyperactivity disorder (ADHD) medication use trajectories among women in the perinatal period. CNS Drugs. 2024;38:303–14.

Bayrampour H, Kapoor A, Bunka M, Ryan D. The risk of relapse of depression during pregnancy after discontinuation of antidepressants: a systematic review and meta-analysis. J Clin Psychiatry. 2020;81

Bénard-Laribière A, Pambrun E, Sutter-Dallay AL, Gautier S, Hurault-Delarue C, Damase-Michel C, Lacroix I, Bégaud B, Pariente A. Patterns of antidepressant use during pregnancy: a nationwide population-based cohort study. Br J Clin Pharmacol. 2018;84:1764–75.

Berard A, Zhao JP, Sheehy O. Success of smoking cessation interventions during pregnancy. Am J Obstet Gynecol. 2016;215:611.e1–8.

Bérard A, Sheehy O, Zhao JP, Vinet É, Bernatsky S, Abrahamowicz M. SSRI and SNRI use during pregnancy and the risk of persistent pulmonary hypertension of the newborn. Br J Clin Pharmacol. 2017a;83:1126–33.

Bérard A, Zhao JP, Sheehy O. Antidepressant use during pregnancy and the risk of major congenital malformations in a cohort of depressed pregnant women: an updated analysis of the Quebec pregnancy cohort. BMJ Open. 2017b;7:e013372.

Bérard A, Abbas-Chorfa F, Kassai B, Vial T, Nguyen KA, Sheehy O, Schott AM. The French pregnancy cohort: medication use during pregnancy in the French population. PLoS One. 2019;14:e0219095.

Bergink V, Laursen TM, Johannsen BM, Kushner SA, Meltzer-Brody S, Munk-Olsen T. Preeclampsia and first-onset postpartum psychiatric episodes: a Danish population-based cohort study. Psychol Med. 2015;45:3481–9.

Blotière PO, Miranda S, Weill A, Mikaeloff Y, Peyre H, Ramus F, Mahmoud Z, Coste J, Dray-Spira R. Risk of early neurodevelopmental outcomes associated with prenatal exposure to the antiepileptic drugs most commonly used during pregnancy: a French nationwide population-based cohort study. BMJ Open. 2020;10:e034829.

Boden R, Lundgren M, Brandt L, Reutfors J, Andersen M, Kieler H. Risks of adverse pregnancy and birth outcomes in women treated or not treated with mood stabilisers for bipolar disorder: population based cohort study. BMJ. 2012;345:e7085.

Boukhris T, Sheehy O, Berard A. Antidepressant use in pregnancy and the risk of attention deficit with or without hyperactivity disorder in children. Paediatr Perinat Epidemiol. 2017;31:363–73.

Brody DJ, Gu Q. Antidepressant use among adults: United States, 2015–2018. In: NCHS data brief. Hyattsville: National Center for Health Statistics; 2020.

Broeks SC, Thisted Horsdal H, Glejsted Ingstrup K, Gasse C. Psychopharmacological drug utilization patterns in pregnant women with bipolar disorder – a nationwide register-based study. J Affect Disord. 2017;210:158–65.

Brown HK, Ray JG, Wilton AS, Lunsky Y, Gomes T, Vigod SN. Association between serotonergic antidepressant use during pregnancy and autism Spectrum disorder in children. JAMA. 2017;317:1544–52.

Caparros-Gonzalez RA, Torre-Luque A, Romero-Gonzalez B, Quesada-Soto JM, Alderdice F, Peralta-Ramírez MI. Stress during pregnancy and the development of diseases in the offspring: a systematic-review and meta-analysis. Midwifery. 2021;97:102939.

Charlton RA, Jordan S, Pierini A, Garne E, Neville AJ, Hansen AV, Gini R, Thayer D, Tingay K, Puccini A, Bos HJ, Nybo Andersen AM, Sinclair M, Dolk H, Den Berg DJ-V, L. T. Selective serotonin reuptake inhibitor prescribing before, during and after pregnancy: a population-based study in six European regions. BJOG. 2015;122:1010–20.

Cooper WO, et al. Increasing use of antidepressants in pregnancy. Am J Obstet Gynecol. 2007;196:544–5.

Coughlin CG, Blackwell KA, Bartley C, Hay M, Yonkers KA, Bloch MH. Obstetric and neonatal outcomes after antipsychotic medication exposure in pregnancy. Obstet Gynecol. 2015;125:1224–35.

Creeley CE, Denton LK. Use of prescribed Psychotropics during pregnancy: a systematic review of pregnancy, neonatal, and childhood outcomes. Brain Sci. 2019;9:235.

Danielson MLB et al. Trends in stimulant prescription fills among commercially insured children and adults – United States, 2016–2021. MMWR Morb Mortal Wkly Rep; 2023.

De Vries C, Gadzhanova S, Sykes MJ, Ward M, Roughead E. A systematic review and meta-analysis considering the risk for congenital heart defects of antidepressant classes and individual antidepressants. Drug Saf. 2021;44:291–312.

Deierlein AL, Park C, Patel N, Gagnier R, Thorpe M. Mental health outcomes across the reproductive life course among women with disabilities: a systematic review. Arch Womens Ment Health. 2024;

Denton LK, Creeley CE, Stavola B, Hall K, Foltz BD. An analysis of online pregnancy message boards: mother-to-mother advice on medication use. Women Birth. 2020;33:e48–58.

Donald S, Sharples K, Barson D, Horsburgh S, Parkin L. Antidepressant dispensing before, during, and after pregnancy in New Zealand, 2005-2014. Aust N Z J Obstet Gynaecol. 2021;61:837–45.

Edinoff AN, Sathivadivel N, McNeil SE, et al. Antipsychotic use in pregnancy: patient mental health challenges, teratogenicity, pregnancy complications, and postnatal risks. Neurol Int. 2022;14:62–74.

Forsberg L, Navér L, Gustafsson LL, Wide K. Neonatal adaptation in infants prenatally exposed to antidepressants – clinical monitoring using neonatal abstinence score. PLoS One. 2014;9:e111327.

FrayNE J, Ellies R, Nguyen T. Experiences of decision making about psychotropic medication during pregnancy and breastfeeding in women living with severe mental illness: a qualitative study. Arch Womens Ment Health. 2023;26:379–87.

Furu K, Kieler H, Haglund B, Engeland A, Selmer R, Stephansson O, Valdimarsdottir UA, Zoega H, Artama M, Gissler M, Malm H, Nørgaard M. Selective serotonin reuptake inhibitors and venlafaxine in early pregnancy and risk of birth defects: population based cohort study and sibling design. BMJ. 2015;350:h1798.

Grigoriadis S, Graves L, Peer M, Mamisashvili L, Dennis CL, Vigod SN, Steiner M, Brown C, Cheung A, Dawson H, Rector N, Guenette M, Richter M. Benzodiazepine use during pregnancy alone or in combination with an antidepressant and congenital malformations: systematic review and meta-analysis. J Clin Psychiatry. 2019;80

Guo N, Robakis T, Miller C, Butwick A. Prevalence of depression among women of reproductive age in the United States. Obstet Gynecol. 2018;131:671–9.

Habermann F, Fritzsche J, Fuhlbruck F, Wacker E, Allignol A, Weber-Schoendorfer C, Meister R, Schaefer C. Atypical antipsychotic drugs and pregnancy outcome: a prospective, cohort study. J Clin Psychopharmacol. 2013;33:453–62.

Hagatulah N, Bränn E, Oberg AS, Valdimarsdóttir UA, Shen Q, Lu D. Perinatal depression and risk of mortality: nationwide, register based study in Sweden. BMJ. 2024;384:e075462.

Hall SV, Pangori A, Tilea A, Schroeder A, Admon LK, Zivin K. Antidepressant prescriptions increased for privately insured people with perinatal mood and anxiety disorder, 2008-20. Health Aff (Millwood). 2024;43:514–22.

Hanley GE, Mintzes B. Patterns of psychotropic medicine use in pregnancy in the United States from 2006 to 2011 among women with private insurance. BMC Pregnancy Childbirth. 2014;14:242.

Hanley GE, Miller T, Mintzes B. A cohort study of psychotropic prescription drug use in pregnancy in British Columbia, Canada from 1997 to 2010. J Womens Health (Larchmt). 2020;29:1339–49.

Harman JS, Edlund MJ, Fortney JC. Trends in antidepressant utilization from 2001 to 2004. Psychiatr Serv. 2009;60:611–6.

Hartz I, Madsstuen NHH, Andersen PN, Handal M, Odsbu I. Nationwide trends in the use of ADHD medications in the period 2006-2022: a study from the Norwegian prescription database. BMC Psychiatry. 2024;24:767.

Hastie R, Tong S, Hiscock R, Lindquist A, Lindström L, Wikström AK, Sundström-Poromaa I. Maternal lithium use and the risk of adverse pregnancy and neonatal outcomes: a Swedish population-based cohort study. BMC Med. 2021;19:291.

Heinonen E, Tötterman K, Bäck K, Sarman I, Svedenkrans J, Forsberg L. Lithium use during breastfeeding was safe in healthy full-term infants under strict monitoring. Acta Paediatr. 2022;111:1891–8.

Hiemke C, Hartter S. Pharmacokinetics of selective serotonin reuptake inhibitors. Pharmacol Ther. 2000;85:11–28.

Hogue AN, Temple-Cooper ME, Lagzdins M, Worley S, Scwersenski J, Floyd R, Saker F. Effects of in-utero exposure to selective serotonin reuptake inhibitors and venlafaxine on term and preterm infants. J Neonatal Perinatal Med. 2017;10:371–80.

Huybrechts KF, Palmsten K, Mogun H, Kowal M, Avorn J, Setoguchi-Iwata S, Hernandez-Diaz S. National trends in antidepressant medication treatment among publicly insured pregnant women. Gen Hosp Psychiatry. 2013;35:265–71.

Huybrechts KF, Bateman BT, Hernandez-Diaz S. Maternal antidepressant use and persistent pulmonary hypertension of the newborn – reply. JAMA. 2015;314:1294.

Iqbal MM, Sobhan T, Ryals T. Effects of commonly used benzodiazepines on the fetus, the neonate, and the nursing infant. Psychiatr Serv. 2002;53:39–49.

James H, Smith S, Rai D, Culpin I, Turner K. Making decisions about antidepressant use during pregnancy: a qualitative interview study of a sample of women in the United Kingdom. Br J Gen Pract. 2024;75:e440.

Jimenez-Solem E, Andersen JT, Petersen M, Broedbaek K, Andersen NL, Torp-Pedersen C, Poulsen HE. Prevalence of antidepressant use during pregnancy in Denmark, a nation-wide cohort study. PLoS One. 2013;8:e63034.

Johnson KC, Laprairie JL, Brennan PA, Stowe ZN, Newport DJ. Prenatal antipsychotic exposure and neuromotor performance during infancy. Arch Gen Psychiatry. 2012;69:787–94.

Kacirova I, Grundmann M, Brozmanova H. Valproic acid concentrations in nursing mothers, mature milk, and breastfed infants in monotherapy and combination therapy. Epilepsy Behav. 2019;95:112–6.

Kallen B, Borg N, Reis M. The use of central nervous system active drugs during pregnancy. Pharmaceuticals. 2013;6:1221–86.

Kaplan YC, Keskin-Arslan E, Acar S, Sozmen K. Maternal SSRI discontinuation, use, psychiatric disorder and the risk of autism in children: a meta-analysis of cohort studies. Br J Clin Pharmacol. 2017;83:2798–806.

Kappel D, Sahin L, Yao L, Thor S, Kweder S. A comparison of FDA and EMA pregnancy and lactation labeling. Clin Pharmacol Ther. 2023;113:1251–7.

Kim JJ, Silver RK. Perinatal suicide associated with depression diagnosis and absence of active treatment in 15-year UK national inquiry. Evid Based Ment Health. 2016;19:122.

Kolding L, Ehrenstein V, Pedersen L, Sandager P, Petersen OB, Uldbjerg N, Pedersen LH. Antidepressant use in pregnancy and severe cardiac malformations: Danish register-based study. BJOG. 2021;128:1949–57.

Koukopoulos AE, Angeletti G, Sani G, Janiri D, Manfredi G, Kotzalidis GD, De Chiara L. Perinatal mixed affective state: wherefore art thou? Psychiatr Clin North Am. 2020;43:113–26.

Kozhimannil KB, Pereira MA, Harlow BL. Association between diabetes and perinatal depression among low-income mothers. JAMA. 2009;301:842–7.

Kummerlowe MN, Leung JG, Kummer LA, Moore KM, Huppert RL, Betcher HK. Retrospective review of postpartum lithium use including during lactation. Breastfeed Med. 2024;19:796–800.

Lemelin M, Boukhris T, Zhao JP, Sheehy O, Bérard A. Prevalence and determinants of attention deficit/hyperactivity disorder (ADHD) medication use during pregnancy: results from the Quebec pregnancy/children cohort. Pharmacol Res Perspect. 2021;9:e00781.

Leong C, Raymond C, Château D, Dahl M, Alessi-Severini S, Falk J, Bugden S, Katz A. Psychotropic drug use before, during, and after pregnancy: a population-based study in a Canadian cohort (2001-2013). Can J Psychiatr. 2017;62:543–50.

Lin HC, Chen IJ, Chen YH, Lee HC, Wu FJ. Maternal schizophrenia and pregnancy outcome: does the use of antipsychotics make a difference? Schizophr Res. 2010;116:55–60.

Liu X, Molenaar N, Agerbo E, Momen NC, Rommel AS, Lupattelli A, Bergink V, Munk-Olsen T. Antidepressant discontinuation before or during pregnancy and risk of psychiatric emergency in Denmark: a population-based propensity score-matched cohort study. PLoS Med. 2022;19:e1003895.

Louik C, Kerr S, Mitchell AA. First-trimester exposure to bupropion and risk of cardiac malformations. Pharmacoepidemiol Drug Saf. 2014;23:1066–75.

Maan JS, Ershadi M, Khan I, Saadabadi A. Quetiapine. Treasure Island: StatPearls Publishing; 2025.

Margulis AV, Kang EM, Hammad TA. Patterns of prescription of antidepressants and antipsychotics across and within pregnancies in a population-based UK cohort. Matern Child Health J. 2014;18:1742–52.

Martin FZ, Sharp GC, Easey KE, Madley-Dowd P, Bowen L, Nimmo-Smith V, Sadik A, Richardson JL, Rai D, Forbes H. Patterns of antidepressant prescribing in and around pregnancy: a descriptive analysis in the UK Clinical Practice Research Datalink; 2024. medRxiv, 2024.08.08.24311553.

Masters GA, Hugunin J, Xu L, Ulbricht CM, Moore Simas TA, Ko JY, Byatt N. Prevalence of bipolar disorder in perinatal women: a systematic review and meta-analysis. J Clin Psychiatry. 2022;83

McCrea RL, Nazareth I, Evans SJ, Osborn DP, Pinfold V, Cowen PJ, Petersen I. Lithium prescribing during pregnancy: a UK primary care database study. PLoS One. 2015;10:e0121024.

Mohamed MA, Elhelbawy A, Khalid M, Abdallatif LA, Lialy HE. Effects of bipolar disorder on maternal and fetal health during pregnancy: a systematic review. BMC Pregnancy Childbirth. 2023;23:617.

Molenaar NM, Bais B, Lambregtse-Van Den Berg MP, Mulder CL, Howell EA, Fox NS, Rommel AS, Bergink V, Kamperman AM. The international prevalence of antidepressant use before, during, and after pregnancy: a systematic review and meta-analysis of timing, type of prescriptions and geographical variability. J Affect Disord. 2020;264:82–9.

Molenaar NM, Maegbaek ML, Rommel AS, Ibroci E, Liu X, Munk-Olsen T, Bergink V. The incidence of depressive episodes is different before, during, and after pregnancy: a population-based study. J Affect Disord. 2023;322:273–6.

Monk C, Webster RS, McNeil RB, Parker CB, Catov JM, Greenland P, Bairey Merz CN, Silver RM, Simhan HN, Ehrenthal DB, Chung JH, Haas DM, Mercer BM, Parry S, Polito L, Reddy UM, Saade GR, Grobman WA. Associations of perceived prenatal stress and adverse pregnancy outcomes with perceived stress years after delivery. Arch Womens Ment Health. 2020;23:361–9.

Morrison JL, Riggs KW, Rurak DW. Fluoxetine during pregnancy: impact on fetal development. Reprod Fertil Dev. 2005;17:641–50.

Mota NP, Chartier M, Ekuma O, Nie Y, Hensel JM, Macwilliam L, McDougall C, Vigod S, Bolton JM. Mental disorders and suicide attempts in the pregnancy and postpartum periods compared with non-pregnancy: a population-based study. Can J Psychiatr. 2019;64:482–91.

Murugappan MN, Westberg SM, Contag S, Melnik TE, Kumar A, Rajpurohit A, Thorsness K, Farley JF. Maternal ADHD and perinatal prescription stimulant use. J Atten Disord. 2022;26:1347–56.

Nikfar S, Rahimi R, Hendoiee N, Abdollahi M. Increasing the risk of spontaneous abortion and major malformations in newborns following use of serotonin reuptake inhibitors during pregnancy: a systematic review and updated meta-analysis. DARU J Pharma Sci. 2012;20:75.

Noh Y, Choe SA, Kim WJ, Shin JY. Discontinuation and re-initiation of antidepressants during pregnancy: a nationwide cohort study. J Affect Disord. 2022;298:500–7.

Olfson M, Blanco C, Liu SM, Wang S, Correll CU. National trends in the office-based treatment of children, adolescents, and adults with antipsychotics. Arch Gen Psychiatry. 2012;69:1247–56.

Park Y, Huybrechts KF, Cohen JM, Bateman BT, Desai RJ, Patorno E, Mogun H, Cohen LS, Hernandez-Diaz S. Antipsychotic medication use among publicly insured pregnant women in the United States. Psychiatr Serv. 2017;68:1112–9.

Patorno E, Huybrechts KF, Hernandez-Diaz S. Lithium use in pregnancy and the risk of cardiac malformations. N Engl J Med. 2017;377:893–4.

Patton SW, Misri S, Corral MR, Perry KF, Kuan AJ. Antipsychotic medication during pregnancy and lactation in women with schizophrenia: evaluating the risk. Can J Psychiatr. 2002;47:959–65.

Payne JL. Psychiatric medication use in pregnancy and breastfeeding. Obstet Gynecol Clin N Am. 2021;48:131–49.

Peng M, Gao K, Ding Y, Ou J, Calabrese JR, Wu R, Zhao J. Effects of prenatal exposure to atypical antipsychotics on postnatal development and growth of infants: a case-controlled, prospective study. Psychopharmacology. 2013;228:577–84.

Perry A, Gordon-Smith K, Di Florio A, Craddock N, Jones L, Jones I. Mood episodes in pregnancy and risk of postpartum recurrence in bipolar disorder: the bipolar disorder research network pregnancy study. J Affect Disord. 2021;294:714–22.

Poels EMP, Bijma HH, Galbally M, Bergink V. Lithium during pregnancy and after delivery: a review. Int J Bipolar Disord. 2018;6:26.

Qato DM, Gandhi AB. Opioid and benzodiazepine dispensing and co-dispensing patterns among commercially insured pregnant women in the United States, 2007–2015. BMC Pregnancy Childbirth. 2021;21:350.

Richardson JL, Martin F, Dunstan H, Greenall A, Stephens S, Yates LM, Thomas SHL. Pregnancy outcomes following maternal venlafaxine use: a prospective observational comparative cohort study. Reprod Toxicol. 2019;84:108–13.

Robiyanto R, Schuiling-Veninga CCM, Bos JHJ, Hak E, Van Puijenbroek EP. Exposure to psychotropic drugs before and during pregnancy: what has changed over the last two decades? Arch Womens Ment Health. 2023;26:39–48.

Rusner M, Berg M, Begley C. Bipolar disorder in pregnancy and childbirth: a systematic review of outcomes. BMC Pregnancy Childbirth. 2016;16:331.

Sheehy O, Zhao JP, Bérard A. Association between incident exposure to benzodiazepines in early pregnancy and risk of spontaneous abortion. JAMA Psychiatry. 2019;76:948–57.

Smith B, Dubovsky SL. Pharmacotherapy of mood disorders and psychosis in pre- and post-natal women. Expert Opin Pharmacother. 2017;18:1703–19.

Stevenson F, Hamilton S, Pinfold V, Walker C, Dare CR, Kaur H, Lambley R, Szymczynska P, Nicolls V, Petersen I. Decisions about the use of psychotropic medication during pregnancy: a qualitative study. BMJ Open. 2016;6:e010130.

Straub L, Hernández-Díaz S, Bateman BT, Wisner KL, Gray KJ, Pennell PB, Lester B, Mcdougle CJ, Suarez EA, Zhu Y, Zakoul H, Mogun H, Huybrechts KF. Association of Antipsychotic Drug Exposure in pregnancy with risk of neurodevelopmental disorders: a National Birth Cohort Study. JAMA Intern Med. 2022;182:522–33.

Sujan AC, Rickert ME, Öberg AS, Quinn PD, Hernández-Díaz S, Almqvist C, Lichtenstein P, Larsson H, D'onofrio BM. Associations of maternal antidepressant use during the first trimester of pregnancy with preterm birth, small for gestational age, autism spectrum disorder, and attention-deficit/hyperactivity disorder in offspring. JAMA. 2017;317:1553–62.

Sun Y, Dreier JW, Liu X, Glejsted Ingstrup K, Maegbaek ML, Munk-Olsen T, Christensen J. Trend of antidepressants before, during, and after pregnancy across two decades-a population-based study. Brain Behav. 2019;9:e01441.

Ter Horst PG, Van Der Linde S, Smit JP, Den Boon J, Van Lingen RA, et al. Clomipramine concentration and withdrawal symptoms in 10 neonates. Br J Clin Pharmacol. 2012;73:295–302.

Terrana N, Koren G, Pivovarov J, Etwel F, Nulman I. Pregnancy outcomes following in utero exposure to second-generation antipsychotics: a systematic review and meta-analysis. J Clin Psychopharmacol. 2015;35:559–65.

Thyagarajan V, Robin Clifford C, Wurst KE, Ephross SA, Seeger JD. Bupropion therapy in pregnancy and the occurrence of cardiovascular malformations in infants. Pharmacoepidemiol Drug Saf. 2012;21:1240–2.

Toh S, Li Q, Cheetham TC, Cooper WO, Davis RL, Dublin S, Hammad TA, Li DK, Pawloski PA, Pinheiro SP, Raebel MA, Scott PE, Smith DH, Bobo WV, Lawrence JM, Dashevsky I, Haffenreffer K, Avalos LA, Andrade SE. Prevalence and trends in the use of antipsychotic medications during pregnancy in the U.S., 2001-2007: a population-based study of 585,615 deliveries. Arch Womens Ment Health. 2013;16:149–57.

Tong VT, England LJ, Dietz PM, Asare LA. Smoking patterns and use of cessation interventions during pregnancy. Am J Prev Med. 2008;35:327–33.

Trost SL, Beauregard JL, Smoots AN, Ko JY, Haight SC, Moore Simas TA, Byatt N, Madni SA, Goodman D. Preventing pregnancy-related mental health deaths: insights from 14 US maternal mortality review committees, 2008-17. Health Aff (Millwood). 2021;40:1551–9.

U.S. Food And Drug Administration. DA drug safety communication: selective serotonin reuptake inhibitor (SSRI) antidepressant use during pregnancy and potential risk of persistent pulmonary hypertension of the newborn (PPHN) [Online]; 2011. Available: https://www.fda.gov/drugs/drug-safety-and-availability/fda-drug-safety-communication-selective-serotonin-reuptake-inhibitor-ssri-antidepressant-use-during. Accessed 28 Feb 2025

Uguz F. A new safety scoring system for the use of psychotropic drugs during lactation. Am J Ther. 2021;28:e118–26.

UNFPA. Nearly half of all pregnancies are unintended – a global crisis, says new UNFPA report [Online]; 2022. Available: https://www.unfpa.org/press/nearly-half-all-pregnancies-are-unintended-global-crisis-says-new-unfpa-report?utm_source=chatgpt.com. Accessed 27 Feb 2025.

Van Boekholt AA, Hartong EG, Huntjens-Fleuren H, Grootens KP, Semmekrot BA. Quetiapine concentrations during exclusive breastfeeding and maternal quetiapine use. Ann Pharmacother. 2015;49:743–4.

Vigod SN, Kurdyak PA, Dennis CL, Gruneir A, Newman A, Seeman MV, Rochon PA, Anderson GM, Grigoriadis S, RAY, J. G. Maternal and newborn outcomes among women with schizophrenia: a retrospective population-based cohort study. BJOG. 2014;121:566–74.

Viguera AC, Newport DJ, Ritchie J, Stowe Z, Whitfield T, Mogielnicki J, Baldessarini RJ, Zurick A, Cohen LS. Lithium in breast milk and nursing infants: clinical implications. Am J Psychiatry. 2007;164:342–5.

Walsh K, McCormack CA, Webster R, Pinto A, Lee S, Feng T, Krakovsky HS, et al. Maternal prenatal stress phenotypes associate with fetal neurodevelopment and birth outcomes. Proc Natl Acad Sci USA. 2019;116:23996–4005.

Wesseloo R, Kamperman AM, Munk-Olsen T, Pop VJ, Kushner SA, Bergink V. Risk of postpartum relapse in bipolar disorder and postpartum psychosis: a systematic review and meta-analysis. Am J Psychiatry. 2016;173:117–27.

Wisner KL, Perel JM. Serum levels of valproate and carbamazepine in breastfeeding mother-infant pairs. J Clin Psychopharmacol. 1998;18:167–9.

Wohrer F, Ngo H, Didomenico J, et al. Potentially modifiable risk and protective factors affecting mental and emotional wellness in pregnancy. Front Hum Neurosci. 2024;18:1323297.

Zoega H, Kieler H, Nørgaard M, Furu K, Valdimarsdottir U, Brandt L, Haglund B. Use of SSRI and SNRI antidepressants during pregnancy: a population-based study from Denmark, Iceland, Norway and Sweden. PLoS One. 2015;10:e0144474.

Maternal and Infant Pharmacokinetics of Psychotropic Medications During Pregnancy and Lactation

2

Nikolaos Kokras, Eleni Poulogiannopoulou, Marinos G. Sotiropoulos, and Christina Dalla

2.1 Pharmacokinetics of the Pregnancy

Pregnant women often take over-the-counter, herbal, or prescribed medications, and there is a trend for increased medication consumption by pregnant women over the last decades. Moreover, pregnancy and the postpartum period is now clearly recognized as a risk situation for the development or exacerbation of many psychiatric disorders. Consequently, there is an increased possibility that a pregnant woman will require pharmacological treatment involving a psychotropic medication. However, there is limited evidence regarding the safe use of medications in pregnancy and during lactation. From a pharmacokinetic perspective, few studies focus on the physiological changes that take place during pregnancy, and even fewer attempt to link pharmacokinetics to pharmacodynamics. Unfortunately, despite the growing need, there is modest incentive from the industry to invest in improving our knowledge about the pharmacokinetics and pharmacodynamics of psychotropics during pregnancy and the lactating period (Pariente et al. 2016; Ansari et al. 2016).

N. Kokras
First Department of Psychiatry, Eginition Hospital, Medical School, National & Kapodistrian University of Athens, Athens, Greece

E. Poulogiannopoulou
Second Department of Anaesthesiology, Medical School, National & Kapodistrian University of Athens, Athens, Greece

M. G. Sotiropoulos
Department of Neurology, Mass General Brigham, Harvard Medical School, Boston, MA, USA

C. Dalla (✉)
Second Department of Obstetrics & Gynecology, Aretaieio Hospital, Medical School, National & Kapodistrian University of Athens, Athens, Greece
e-mail: cdalla@med.uoa.gr

F. Uguz, L. Orsolini (eds.), *Perinatal Psychopharmacology*,
https://doi.org/10.1007/978-3-031-99720-4_2

2.1.1 Pharmacokinetics of the Pregnant Woman

Dynamic changes in female physiology during pregnancy affect several pharmacokinetic parameters and further amplify the already present sex differences in drug absorption, distribution, metabolism, and elimination of psychotropics, especially when interacting with the altered hormonal milieu (Kokras et al. 2011; Damoiseaux et al. 2014). Such complex changes often result in counteracting effects, which create difficulties in assessing the net effect on drug pharmacokinetics. Pregnancy decelerates gastric emptying, as well as the small bowel and colonic transit time of the drug. Therefore, drug absorption is generally decreased (Deligiannidis et al. 2014). However, in some cases, genetic polymorphisms of transporters responsible to limit maternal gastrointestinal drug absorption, such as the P-glycoprotein (Pgp), may lead to a reduced transport activity, and thus higher plasma drug concentrations (DeVane et al. 2006). During gestation there is an escalation of the maternal plasma volume, which reaches a 50% increase during the third semester. The protein-binding capacity undergoes changes as albumin levels are lowered, and the ratio of lean muscle to adipose tissue is decreased resulting in a greater volume of drug distribution. Moreover, the free fraction of drugs is increased. Most psychotropic drugs have a lipophilic profile and show a greater volume of distribution during pregnancy, which may lead to lower peak plasma concentrations (Deligiannidis et al. 2014; Eberhard-Gran et al. 2005; Chisolm and Payne 2016). Due to a simultaneous higher clearance, the plasma concentration of drugs is often lower than that of healthy adults (Goldberg and Nissim 1994). As gestation progresses, the renal blood flow and the glomerular filtration rate (GFR) are increased, and this results in acceleration of drug elimination. Although data is still inconclusive, hepatic blood flow seems to increase as well, leading to high drug extraction ratios (Deligiannidis et al. 2014; Chisolm and Payne 2016; Goldberg and Nissim 1994).

Nevertheless, the most complex and pronounced changes in the pharmacokinetics of psychotropic medications during pregnancy are due to the hormonal induction or inhibition of metabolic processes. Both the cytochrome P450 (CYP) family, which plays a key role in the phase 1 drug metabolism, as well as the phase 2 metabolism enzymes, such as uridine diphosphate glucuronosyltransferase (UGT) and n-acetyltransferase, are modulated by sex hormones during the gestation period. CYP3A4, which is already more active in female than male adults, is further induced during gestation due to progesterone. Sex hormones also induce CYP2A6, CYP2D6, and increase glucuronidation by upregulating UGT1A4 and possibly UGT2B7. On the other hand, CYP1A2 and CYP2C19 are inhibited by increased levels of sex steroids during pregnancy. During the late stages of gestation, CYP1A2 activity is reduced by 65–70% and CYP2C19 activity is reduced by 50% in comparison to the postpartum period. However, it is important to mention that the maternal metabolic phenotype (poor, intermediate, extensive, or ultra-rapid) plays a key role in the final metabolic rate and that, for every enzyme phenotype, the metabolic rate is affected at a different extent. Therefore, many drugs require close and personalized dose monitoring during pregnancy (Deligiannidis et al. 2014; Chisolm and Payne 2016). Moreover, drug plasma concentration may increase in women with a poor metabolizer genotype, and as a result a greater amount of the drug is transferred to the fetus through the placenta (DeVane et al. 2006).

After delivery, sex hormone levels in the maternal plasma decrease rapidly. During the postpartum period the plasma volume is normalized, and the hepatic enzyme activity returns to baseline after a short period of time. There is also a decrease in the renal blood flow and glomerular filtration rate which also return to normal range. Thus, after delivery this rapid normalization of previously modified factors may lead to high drug maternal plasma concentrations, especially if the drug dose administered during pregnancy is not closely monitored and modified during the postpartum period (Deligiannidis et al. 2014).

2.1.2 Pharmacokinetics of the Fetus and the Neonate

The modified maternal drug pharmacokinetics in combination with the placental transfer potential and the fetal drug metabolic rate determine the fetal psychotropic drug exposure (Deligiannidis et al. 2014). Fetal exposure depends on the drug dose, the maternal absorption, distribution and elimination, the placental transfer and the fetal distribution and elimination of the drug. Three main factors determine the drug's placental transfer rate: the lipophilicity of the drug, the pH gradient across the placenta, and the drug's protein binding characteristics.

It is known that nonionized, low molecular weight, lipid-soluble drugs are well absorbed. The concentration of a lipophilic drug tends to reach an equilibrium across the two sides of the placental barrier, and therefore the rate of drug transfer is largely dependent upon the concentration gradient (indicated by the fetal/maternal ratio) and the placental blood flow (Goldberg and Nissim 1994). Most psychotropic drugs administered to pregnant women are highly lipophilic, cross the placental barrier, reach and distribute to the fetal compartment with varying transfer rates, possibly causing teratogenic effects, neonatal toxicity, withdrawal syndromes, or long-term neurobehavioral effects (DeVane et al. 2006; Eberhard-Gran et al. 2005; Chisolm and Payne 2016; Goldberg and Nissim 1994). After delivery, the previous equilibrium between the fetus and its mother via the placenta does not apply to the neonate. For this reason, high concentrations of a particular drug in the fetus may result to significantly prolonged effects postnatally (Goldberg and Nissim 1994).

Another determinant of placental crossing of psychotropic drugs is their affinity for drug transporters. Transplacental passage is moderated by these transporters. Several ATP-binding cassette (ABC) transporters, such as P-glycoprotein (P-gp), multidrug resistance proteins 1–3 (e.g., ABCC2, MRP2), and breast cancer resistance protein (ABCG2, BCRP) significantly reduce the transplacental passage of drugs, therefore limiting their disposition into the fetal compartment (DeVane et al. 2006). After a drug has crossed the placental barrier, the total concentration of plasma proteins, as well as the protein-binding affinity for drugs are low in the fetus in comparison to the mother. This results to a higher free fraction of the drugs in the fetus, which facilitates tissue distribution. On top of that, the permeability of the fetal blood-brain barrier is relatively high and the immature central nervous system appears generally more sensitive to drug effects (Goldberg and Nissim 1994; Menon 2008).

Moreover, the hepatic mechanisms of drug elimination are not mature in the fetus (less activity and a smaller concentration of certain microsomal enzymes), and this results in a reduced rate of drug metabolism, as well as an increased drug accumulation in the fetal compartment. However, drug metabolism in the fetal liver is more likely to be more active than the drug metabolism in the placenta (Goldberg and Nissim 1994). In the late stages of gestation, and approximately during the first 3 months of life, the metabolic capacity of the fetus/newborn is relatively low, exposing it to high quantities of almost any drug administered to the mother (Jain and Lacy 2005; Harding and Timko 1999). The drug metabolites in the fetus are either products of the limited fetal metabolism, or compounds of maternal origin. Once these metabolites are present in the fetus, they cannot be easily transferred back to the maternal blood (Menon 2008). After delivery, the physiologic mechanisms of the newborn also undergo changes. After the first 3 months of life, the hepatic enzymes have developed, although the maturation rate seems to vary among subjects (Jain and Lacy 2005). Lastly, for the majority of drugs, excretion is reduced as the neonate's glomerular filtration rate is proportionally lower in comparison to adults (Goldberg and Nissim 1994).

2.1.3 Pharmacokinetics of Anxiolytics in Pregnancy

Benzodiazepines cross the placenta and reach fetus through diffusion, which is not constant throughout pregnancy. In late pregnancy, changes in the placental circulation, size, permeability, and lipid content lead to an increased diffusion in comparison to early pregnancy. In addition, some benzodiazepines have long half-lives, and long-term administration may lead to drug accumulation in the maternal and fetal compartment. Even after a single dose or until a steady-state is achieved, the fetal levels of benzodiazepines may be even higher than maternal levels, due to the rapid maternal drug distribution. For instance, after an intravenous or oral single dose of diazepam the fetomaternal ratio increases from 1.2 (i.v.) and 0.4 (oral) in early pregnancy to 1.8 (i.v.) and 0.8 (oral) in late pregnancy (Kanto 1982).

Regarding diazepam, the fetus is able to metabolize it from the 13th week of gestation. However, in the early pregnancy stages, the metabolic rates are really low for both the placenta and the fetus. As a result, diazepam and its metabolites accumulate in the fetus (Mandelli et al. 1978; Jørgensen et al. 1988). Thus, after administration of high diazepam doses in late pregnancy, newborns are affected, and high levels of the drug are detected in their circulation.

On the other hand, oxazepam has a relatively short half-life and lacks active metabolites. Pregnant women have a shorter oxazepam half-life and higher clearance. After oral oxazepam administration the fetomaternal ratio is 0.6 and 1.1 in early and late pregnancy, respectively. During the late stages of gestation, fetal levels are higher than the maternal ones. This indicates that during this period there is increased diffusion of benzodiazepines through the placenta, high maternal volume drug distribution, and high maternal metabolic and elimination rates (Jørgensen et al. 1988). Regarding the neonate, oxazepam has three to four times longer half-life, in comparison to the mother, but after the first few days of life, oxazepam elimination in the infant is increased, probably due to more effective glucuronidation and renal excretion (Kanto 1982; Gaillot et al. 1983).

Chlordiazepoxide was primarily used as a labor sedative, and it has been shown that after a single dose of chlordiazepoxide during labor, the fetomaternal drug ratio is near one. Chlordiazepoxide's half-life in the newborn is 20% higher than normal, but no symptoms of sedation have been reported in neonates (Kanto 1982; McElhatton 1994).

Regarding lorazepam, moderate perinatal doses are considered safe for the mother and the newborn. Lorazepam diffuses rapidly across the placenta, and fetal concentrations are similar to the maternal concentrations. The infant metabolism of lorazepam does not differ significantly from the mother's, it has no active metabolites, and plasma levels are reduced within 7 days (Kanto 1982; McElhatton 1994). Similarly, it has been shown that the flunitrazepam fetomaternal ratio is 0.22 after a single dose of oral flunitrazepam administered in late pregnancy. Drug concentrations in cord, umbilical vein, and artery plasma are lower than those in maternal venous plasma, and amniotic fluid levels are negligible. However, long-term use of flunitrazepam during pregnancy is associated with a high possibility of accumulation in the fetus due to the drug's long elimination half-life. Likewise, a single dose of oral nitrazepam during delivery or in early pregnancy results in a fetomaternal plasma concentration ratio between 0.4 and 0.9. Maternal plasma levels of nitrazepam do not differ between early and late pregnancy, but fetal plasma levels are higher in late stages of gestation (Kanto 1982).

Trazodone, a triazolopyridine antidepressant commonly used for anxiety and insomnia, and its active metabolite 1-m-chlorophenylpiperazine (mCPP), both readily cross the placenta: cord blood levels are comparable to maternal serum levels, although this is not known to lead to major birth defects (Saito et al. 2021). Finally, zopiclone and its metabolites pass through the placental barrier to a limited degree. One study in pregnant rats showed that concentrations of total radioactivity and concentrations of the unchanged compound in fetal tissues were 3–4 times lower than those in the placenta. Amniotic fluid concentrations of total radioactivity were also low (Gaillot et al. 1983).

2.1.4 Pharmacokinetics of Antidepressants in Pregnancy

During pregnancy—and especially the third trimester –, increased metabolism, as described above, reduces the plasma concentrations of many antidepressants, including trimipramine, fluvoxamine, nortriptyline and to a lesser extent citalopram, clomipramine, imipramine, paroxetine, escitalopram, fluoxetine and venlafaxine, and thus their overall availability (Schoretsanitis et al. 2020a) (Pariente et al. 2016). However, because some antidepressants have active metabolites (as other psychotropics as well), fetal exposure to an active metabolite may unpredictably increase due to the increased metabolism of the parent drug during pregnancy. Indeed, whereas sertraline, citalopram, and fluoxetine levels are reduced during pregnancy, a higher metabolite to parent drug ratio is found during late pregnancy (Deligiannidis et al. 2014). Likewise, buproprion levels decrease during pregnancy and the drug is undetectable in the fetus. However its active metabolite reaches significant levels in the pregnant mother and can be detected in the fetus, with potentially hazardous consequences (Fokina et al. 2016; Neuman et al. 2014). Paroxetine levels may also decrease, especially if the pregnant woman is an extensive or ultrarapid metabolizer. On the contrary, in pregnant women with intermediate and poor metabolizing genotypes, increased plasma levels can be observed, with potential consequences to the fetus (Deligiannidis et al. 2014). Moreover, the elimination half-life (short or long) of the antidepressant administered will determine whether it is more likely to observe fetal withdrawal symptoms or toxicity (Kieviet et al. 2013). Another important issue regards the transport proteins during pregnancy. Some antidepressants may further inhibit the already downregulated P-gp in pregnancy, and P-gp genetic polymorphisms may result in significant individual differences in drug exposure to the mother and the fetus (DeVane et al. 2006; Feghali et al. 2015). Fluoxetine, paroxetine, and sertraline are especially prone to P-gp-related effects. Regarding other classes of antidepressants, clomipramine has an increased elimination half-life and along with its active metabolite they have a F/P ratio of 0.5 to 0.8 (ter Horst et al. 2012). Although venlafaxine levels may decrease during pregnancy (ter Horst et al. 2014), the degree is considered insignificant and concentration of its active metabolite (O-desmethylvenlafaxine) remains stable (ter Horst et al. 2014; Westin et al. 2017).

2.1.5 Pharmacokinetics of Antipsychotics in Pregnancy

Examining antipsychotic drug fetal exposure during pregnancy, a study indicated that olanzapine and haloperidol had the highest placental passage ratio (mean of 72.1% and 65.5% respectively). Risperidone follows (mean = 49.2%), as well as quetiapine, with the latter having the lowest passage ratio of all antipsychotics (mean = 23.8%). Notably, quetiapine and risperidone are atypical antipsychotics found to share a good P-glycoprotein (P-gp) affinity, and as a result placental P-gp is able to reduce the placental passage of these drugs. On the other hand, olanzapine and clozapine are intermediate and poor substrates, respectively. Their low affinity for the P-gp efflux transporter results to an easier passage through placental barrier, due to their lipid solubility, without being hindered by the P-gp efflux transport (Babu et al. 2015). Moreover, quetiapine is metabolized primarily by CYP3A4, which is induced in pregnancy. This explains the rapid elimination and low plasma concentration of quetiapine in most pregnant women. In fact, a dose increase may be required during pregnancy and a post-partum decrease would avoid toxic side-effects, as quetiapine's bioavailability is much higher in the postpartum period than in gestation (Pinheiro et al. 2018; Klier et al. 2007).

2.1.6 Pharmacokinetics of Mood Stabilizers in Pregnancy

Most mood stabilizing drugs (lithium, valproic acid, carbamazepine, and lamotrigine) cross the placenta, a fact proven by either detectable levels in cord blood or by their teratogenic and fetotoxic effects in animals (Iqbal et al. 2001a). Even in the early stages of pregnancy, the lithium clearance increases by 50–100%, because of the increased renal function. As a result, serum lithium concentration decreases significantly. In the postpartum period, lithium clearance rapidly returns to baseline values and along with the normalization of other pregnancy-related pharmacokinetic parameters, the dose adjustment of lithium becomes of significant importance (Iqbal et al. 2001b; Schou et al. 1973). The relative lithium concentration in umbilical cord blood to maternal blood is 1,05, a ratio that remains constant for a wide range of lithium serum concentrations (Ohman et al. 2000).

Regarding valproate, its absorption does not seem to change in pregnancy, but the total blood levels apparently decrease in pregnancy along with an increased volume of distribution. However, the unbound, active fraction (normally 10%) may not change. This happens because, on one hand, there is increased clearance of the unbound valproate due to increased renal clearance and lower protein binding sites in pregnancy. On the other hand, this effect is compensated by increased binding in tissues and altered drug metabolism. The total effect of all these complex pharmacokinetic changes may not result in significant difference in free valproate levels during pregnancy. However, postpartum levels may increase rapidly, requiring dose adjustment. Moreover, valproate and its metabolites are found in higher concentrations in the fetus than maternal blood, as the neonate/maternal blood ratio has been estimated at 1.3–4.6 (Iqbal et al. 2001b; Johannessen 1992; Hendrickx et al. 1988). These increased valproate concentrations suggest that the fetus may function as a deep compartment for the drug's distribution, the drug is actively transported through the placenta, or valproate binds fetal serum proteins with higher affinity. In any case, valproate is clearly contraindicated not only for pregnant women, but generally for women of reproductive age and their male partners as well (PMID 38228350).

Lamotrigine binding to plasma proteins is only 55%, and this does not change in pregnant women (Franco et al. 2008). However, lamotrigine metabolism is significantly affected in pregnancy, albeit with significant variations among women. In pregnancy, metabolism and clearance of lamotrigine increases, resulting in lower plasma levels and a 40–300% higher dose-to-plasma concentration ratio. However the lower plasma concentrations are observed when lamotrigine is administered alone, and not when co-administered with valproate (Tomson et al. 2006; De Haan et al. 2004). Plasma lamotrigine levels also display pulsatile variations within the day, possibly due to hormonal or other physiological changes in pregnant women, but this phenomenon has not yet been studied thoroughly. After delivery, lamotrigine clearance quickly reverts to its pre-pregnancy levels (Franco et al. 2008; Grover and Avasthi 2015). Notably, lamotrigine is extensively transferred to the newborn, reaching levels similar or greater than the maternal ones (Iqbal et al. 2001a; De Haan et al. 2004; Grover and Avasthi 2015). After birth, the newborn clears the drug at a slow rate, because of immature glucuronidation and undeveloped renal excretion (Grover and Avasthi 2015).

Carbamazepine, oxcarbazepine, and their metabolites' plasma levels also decrease during pregnancy but their concentration in cord blood equals maternal serum levels. The placenta metabolizes oxcarbazepine into its active metabolite (10-OH-CBZ), but it does not metabolize carbamazepine or 10-OH-CBZ. Moreover, carbamazepine's induction of CYP3A4, resulting in induction of its own metabolism, does not take place into the placenta, which lacks CYP3A4 activity. Finally, all substances readily cross the placenta and affect the fetus, with 10-OH-CBZ showing a slower transfer due to its lower liposolubility (Franco et al. 2008; Pienimäki et al. 1997).

2.1.7 Pharmacokinetics of Opioids in Pregnancy

Opioid pharmacokinetics depend heavily on the observed metabolism changes induced by pregnancy, importantly changes in the CYP and the P-gp enzyme function, whose substrates include many opioids. Pregnancy progression alters the concentration of plasma binding proteins, but for most opioids, the associated differences in the unbound drug fractions are not statistically significant. However, the activity of various opioid metabolizing cytochrome P450 (CYP) enzymes is widely affected. Because of several genetic CYP2D6 polymorphisms, resulting in poor, intermediate, extensive, and ultrarapid metabolizers, opioid pharmacokinetics are difficult to predict in pregnancy. Generally, throughout gestation, CYP2D6 activity gradually increases in ultrarapid and extensive metabolizers, and decreases in poor and intermediate metabolizers. CYP3A4 enzyme (involved in the metabolism of buprenorphine, oxycodone, fentanyl) and CYP2B6 (the main enzyme involved in methadone metabolism) are also induced during gestation. Normally, from an oxycodone dose, 45% is metabolized by CYP3A4 to the weak analgesic metabolite noroxycodone and 11% is metabolized by CYP2D6 to oxymorphone (pharmacologically active, ten-fold higher antinociceptive potency than morphine). More clinical studies are needed to determine which enzyme (CYP3A4 or CYP2D6) undergoes greater induction during pregnancy and, subsequently, which is the predominant oxycodone metabolite (active or inactive). UGT2B7 (involved in the glucuronidation of morphine, buprenorphine, and its metabolite norbuprenorphine) is also induced during pregnancy. Moreover, pregnancy increases renal P-gp activity and thus urine excretion of morphine's potent metabolite (MG6) and methadone. In fact, the placenta itself has also been proven to express P-glycoprotein (Madadi et al. 2012; de Barros et al. 2009). Oral methadone clearance is accelerated by 1,5- to two-fold. Women in methadone maintenance have lower plasma levels and lower half-life (19 vs 30 hours) possibly due to the enhanced CYP3A4 and CYP2B6 activity, the higher plasma volume, the larger tissue reservoir, the metabolism occurring in the fetus and the placenta, as well as due to the increased renal excretion. Those changes require the administration of increased and more frequent methadone doses in pregnant women (Dickmann and Isoherranen 2012; Drozdick et al. 2002; Pond et al. 1985; Jarvis et al. 1999; van Hoogdalem et al. 2022).

During labor and caesarean delivery, opioids are administered as a co-adjuvant to local anesthetics via the epidural and/or intrathecal route for obstetric pain management (Kesavan et al. 2018; Reynolds et al. 2002; Grangier et al. 2020; Wang et al. 2014; Practice Guidelines for Obstetric Anesthesia 2016). Fentanyl epidural administration results in slower onset of action and longer duration than its intravenous administration (3–5 fold slower onset and 3–6 fold longer duration) (Moises et al. 2005). After an epidural injection, fentanyl diffuses freely from the epidural space into the maternal circulation, crosses the placental barrier, and has been detected in the umbilical vein (UV) within 30 min of an epidural dose to parturient women (Moises et al. 2005; Desprats et al. 1991, 1995; Haidl et al. 2018). The UV to maternal vein (MV) plasma concentration ratio can vary widely during labor depending on the route of administration (iv or epidural), the drug dose and type of administration (bolus or infusion), the stage of pregnancy, as well as the rapid changes occurring in maternal and fetal plasma concentrations (fentanyl UV/MV ratios: 0.3–3.4 within an hour after epidural bolus dose (de Barros et al. 2009; Moises et al. 2005; Desprats et al. 1991; Desprats et al. 1995), 0.3–1.9 within an hour after intravenous dosing (Morley-Forster et al. 2000), 0.6–3.1 at 1–15 hours after epidural infusion) (Haidl et al. 2018; Loftus et al. 1995; Bader et al. 1995). Intrathecal morphine is also used for pain relief during a caesarean delivery, usually as a part of regional anesthesia (administration in the subarachnoid and/or epidural space) (Practice Guidelines for Obstetric Anesthesia 2016). After neuraxial administration, morphine is rapidly absorbed in the maternal circulation, is metabolized, and then undergoes renal excretion (Zakowski et al. 1993). Although exhibiting modest labor pain relief, patient-controlled analgesia with intravenous opioids is an alternative when neuraxial anesthesia is contraindicated (fentanyl, morphine, nalbuphine, or remifentanil). Remifentanyl is usually preferred as it has both a rapid onset of action and a rapid offset (half-life 4 min). It is metabolized by non-specific tissue and plasma esterases to non-active metabolites. Remifentanil rapidly crosses the placenta (UV/MA concentration: 0.88) and is quickly metabolized and redistributed in the fetus (UA/UV concentration 0.29) (Anderson 2011; Van de Velde and Carvalho 2016). It is worth mentioning that the method used by most studies to assess transplacental drug permeability (measurement of UV/MV ratios) might lead to systematic errors, as the placenta is perfused with maternal arterial blood instead of venous blood. The main determinant of drug distribution kinetics across the placenta is the maternal arterial blood concentration. The maternal arteriovenous concentration difference could vary depending on each drug's pharmacokinetic properties (Huang and Isoherranen 2020) resulting in very different UV/MV and UV/MA concentration ratios. For example, fentanyl's high UV/MV ratio might reflect the maternal arteriovenous distribution kinetics, rather than a rapid transplacental transfer of the drug (Shum et al. 2021). Moreover, there is evidence suggesting that the placental intervillous space might be a fentanyl deposit site due to the possible role of placental P-glycoprotein (P-gp), which might prevent a large amount of the drug from moving into the fetal compartment (de Barros et al. 2009).

2.2 Pharmacokinetics of Lactation

Many women require psychotropic medication during the postpartum and lactation periods. As a result, there is concern for the potential infant exposure through the breast milk. The pharmacokinetics of psychotropic drugs in lactation are examined in three distinct stages: (a) pharmacokinetics in the lactating mother, (b) drug excretion into the breast milk, and (c) pharmacokinetics in the newborn that receives the drug through breastfeeding (Buist et al. 1990). Few studies have focused on the pharmacokinetics of psychotropics during lactation, and even fewer have employed high-quality methodology (Buist et al. 1990; Llewellyn and Stowe 1998). Ethical issues, the process of taking frequent samples from mothers and infants, carrying out a long-term prospective study, and measuring concentrations, are difficulties that have contributed to the lack of adequate studies. The results are often contradictory, and the conduction of a meta-analysis would be impossible due to the heterogeneity in the measuring methods (Yoshida et al. 1999). As a result, the strong suspicion that most psychotropic drugs enter breast milk, and the lack of substantial evidence on infant dose, kinetics, and safety, have pushed clinicians toward a conservative attitude toward breastfeeding for women on psychotropic medication. Nonetheless, there is some methodology in place and some knowledge that should allow more informed decisions. Breast milk pumping at regular intervals within 24 h is a method that simulates normal feeding. Psychotropic drugs can be measured in the breast milk, with concentrations corresponding to an infant's daily ingested dose. If blood is drawn from the mother, preferably at the same time as milk pumping, the milk-to-plasma concentration ratio can be calculated. The M/P ratio for each drug varies, depending on dosage interval and time of sampling. The estimated drug exposure of the infant can be expressed as a percentage of the normal dose adjusted for weight and age (in mg/kg), or more frequently as a percentage of the maternal dose (Pons et al. 1994; Spigset and Hägg 1998). A M/P ratio of less than 1 suggests negligible excretion to the milk, and a drug is generally considered safe if the relative infant dose is less than 10% of the maternal dose (Kronenfeld et al. 2017; Burkey and Holmes 2013).

2.2.1 Pharmacokinetics in the Lactating Mother

The effects of lactation on pharmacokinetics have not been studied and remain largely unknown. All the physiologic changes of pregnancy (e.g., increased plasma volume, decreased plasma proteins, increased renal function) revert to normal after delivery, but this return may be gradual, affecting drug concentrations in the postpartum period. For instance, while maternal caffeine clearance reverts to baseline within days, phenytoin clearance takes months to reach its pre-pregnancy levels. Labor and delivery may also impact pharmacokinetics, as they result in physiologic stress, decreased plasma volume, and other changes (Pons et al. 1994).

2.2.2 Drug Excretion to the Breast Milk

A drug's concentration in breast milk varies, and depends on its chemical properties (lipophilicity, molecular weight, degree of ionization), the characteristics of the milk (pH, protein and lipid content), as well as the maternal pharmacokinetics (dose, frequency, absorption, blood flow to the breast, and drug metabolism by the mammary tissue). Breast milk is not a reservoir where drugs accumulate, but rather a compartment where drugs undergo bidirectional transfer, being in a continuous equilibrium with blood plasma. In order to calculate an infant's drug exposure, milk yield and intake, drug concentration, and the presence of active metabolites must be measured. There are also differences in drug concentrations when the two breasts are compared, as previous feeding may affect milk yield and drug excretion (Pons et al. 1994). The timing of the dose is also important, as the infant will be exposed to smaller drug quantities if feeding and medication times are arranged correctly. Immediate release drugs taken immediately after breastfeeding will have lower concentrations in breast milk after a few hours (Kronenfeld et al. 2017). Psychotropic drugs are lipophilic—as they need to cross the blood-brain barrier to reach their site of action—and can easily penetrate into breast milk via passive diffusion (Shah and Aftab 2015). Highly lipid-soluble and unionized molecules diffuse more rapidly through the membrane, and this is shown by a measured milk-to-plasma concentration ratio approaching one. A milk-to-plasma ratio of one or higher is generally considered significant exposure for the infant (Menon 2008). Breast milk has a higher lipid content than plasma, resulting in high concentrations of psychotropic drugs, most of which are lipid-soluble. Colostrum, which is produced from day 1 to day 5 postpartum, has a mean lipid concentration of 29 g/L, and mature milk has a 42 g/L concentration. Hindmilk also has more fat than foremilk, and thus contains larger quantities of psychotropic drugs. The main drug-binding proteins in breast milk are α-lactalbumin, casein, and lactoferrin. Colostrum has a total protein concentration of 23 g/L, mature milk (>30 days postpartum) has 9 g/L of protein, while blood plasma has more than 60 g/L. Hindmilk (at the end of a feeding) has a 50% higher protein content than foremilk. Concentrations of protein-bound drugs follow these fluctuations. The percentage of unbound drug in the milk remains stable regardless of its concentration, and depends on the milk's pH (Goldberg and Nissim 1994; Buist et al. 1990; Pons et al. 1994). Milk pH is usually lower than plasma pH. It varies from 6.35 to 7.65, and gradually decreases as the milk matures. Most psychotropic drugs are weak bases, and thus diffuse readily down the pH gradient. Once in the breast milk, the low pH induces ionization and ionized drugs become more water soluble and may be trapped in the breast milk (Menon 2008; Pons et al. 1994; Spigset and Hägg 1998; Kronenfeld et al. 2017; Kohen 2005). Finally, ingredients such as lactose, serum albumin, calcium, phosphates, and various enzymes also affect drug concentrations in breast milk (Burt et al. 2001).

2.2.3 Pharmacokinetics of Nursing Infant

An infant's drug exposure depends not only on the dose ingested with breast milk, but also on its own pharmacokinetics, for which infant age is the determining factor (Spigset and Hägg 1998). The particulars of breastfeeding (suckling, time on each breast, amount of milk ingested, and feeding intervals) also play an important role (Buist et al. 1990). In studies assessing drug safety, a 100% oral bioavailability with no first-pass metabolism is usually assumed, so as to examine the "worst-case scenario". However, gastrointestinal absorption of drugs has not been studied adequately in infants. It is believed that irregular motility and slow gastric emptying affect absorption rate. Stomach acidity is developed within the first day of life. For the next 8 days, pH returns to neutral, and then descends to adult levels within 2 years. For all these reasons, the total amount that is eventually absorbed may be smaller, equal to, or larger than the equivalent amount in adults (Yoshida et al. 1999; Spigset and Hägg 1998).

Drug distribution also displays significant differences between infants and adults, because of differences in total body water, extracellular fluid, fat and muscle content, pH, and protein binding. The protein-bound fraction of drugs is lower in infants, owing to a different albumin structure, decreased albumin and globulin concentration in the first year of life, and increased bilirubin and free fatty acids, which bind to the available binding sites. Thus, drugs binding to albumin have a higher free, active fraction in infants (Buist et al. 1990; Yoshida et al. 1999; Pons et al. 1994; Spigset and Hägg 1998). Newborns also have an immature blood-brain barrier, and CSF concentrations of lipid-soluble drugs can be 10–30 times higher than plasma concentrations. Fat quantity is also decreased, and lipid-soluble drugs have fewer storage sites, thus accumulating in the nervous system in higher concentrations (Burt et al. 2001).

Drug metabolism and excretion occur at a slower rate in neonates. Preterm infants have even slower metabolism and excretion rates, and should not be exposed to psychotropic drugs through lactation (Kohen 2005). Cytochrome P-450 is an important enzyme for the metabolism of certain psychotropic drugs. The newborn has only one-half of the enzymatic activity of an adult, and this can influence drug metabolism. Especially, during the first 2 weeks of life, enzymatic activity in the liver is estimated at 20% of adult activity. Like all liver enzymes, CYP matures after birth, slowly reaching maximum activity (Kronenfeld et al. 2017). The enzymes that take part in phase 1 reactions (oxidation, reduction, and hydrolysis) mature quickly, and reach higher levels of capacity during years 0–3 than they do in adult life. Stable levels are not reached until puberty. Isozymes of CYP mature at different rates: CYP1A2, CYP2C19, and CYP2D6 have low capacity in infants, while CYP3A has higher capacity. Genetic polymorphisms leading to high or low enzyme activity in adults ("poor" vs "extensive metabolizers") have the same effects in infant age (Spigset and Hägg 1998). Moreover, unique metabolic products produced only in infants have also been documented, as is the case with chlorpromazine (Buist et al. 1990). Phase 2 reactions (conjugation and glycine sulphate formation) are known to exhibit high interindividual variability because of genetic polymorphisms, and reach adult capacity at 1,5–2 years of life. If glucuronidation is the only metabolic pathway available for a drug (e.g., oxazepam), infant concentrations will be significantly increased. As mentioned before, each enzyme develops the ability to metabolize different substrates at different time points during maturation. For instance, glucuronyl transferase can metabolize bilirubin on day 3, but cannot fully metabolize chloramphenicol before day 10. Premature infants have even more pronounced enzyme immaturity (Yoshida et al. 1999; Spigset and Hägg 1998; Kohen 2005; Burt et al. 2001).

Despite having proportionally larger kidneys, neonates exhibit a glomerular filtration rate of 2–4 ml/min, i.e., only 30–40% of the adult GFR, and 20–30% of the adult tubular secretion. Drugs are thus excreted more slowly and can easily accumulate and reach toxic levels. Preterm infants' kidneys are even less developed. The GFR and tubular secretion mature to adult levels within 2–5 months and 5–9 months of life, respectively (Buist et al. 1990; Burt et al. 2001). However, renal excretion is not the primary route of elimination for most psychotropic drugs (with some notable exceptions, like lithium, pregabalin, risperidone/paliperidone) (Spigset and Hägg 1998). Moreover, breastfeeding is usually fully initiated after the second day of life (when the GFR has already tripled), decreasing the danger of toxic drug accumulation (Yoshida et al. 1999). In general, drug exposure through breast milk is lower (and thus safer) than exposure through transplacental transfer, unless the infant is premature or has a metabolic defect (Eberhard-Gran et al. 2006).

2.2.4 Pharmacokinetics of Anxiolytics and Hypnotics During Lactation

Most anxiolytics are passively diffused into breast milk due to their lipophilic, unionized, and highly protein-bound profile. Clinicians tend to prefer short-acting benzodiazepines and avoid repeated administration that would lead to steady-state pharmacokinetics and increased infant exposure (Fortinguerra et al. 2009). For example, oxazepam has a short half-life, does not undergo liver demethylation or hydroxylation, and has no active metabolites. Whereas conjugation occurs more slowly in neonates, oxazepam conjugation is sufficiently effective within 1 week of life (Spigset and Hägg 1998). Milk to plasma (M/P) ratio varied from 0.1 to 0.3, and the infant exposure was found to be less than 1/1000th of the maternal dose (Oo et al. 1995; Ram and Gandotra 2015). Lorazepam's M/P ratio varies from 0.15 to 0.26, and its milk concentration is negligible (Oo et al. 1995). B-glucuronidase activity reduces lorazepam ingested by the infant to 6.1% of the weight-adjusted maternal daily dose (McElhatton 1994), and only mild sedation of the infant has been reported in a study of 51 lactating women (Ram and Gandotra 2015). Midazolam's M/P ratio is 0.09–0.16, and the exposure of the infant is 0.1% of the adjusted maternal single dose (McElhatton 1994; Oo et al. 1995). Prazepam and temazepam M/P ratios ranged from 0.10 to 0.14, and they are not detectable in the infants' serum during lactation (Menon 2008; Oo et al. 1995). On the contrary, lormetazepam is detected in both breast milk and plasma of nursing infants, and milk concentrations increase with each day of administration (Spigset and Hägg 1998). Alprazolam's milk to maternal plasma ratio was approximately 0.36, and the infant exposure was 3% of the maternal dose (Oo et al. 1995). Clorazepate and its metabolite nordiazepam are transferred into milk during lactation. The drug's very short half-life indicates that the detected product is most probably nordiazepam. Total clorazepate concentration found in the milk accounted for 15–30% of maternal plasma levels, and infant plasma levels accounted for 50% of the milk drug concentration (Rey et al. 1979). Diazepam and its metabolites are found in the breast milk, and infants exposed to diazepam may have longer lasting neonatal jaundice because of decreased bilirubin conjugation (Goldberg and Nissim 1994). Even after a single high postpartum dose administered to the mother, diazepam and its active metabolites can be detected in the breast milk, maternal and infant plasma for 6 days, following an accumulation pattern. The relative dose (diazepam and demethyl-diazepam) ranges from 2.6% to 13.4% of the mother's dose, and 4–5% of the pediatric dose. Plasma concentrations in newborns range from 35% (diazepam) and 71% (demethyl-diazepam) of the maternal concentration after 4 days of life, to 12% (diazepam) and 6% (demethyl-diazepam) (Spigset and Hägg 1998). Niitrazepam also accumulates in the maternal plasma and breast milk, and repeated administration or higher doses should be of concern (Kanto 1982). Interestingly, zopiclone, zolpidem, and zaleplone have very short half-lives, as well as fast elimination, making them less likely to accumulate in infant tissues. Their M/P ratio varies between 0.13 (zolpidem) and 0.6 (zopiclone), and the estimated infant exposure through breastfeeding should be less than 5% (Gaillot et al. 1983; Pons et al. 1994; Kohen 2005; Ram and Gandotra 2015; Aleksy and Smith 1998). Trazodone (not a benzodiazepine but an antidepressant commonly used off-label for sleep disorders) has been shown to have a milk:plasma ratio of 0.14, leading to minimal infant exposure amounting to 0.65–0.8% of the maternal weight-adjusted dose (Verbeeck et al. 1986).

2.2.5 Pharmacokinetics of Antidepressants During Lactation

Regarding all selective serotonin re-uptake inhibitors (SSRIs), the lactating infant is exposed to less than 10% when the relative infant dose is expressed as a percentage of the maternal dose (Sie et al. 2012). Such exposure is considered to be lower than the in utero exposure of the fetus. As a result, blood measurements of SSRI in lactating infants often show concentrations that are negligible or below the detection limit of the employed method. However, significant variations are reported in the literature. In fact, the relative infant dose ranges are 5–7% for citalopram and escitalopram, 3–6% for fluoxetine and norfluoxetine, 0–1% for fluvoxamine, 0–1% for paroxetine, and 0–3% for sertraline. When researchers found detectable levels of an antidepressant in lactating infants, the calculated M/P concentration ratio was also low. For example, the fluoxetine ratio was 0.3 and the ratio of its metabolite norfluoxetine was 0.2 (Burt et al. 2001; Weisskopf et al. 2015; Andrade 2014; Craig and Abel 2001).

Regarding the serotonin-norepinephrine reuptake inhibitors, duloxetine displayed a 0–1% relative infant dose and venlafaxine showed some accumulation in the milk with a relative infant dose of 3.2% (Kohen 2005). Current evidence taken together suggests that fluoxetine and mostly citalopram (and escitalopram) may result in higher risk for the lactating infant, whereas sertraline, paroxetine, and fluvoxamine probably carry the lowest risk (Burt et al. 2001; Fortinguerra et al. 2009). An additional benefit of sertraline is that it has a relatively short half-life and thus it can be administered once daily in a lactating mother, who can time the breastfeeding (or pumping) accordingly. Regarding the tricyclic antidepressants, most of them are detected in breast milk as they are bases and can be trapped in it. Tricyclics have large volumes of distribution and variable serum levels in lactating infants, ranging from nondetectable to notable. Indeed, the relative infant exposure for clomipramine was calculated at 3–4%, whereas for amitriptyline and nortriptyline it was approximately 2% (Pons et al. 1994; Burt et al. 2001). Nowadays use of tricyclic antidepressants is limited in most countries, but if they need to be prescribed, amitriptyline and imipramine are recommended (Kohen 2005). Concerning mirtazapine, the reported absolute and relative infant dose ranges from undetectably low to 2.86%, with no infant adverse effects detected (Smit et al. 2016).

2.2.6 Pharmacokinetics of Antipsychotics During Lactation

Milk/plasma ratios for first- and second-generation antipsychotics are mostly below 1, and with a few notable exceptions, infant exposure is generally modest. Thus, accumulation of antipsychotics in the newborns is unlikely, as infant plasma and urine drug levels are low (Babu et al. 2015). Breast milk levels of zuclopenthixol, perphenazine, trifluoperazine, haloperidol, and chlorpromazine were 1–3% of the maternal daily dose (Kronenfeld et al. 2017; Patton et al. 2002). The milk-to-plasma ratio for haloperidol was 0.67, for chlorpromazine between 0.5 to 1, and for perphenazine closer to 1. However, mothers on combined haloperidol and chlorpromazine treatment had increased blood and milk levels of both drugs (Pons et al. 1994; Spigset and Hägg 1998; Kohen 2005; Yoshida et al. 1998).

Regarding second-generation antipsychotic agents, infant estimated exposure to olanzapine, risperidone, and quetiapine during lactation is not considered significant and these drugs have very low concentration in the plasma of the lactating newborn. Olanzapine levels in infant plasma are undetectable, and infant exposure has been estimated to 1.8% of the maternal dosage (Kohen 2005). Risperidone and its active metabolite 9-hydroxyrisperidone (paliperidone) have M/P ratios of 0.42 and 0.24 respectively, and the estimated infant exposure is 4.3% of weight-adjusted maternal daily dosage (Patton et al. 2002). Infant exposure to quetiapine is probably modest, as doses of 75 mg or less are generally not detected in the breast milk, but in one case, a dose of 400 mg showed significantly higher milk drug concentrations (Misri et al. 2006). On the other hand, clozapine is known to accumulate in breast milk and fetal serum, and is contraindicated in breastfeeding women (Kohen 2005). In fact, measured clozapine levels in the lactating infant were 2.8–4.3 times higher than in the maternal plasma (Babu et al. 2015; Patton et al. 2002). Very few and inconclusive data exist on amisulpride, aripiprazole, ziprasidone, asenapine, and sertindole (Babu et al. 2015; Kronenfeld et al. 2017). A note of concern is that following an evaluation by Hummels et al., very few studies regarding antipsychotics and lactation correctly reported the M/P ratio, the Absolute Infant Dose (AID), and the Relative Infant Dose (RID), thus raising some concerns about the quality of the evidence so far (Hummels et al. 2016). Moreover, a most recent systematic review by Schoretsanitis et al. reports that there is a variability on milk penetration ratio for many antipsychotics. This might be explained by the differences between foremilk and hindmilk drug concentrations, as well as differences/errors in sample collection. Caution is required when using this pharmacokinetic evidence to assess infant antipsychotic exposure. The weight-adjusted relative infant dose and the infant serum drug concentration are expected to be more relatable indicators of infant drug exposure (Schoretsanitis et al. 2020b).

2.2.7 Pharmacokinetics of Mood Stabilizers During Lactation

The free, unbound fraction of mood stabilizing drugs can be excreted into breast milk, where no protein binding occurs (Johannessen 1992). Importantly, if a lactating mother is treated with lithium, the drug is detected in both breast milk and infant serum. Milk levels highly correlate with plasma levels in low lithium concentrations, but can reach 1.5 times the plasma level, in higher concentrations. Consequently, mean breast milk levels are approximately 40% of the maternal serum levels, but levels higher than 50% have also been observed. Accordingly, infant plasma concentrations are between 10% and 50% of maternal levels, and 80% of the weight-adjusted dose. In addition, infants might lack the ability to excrete large lithium quantities, and infection or dehydration can exacerbate this inability, thereby increasing lithium concentrations (Iqbal et al. 2001a, b; Spigset and Hägg 1998; Craig and Abel 2001). However, a recent study on breastfeeding neonates (mothers on lithium therapy) showed that even after 53–60 days of exclusive breastfeeding, lithium did not accumulate in the infants and, during the lactation follow-up, there was no acute growth or developmental delay (Imaz et al. 2021). Overall, lithium's relative infant dose has been reported to be 12.2% (ranging between 10 and 25%) and the average M/P ratio is 0.49 (Imaz et al. 2019).

Valproate levels in breast milk are low, corresponding to 5% or less of maternal serum concentrations, as shown by various studies (Grover and Avasthi 2015; Von Unruh et al. 1984; Nau et al. 1981). The dose found in infants corresponds to less than 6% of the initial pediatric dose for epilepsy (Spigset and Hägg 1998). Despite low levels of valproate, there is some risk involved, because of potential fetal hepatotoxicity (Goldberg and Nissim 1994). Regarding carbamazepine, the milk-to-plasma ratios are found between 0.4 and 1.8, and infant blood levels range from 6% to 65% of maternal blood concentration (Grover and Avasthi 2015; Yoshida et al. 1999). However, carbamazepine is considered to have a more favorable pharmacokinetic profile than lithium, as the final exposure of the lactating infant corresponds to only a fraction of the lowest therapeutic dose after weight-adjustment (Iqbal et al. 2001b; Spigset and Hägg 1998). Finally, lamotrigine is also excreted, and the breast milk/maternal plasma ratio may vary considerably, between 40% and 60%, and even as high as 150%, as shown by several studies (Iqbal et al. 2001a; Ohman et al. 2000; De Haan et al. 2004; Grover and Avasthi 2015). Lactating infants eliminate lamotrigine slower, therefore are prone to display enhanced lamotrigine levels. Moreover, it should be highlighted that lamotrigine serum levels in the mother undergo a rapid increase immediately after delivery, thus loading the breast milk with high lamotrigine concentrations (Ohman et al. 2000).

2.2.8 Opioid Pharmacokinetics During Lactation

Opioid relative infant dose is generally low (1–5%), however long-term maternal use (more than 3–4 days) potentially leads to drug accumulation in the infant, especially if the newborn's renal clearance is impaired. Morphine and M6G are excreted into milk and can be detected in the colostrum. Without counting in MG6, the relative infant dose of morphine is 2–3% of the weight-adjusted maternal morphine dose. However, MG6, especially in the early postpartum period, might reach high maternal plasma levels and its bioavailability in the infant still remains unknown (Ito 2018). Regarding codeine, the related infant dose is 1.2% of the maternal codeine dose. Despite the apparent safety of codeine and morphine, caution should be exerted as a rapid/ultrarapid metabolizing mother can transform increased amounts of codeine to morphine, thus overdosing the lactating infant which has low capacity of morphine glucuronidation. CYP2D6 genotype status crucially affects codeine/morphine disposition in milk making it difficult to predict. Moreover, these relative infant dose calculations for codeine do not include MG6 infant exposure. Overall, short-term postpartum administration of morphine is compatible with breastfeeding, but codeine should be avoided according to the FDA (Madadi et al. 2012; Ito 2018). Fentanyl excretion in the colostrum is very low both after epidural and intravenous administration during delivery. Following transdermal fentanyl administration to the lactating mother, fentanyl and its metabolite, norfentanyl, are undetectable in the infant's blood (relative infant dose 2–3%). Fentanyl exposure of the lactating infant corresponds to 10% of the one-time oral dose recommended for anesthesia in children. Such low doses are unlikely to exert any effects, and short-term fentanyl use during breastfeeding is considered relatively safe (Ito 2018; Cohen 2009). Tramadol is frequently used for labor analgesia, and its kinetics in the newborn and breast milk are relatively well-studied. The relative infant dose of tramadol and its metabolite, O-desmethyltramadol combined, is calculated to approximately 3% (Salman et al. 2011). Tramadol metabolism in the neonate is adequate and becomes substantial over the first year of life, but in return, accumulation of its metabolite can take place due to its limited excretion (Bloor et al. 2012). Overall, tramadol, due to its complex mechanism of action and its contraindication for children younger than 12 years of age, is not yet recommended for breastfeeding women (Ito 2018). Regarding methadone, its breast milk levels are modest. Ingested methadone through breastfeeding is calculated to be 0,1–0.3 mg daily, and the weight-adjusted dose for the infant is low, approximately 2,8% of the maternal dose. However, there have been scarce reports of neonatal abstinence syndrome after breastmilk feeding was discontinued (Jansson et al. 2008; Jansson et al. 2004). The relative infant dose of buprenorphine has been reported less than 1–2% of the maternal sublingual dose. For both methadone and buprenorphine, uneventful breastfeeding cases have been reported, although close infant monitoring should take place to treat infant opioid withdrawal syndrome (Ito 2018). There is limited evidence of oxycodone milk pharmacokinetics. The relative infant dose might vary from 0.1% to 3%. However, oxycodone can accumulate in breast milk if the nursing mother uses the drug for a prolonged period of time (more than 3 days) and/or if the newborn's drug clearance is impaired (Ito 2018).

2.3 Conclusions

Pregnancy results in a myriad of physiological changes, and unavoidably this leads to significant changes in the pharmacokinetics of nearly all psychotropics. Unfortunately, whether these changes are clinically important or not has not been clarified yet (Pariente et al. 2016). Moreover, it becomes immensely more difficult to clarify the final net effect of those changes, as many alterations have effects that cancel each other. Notably, although the placenta barrier normally protects the fetus, this does not apply to psychotropic medications, which are designed to penetrate human barriers, such as the blood-brain barrier and thus also the placenta. As a result, there is no "safe" drug in pregnancy, and pharmacokinetic data should merely be interpreted as aids in the "risk to benefit" decision-making processes made by clinicians. Randomized trials and well-designed pharmacokinetic studies in pregnant and lactating women would significantly improve our knowledge. Both kinds of studies are unlikely to occur, even for psychotropic medications routinely or widely used, as the pharmaceutical industry lacks the financial incentive to study those special populations and the regulatory framework is, righteously, very strict. Even if all these obstacles were overcome, the recruitment for such studies would be very problematic (Thomas and Yates 2012).

Based on current limited data, some prescribing strategies based on pharmacokinetics can be concluded: dose reduction during pregnancy is not always as attractive a strategy as it intuitively sounds, except for very specific cases. Pregnancy itself results in a reduced bioavailability of many medications and for many psychotropics there is not a clear or linear dose-response curve (W't Jong and Einarson 2017). As a result, clinicians should carefully assess the risk of disease exacerbation or recurrence, and even consider a dose increase if required. From a pharmacokinetics point of view, in order to minimize the exposure of the fetus to a psychotropic medication, higher protein binding, smaller distribution volume, shorter half-life, and ideally good affinity with efflux transporters are characteristics that would make one psychotropic medication more suitable than others for pregnant women. In any case, combinations of drugs should be avoided, especially those involving extensive

P450 metabolism, as the cytochrome is heavily modulated by pregnancy and interactions cannot be easily predicted.

Regarding breastfeeding, traditionally women on psychotropic medications were discouraged from it, a recommendation mostly based on principle rather than firm evidence. Alternatively, psychotropic medications were discontinued if breastfeeding was chosen, but this practice also ignores the individual characteristics and pharmacokinetic profile of each psychotropic medication. It is considered that infant drug concentration of 10% or less of the maternal drug therapeutic dose is a safe infant exposure, and for several psychotropic medications there is evidence (though still not unequivocally firm) that they have nearly undetectable levels in the lactating infant (W't Jong and Einarson 2017). A word of caution for those drugs that display low to moderate levels in the systemic circulation of a lactating infant is that brain concentrations can be significantly higher, or more impactful, due to the immature blood-brain barrier and brain tissue (Craig and Abel 2001). Specific strategies can be implemented to further reduce the exposure of the infant, i.e., selection of psychotropics with shorter half-life, administration at the lowest effective dose, breast-feeding and/or pumping milk (for later feeding), just before the scheduled time to take the medication (Menon 2008; Burt et al. 2001).. Pharmacogenomic considerations may enter clinical practice in the future, as, for example, CYP metabolizer status could guide drug dose adjustments during pregnancy and lactation (Betcher and George Jr. 2020). Breastfeeding mothers should be well-informed and educated, in order to observe for potential adverse effects (Harding and Timko 1999; Fortinguerra et al. 2009). Infant age should also be taken into consideration, as the potential risks progressively diminish with the maturation of the infant's hepatic metabolism and renal clearance. In any case, premature infants should not be exposed to psychotropics (Craig and Abel 2001).

References

Aleksy LM, Smith MAM. Sedatives and hypnotics in lactation. J Hum Lact. 1998;14(1):61–4.

Anderson D. A review of systemic opioids commonly used for labor pain relief. J Midwifery Womens Health. 2011;56(3):222–39.

Andrade C. The safety of duloxetine during pregnancy and lactation. J Clin Psychiatry. 2014;75(12):1423–7.

Ansari J, Carvalho B, Shafer SL, Flood P. Pharmacokinetics and pharmacodynamics of drugs commonly used in pregnancy and parturition. Anesth Analg. 2016;122(3):786–804.

Babu GN, Desai G, Chandra PS. Antipsychotics in pregnancy and lactation. Indian J Psychiatry. 2015;57(Suppl 2):S303.

Bader AM, Fragneto R, Terui K, Arthur GR, Loferski B, Datta S. Maternal and neonatal fentanyl and bupivacaine concentrations after epidural infusion during labor. Anesth Analg. 1995;81(4):829–32.

Betcher HK, George AL Jr. Pharmacogenomics in pregnancy. Semin Perinatol. 2020;44(3):151222.

Bloor M, Paech M, Kaye R. Tramadol in pregnancy and lactation. Int J Obstet Anesth. 2012;21(2):163–7.

Buist A, Norman TR, Dennerstein L. Breastfeeding and the use of psychotropic medication: a review. J Affect Disord. 1990;19(3):197–206.

Burkey BW, Holmes AP. Evaluating medication use in pregnancy and lactation: what every pharmacist should know. J Pediatr Pharmacol Ther. 2013;18(3):247–58.

Burt VK, Suri R, Altshuler L, Stowe Z, Hendrick VC, Muntean E. The use of psychotropic medications during breast-feeding. Am J Psychiatry. 2001;158(7):1001–9.

Chisolm MS, Payne JL. Management of psychotropic drugs during pregnancy. BMJ. 2016;532:h5918.

Cohen RS. Fentanyl transdermal analgesia during pregnancy and lactation. J Hum Lact. 2009;25(3):359–61.

Craig M, Abel K. Prescribing for psychiatric disorders in pregnancy and lactation. Best Pract Res Clin Obstet Gynaecol. 2001;15(6):1013–30.

Damoiseaux VA, Proost JH, Jiawan VC, Melgert BN. Sex differences in the pharmacokinetics of antidepressants: influence of female sex hormones and oral contraceptives. Clin Pharmacokinet. 2014;53(6):509–19.

de Barros DL, Moises EC, Carvalho Cavalli R, Lanchote VL, Duarte G, da Cunha SP. Distribution of fentanyl in the placental intervillous space and in the different maternal and fetal compartments in term pregnant women. Eur J Clin Pharmacol. 2009;65(8):803–8.

De Haan G-J, Edelbroek P, Segers J, Engelsman M, Lindhout D, Devile-Notschaele M, et al. Gestation-induced changes in lamotrigine pharmacokinetics: a monotherapy study. Neurology. 2004;63(3):571–3.

Deligiannidis KM, Byatt N, Freeman MP. Pharmacotherapy for mood disorders in pregnancy: a review of pharmacokinetic changes and clinical recommendations for therapeutic drug monitoring. J Clin Psychopharmacol. 2014;34(2):244.

Desprats R, Dumas JC, Giroux M, Campistron G, Faure F, Teixeira MG, et al. Maternal and umbilical cord concentrations of fentanyl after epidural analgesia for cesarean section. Eur J Obstet Gynecol Reprod Biol. 1991;42(2):89–94.

Desprats R, Giroux M, Dumas JC, Campistron G, Teixeira MG, Houin G, et al. Effect of adrenaline on plasma concentrations of fentanyl during epidural anaesthesia for caesarean section. Int J Obstet Anesth. 1995;4(4):225–9.

DeVane CL, Stowe ZN, Donovan JL, Newport DJ, Pennell PB, Ritchie JC, et al. Therapeutic drug monitoring of psychoactive drugs during pregnancy in the genomic era: challenges and opportunities. J Psychopharmacol. 2006;20(4_suppl):54–9.

Dickmann LJ, Isoherranen N. Quantitative prediction of CYP2B6 induction by estradiol during pregnancy, potential explanation for increased methadone clearance during pregnancy. Drug Metab Dispos. 2012;41:270.

Drozdick J, Berghella V, Hill M, Kaltenbach K. Methadone trough levels in pregnancy. Am J Obstet Gynecol. 2002;187(5):1184–8.

Eberhard-Gran M, Eskild A, Opjordsmoen S. Treating mood disorders during pregnancy. Drug Saf. 2005;28(8):695–706.

Eberhard-Gran M, Eskild A, Opjordsmoen S. Use of psychotropic medications in treating mood disorders during lactation. CNS Drugs. 2006;20(3):187–98.

Feghali M, Venkataramanan R, Caritis S. Pharmacokinetics of drugs in pregnancy. In: Seminars in perinatology, vol. 39. Elsevier; 2015. p. 512.

Fokina VM, Xu M, Rytting E, Abdel-Rahman SZ, West H, Oncken C, et al. Pharmacokinetics of bupropion and its pharmacologically active metabolites in pregnancy. Drug Metab Dispos. 2016;44(11):1832–8.

Fortinguerra F, Clavenna A, Bonati M. Psychotropic drug use during breastfeeding: a review of the evidence. Pediatrics. 2009;124(4):e547–e56.

Franco V, Mazzucchelli I, Gatti G, Specchio LM, La Neve A, Papantonio A, et al. Changes in lamotrigine pharmacokinetics during pregnancy and the puerperium. Ther Drug Monit. 2008;30(4):544–7.

Gaillot J, Heusse D, Hougton G, Aurele JM, Dreyfus J. Pharmacokinetics and metabolism of zopiclone. Pharmacology. 1983;27(Suppl. 2):76–91.

Goldberg HL, Nissim R. Psychotropic drugs in pregnancy and lactation. Int J Psychiatry Med. 1994;24(2):129–47.

Grangier L, Martinez de Tejada B, Savoldelli GL, Irion O, Haller G. Adverse side effects and route of administration of opioids in combined spinal-epidural analgesia for labour: a meta-analysis of randomised trials. Int J Obstet Anesth. 2020;41:83–103.

Grover S, Avasthi A. Mood stabilizers in pregnancy and lactation. Indian J Psychiatry. 2015;57(Suppl 2):S308.

Haidl F, Rosseland LA, Spigset O, Dahl V. Effects of adrenaline on maternal and fetal fentanyl absorption in epidural analgesia: a randomized trial. Acta Anaesthesiol Scand. 2018;62(9):1267–73.

Harding JJ, Timko JV. The use of psychotropic medications during pregnancy and lactation. The Foundation for The Global Library of Women's Medicine. 1999.

Hendrickx A, Nau H, Binkerd P, Rowland J, Rowland J, Cukierski M, et al. Valproic acid developmental toxicity and pharmacokinetics in the rhesus monkey: an interspecies comparison. Teratology. 1988;38(4):329–45.

Huang W, Isoherranen N. Sampling site has a critical impact on physiologically based pharmacokinetic modeling. J Pharmacol Exp Ther. 2020;372(1):30–45.

Hummels H, Bertholee D, van der Meer D, Smit JP, Wilffert B, ter Horst P. The quality of lactation studies including antipsychotics. Eur J Clin Pharmacol. 2016;72(12):1417–25.

Imaz ML, Torra M, Soy D, Garcia-Esteve L, Martin-Santos R. Clinical lactation studies of lithium: a systematic review. Front Pharmacol. 2019;10:1005.

Imaz ML, Langohr K, Torra M, Soy D, Garcia-Esteve L, Martin-Santos R. Neonatal feeding trajectories in mothers with bipolar disorder taking lithium: pharmacokinetic data. Front Pharmacol. 2021;12:752022.

Iqbal MM, Gundlapalli SP, Ryan WG, Ryals T, Passman TE. Effects of antimanic mood-stabilizing drugs on fetuses, neonates, and nursing infants. South Med J. 2001a;94(3):304–22.

Iqbal MM, Sohhan T, Mahmud SZ. The effects of lithium, valproic acid, and carbamazepine during pregnancy and lactation. J Toxicol Clin Toxicol. 2001b;39(4):381–92.

Ito S. Opioids in breast milk: pharmacokinetic principles and clinical implications. J Clin Pharmacol. 2018;58(Suppl 10):S151–S63.

Jain AE, Lacy T. Psychotropic drugs in pregnancy and lactation. J Psychiatr Pract. 2005;11(3):177–91.

Jansson LM, Velez M, Harrow C. Methadone maintenance and lactation: a review of the literature and current management guidelines. J Hum Lact. 2004;20(1):62–71.

Jansson LM, Choo R, Velez ML, Lowe R, Huestis MA. Methadone maintenance and long-term lactation. Breastfeed Med. 2008;3(1):34–7.

Jarvis MA, Wu-Pong S, Kniseley JS, Schnoll SH. Alterations in methadone metabolism during late pregnancy. J Addict Dis. 1999;18(4):51–61.

Johannessen SI. Pharmacokinetics of valproate in pregnancy: mother-foetus-newborn. Pharm World Sci. 1992;14(3):114–7.

Jørgensen N, Thurmann-Nielsen E, Walstad R. Pharmacokinetics and distribution of diazepam and oxazepam in early pregnancy. Acta Obstet Gynecol Scand. 1988;67(6):493–7.

Kanto JH. Use of benzodiazepines during pregnancy, labour and lactation, with particular reference to pharmacokinetic considerations. Drugs. 1982;23(5):354–80.

Kesavan R, Rajan S, Kumar L. Effect and safety of labor epidural analgesia with intermittent boluses of 0.1% bupivacaine with fentanyl on fetal and maternal outcomes and wellbeing. Anesth Essays Res. 2018;12(4):769–73.

Kieviet N, Dolman KM, Honig A. The use of psychotropic medication during pregnancy: how about the newborn? Neuropsychiatr Dis Treat. 2013;9:1257.

Klier CM, Mossaheb N, Saria A, Schloegelhofer M, Zernig G. Pharmacokinetics and elimination of quetiapine, venlafaxine, and trazodone during pregnancy and postpartum. J Clin Psychopharmacol. 2007;27(6):720–2.

Kohen D. Psychotropic medication and breast-feeding. Adv Psychiatr Treat. 2005;11(5):371–9.

Kokras N, Dalla C, Papadopoulou-Daifoti Z. Sex differences in pharmacokinetics of antidepressants. Expert Opin Drug Metab Toxicol. 2011;7(2):213–26.

Kronenfeld N, Berlin M, Shaniv D, Berkovitch M. Use of psychotropic medications in breastfeeding women. Birth Defects Res. 2017;109(12):957–97.

Llewellyn A, Stowe ZN. Psychotropic medications in lactation. J Clin Psychiatry. 1998;59(Suppl 6):57.

Loftus JR, Hill H, Cohen SE. Placental transfer and neonatal effects of epidural sufentanil and fentanyl administered with bupivacaine during labor. Anesthesiology. 1995;83(2):300–8.

Madadi P, Avard D, Koren G. Pharmacogenetics of opioids for the treatment of acute maternal pain during pregnancy and lactation. Curr Drug Metab. 2012;13(6):721–7.

Mandelli M, Tognoni G, Garattini S. Clinical pharmacokinetics of diazepam. Clin Pharmacokinet. 1978;3(1):72–91.

McElhatton PR. The effects of benzodiazepine use during pregnancy and lactation. Reprod Toxicol. 1994;8(6):461–75.

Menon SJ. Psychotropic medication during pregnancy and lactation. Arch Gynecol Obstet. 2008;277(1):1–13.

Misri S, Corral M, Wardrop AA, Kendrick K. Quetiapine augmentation in lactation: a series of case reports. J Clin Psychopharmacol. 2006;26(5):508–11.

Moises EC, de Barros DL, de Carvalho CR, Lanchote VL, Duarte G, da Cunha SP. Pharmacokinetics and transplacental distribution of fentanyl in epidural anesthesia for normal pregnant women. Eur J Clin Pharmacol. 2005;61(7):517–22.

Morley-Forster PK, Reid DW, Vandeberghe H. A comparison of patient-controlled analgesia fentanyl and alfentanil for labour analgesia. Can J Anaesth. 2000;47(2):113–9.

Nau H, Koch S, Häuser I, Helge H. Valproic acid and its metabolites: placental transfer, neonatal pharmacokinetics, transfer via mother's milk and clinical status in neonates of epileptic mothers. J Pharmacol Exp Ther. 1981;219(3):768–77.

Neuman G, Colantonio D, Delaney S, Szynkaruk M, Ito S. Bupropion and escitalopram during lactation. Ann Pharmacother. 2014;48(7):928–31.

Ohman I, Vitols S, Tomson T. Lamotrigine in pregnancy: pharmacokinetics during delivery, in the neonate, and during lactation. Epilepsia. 2000;41(6):709–13.

Oo C, Kuhn R, Desai N, Wright C, McNamara P. Pharmacokinetics in lactating women: prediction of alprazolam transfer into milk. Br J Clin Pharmacol. 1995;40(3):231–6.

Pariente G, Leibson T, Carls A, Adams-Webber T, Ito S, Koren G. Pregnancy-associated changes in pharmacokinetics: a systematic review. PLoS Med. 2016;13(11):e1002160.

Patton SW, Misri S, Corral MR, Perry KF, Kuan AJ. Antipsychotic medication during pregnancy and lactation in women with schizophrenia: evaluating the risk. Can J Psychiatry. 2002;47(10):959–65.

Pienimäki P, Lampela E, Hakkola J, Arvela P, Raunio H, Vähäkangas K. Pharmacokinetics of oxcarbazepine and carbamazepine in human placenta. Epilepsia. 1997;38(3):309–16.

Pinheiro EA, Wisner KL, Clark CT. Quetiapine dose adjustments in pregnant and postpartum women with bipolar disorder. J Clin Psychopharmacol. 2018;38(1):89–91.

Pond SM, Kreek MJ, Tong TG, Raghunath J, Benowitz NL. Altered methadone pharmacokinetics in methadone-maintained pregnant women. J Pharmacol Exp Ther. 1985;233(1):1–6.

Pons G, Rey E, Matheson I. Excretion of psychoactive drugs into breast milk. Clin Pharmacokinet. 1994;27(4):270–89.

Practice Guidelines for Obstetric Anesthesia. An updated report by the American Society of Anesthesiologists Task Force on obstetric anesthesia and the Society for Obstetric Anesthesia and Perinatology. Anesthesiology. 2016;124(2):270–300.

Ram D, Gandotra S. Antidepressants, anxiolytics, and hypnotics in pregnancy and lactation. Indian J Psychiatry. 2015;57(Suppl 2):S354.

Rey E, Giraux P, d'Athis P, Turquais J, Chavinie J, Olive G. Pharmacokinetics of the placental transfer and distribution of clorazepate and its metabolite nordiazepam in the feto-placental unit and in the neonate. Eur J Clin Pharmacol. 1979;15(3):181–5.

Reynolds F, Sharma SK, Seed PT. Analgesia in labour and fetal acid-base balance: a meta-analysis comparing epidural with systemic opioid analgesia. BJOG. 2002;109(12):1344–53.

Saito J, Ishii M, Mito A, Yakuwa N, Kawasaki H, Tachibana Y, et al. Trazodone levels in maternal serum, cord blood, breast Milk, and neonatal serum. Breastfeed Med. 2021;16(11):922–5.
Salman S, Sy SK, Ilett KF, Page-Sharp M, Paech MJ. Population pharmacokinetic modeling of tramadol and its O-desmethyl metabolite in plasma and breast milk. Eur J Clin Pharmacol. 2011;67(9):899–908.
Schoretsanitis G, Spigset O, Stingl JC, Deligiannidis KM, Paulzen M, Westin AA. The impact of pregnancy on the pharmacokinetics of antidepressants: a systematic critical review and meta-analysis. Expert Opin Drug Metab Toxicol. 2020a;16(5):431–40.
Schoretsanitis G, Westin AA, Deligiannidis KM, Spigset O, Paulzen M. Excretion of antipsychotics into the amniotic fluid, umbilical cord blood, and breast Milk: a systematic critical review and combined analysis. Ther Drug Monit. 2020b;42(2):245–54.
Schou M, Amdisen A, Steenstrup OR. Lithium and pregnancy. II. Hazards to women given lithium during pregnancy and delivery. Br Med J. 1973;2(5859):137–8.
Shah AA, Aftab A. Are psychotropic drugs safe to use during lactation? Psychiatr Ann. 2015;45(2):77–82.
Shum S, Shen DD, Isoherranen N. Predicting maternal-fetal disposition of fentanyl following intravenous and epidural administration using physiologically based pharmacokinetic modeling. Drug Metab Dispos. 2021;49(11):1003–15.
Sie SD, Wennink JM, van Driel JJ, te Winkel AG, Boer K, Casteelen G, et al. Maternal use of SSRIs, SNRIs and NaSSAs: practical recommendations during pregnancy and lactation. Arch Dis Child Fetal Neonatal Ed. 2012;97(6):F472–6.
Smit M, Dolman KM, Honig A. Mirtazapine in pregnancy and lactation – a systematic review. Eur Neuropsychopharmacol. 2016;26(1):126–35.
Spigset O, Hägg S. Excretion of psychotropic drugs into breast milk. CNS Drugs. 1998;9(2):111–34.
ter Horst PG, van der Linde S, Smit JP, den Boon J, van Lingen RA, Jansman FG, et al. Clomipramine concentration and withdrawal symptoms in 10 neonates. Br J Clin Pharmacol. 2012;73(2):295–302.
ter Horst PG, Larmene-Beld KH, Bosman J, van der Veen EL, Wieringa A, Smit JP. Concentrations of venlafaxine and its main metabolite O-desmethylvenlafaxine during pregnancy. J Clin Pharm Ther. 2014;39(5):541–4.
Thomas SHL, Yates LM. Prescribing without evidence – pregnancy. Br J Clin Pharmacol. 2012;74(4):691–7.
Tomson T, Luef G, Sabers A, Pittschieler S, Öhman I. Valproate effects on kinetics of lamotrigine in pregnancy and treatment with oral contraceptives. Neurology. 2006;67(7):1297–9.
Van de Velde M, Carvalho B. Remifentanil for labor analgesia: an evidence-based narrative review. Int J Obstet Anesth. 2016;25:66–74.
van Hoogdalem MW, Wexelblatt SL, Akinbi HT, Vinks AA, Mizuno T. A review of pregnancy-induced changes in opioid pharmacokinetics, placental transfer, and fetal exposure: towards fetomaternal physiologically-based pharmacokinetic modeling to improve the treatment of neonatal opioid withdrawal syndrome. Pharmacol Ther. 2022;234:108045.
Verbeeck RK, Ross SG, McKenna EA. Excretion of trazodone in breast milk. Br J Clin Pharmacol. 1986;22(3):367–70.
Von Unruh G, Froescher W, Hoffmann F, Niesen M. Valproic acid in breast milk: how much is really there? Ther Drug Monit. 1984;6(3):272–6.
Wang K, Cao L, Deng Q, Sun LQ, Gu TY, Song J, et al. The effects of epidural/spinal opioids in labour analgesia on neonatal outcomes: a meta-analysis of randomized controlled trials. Can J Anaesth. 2014;61(8):695–709.
Weisskopf E, Fischer CJ, Bickle Graz M, Morisod Harari M, Tolsa J-F, Claris O, et al. Risk-benefit balance assessment of SSRI antidepressant use during pregnancy and lactation based on best available evidence. Expert Opin Drug Saf. 2015;14(3):413–27.
Westin AA, Brekke M, Molden E, Skogvoll E, Spigset O. Selective serotonin reuptake inhibitors and venlafaxine in pregnancy: changes in drug disposition. PLoS One. 2017;12(7):e0181082.
W't Jong G, Einarson A. Maternal use of SSRIs, SNRIs and NaSSAs: practical recommendations during pregnancy and lactation. 2017.

Yoshida K, Smith B, Craggs M, Kumar R. Neuroleptic drugs in breast-milk: a study of pharmacokinetics and of possible adverse effects in breast-fed infants. Psychol Med. 1998;28(1):81–91.

Yoshida K, Smith B, Kumar R. Psychotropic drugs in mothers' milk: a comprehensive review of assay methods, pharmacokinetics and of safety of breast-feeding. J Psychopharmacol. 1999;13(1):64–80.

Zakowski MI, Ramanathan S, Turndorf H. A two-dose epidural morphine regimen in cesarean section patients: pharmacokinetic profile. Acta Anaesthesiol Scand. 1993;37(6):584–9.

Safety Parameters and Risk Categories Used for Psychotropic Drugs in Pregnancy and Lactation

3

Yusuf Cem Kaplan, Hilal Erol, and Elif Keskin-Arslan

3.1 Introduction

The perinatal period is associated with an increased risk of psychiatric disorders which may necessitate maternal pharmacotherapy. In this chapter, we aim to provide the reader with the basics of safety assessment regarding medication use during pregnancy and breastfeeding.

3.2 Pregnancy Risk Categories

The Thalidomide disaster of the 1960s caused a drastic change in our understanding of risks associated with medication use during pregnancy. One of the key consequences of this incident, apart from the changes in regulations regarding preclinical trials, was the emergence of a need to develop a categorization for the medications based on the risks they pose to the fetus and this need led to the introduction of the various pregnancy risk categories across different countries.

The first risk categorization system regarding medication use in pregnancy was developed and introduced in Sweden in 1978, named as The Swedish Catalogue of Approved Drugs (FASS) and 4 risk categories (A, B, C, D) have been proposed

Y. C. Kaplan (✉)
Department of Pharmacology, Izmir Katip Celebi University Faculty of Medicine, Izmir, Turkey

Terafar – Izmir Katip Celebi University Teratology Information, Research and Training Center, Izmir, Turkey

H. Erol
Independent Researcher, Izmir, Turkey

E. Keskin-Arslan
Department of Pharmacology, Izmir Bakırcay University Faculty of Medicine, Izmir, Turkey

F. Uguz, L. Orsolini (eds.), *Perinatal Psychopharmacology*,
https://doi.org/10.1007/978-3-031-99720-4_3

Table 3.1 Short summary of pregnancy warning classification systems in Sweden, the United States, and Australia

Category
Sweden
A No known risk
B Human data insufficient
B1 no fetal effects in animal data
B2 incomplete animal data
B3 fetal effects in animal data
C Pharmacological effects on fetus
D Causes or is suspected of causing fetal damage in humans
United States
A Controlled studies show no risk
B No evidence of human risk (controlled studies show no risk or animal studies indicate no risk)
C Risk cannot be ruled out
D Positive evidence of risk but potential benefit may outweigh potential risk
X Contraindicated in pregnancy
Australia
A-D As in Sweden
X Should not be used in pregnancy

From Källén (1999) with permission

(Källén 1999). Category A denotes the safest drugs and the possible risk of the medication is expected to increase from A to D. Category B comprises 3 subgroups (B1, B2, B3).

The following year (1979), the US Food and Drug Administration (FDA) introduced its own pregnancy risk categorization system which was composed of 5 subgroups. Similar to the FASS system, categories ranged from A to D, with the additional subgroup, Category X, which represents contraindicated drugs (Addis et al. 2000). The Australian Drug Evaluation Committee (ADEC) classification was developed in 1989. ADEC can be regarded as a combination of both previous categories since it comprises subcategories B1, B2, B3, and X (Addis et al. 2000). Table 3.1 presents a short summary of these 3 systems. Significant differences in the classification of similar medications between these 3 systems were previously reported by Addis et al. in 2000 (Addis et al. 2000).

3.3 Criticisms Regarding the FDA Pregnancy Risk Categories

The primary aim of the FDA pregnancy risk categorization system was to provide evidence-based risk assessment to help physicians in counseling the women who are planning a pregnancy. However, it was generally misunderstood by the healthcare providers, as a tool for assessing exposure risks that happened during an inadvertent pregnancy. At the time the risk categories were designed, pregnant women were generally considered to be young, healthy individuals who were free of diseases. However, this perception has been changed since the last two decades witnessed an increasing rate of pregnancy in women aged 35 and older (Dunlop et al. 2008), which consequently led to an increase in the number of pregnant women who are entering pregnancy with a pre-existing chronic disease that necessitates pharmacotherapy. For instance, approximately 40% of women in reproductive age (19–45) are reported to be diagnosed with a chronic disease in the United States (Chatterjee et al. 2008) and one in five pregnant women is reported to have at least one chronic disease in Germany (Kersten et al. 2014).

Toward the end of the 1990s, the FDA recognized the important limitations and shortcomings of the 1979 categorization system which may misguide clinical practice. A public hearing resulted in the following implications (Feibus 2008):

1. Categories are inadequate in conveying the risk because of the oversimplified narrative.
2. Categories indicate that the teratogenic potencies of drugs in the same category are similar, which is a false perception.
3. Categories do not differentiate between the possible severity and incidence of the fetal adverse effects. They also do not distinguish between the time, dose, route, duration, and frequency of the exposure.
4. Categories focus on drug use in planned pregnancies. They are insufficient in identifying risks for the exposures during an inadvertent pregnancy.
5. Categories lack sufficient distinction to provide meaningful interpretations between animal and human data.

Following extensive reviews and thorough discussions with key stakeholders, the FDA decided to remove the pregnancy letter categories A, B, C, D and X from the product labeling and replace with the Pregnancy and Lactation Labeling Rule (PLLR) which is the narrative summary of the risk associated with the use of a medication during pregnancy and lactation. The new pregnancy labeling includes three sections: (1) Fetal Risk Summary, (2) Clinical considerations, and (3) Data (Frederiksen 2011). Each pregnancy label begins with contact information for relevant pregnancy exposure registries and, when available, includes a standard statement about the baseline risk of major congenital malformations and other adverse pregnancy outcomes that exist for all pregnancies regardless of medication exposure (Feibus 2008). The Fetal Risk Summary section also provides a conclusion describing the likelihood that the medication increases risk to the fetus. It covers the possible fetal adverse effects of the medication such as structural malformations, fetal and infant death, physiological dysfunctions, and fetal growth abnormalities and their incidence, seriousness, reversibility, and correctability. The summary also considers possible fetal risks with regard to the dose, duration, and time window of the medication exposure (Frederiksen 2011). The Clinical Consideration section includes information regarding inadvertent exposure such as dose, critical time window for the possible risks, and the possible risks of underlying maternal clinical condition, if present. It also addresses neonatal concerns, and their severity and reversibility, associated with the use of medication. The possible effects of the medication on the duration of labor and birth will also be included. Finally, the data section discusses available human and animal data. Animal data are reviewed in terms of species, dose ranges, human dose equivalents, and possible mechanisms of action (Feibus 2008).

This rule took effect on June 30, 2015, and requires medications and biological products approved after June 30, 2001, to revise the information found in the Pregnancy and Nursing Mothers subsections of product labeling (Sahin et al. 2016). Between 2000 and 2022, 488 new drug applications (NDAs) approved by the FDA were assessed for post-marketing commitments, breastfeeding, and pregnancy requirements. Of the 59 approved NDAs, 41 included requirements for pregnancy, 4 for lactation, and 14 for both (Avachat et al. 2023).

The new PLLR labeling was evaluated in a survey carried out in 2018. The results of this survey indicate that despite the extremely low response rate, the majority of clinicians were unaware of the new PLLR format and were still utilizing the pregnancy letter category system (Namazy et al. 2020).

3.4 Assessing the Possible Teratogenic Risk of Medications

3.4.1 Variables Related with the Administration of the Medication

3.4.1.1 Time of Administration

The time after conception to implantation (8–10 days) is considered as the "all or none" period which implies the exposure to any harmful agent of the embryo would either yield to spontaneous abortion or intact survival. The embryonic period, in which the organogenesis takes place, starts after the implantation and lasts 54–60 days after conception. This period where a set of complex cellular events take place, such as cellular migration and differentiation, is the most sensitive period of embryo to teratogenic insults resulting in structural malformations. The fetal period just starts after the organogenesis and continues to term. Growth and functional maturation of organs occur in this phase and teratogenic exposure during this period usually ends up with the disruption in function or size of the organs rather than structural anomalies.

For most drugs, the main concern is the first trimester of pregnancy (Brent 2004a), however there may be exceptions. For instance, exposure to selective serotonin reuptake inhibitors (SSRIs) in late pregnancy was shown to be significantly associated with persistent pulmonary hypertension of the newborn whereas a significant association with early pregnancy exposure was not apparent (Grigoriadis et al. 2014).

3.4.1.2 Dose of Medication

Valproic acid (VPA) constitutes an important example of dose-related teratogenicity. Studies report different dose categories in which the rates of structural malformations with VPA monotherapy are significantly increased; the largest increased risk is demonstrated with doses greater than 1000 mg per day (Diav-Citrin et al.

2008; Kaneko et al. 1999). Tomson et al. reported the malformation rates regarding VPA monotherapy in pregnancy as 5.6%, 10.4%, and 24.2% with doses <700 mg/day, ≥ 700 to <1500, and ≥ 1500 mg per day, respectively (Tomson et al. 2011). Regarding the neurodevelopmental abnormalities, a VPA dose greater than 900 mg per day and 1000 mg per day is associated with a decreased total development score and IQ, respectively (Bromley et al. 2010; Meador et al. 2009).

3.4.1.3 Route of Administration

Route of administration is one of the major determinants of drug bioavailability, which is the ability of a drug to reach the systemic circulation and therefore the fetus. Retinoids are potent and well-established teratogens which constitute a good example for this issue. Systemic retinoid exposure has been demonstrated to increase the rates or major malformations up to 35% (Lammer et al. 1985). This high figure, which is only comparable to that of thalidomide, and some case reports with major malformations (Lipson et al. 1993; Camera and Pregliasco 1992) in the 1990s led to an increased teratogenic risk perception regarding topical retinoids. However, cohort studies (Panchaud et al. 2012; Loureiro et al. 2005; Shapiro et al. 1997; Jick et al. 1993) and a recent meta-analysis (Kaplan et al. 2015b) demonstrated that inadvertent exposure to topical retinoids does not seem to increase the rate of major malformations which is in line with in vivo and in vitro pharmacokinetic data suggesting that their dermal absorption is minimal and unlikely to result in fetal harm (Jensen et al. 1991; Lehman et al. 1988). However, a rare association suggested by the case reports still cannot be excluded and contraindicates their use during pregnancy.

3.4.1.4 Monotherapy Versus Polytherapy

Psychotropic drug polytherapy in pregnant women is a common practice (Sadowski et al. 2013). However, data regarding the teratogenicity risk of polytherapy vs monotherapy with psychotropic drugs are very limited, however, a few studies are worth mentioning. Tomson et al. reported that VPA is a primary determinant of the risk of major malformations regarding the combination therapy in pregnant women using antiepileptic drugs (Tomson et al. 2011). This finding confirmed the results of the previous studies which suggested that it was VPA and not the number of antiepileptic drugs in the combinations that was associated with the increased risk for major malformations (Vajda 2010; Vajda et al. 2010). However, a recent study questioned this finding and suggested that topiramate, when used in polytherapy, is also associated with an increased risk of major malformations (Vajda et al. 2016). Second-generation antipsychotic monotherapy appears to pose less risk to the fetus when compared with polytherapy (Sadowski et al. 2013). Nevertheless, this area remains to be further investigated.

3.4.2 Evaluating the Data

As previously mentioned, lack of available data regarding a particular drug's effects during pregnancy is one of the biggest challenges we face in the clinical setting.

Because ethical concerns limit the availability of pregnant women for randomized-controlled trials, data regarding the effects of a drug on fetus is not usually available at the time of its launch. It has been shown that 92.1% of the drugs which have been approved by FDA between years 1980 and 2000, and 97.7% of the drugs that have been approved between 2000 and 2010 lack adequate data at the time of their approval (Adam et al. 2011; Lo and Friedman 2002). It takes at least 6.0 ± 4.1 years to determine the teratogenic effect of a drug after its approval, while ruling out even takes much longer (9.1 ± 4.5 years) (Lo and Friedman 2002). Knowing how to interpret animal and human data therefore becomes more critical.

3.4.2.1 Experimental Studies

Animal Studies

Although there are difficulties in extrapolating the results to humans, animal studies can provide important information regarding the teratogenic effects of drugs. However, their protocols should be well-planned and results need to be reported and interpreted carefully in order to rule out any bias (Brent 2004b). Detected malformations should be interpreted regarding the type and rate, since some malformations are common in some species. Variations, definition of which depends on different factors such as animal species, strain, supplier, and laboratory environment, should not be reported and/or interpreted as major malformations. It should also be kept in mind that excessive maternal toxicity induced by the drug may lead to non-specific developmental toxicity in the offspring (Guittina et al. 2000).

3.4.2.2 Human Studies

Case Reports

Case reports are very useful tools in the field of teratology if used properly. Observation of a repetitive "rare defect" appearing after a "rare environmental exposure" (Shepard 1994) by the "astute clinicians" (Carey et al. 2009) has been a very effective way to detect teratogens. The identification of warfarin (Holzgreve et al. 1976; Fourie and Hay 1975), diethylstilbestrol (Herbst and Scully 1970), isotretinoin (Rosa 1983), fluconazole (only with high dose and prolonged use for systemic infections) (Pursley et al. 1996; Lee et al. 1992), and mycophenolate mofetil (Sifontis et al. 2006; Le Ray et al. 2004) as human teratogens was originally based on case reports. However, case reports cannot provide any estimates regarding the absolute risk since they lack a denominator. Because it is quite common to report and publish the positive findings (Song et al. 2013), case reports trying to associate drug exposure in pregnancy with relatively common major malformations, the background risk of which is 3% in the general population regardless of any exposure, exist in the literature. The clinician should be careful in interpreting those findings and should only consider the ones reporting a unique and repeating pattern of malformations with a particularly rare exposure during pregnancy as a signal.

Epidemiologic Studies

The ethical barriers that exist for enrolling pregnant women in randomized-controlled trials make the observational cohort and case-control studies the primary sources of information for drug use during pregnancy. Both studies are mutually complementary in assessing the teratogenic risk of drugs.

The development of teratology information services (TISes), which counsel hundreds of pregnant women every year about drug use in pregnancy, and their networks such as MotherToBaby (formerly OTIS, Organisation of Teratology Information Services) (Leen-Mitchell et al. 2000) and European Network of Teratology Information Services (ENTIS) (Schaefer 2011) contributed significantly to the field of teratology by enabling the implementation of multicentral prospective cohort studies. Prospective cohort studies undertaken by TISes have important strengths such as assigning the subjects before the outcome is known, identifying the precise exposure time and minimizing the risk of recall bias by prospectively collected data, and being able to match the subjects in the exposed and control groups with regard to potential confounders mentioned below (Källén 2012; Irl and Hasford 2000).

Recent developments in the information technology have also enabled national medical databases and birth registries as sources of data for conducting prospective cohort studies. Medicaid and private insurance claims databases in the United States, Saskatchewan Health Services Database in Canada, The General Practice Research Database in UK and Population Medical Databases in Nordic Countries are important examples which enables relatively quick and inexpensive analysis of a data from a large population that is prospectively collected for routine purposes (Ehrenstein et al. 2010). Among other things, pregnancy registries may be product- or disease-specific, like the "Epilepsy Pregnancy Register" or the "National Pregnancy Registry for Atypical Antipsychotics" (EMA 2012).

Case-control studies are designed to assess whether a specific type exposure is associated with a specific outcome by evaluating both subjects with and those without the specific outcome. A major strength of these studies is their increased statistical power which is usually adequate to detect moderate increases in the rate of specific malformations (Mitchell 2003). Case-control surveillance systems offer a convenient approach to carry out these studies. "Slone Epidemiology Unit Birth Defects Study" in the United States and Canada, "National Birth Defects Prevention Study" in the United States, and "Hungarian Case-control of Congenital Abnormalities Study" in Hungary are noteworthy surveillance systems (EMA 2012).

Meta-Analysis

Meta-analysis emerged as a powerful tool of epidemiology enabling the pooling of results from individual, yet comparable, studies (Egger et al. 2002). This method is useful in assessing the possible teratogenic effects of drugs, by combining the data from observational studies, with an increased sample size and power. It may also offer subgroup analyses, such as organ-specific malformations, which are reported but not evaluated in individual studies.

3.4.2.3 Methodological Issues

Sample Size, Characteristics, Follow-Up

The background rate for major congenital malformations is 3%. Very few teratogens (thalidomide, isotretinoin, valproic acid) increase this rate by a factor of more than two, while most only increase a specific malformation rate. At least 220 exposed and controlled (unexposed) pregnancies will be required to show that the major congenital malformation risk is increased by a factor of 2.5, with a power of 80 percent. Prospective cohort studies, which are usually conducted by TISes, include a relatively small number of patients (<300). Although this number makes it difficult to detect a specific malformation rate, it is adequate to rule out the particular drug being a major teratogen. Another issue with these studies is that the pregnant women who call TISes voluntarily may not be the representative of the general population. The follow-up period of the infants is usually 1 year and limits the inclusion of the malformations which are identified later. The loss-to-follow-up of pregnant patients due to technical reasons may also be a concern in some of these studies (Chambers 2011).

Recall Bias

Recall of drug use is a potential limitation of case-control studies due to the reason that mothers with malformed children may be better at remembering their drug use and course of pregnancies (Mitchell 2003). Selecting the children with different malformations in the control group is suggested to overcome this problem.

Confounders

Maternal age, parity, gestational week, previous miscarriages or birth of malformed infants, folic acid use, body mass index, maternal smoking, alcohol or illicit drug use are important confounders in studies evaluating the association of structural malformations with drugs used in pregnancy (Källén 2012). Maternal and paternal IQ, socioeconomic status, and level of education are important for the studies which assess long-term neurodevelopmental outcomes in children. A recent study suggested that severity of maternal depression, and not selective reuptake inhibitor antidepressants, was a significant predictor of a decreased behavioral score in infants aged 3–6 years (Nulman et al. 2015).

Confounding by Indication

The risk of major and/or organ-specific congenital malformations has been demonstrated to increase in some chronic diseases regardless of drug use. For instance, diabetes and chronic hypertension in the mother have been associated with an increased rate of congenital malformations (Bateman et al. 2015; Correa et al. 2008). Studies evaluating the possible teratogenic medications should consider and control, if possible, the effect of underlying diseases. Including an untreated disease group may be beneficial, however the severity of the disease in such a group may also be lower since treatment is not required (Källén 2005).

Meta-Analysis

Although considered as the evidence of highest quality, meta-analysis may include different forms of bias and limitations (Egger et al. 2002). Search should include different medical databases and languages while validated methods of quality assessment for the included studies should be chosen. In the context of observational studies, a rigorous systematic review of the included studies should be conducted, and results of the meta-analysis should be discussed with regard to possible confounders and limitations. It is now generally accepted that studies reporting positive findings are more likely to get published than studies reporting negative ones, which is called publication bias or bias against the null hypothesis and discussed elsewhere (Koren et al. 2014; Song et al. 2013), and may lead to erroneous interpretations regarding drug safety.

3.4.2.4 Important Points to Consider for Medication Use During Pregnancy

The background frequency of major congenital malformations is approximately 3%. Unfortunately, no consensus is available in scientific literature regarding the safety of a drug during pregnancy in terms of the exposed number of pregnancies without a detectable teratogenic signal. As Larsen et al. pointed out in their recent review, 200 first trimester exposures without any signs of increase in risk of malformations (80% power, 5% level of significance) would mean that the real risk is not more than three times higher than the background risk (Larsen et al. 2015). If the exposure number is increased to 700, the real risk factor would decrease to two. In order to provide a real risk factor of 1.5, the number of exposed pregnancies without any detectable increase in risk would be 2000. However, these numbers of exposures are not available for most of the drugs on the market. Further complicating the issue is that those estimates are identified for the general risk and specific rare malformations, neonatal complications, and possible long-term effects are not considered in the computations above. Nevertheless, the European Medicine Agency considers 1000 prospective exposed pregnancies with known outcome in the first trimester without any detectable signal as strong evidence suggesting that the malformation risk is unlikely (EMA 2008). If this data volume cannot be reached, then the risk assessment should be made according to the available amount of data. The clinician should always weigh the possible fetal risks of the medication against the consequences of untreated maternal psychiatric illness. A discussion regarding those issues, as well as the medical and personal priorities should be held between the physician and pregnant patient before deciding to start, continue, or quit the pharmacotherapy.

3.5 Lactation

3.5.1 Factors Influencing the Passage of the Medication into the Breastmilk and Infant Exposure

3.5.1.1 Maternal Plasma Concentration and Plasma Protein Binding

Because passive diffusion is the primary pathway of medications entering the breast milk, the maternal plasma concentration of the medication usually shows good correlation with the concentration of the medication in the breast milk depending on the other pharmacokinetic variables such as the plasma protein binding. A high volume of the distribution and plasma protein binding leads to a lower maternal plasma concentration and unbound (free) medication levels which results in lower breast milk concentrations. For instance, sertraline has a relatively high volume of distribution and plasma protein binding which leads to a lower maternal plasma and breast milk concentration (LactMed 2018). On the other hand, lamotrigine's lower volume of distribution and plasma protein binding capacity leads to higher breast milk levels (LactMed 2018).

3.5.1.2 Size of the Molecule

Most medications, and so do the psychotropic drugs, are small enough to enter the breast milk. Exceptions are the larger molecules such as heparin.

3.5.1.3 Degree of Ionization

Medications should be nonionized in order to cross membranes and enter the milk. Of importance, breast milk is relatively more acidic (pH 7.2) compared to the maternal plasma (pH 7.4) (Hotham and Hotham 2015). Weak bases such as codeine and amphetamines become ionized at this pH and may accumulate in the milk (Hotham and Hotham 2015; Hale 2012).

3.5.1.4 Lipid Solubility

Mature milk, which has a relatively stable composition and is produced by 2–3 weeks after birth, is composed of ions, proteins, and lipids. Some lipid-soluble drugs, such as citalopram, may become dissolved in the lipid droplets and be co-secreted which may lead to a higher concentration in a milk with high fat content (hind-milk) compared to the milk with low fat content (fore-milk) (Ilett and Kristensen 2005). However, the practical implications of this issue are unclear and unlikely to influence the choice of pharmacotherapy (Hotham and Hotham 2015).

3.5.1.5 Pharmacogenomics

Pharmacogenomics of mother and the infant may affect the exposure of the infant to the drugs in breast milk. This is particularly highlighted for opioids (Madadi et al. 2012). As one study reported, the adverse outcomes in the breastfeeding mother-infant pairs are significantly associated with the maternal risk genotypes in CYP2D6 and ABCB1 (Sistonen et al. 2012). However, this domain should be further explored.

3.5.1.6 Oral Bioavailability

A drug with low bioavailability in adults is usually expected to behave similarly in neonates. For instance, drugs with large molecules, protein or peptide drugs (unstable in the gut) exhibit limited transfer to the milk and therefore suggest limited bioavailability of the orally ingested drug in the infant through the breast milk (Ilett and Kristensen 2005).

3.5.1.7 The Age of the Infant

The first 3 days of postpartum is the period in which many drugs and immunoglobulin, lymphocyte, leukocyte, macrophage, and maternal proteins are able to pass to the colostrum due to alveolar intercellular gaps. These gaps are closed after a week, and passage of most drugs and molecules is reduced. Although colostrum is able to contain higher drug concentrations than the mature milk, the amount of colostrum produced in the early postpartum period is expected to be low (30–100 ml/day). Clinicians should be more careful at this stage, because of the possibility of the high drug concentration in the milk and premature or unstable newborns may have insufficient capacity to metabolize medications. The amount of milk taken by babies over 1 year of age is usually reduced, and consequently the drug intake will be less (Hale and Rowe 2017). In a review investigating the adverse drug reactions seen in the breastfed infants whose mothers are using medications, 63% of the cases were observed in the first month (newborn) and 16% were in the second month of life which means that almost 80% of the adverse events occurred during the first 2 months. Therefore, careful monitoring is particularly needed for this period (Anderson et al. 2016).

3.5.2 Effect of Medications on Milk Production

Prolactin released from the anterior pituitary gland is the most important hormone that provides milk production. Drugs may cause an increase in milk production through dopamine-blocking actions which result in stimulation of prolactin production and release. Amisulpiride, phenothiazines, and risperidone are the antipsychotics with potent dopamine blocking actions which may cause galactorrhea (Ilett and Kristensen 2005). In addition, TRH, serotonin, vasopressin, oxytocin, prostaglandins, opioids, histamine, and noradrenaline stimulate prolactin secretion (Richards and Williams 1976). On the other hand, drugs may interfere with the milk production through decreasing prolactin release or local blood flow to the breast tissue. Bromocriptine, cabergoline, ergotamine, estrogens, and pseudoephedrine can cause a reduction in breast milk supply.

3.5.3 Calculating and Interpreting Infant Exposure

3.5.3.1 Milk Plasma Ratio (M/P Ratio)

The milk plasma (M/P) ratio is the comparison of milk and maternal plasma drug concentrations. This ratio lets us determine the dose of the ingested drug by the infant and whether the amount of drug being exposed is within the therapeutic range via the average amount of milk (150 ml/kg/day) taken per day of the infant. A M/P ratio > 1 indicates that the medication passes to the milk in high levels whereas a M/P ratio < 1 indicates that the medication has passed to the milk at low levels (Hale and Rowe 2017). For instance, the concentration of SSRIs, tricyclic, or other antidepressants such as bupropion, nefazodone, and venlafaxine in the milk is between 1% and 10% of the maternal plasma concentration (Ito 2014).

3.5.3.2 Relative Infant Dose

The relative infant dose (RID) is the key parameter to assess potential risks of medication use during breastfeeding for infants. RID is calculated by dividing the dose the infant ingests per kilogram of body weight by the maternal dose per kilogram of body weight and expressed as a percentage. Infant exposure is considered as minimal when the relative dose is below 2%, small when the relative dose is 2–5%, moderate when the relative dose is 5–10% and high when the relative dose is above 10% (Larsen et al. 2015). If the RID <10%, breastfeeding is usually considered as safe (Hale and Rowe 2017) although infrequent cases of possible adverse effects in the infants are reported even with relative doses below but close to 10% such as aripiprazole. Nevertheless, breastfeeding does not need to be contraindicated during the maternal treatment with some drugs of which RID are above 10%, such as fluconazole (Kaplan et al. 2015a). The RID is above 5% for most neuroactive drugs because of their high lipid solubility.

3.5.3.3 Infant Plasma Concentration

Although it is an invasive and painful method, infant plasma concentration is the most direct method of evaluating infant exposure. It can also be used to assess a suspicious adverse reaction related with medication use during lactation in individual infants. An estimate of the average infant plasma concentration can be made using the following equation (Anderson and Sauberan 2016):

$$Cp = F \text{ X daily concentration in milk x daily volume of milk ingested} / CL$$

F is the bioavailability and CL is the clearance of the medication. A thorough discussion of limitations of this method can be found elsewhere (Anderson and Sauberan 2016).

3.5.3.4 The Ratio of Infant Plasma Concentration to the Maternal Plasma Concentration

This ratio might be more advantageous in terms of minimizing the variables such as the bioavailability and the differences in clearances between the infant and the mother (Anderson and Sauberan 2016). It would be more accurate for the medications with relatively long half-lives since the fluctuations regarding medication levels would be minimal. WHO Working Group considers a medication unacceptable if a steady-state infant plasma concentration is greater than 25% of the lower end of the therapeutic concentration range although this is an arbitrary cut-off point (Anderson and Sauberan 2016). A ratio over 10% is accepted as a cause for concern by the American Academy of Pediatrics (AAP) (Sachs 2013). The choice of the cut-off points, and the time for the sampling (the effect of transplacental passage) is very important in the assessment of the data (Anderson and Sauberan 2016).

3.5.3.5 Lactation Categories

A lactation risk categorization system was developed by Hale et al. to determine whether a drug is compatible with breastfeeding (Hale and Rowe 2017). Five categories are described as follows:

L1-compatible: No adverse effects have been observed in the baby of many lactating mothers, or no increase in risk has been detected during controlled studies, or the oral bioavailability of the drug is absent or very low.

L2-probably compatible: Studies with a limited number of lactating mothers have not found an increase in adverse effects and/or evidence is far from possible adverse effects.

L3-probably compatible: There are no controlled studies but there is a possibility that adverse effects may occur on infants or minimal, non-life-threatening adverse effects have been reported in controlled studies. The drugs in this group should only be used if necessary, taking into account the risk-benefit ratio. Also new drugs that have no data are included in this group.

L4-potentially hazardous: There is evidence that it is risky for infant or mother's milk production, but breastfeeding may be acceptable if the benefits of the medication are taken into consideration (if the mother cannot be treated with other medications which are compatible with breastfeeding in the presence of a life-threatening serious condition).

L5-hazardous: Studies conducted with breastfeeding mothers have shown that there is a significant risk for infant, or the risk of harm to the infant is high. Breastfeeding while using these drugs is contraindicated.

A proposed safety scoring system assessed six key parameters for the safe use of psychotropic drugs during breastfeeding. The proposed parameters include the reported total sample size, the reported maximum relative infant dose, the reported sample size for relative infant dose, infant plasma drug levels, the prevalence of any reported adverse effect, and the reported serious adverse effects. The sum of the scores is between 0 and 10. Increased ratings indicate a higher level of safety (Uguz 2021).

3.5.4 Important Points to Consider for Medication Use During Lactation

Drug use during breastfeeding should be avoided unless it is necessary. If clinically indicated, the medications with more documented experience should be preferred to relatively new drugs. The risks and benefits of each medicine for the mother and the infant should be evaluated. Most drugs are compatible with breastfeeding because they do not reach therapeutic doses in an infant's plasma, but for some drugs, taking off breastfeeding for a few hours, or to completely stop breastfeeding may be recommended. If possible, drugs with low oral bioavailability, short half-lives, high protein binding, or high molecular weight should be preferred (Hale and Rowe 2017). Before the drug is administered to the mother, the infant's age and clinical condition should also be assessed. Medications that are safe to use in infants are generally safe to use in breastfeeding women. It could be required to monitor maternal and infant serum drug levels when using certain medications, as is the case with lithium (Imaz et al. 2019). Infants should be monitored for adverse effects similar to those seen in the mother for antiepileptics, antidepressants, and antipsychotics (Hale and Rowe 2017).

Studies suggest a link between antidepressant use in late pregnancy and lower rates of breastfeeding initiation. Thus, it is important to support mothers in promoting breastfeeding (Grzeskowiak et al. 2022; Leggett et al. 2017).

3.6 Information Sources Regarding Medication Use During Pregnancy and Lactation

Teratology Information Services (TIS) are the most important sources of evidence-based information regarding medication use during pregnancy and lactation since they provide an individualized risk assessment for the particular patients. TIS are important sources of evidence since they conduct prospective cohort studies. The European Network of Teratology Information Services (ENTIS) (Schaefer 2011) and Mother To Baby (Organization of Teratology Information Specialists, OTIS) (Leen-Mitchell et al. 2000) are TIS societies, of which members in individual countries counsel thousands of patients regarding medication use during pregnancy and lactation every year. According to a survey conducted with practitioners in Melbourne, Australia in 2009, most of the physicians (73%) stated that they used software programs or books in this

Table 3.2 Information sources (Holmes 2011)

1. PubMed and other evidence-based databases
2. Review resources (a) Micromedex® solutions (b) Reprotox (http://reprotox.org) (c) Clinical teratology web—TERIS, http://depts.washington.edu/terisdb/terisweb/index.html (d) LactMed, https://toxnet.nlm.nih.gov/newtoxnet/lactmed.htm (e) Catalog of teratogenic agents (13thed). Shepard TH, Lemire RJ, Baltimore, MD: Johns Hopkins University Press, 2010.
3. Reference books (a) Briggs GG, towers CV, Forinash AB. Briggs drugs in pregnancy and lactation: A reference guide to fetal and neonatal risk. 12th edition. Lippincott Williams & Wilkins, a Wolters Kluwer business; 2021. (b) Schaefer C, Peters P, miller RK. Drugs during pregnancy and lactation. 3rd ed. academic press; 2014 Dec 10. (c) Koren G. Medication safety in pregnancy and breastfeeding: The evidence-based A-to-Z clinician's pocket guide. New York: McGraw-Hill Medical; 2007. (d) Koren G. Medication safety in pregnancy and breastfeeding. New York: McGraw-Hill, health professions division; 2007. (e) Hale TW, Krutsch K. Hale's Medications & Mothers' Milk 2023: A Manual of Lactational Pharmacology. 20th ed. Springer Publishing; 2023.
4. Websites of teratology information service networks (a) OTIS (Organization of Teratology Information Services) in the United States and Canada, http://www.mothertobaby.org (b) ENTIS (European network teratology information services), http://www.entis-org.eu

subject as information sources and 51% of the physicians reached information by phone (Amir and Pirotta 2009). Reprotox® and TERIS are the most known online databases which require a modest annual fee for the membership. Lactmed is a peer-reviewed online source with free access which focuses on drug use during breastfeeding (LactMed 2018). A summary of information sources for drug use during pregnancy and breastfeeding is shown in Table 3.2.

3.7 Conclusion

The risk assessment of psychotropic medication use during the perinatal period requires the critical appraisal skills that enable us to assess the up-to-date information emerging from the observational studies. The decision whether to use the medication or not should be made on a case-by-case basis, weighing the possible risks of the untreated maternal psychiatric disorder on mother, fetus, and growing child against the possible adverse effects of the medication on fetus or child. The decision-making process should involve the patient while the mutual understanding of physicians' and patients' priorities should be ensured.

References

Adam MP, Polifka JE, Friedman JM. Evolving knowledge of the teratogenicity of medications in human pregnancy. Am J Med Genet C Semin Med Genet. 2011;157(3):175–82.

Addis A, Sharabi S, Bonati M. Risk classification systems for drug use during pregnancy: are they a reliable source of information? Drug Saf. 2000;23(3):245–53.

Amir LH, Pirotta MV. Medicines for breastfeeding women: a postal survey of general practitioners in Victoria. Med J Aust. 2009;191(2):126.

Anderson PO, Sauberan JB. Modeling drug passage into human milk. Clin Pharmacol Ther. 2016;100(1):42–52.

Anderson PO, Manoguerra AS, Valdés V. A review of adverse reactions in infants from medications in breastmilk. ClinPediatr (Phila). 2016;55(3):236–44.

Avachat C, Younis IR, Birnbaum AK. Characterization of the US Food and Drug Administration post-marketing commitments and requirements for pregnancy and lactation. Clin Pharmacol Ther. 2023 Dec;114(6):1238–42.

Bateman BT, Huybrechts KF, Fischer MA, Seely EW, Ecker JL, Oberg AS, Franklin JM, Mogun H, Hernandez-Diaz S. Chronic hypertension in pregnancy and the risk of congenital malformations: a cohort study. Am J Obstet Gynecol. 2015;212(3):337–14.

Brent RL. Utilization of animal studies to determine the effects and human risks of environmental toxicants (drugs, chemicals, and physical agents). Pediatrics. 2004a;113(4 Suppl):984–95.

Brent RL. Environmental causes of human congenital malformations: the pediatrician's role in dealing with these complex clinical problems caused by a multiplicity of environmental and genetic factors. Pediatrics. 2004b;113(4 Suppl):957–68.

Bromley RL, Mawer G, Love J, Kelly J, Purdy L, McEwan L, Briggs M, Clayton-Smith J, Shi X, Baker GA. Liverpool and Manchester neurodevelopment group (LMNDG): early cognitive development in children born to women with epilepsy: a prospective report. Epilepsia. 2010;51:2058–65.

Camera G, Pregliasco P. Ear malformation in baby born to mother using tretinoin cream. Lancet. 1992;339(8794):687.

Carey JC, Martinez L, Balken E, Leen-Mitchell M, Robertson J. Determination of human teratogenicity by the astute clinician method: review of illustrative agents and a proposal of guidelines. Birth Defects Res A Clin Mol Teratol. 2009;85(1):63–8.

Chambers C. The role of teratology information services in screening for teratogenic exposures: challenges and opportunities. Am J Med Genet C Semin Med Genet. 2011;157C(3):195–200.

Chatterjee S, Kotelchuck M, Sambamoorthi U. Prevalence of chronic illness in pregnancy, access to care, and health care costs: implications for interconception care. Womens Health Issues. 2008;18(6 Suppl):S107–16.

Correa A, Gilboa SM, Besser LM, Botto LD, Moore CA, Hobbs CA, Cleves MA, Riehle-Colarusso TJ, Waller DK, Reece EA. Diabetes mellitus and birth defects. Am J Obstet Gynecol. 2008;199(237):e1–9.

Diav-Citrin O, Shechtman S, Bar-Oz B, Cantrell D, Arnon J, Ornoy A. Pregnancy outcome after in utero exposure to valproate: evidence of dose relationship in teratogenic effect. CNS Drugs. 2008;22:325–234.

Drugs and Lactation Database (LactMed). Toxnet. National Institutes of Health. 2018. https://toxnet.nlm.nih.gov/newtoxnet/lactmed.htm. Accessed 12 Feb 2018.

Dunlop AL, Jack BW, Bottalico JN, Lu MC, James A, Shellhaas CS, Hallstrom LH, Solomon BD, Feero WG, Menard MK, Prasad MR. The clinical content of preconception care: women with chronic medical conditions. Am J Obstet Gynecol. 2008;199(6 Suppl 2):S310–27.

Egger M, Ebrahim S, Smith GD. Where now for meta-analysis? Int J Epidemiol. 2002;31(1):1–5.

Ehrenstein V, Sørensen HT, Bakketeig LS, Pedersen L. Medical databases in studies of drug teratogenicity: methodological issues. Clin Epidemiol. 2010;2:37–43.

European Medicines Agency. Guideline on risk assessment of medicinal products on human reproduction and lactation: from data to labelling. 2008. http://www.ema.europa.eu/docs/en_GB/document_library/Scientific_guideline/2009/09/WC500003307.pdf. Accessed 12 Feb 2018.
European Medicines Agency (EMA). Systematic overview of data sources for drug safety in pregnancy research. Consultancy EMA/2010/29/CN prepared for the European Medicines Agency, June 2012. Updated for ENCePP June 2016. https://encepp.europa.eu/publications/systematic-overview-data-sources-drug-safety-pregnancy-research_en?prefLang=sv#details
Feibus KB. FDA's proposed rule for pregnancy and lactation labeling: improving maternal child health through well-informed medicine use. J Med Toxicol. 2008;4:284–8.
Fourie DT, Hay IT. Warfarin as a possible teratogen. S Afr Med J. 1975;49(50):2081–3.
Frederiksen MC. The new FDA pregnancy labeling requiremens for drugs. J Midwifery Womens Health. 2011;56:303–7.
Grigoriadis S, Vonderporten EH, Mamisashvili L, Tomlinson G, Dennis CL, Koren G, Steiner M, Mousmanis P, Cheung A, Ross LE. Prenatal exposure to antidepressants and persistent pulmonary hypertension of the newborn: systematic review and meta-analysis. BMJ. 2014;14(348):f6932.
Grzeskowiak LE, Saha MR, Nordeng H, Ystrom E, Amir LH. Perinatal antidepressant use and breastfeeding outcomes: findings from the Norwegian mother, father and child cohort study. Acta Obstet Gynecol Scand. 2022;101(3):344–54.
Guittina P, Eléfant E, Saint-Salvi B. Hierarchization of animal teratology findings for improving the human risk evaluation of drugs. Reprod Toxicol. 2000;14:369–75.
Hale TW. Medications and mothers' milk. 15th ed. Amarillo: Hale Publishing; 2012.
Hale TW, Rowe HE. Medications and mothers milk. 17th ed. New York: Springer Publishing Company; 2017.
Herbst AL, Scully RE. Adenocarcinoma of the vagina in adolescence: a report of 7 cases including 6 clear-cell carcinomas. Cancer. 1970;25:745–57.
Holmes LB. Human teratogens: update 2010. Birth Defects Res A Clin Mol Teratol. 2011;91:1–7.
Holzgreve W, Carey JC, Hall BD. Warfarin-induced fetal abnormalities. Lancet. 1976;2(7991):914–5.
Hotham N, Hotham E. Drugs in breastfeeding. Aust Prescr. 2015;38:156–9.
Ilett KF, Kristensen JH. Drug use and breastfeeding. Expert Opin Drug Saf. 2005;4:745–68.
Imaz ML, Torra M, Soy D, García-Esteve L, Martin-Santos R. Clinical lactation studies of lithium: a systematic review. Front Pharmacol. 2019;10:1005.
Irl C, Hasford J. Assessing the safety of drugs in pregnancy: the role of prospective cohort studies. Drug Saf. 2000;22(3):169–77.
Ito S. Chronic illness and the breastfeeding mother. J Popul Ther Clin Pharmacol. 2014;21(3):e565–8.
Jensen BK, McGann LA, Kachevsky V, Franz TJ. The negligible systemic availability of retinoids with multiple and excessive topical application of isotretinoin 0.05% gel (Isotrex) in patients with acne vulgaris. J Am Acad Dermatol. 1991;24:425–8.
Jick SS, Terris BZ, Jick H. First trimester topical tretinoin and congenital disorders. Lancet. 1993;341(8854):1181–2.
Källén B. Drugs in pregnancy – the dilemma of labeling. Drug Inform J. 1999;33:1135–43.
Källén BA. Methodological issues in the epidemiological study of the teratogenicity of drugs. CongenitAnom (Kyoto). 2005;45(2):44–51.
Källén B. The problem of confounding in studies of the effect of maternal drug use on pregnancy outcome. Obstet Gynecol Int. 2012;2012:148616.
Kaneko S, Battino D, Andermann E, Wada K, Kan R, Takeda A, Nakane Y, Ogawa Y, Avanzini G, Fumarola C, Granata T, Molteni F, Pardi G, Minotti L, Canger R, Dansky L, Oguni M, Lopes-Cendas I, Sherwin A, Andermann F, Seni MH, Okada M, Teranishi T. Congenital malformations due to antiepileptic drugs. Epilepsy Res. 1999;33(2–3):145–58.
Kaplan YC, Koren G, Ito S, Bozzo P. Fluconazole use during breastfeeding. Can Fam Physician. 2015a;61(10):875–6.

Kaplan YC, Ozsarfati J, Etwel F, Nickel C, Nulman I, KorenG. Pregnancy outcomes following first trimester exposure to topical Retinoids : a systematic review and meta-analysis. Br J Dermatol. 2015b;173(5):1132–41.

Kersten I, Lange AE, Haas JP, Fusch C, Lode H, Hoffmann W, Thyrian JR. Chronic diseases in pregnant women: prevalence and birth outcomes based on the SNiP-study. BMC Pregnancy Childbirth. 2014;14:75.

Koren G, Madjunkova S, Maltepe C. Bias against the null hypothesis: scaring pregnant women about drugs in pregnancy. Can Fam Physician. 2014;60(5):441–2.

Lammer EJ, Chen DT, Hoar RM, Agnish ND, Benke PJ, Braun JT, Curry CJ, Fernhoff PM, Grix AW Jr, Lott IT, Richard JM, Sun SC. Retinoic acid embryopathy. N Engl J Med. 1985;313(14):837–41.

Larsen ER, Damkier P, Pedersen LH, Fenger-Gron J, Mikkelsen RL, Nielsen RE, et al. Use of psychotropic drugs during pregnancy and breast-feeding. Acta Psychiatr Scand Suppl. 2015;445:1–28.

Le Ray C, Coulomb A, Elefant E, Frydman R, Audibert F. Mycophenolate mofetil in pregnancy after renal transplantation: a case of major fetal malformations. Obstet Gynecol. 2004;103(5 Pt 2):1091–4.

Lee BE, Feinberg M, Abraham JJ, Murthy AR. Congenital malformations in an infant born to a woman treated with fluconazole. Pediatr Infect Dis J. 1992;11(12):1062–4.

Leen-Mitchell M, Martinez L, Gallegos S, Robertson J, Carey JC. Mini-review: history of organized teratology information services in North America. Teratology. 2000;61:314–7.

Leggett C, Costi L, Morrison JL, Clifton VL, Grzeskowiak LE. Antidepressant use in late gestation and breastfeeding rates at discharge from hospital. J Hum Lact. 2017;33(4):701–9.

Lehman PA, Slattery JT, Franz TJ. Percutaneous absorption of retinoids: influence of vehicle, light exposure, and dose. J Invest Dermatol. 1988;91:56–61.

Lipson AH, Collins F, Webster WS. Multiple congenital defects associated with maternal use of topical tretinoin. Lancet. 1993;341(8856):1352–3.

Lo WY, Friedman JM. Teratogenicity of recently introduced medications in human pregnancy. Obstet Gynecol. 2002;100(3):465–73.

Loureiro KD, Kao KK, Jones KL, Alvarado S, Chavez C, Dick L, Felix R, Johnson D, Chambers CD. Minor malformations characteristic of the retinoic acid embryopathy and other birth outcomes in children of women exposed to topical tretinoin during early pregnancy. Am J Med Genet A. 2005;136(2):117–21.

Madadi P, Avard D, Koren G. Pharmacogenetics of opioids for the treatment of acute maternal pain during pregnancy and lactation. Curr Drug Metab. 2012;13(6):721–7.

Meador KJ, Baker GA, Browning N, Clayton-Smith J, Combs-Cantrell DT, Cohen M, Kalayjian LA, Kanner A, Liporace JD, Pennell PB, Privitera M, Loring DW. Cognitive function at 3 years of age after fetal exposure to antiepileptic drugs. N Engl J Med. 2009;360:1597–605.

Mitchell AA. Systematic identification of drugs that cause birth defects – a new opportunity. N Engl J Med. 2003;349(26):2556–9.

Namazy J, Chambers C, Sahin L, Johnson T, Dinatale M, Lappin B, Schatz M. Clinicians' perspective of the new pregnancy and lactation labeling rule (PLLR): results from an AAAAI/FDA survey. J Allergy Clin Immunol Pract. 2020;8(6):1947–52.

Nulman I, Koren G, Rovet J, Barrera M, Streiner DL, Feldman BM. Neurodevelopment of children prenatally exposed to selective reuptake inhibitor antidepressants: Toronto sibling study. J Clin Psychiatry. 2015;76(7):e842–7.

Panchaud A, Csajka C, Merlob P, Schaefer C, Berlin M, De Santis M, Vial T, Ieri A, Malm H, Eleftheriou G, Stahl B, Rousso P, Winterfeld U, Rothuizen LE, Buclin T. Pregnancy outcome following exposure to topical retinoids: a multicenter prospective study. J Clin Pharmacol. 2012;52(12):1844–51.

Pursley TJ, Blomquist IK, Abraham J, Andersen HF, Bartley J. Fluconazole-induced congenital anomalies in three infants. Clin Infect Dis. 1996;22(2):336–40.

Richards JS, Williams JJ. Luteal cell receptor content for prolactin (PRL) and luteinizing hormone (LH): regulation by LH and PRL. Endocrinology. 1976;99:1571–81.

Rosa FW. Teratogenicity of isotretinoin. Lancet. 1983;2:513.

Sachs HC. The transfer of drugs and therapeutics into human breast milk: an update on selected topics. Pediatrics. 2013;132:e796–809.

Sadowski A, Todorow M, Yazdani Brojeni P, Koren G, Nulman I. Pregnancy outcomes following maternal exposure to second-generation antipsychotics given with other psychotropic drugs: a cohort study. BMJ Open. 2013;3(7):e003062.

Sahin L, Nallani SC, Tassinari MS. Medication use in pregnancy and the pregnancy and lactation labeling rule. Clin Pharmacol Ther. 2016;100(1):23–5.

Schaefer C. Drug safety in pregnancy: utopia or achievable prospect? Risk information, risk research and advocacy in teratology information services. Congenit Anom (Kyoto). 2011;51:6–11.

Shapiro L, Pastuszak A, Curto G, Karen G. Safety of first-trimester exposure to topical tretinoin: prospective cohort study. Lancet. 1997;350(9085):1143–4.

Shepard TH. Proof of human teratogenicity. Teratology. 1994;50:97–8.

Sifontis NM, Coscia LA, Constantinescu S, Lavelanet AF, Moritz MJ, Armenti VT. Pregnancy outcomes in solid organ transplant recipients with exposure to mycophenolate mofetil or sirolimus. Transplantation. 2006;82(12):1698–7102.

Sistonen J, Madadi P, Ross CJ, et al. Prediction of codeine toxicity in infants and their mothers using a novel combination of maternal genetic markers. Clin Pharmacol Ther. 2012;91(4):692–9.

Song F, Hooper L, Loke YK. Publication bias: what is it? How do we measure it? How do we avoid it? Open Access J Clin Trials. 2013;5(1):51–81.

Tomson T, Battino D, Bonizzoni E, Craig J, Lindhout D, Sabers A, Perucca E, Vajda F, EURAP study group. Dose-dependent risk of malformations with antiepileptic drugs: an analysis of data from the EURAP epilepsy and pregnancy registry. Lancet Neurol. 2011;10(7):609–17.

Uguz F. A new safety scoring system for the use of psychotropic drugs during lactation. Am J Ther. 2021;28(1):e118–26.

Vajda FJ. The Australian pregnancy register of antiepileptic drugs: 10 years of progress. J Clin Neurosci. 2010;17:1485–8.

Vajda FJ, Hitchcock AA, Graham J, O'Brien TJ, Lander CM, Eadie MJ. The teratogenic risk of antiepileptic drug polytherapy. Epilepsia. 2010;51:805–10.

Vajda FJ, O'Brien TJ, Lander CM, Graham J, Eadie MJ. Antiepileptic drug combinations not involving valproate and the risk of fetal malformations. Epilepsia. 2016;57(7):1048–52.

General Approach to Psychopharmacological Treatment During the Perinatal Period

4

Cesario Bellantuono

4.1 Introduction

Psychiatrists are usually worried to prescribe psychotropic drugs (PDs) during the perinatal period and particularly in early pregnancy. The reason of such "*psychopharmacotheratophobia*" is mainly due to the fear that PDs could interfere with the physiological development of the fetus. As a consequence, during the pregnancy and particularly during the organogenesis period (first 12 weeks), the risk of congenital major malformations (MM) is a matter of great concern. On the other hand, even in late pregnancy, the risks associated with PDs exposure concern some gestational adverse events, such as spontaneous abortion, preterm birth, and neonatal complications after delivery. Another reason for further concern is the long-term impact that fetal exposure to PDs can have on the infant's neurodevelopment and/or cognitive functions. Nonetheless, recent clinical guidelines as well as the consensus panel recommendations, from European and North-American countries, provide psychiatrists with reassuring and reliable data to ensure a *good clinical practice* in prescribing psychotropic medications during the antenatal and the postpartum period.

One of such guidelines is the *Consensus guidance on the use of psychotropic medications in pregnancy and postpartum* endorsed by the British Association of Psychopharmacology (BAP) (McAllister-Williams et al. 2017).

More recently in Italy an updated *Consensus panel recommendation for pharmacological management of pregnant women with depressive disorders* has also been published (Eleftheriou et al. 2023).

In this overview, 112 studies were analyzed including original studies, systematic reviews, and meta-analyses. This relevant investigation has substantially

C. Bellantuono (✉)
DeGra Clinic for Perinatal Mental Disorders, Verona, Italy;
http://www.depressionegravidanza.it

F. Uguz, L. Orsolini (eds.), *Perinatal Psychopharmacology*,
https://doi.org/10.1007/978-3-031-99720-4_4

confirmed that the majority of antidepressants, particularly selective serotonin reuptake inhibitors (SSRIs), benzodiazepines as a class and the so-called Z-drugs can be considered relatively safe during gestation, even though some neonatal complications, such the neonatal adaptation syndrome (NAS) or the withdrawal reactions should be taking into account, particularly in very preterm newborns.

Nevertheless, as reported by the National Institute of Clinical Evidence (NICE) guidelines in the 1914 "*No psychotropic medication has a UK marketing authorization specifically for women who are pregnant or breastfeeding. The prescriber should follow relevant professional guidance, taking full responsibility for the decision. The woman should provide informed consent, which should be documented*"; a statement that, even though understandable from a medico-legal point of view, is still a further reason of concern for clinicians who need to prescribe PDs during the perinatal period.

An editorial published more than 10 years ago emphasized that pregnant woman can be considered as the "*The last true therapeutic orphan*", because due to the ethical, medico-legal, and infant safety concerns during pregnancy, few pharmacokinetic, pharmacodynamic, or randomized controlled clinical trials (RCT) are conducted during the pregnancy as well as during the breastfeeding (Wisner 2012).

However, despite the concern still present in the area of perinatal psychopharmacotherapy, in some European and north-American countries a significant increase in the prescriptions of PDs during pregnancy, particularly concerning the antidepressants belonging to the SSRI class, was reported (Huybrechts et al. 2013). The reasons that may explain such increase in the prescription rate of SSRI are likely due to:

(a) High prevalence rate in the identification of major depressive disorders and/or anxiety disorders during the perinatal period in the routine clinical practice.
(b) Recommendations that untreated depressive and/or anxiety disorders, as well as other psychiatric illnesses (e.g., bipolar disorder) must be timely and effectively treated to avoid severe risks for the mother, the gestation, and the newborn even in the long term.
(c) Clinical experience and data from international literature that have well established the efficacy and safety of SSRI in major depressive and general anxiety disorders during the perinatal period.

It is also well-known from psychiatric practice that, among women affected by severe and persistent psychiatric disorders, psychological strategies alone can be in most patients only partially effective. It goes without saying that the final goal in the field of perinatal mental health is to treat the women, with any effective therapeutic option available, to decrease the burden of maternal psychiatric disorders on the mother, fetus, newborn, and her family.

4.2 Risks of Untreated Mental Illnesses During the Perinatal Period

Although the perinatal period has been usually considered as a period of "*well-being and happiness*" for women and a time of relative psychological stability, depressive and/or anxiety disorders occurring in pregnancy and during the postpartum are much more frequent than those observed in the general population.

4.2.1 Risks of Adverse Pregnancy and Neonatal Outcomes

Many studies, including original investigations, systematic reviews, and meta-analyses, well documented that an untreated severe psychiatric disorder can be associated with some gestational and neonatal complications. Moreover, it should be noted that, while most studies focused on patients with anxiety and/or depressive disorders, less information is available for other severe psychopathological conditions, such as psychotic, obsessive-compulsive, eating, and personality disorders.

A severe maternal mental illness has been associated with adverse perinatal outcomes, including spontaneous abortion, newborns small for gestational age, low birth weight, fetal distress, preterm delivery, adverse neurodevelopmental outcomes, and changes in the fetus-mother attachment. Pregnant women with untreated mental illness are also more likely to be engaged in high-risk behaviors and unhealthy life-styles, such as smoking, alcohol drinking, drug abuse, inadequate nutrition, and use of folic acid, and can be at risk for gestational diabetes and preeclampsia. Major depression and general anxiety disorders have also been associated with higher rates of neonatal admission to intensive care unit as compared to neonates of the general population. In addition, it should not be underestimated that in the perinatal period the risk of suicide and suicide attempts is not uncommon, since the prevalence rate has been estimated from 5% to 20% of women (Orsolini et al. 2016).

An untreated severe antenatal depression and/or anxiety may also interfere with childhood neuro-development; higher impulsivity, maladaptive social interactions, behavioral and emotional difficulties have been reported in infants of mothers with untreated mental disorders. Women with untreated mental disorders during pregnancy should be considered even at higher risk during the puerperium for depressive disorders, puerperal psychoses, as well as suicide attempt and infanticide. Recent studies also documented that major depression in the perinatal period is associated with relevant alterations in some biological systems, including the hypothalamic-pituitary-adrenal (HPA) axis, immune system, metabolic, and endocrinological dysfunctions. Furthermore, being the pregnancy a phase in which communication between mother and baby is essential, it is not surprising that biological changes, such as high cortisol levels in the mother are transmitted to the developing fetus; after delivery, such increase in neonatal cortisol levels have been also documented up to 12 months after birth (Stein et al. 2014).

In addition, a number of evidences from recent studies have stablished that the intrauterine environment can have an impact on long-term offspring health, the so-called *"fetal programming"*. Among the several environmental stressors which have been studied in humans, maternal mental stress especially if severe and persistent is of particular concern (Stevenson 2020). A systematic review including 13 original studies has supported these findings suggesting that maternal antenatal major depression can be a risk factor for some neuropsychiatric disorders in children (Robinson et al. 2019). Based on the scientific evidences available so far, it can be concluded that there are nowadays enough clinical and biological data to confirm that prenatal maternal major depression and most likely other severe psychiatric illnesses can have significant clinical implications on maternal and offspring's mental health (Bind et al. 2022).

4.2.2 Risks Due to Discontinuation of Psychotropic Drugs

Overall, it has been well established that to discontinue a psychotropic drug treatment before or during pregnancy as well as after delivery, for the fear of adverse events for the fetus, the gestation and the newborn is a decision that needs to be carefully evaluated and obviously adequately discussed with the mother, due to the high risk of relapse/recurrence of a psychiatric disorder during the perinatal period. The discussion should be adequately and comprehensively informed, and the clinician should adequately provide any supportive information to guarantee an informed decision to the mother and her partner.

A large trial published many years ago clearly documented that patients with major depression who discontinued their antidepressant therapy relapsed significantly more frequently as compared to women who maintained their antidepressant therapy during pregnancy. In this study, 68% of patients who discontinued their medication had severe depressive relapse as compared with 26% of those who maintained the drug treatment; moreover, patients who discontinued their medication were 3 times more likely to be hospitalized (Cohen et al. 2006).

Moreover, a higher relapse rate in bipolar women who discontinued their mood stabilizers before or during pregnancy was documented by an original study published several years ago (Viguera et al. 2007). In this study, bipolar patients who discontinued versus those who continued the mood stabilizers, the risk of recurrence was two-fold greater, median time to first recurrence was more than four-fold shorter, and the proportion of weeks ill during pregnancy was five-fold greater. More recently, a systematic review of six studies confirmed that recurrence rate in bipolar women who discontinued their drug treatment during pregnancy was higher (71%) as compared to those who maintained the treatment (24%) (Anya et al. 2019). The risk of relapse following a drug discontinuation has also been reported in other psychopathological conditions, such as schizophrenia, obsessive-compulsive disorder, generalized anxiety, and panic disorders. Therefore, according to the amount of evidence-based data and guidelines, it is strongly recommended that women affected by severe and persistent psychiatric illnesses maintain their drug treatment during pregnancy and postpartum to prevent the risk of relapse.

4.3 Critical Issues in the Evaluation of Safety of PDs During the Perinatal Period

4.3.1 The Evaluation of Safety of PDs During Pregnancy

Despite many studies focusing on the safety of PDs during pregnancy have been published in the last 50 years, the data do not always report univocal results. The reasons are mainly due to the different methodology used in these clinical investigations, such as the kind of experimental design adopted, the sample size, the source of information, the analysis of confounding factors, and the statistical analysis.

A critical issue in this field is that PDs could simply represent an important "marker" and not the cause of an adverse event associated with drug exposure during pregnancy. For example, it has been recently suggested that the exposure to antidepressant treatment during pregnancy should be considered not the cause of some neurodevelopment disorders, such as adult deficit and hyperactivity disorder (ADHD) and/or autism spectrum disorder (ASD), but rather a relevant marker for early screening and intervention in children of mother affected by depressive disorders. (Suarez et al. 2022). Moreover, it should be considered that several risk factors, such as obesity, diabetes, smoking, alcohol, and illicit drugs use, are not uncommon in pregnant women with mental illness and could represent risk factors for congenital birth defects and other adverse pregnancy and neonatal outcomes. Furthermore, it is not surprising that many of the associations lose their statistical significance when "confounders", particularly maternal depression, genetic susceptibility, and other risk factors, are adequately controlled for. Therefore, we must be aware that studies that do not adjust or control for these relevant confounding factors are likely to result in misleading conclusions. Indeed, the biomedical international literature is full of examples of "indication bias", wherein the use of PDs is believed to be associated with a gestational/neonatal adverse event, even though such event is likely to be caused by the clinical condition for which a woman was treated (Smith and Payne 2024). Furthermore, most data concerning the assessment of PDs risks in pregnancy comes from retrospective studies, with associated biases that this entails; so, it is more likely to be reported the occurrence of a congenital birth defect following drug exposure among women taking PDs, as they are usually more often monitored by clinicians (*recall bias*).

Moreover, it is worthwhile to remember that the *Relative Risk* (RR/odds ratio) of specific malformation needs to be evaluated along with data of its *Absolute Risk* (AR), so that the specialist and her patient can better evaluate and also quantify the overall risk of drug exposure in the light of its clinical and epidemiological relevance. This way of communication between doctor and patient can certainly facilitate the decision-making process in taking or not taking a certain drug during pregnancy.

For example, exposure to sertraline during the first trimester of pregnancy was found in a paper published several years ago to be associated with a higher risk (RR = 4,4) of anal atresia. If we consider that anal atresia is a rare defect in general population (5 infants out of 10,000 births, i.e., 0.06%), the AR for a pregnant woman who takes sertraline would be 0.2% of newborns exposed in utero to such drug. This risk, however, has never been highlighted again in other studies (Louik et al. 2007).

As well, a meta-analytic study published more than 10 years ago reported a statistically significant risk of cardiac septal anomalies (RR = 1,5) for infants of women treated with paroxetine. Considering that the rate of cardiac anomalies in the general population is on average 1.1% (from 0.8% to 1.4%), the AR for the newborns exposed in utero to paroxetine would be approximately 1.6% (Grigoriadis et al. 2013). Even in this case, it should be noted that other original well-designed studies and meta-analyses no longer reported such risk of heart defect (Huybrechts et al. 2014).

As general approach, we must be aware that the results of so many studies conducted to assess the risks of PDs exposure in pregnancy, need a careful clinical, statistical and epidemiological evaluation, knowing that in this wide and complex literature, fetal and gestational risks have been found in some investigations but not in many others.

The international literature concerning the perinatal psychopharmacology, which dates back about 50 years, could be considered a sort of "jungle of papers" in which one must critically analyze the methodology adopted in each study and how the results are presented and carefully discussed in term of relative and absolute risk, as well as in the light of their clinical and epidemiological relevance. Many expert clinical researchers have in fact suggested that not all data we found as "statistically significant" are of clinical and/or epidemiological relevance, particularly in the field of perinatal psychopharmacotherapy (Andrade 2020).

4.3.2 The Evaluation of Safety of PDs During Breastfeeding

During the postpartum period, breastfeeding is one of the major problems in women who need to be treated with PDs. It has also been well established by the WHO Guideline that breastmilk is an essential source of nutrition for the baby and that the infant should be exclusively breastfed for at least the first 6 months to achieve optimal growth, development, and health (WHO 2017).

It is common practice that many mothers in maintenance therapy with PDs would like to breastfeed their baby; however, these mothers are rightfully concerned about the transfer of PDs into breast milk and about the potential adverse effects that such medications can induce to breastfed infant. Therefore, information on the safety profile of these drugs during lactation is of great clinical relevance to assist clinicians in the management of such women.

A useful guide to obtain information on the safety of drugs (including PDs) during breastfeeding can be found in *Drugs and Lactation Database—LactMed* (LactMed 2023). However, even in this large database, limited information exists for some drugs, particularly for drugs recently marketed. Moreover, some safety information can be found from case reports or case series. In addition, the majority of such data generally apply to term and healthy infants, while very limited information is available in breastfed premature or sick infants.

An update on *Consensus Panel Recommendations for the Pharmacological Management of Breastfeeding Women with Postpartum Depression* has been recently published (Eleftheriou et al. 2024). In this paper, a panel of 16 Italian clinical research experts, representing eight scientific societies with a keen interest in postpartum depression, has been involved. An extensive review, including 373 studies, was performed to assess the risks associated with untreated maternal depression during breastfeeding and the risk of adverse effects in breastfed infants after the use of antidepressant and anxiolytic drugs during breastfeeding.

The authors strongly suggested, on the basis of the evidence on the safety of these drugs during lactation, to discuss with the patient the risks of untreated illness, as well as the risks and benefits of treatment for the nursed infant. A misleading information can have a significant influence on the woman's decision not to breastfeed their baby, even in the case of drugs considered absolutely safe during breastfeeding. For example, among antidepressants and benzodiazepines, sertraline, paroxetine, lorazepam, and other benzodiazepines oxazepam-like are considered first-line options during lactation as documented by their safety index, particularly the *milk to plasma ratio* (M/P) and *the relative infant dose* (RID).

However, it is clear that further studies are needed to better improve our knowledge on the safety of PDs, particularly of those more recently introduced into the market and for those where the information is still lacking.

4.4 General Approach and Recommendations in PDs Prescription During the Perinatal Period

Planning the drug treatment for women affected by a severe psychopathological condition should be always made before the woman becomes pregnant, that is in the "preconception period". Therefore, it is appropriate that all women affected by psychiatric disorders should be in a good mental health condition for at least 6–8 months before trying to get pregnant. The priority should be to keep the women in a good psychological condition during pregnancy and postpartum period.

Considering that about 50% of pregnancies are unplanned, clinicians often need to make treatment decisions for patients who are already pregnant. Every case should be considered individually, with a careful evaluation on the risks and benefits concerning the prescription of a PDs treatment. The patient's psychiatric history, the severity of symptoms, and the response to treatment all play an important role in planning a course of clinical care during the perinatal period.

Nowadays, there is still a need in routine clinical practice to improve the overall management of women with mental disorders in pregnancy and postpartum. Furthermore, we also need to counteract the stigma still surrounding these women, often considered psychologically inadequate for childbearing and parenting and sometimes even improperly advised to not seek pregnancy.

For many women with severe psychiatric conditions who do not receive adequate social, psychological, and pharmacological support, the motherhood can become a kind of nightmare.

In the following sections, the most relevant clinical recommendations concerning the prescription of PDs before and during the perinatal period have been provided (Orsolini and Bellantuono 2022).

4.4.1 Recommendations in Prescribing PDs in the Preconception Period

- Recent guidelines and the expert opinions recommend that in women of child-bearing age the possibility of becoming pregnant should always be taken into account when a psychotropic treatment is prescribed. It is well established that severe psychopathological disorders, such as major depression, bipolar disorder, and general anxiety, could arise at the first onset of pregnancy or can be exacerbated as a result of significant physiologic and psychosocial changes occurring during the gestational period.
- Contraception and optimization of physical and mental health in potential future pregnancies should therefore be discussed at all stages of care, not just when a woman discovers she is pregnant.
- Women affected by mental illness in their reproductive age should therefore receive updated information from her specialist on the safety profile of drugs they are taking, particularly concerning the fetus development and any gestational and neonatal complications.
- It is documented that about 50% of pregnancies have not been planned.
- Women already taking psychotropic medications for a maintenance therapy should also be adequately informed (before pregnancy) about the high risk of relapse if the drug treatment is discontinued before pregnancy or when they realize they are pregnant, which usually occurs around the 5th/6th week of gestation. This is clinically relevant when the drug prescribed is at risk of teratogenicity, as in case of valproate, whose severe adverse effects (e.g., neural tube defects) can occur precociously, within the first 4th/5th weeks of gestation. In this case could be appropriate to change the drug at risk with an alternative and safe drug treatment, if possible; of course, the new therapeutic option should be evaluated for several months before starting the pregnancy.

4.4.2 Recommendations in Prescribing PDs During Pregnancy

- The prescription of a psychopharmacological treatment during the pregnancy should be reserved to women suffering from a severe mental disorder. The combination of drug treatment, with an effective psychotherapy, such as the cognitive-behavioral therapy CBT), is recommended in patients requiring a psychotherapeutic intervention.
- The management of mental disorders in pregnancy always requires an adequate clinical monitoring of fetal development and maternal mental state, with close liaison among the perinatal mental health professionals (i.e., obstetricians, pedia-

tricians, and midwives). It is also recommended that women treated with PDs should give birth in a general hospital in which there is a neonatal intensive care unit, to provide a timely and effective management of potential neonatal complications, like the "*neonatal adaptation syndrome*" (NAS); a not severe adverse reaction reported in neonates exposed to SSRI late in pregnancy. It was suggested that the discontinuation of drug treatment 2 or 3 weeks before delivery could avoid or attenuate the NAS. Unfortunately, despite the drug discontinuation, such complication can still occur in most newborns, particularly if preterm; in any case the symptoms resolve spontaneously from 1 to 3 weeks. In addition, it should be considered that discontinuing the treatment could pose the mother at risk of an early relapse in a critical period of gestation.

- It is established that formula-fed infants were more likely to develop the NAS than infants who were breastfed; therefore, breastfeeding should always be considered the first-line option, particularly among preterm newborns.
- It is not recommended to stop the medications suddenly after the discovery of pregnancy, because of the risk of relapse or severe maternal withdrawal reaction. It would be much better if the decision to maintain or stop the drug treatment is taken after consulting a specialist in perinatal psychiatry, so that the mother and her partner can share the decision after having updated information about the neonatal possible risks due to drug exposure, as well as about the risks of early relapse in case of drug discontinuation. A written informed consent, in which all available information concerning risks and benefits of drug treatment and non-treatment during pregnancy and postpartum, is strongly suggested.
- During gestation, the prescription of monotherapy is always preferred and the dosage must be individualized, in order to accurately find the "lowest effective dosage" for each patient; hence, polypharmacy should be avoided, if possible. It is also not appropriate to prescribe sub-therapeutic dosages, as this strategy expose in any case the fetus to the risks of a drug and the pregnant to the risk of relapse.
- Drugs with the largest up-to-date evidence of safety for the fetus (e.g., risk of malformations) should be preferred as first-line option; the previous response to drug treatment needs also to be considered in the choice of a psychotropic treatment. For example, agents belonging to SRI (SSRI SNRI) should be preferred as first-line option in depressive and anxiety disorders, because their safety profile has been more investigated during pregnancy than that of other antidepressant drugs.
- All change between psychotropic drugs should be carried out before pregnancy (preconception period); it is better to avoid switching medications during pregnancy, unless the benefits are likely to outweigh the risk; changing the drug once women are pregnant increase also the number of fetal exposures.
- It is recommended not to prescribe PDs which have been recently introduced in the pharmaceutical market, because the data available on their safety profile in pregnancy and breastfeeding is most likely poor.

4.4.3 Recommendations in Prescribing PDs During Breastfeeding

- It is strongly recommended that neonates should be exclusively breastfed during at least the first 6 months of life to achieve optimal growth and development. Thus, clinicians should avoid (if possible) using formula feeding immediately after delivery in infants of women taking PDs, for the fear that these medications can be at risk for the infant. In fact, most drugs are not contraindicated during breastfeeding as their concentration in breast milk is very low or undetectable, such as some SSRIs (e.g., paroxetine or sertraline), some benzodiazepine (e.g., lorazepam, lormetazepam), and some antipsychotic and mood stabilizers (like olanzapine and quetiapine).
- An updated guide for clinicians to get information about the neonatal safety of drugs, including PDs, during breastfeeding can be found in the US above-mentioned database. The LactMed database contains information on drugs to which breastfeeding mothers may be exposed. It includes many data on the levels of such substances in breast milk and infant blood, and the possible adverse effects reported in the nursing infants. Suggested therapeutic alternatives to those drugs are also provided, where appropriate. All data are come from the recent scientific literature and fully referenced. A peer review panel reviews the data to assure scientific validity and currency.
- LactMed database is updated monthly and is free of charge.
- It is strongly recommended that breastfed infants whose mothers have been treated with PDs should be monitored for potential adverse reactions, such the above-mentioned NAS and in case of respiratory distress; this is a are adverse events but particularly frequent in premature or sick newborns and in mothers taking more than one psychotropic medication or taking high dose of these medications in late pregnancy.

4.5 Conclusions

Mental disorders, particularly if severe and persistent, are among the commonest morbidities during the perinatal period and make an important contribution to maternal morbidity and mortality, as well as to adverse neonatal, infant, and child outcomes. Mental health services will always care for women of childbearing age, many of whom will become pregnant, sometimes planned and sometimes unplanned, and have children. Therefore, psychiatrists and other mental health professionals need to be trained to "think family", so that they can deliver care having in mind together pregnancies and families.

It is well established that women with severe mental illness have an increased risk for adverse obstetric and pregnancy outcomes, including preterm births and fetal growth impairments; these women are also at high risk of developing pre-eclampsia, antepartum and postpartum hemorrhage, placental abruption, and stillbirths.

There is a general agreement among psychiatrists that during the antenatal period the prescription of PDs should be always considered in case of women affected by severe psychiatric illness. However, it is also reasonable to prescribe these drugs, as an add-on therapy, in case of women with psychopathological conditions that have only partially responded to non-pharmacological treatments.

The decision to prescribe PDs during the perinatal period is in many cases complex, particularly in early pregnancy and therefore needs a careful assessment of the risks concerning the drug fetal exposure and those concerning the untreated psychiatric illness.

It has been documented by clinical investigations that mental disorders, such as major depression, bipolar disorders, psychotic conditions, have been associated during pregnancy with biological adverse events involving the immune, endocrine, metabolic, and inflammatory system that could significantly interfere in the process of organogenesis and later with child neurodevelopment.

A number of studies focusing on the risks of children of untreated mothers affected by psychopathological condition have reported adverse outcomes including lower IQ, slower language development, increased risk of the ADHD and ASD.

These relevant findings however often seem to get lost in the debate of whether to use or not psychotropic medications during pregnancy (Wang et al. 2022).

Original studies, systematic reviews and meta-analyses have documented that most PDs can be considered safe during early and late pregnancy, as well as during breastfeeding. Therefore, the decision to start, to continue or to stop such drugs, particularly during the antepartum period, need to be taken by the mother and her partner, only after having updated information on the infant risks due to PDs exposure, as well as on the risks of relapse in case of PDs discontinuation.

In women affected by psychiatric illness and being treatment with PDs who wish to have a baby, it would be strongly recommended to consult a specialist in perinatal psychiatry in order to take an evidence-based decision, particularly in the cases concerning drugs at risk.

An excellent overview has been recently published, focusing both on the impact of biological, clinical, and psychosocial effects of mental disorders during the perinatal period and on the safety of the available psychopharmacological treatments (Percudani et al. 2022).

Time has come to consider the *perinatal psychiatry* not simply an “emerging specialty”, but a key issue that should be of interest to all those professional roles working in the field of women’s mental health. The question remains, however, if the amount of so many data published is adequately disseminated and understood to support more broadly the treatment of women in the perinatal period (Freeman 2014).

This is particularly relevant in the field of perinatal clinical psychopharmacology where the results of so many studies published do not always report reliable information about the risks of PDs in pregnancy.

Until now it is not feasible to carry out randomized controlled clinical trials (RCTs) of PDs during pregnancy, due to concerns of the ethics and medico-legal issues related to such trials; nevertheless, it has been suggested, that a challenge might be in the near future, to reach a consensus among researchers, specialists and patients on the group of women for whom there is clinical equipoise that would justify such trials (Howard and Khalifeh 2020).

In addition, it must be observed that the plethora of clinical investigations on PDs use in pregnancy have placed a greater emphasis on the safety of the exposed newborns rather than on their therapeutic efficacy for the mentally unwell new mothers.

This focus on risk of harm to child is well documented in the high rates of psychotropic drug discontinuation in early pregnancy in women with psychiatric disorder, as well documented by several studies in women affected by depressive, anxiety, and bipolar disorders.

A recent investigation was performed to explore the experiences of women living with severe mental illnesses in making decisions concerning psychotropic medication use in pregnancy and breastfeeding and what helped or hindered the decision-making process (Frayne et al. 2023).

The results of this study recommend that the perinatal psychiatrist should provide clear and updated information, giving space for a woman's voice to be heard and guide them from a state of uncertainty and anxiety to one of reassurance and clarification. Collaboration within a multidisciplinary team and external care providers, combined with consistency of care assists this process. A desirable goal would be that the perinatal psychiatry becomes of common interest, not only for psychiatrists and psychologists but also for other clinicians, such as general practitioners, gynecologists, and pediatricians who often deal in their routine clinical practice with problems regarding the motherhood and the children mental health.

It is also worthwhile to remember, according to Viguera, that a proportion of patients during pregnancy are prescribed multiple psychotropic drugs; this practice (polypharmacotherapy) appears to be the norm rather than exception (Viguera 2024). A recent systematic review including 14 studies found that the prevalence of women being prescribed two or more medications during pregnancy ranged from 4.9% to 62.4%, with a median of 22.5% (Anand et al. 2023).

Therefore, reproductive safety data reflecting this clinical practice are crucial, even though remain still inadequate. Closing this research gap is clinically relevant and needs to be addressed in the future studies to enhance maternal and child outcome. This is especially relevant for women with multiple and long-term psychiatric disorders who are most likely to need more than one psychotropic drug.

Finally, it must also be reiterated that the risk of suicide in the perinatal period is not negligible.

It was reported in a large cohort study conducted in Ontario that a high proportion of the pregnant and postpartum women who committed suicide had received mental health care within the last year, predominantly within a primary care setting. The perinatal suicide rate was 2.58 per 100,000 live births, with suicide accounting for 51 (5.3%) of 966 perinatal deaths (Grigoriadis et al. 2017).

For these reasons, it would be important to know more about the type of care provided, particularly what proportion of these women were taking psychotropic drugs when they committed suicide (e.g., antidepressants and/or other drugs?) versus obtaining psychotherapy or other non-drug treatments, and for which psychopathological condition? Even in this case, data are still missing.

As reported by an editorial published many years ago by Robinow, but still quite truthful: "*The stark reality is that pregnancy in the context of a history of mental illness often leaves the mother, the baby, and their doctors between Scylla and Charybdis*" (Robinow 2006).

It would be desirable as well as appropriate that both the investments in clinical psychopharmacological research programs and the dissemination of reliable information on fetal and gestational safety of PDs were seen also as an essential tool for the improvement of women's mental health care during the perinatal period.

References

Anand A, Phillips K, Subramanian A, et al. Prevalence of polypharmacy in pregnancy: a systematic review. BMJ Open. 2023;13:13e067585.

Andrade C. Genes and unmeasured and unknown confounds in studies of neurodevelopmental outcomes after antidepressant prescriptions during pregnancy. J Clin Psychiatry. 2020;81(3):20f–3463.

Anya AWW, Stevens DS, Gossen PJJ, et al. Risk of mood disorders during pregnancy and the impact of medication. A systematic review. J Affect Disorders. 2019;249:96–103.

Bind RH, Sawyer K, Pariante C. Depression in pregnancy: biological, clinical, and psychosocial effects. In: Percudani M, Bramante A, Brenna V, Pariante C, editors. Key topics in perinatal mental health. Springer; 2022.

Cohen LS, Altshuler L, Harlow BL, Nonacs R, Newport DJ, Viguera AC, Suri R, Burt VK, Hendrick V, Reminick AM. Relapse of major depression during pregnancy in women who maintain or discontinue antidepressant treatment. JAMA. 2006;295(5):499–507. Erratum in: *JAMA*. 2006;296(2):170

Eleftheriou G, Zandonella-Callegher R, Butera R. Consensus panel recommendations for the pharmacological management of pregnant women with depressive disorders. J Environ Res Public Health. 2023;20:6565.

Eleftheriou G, Zandonella Gallagher R, Butera R, et al. Consensus panel recommendations for the pharmacological management of breastfeeding women with postpartum depression. Int J Envirom Res Public Health. 2024;21:551.

Frayne J, Ellies R, Nguyen T. Experiences of decision making about psychotropic medication during pregnancy and breastfeeding in women living with severe mental illness: a qualitative study. Arch Womens Ment Health. 2023;26:379–87.

Freeman MP. Perinatal psychiatry: an emerging specialty. J Clin Psychiatry. 2014;75(10):1086–7.

Grigoriadis S, Vonder Porten EH, Mamisashvili L, Roerecke M, Rehm J, Dennis CL, Koren G, et al. Antidepressant exposure during pregnancy and congenital malformations: is there an association? A systematic review and meta-analysis of the best evidence. J Clin Psychiatry. 2013;4(4):e293–308.

Grigoriadis S, Wilton AS, Kurdyak PA, et al. Perinatal suicide in Ontario, Canada: a 15-year population-based study. CMAJ. 2017;189:E1085.

Howard LM, Khalifeh K. Perinatal mental health: a review of progress and challenges. World Psychiatry. 2020;19:313–27.

Huybrechts KF, Palmsten K, Mogun H, Kowal M, Avorn J, Setoguchi-Iwata S, Hernández-Díaz S. National trends in antidepressant medication treatment among publicly insured pregnant women. Gen Hosp Psychiatry. 2013;35(3):265–71.

Huybrechts K, Palmsten K, Avorn J, et al. Antidepressant use in pregnancy and the risk of cardiac defects. N Engl J Med. 2014;370(25):2397–407.

LactMed. Retrieved on 10th January, 2025; 2023. Available at https://www.nlm.nih.gov/pubs/factsheets/lactmedfs.html

Louik C, Lin AE, Werler MM, Hernández-Díaz S, Mitchell AA. First-trimester use of selective serotonin-reuptake inhibitors and the risk of birth defects. N Engl J Medicine. 2007;356(26):2675–83. Erratum in: N Engl J Med 2015; 373(7):686

McAllister-Williams RH, Baldwin DS, et al. Endorsed by the British Association for Psychopharmacology. British Association for Psychopharmacology (BAP). Consensus guidance on the use of psychotropic medication preconception, in pregnancy and postpartum 2017. J Psychopharmacol. 2017;31(5):519–52.

Orsolini L, Bellantuono C. Psychotropic drugs in pregnancy and breastfeeding (chapter 16). In: Percudani M, Bramante A, Brenna V, Pariante C, editors. Key topics in perinatal mental health. Springer Nature Switzerland; 2022.

Orsolini L, Valchera A, Vecchiotti R, Tomasetti C, Iasevoli F, Fornaro M, De Berardis D, Perna G, Pompili M, Bellantuono C. Suicide during perinatal period: epidemiology, risk factors and clinical correlates. Front Psych. 2016;7:138.

Percudani M, Bramante A, Brenna V, Pariante C, editors. Key topics in perinatal mental health. Springer Nature Switzerland; 2022.

Robinow DR. Antidepressant treatment during pregnancy. Between Scylla and Charybdis. Am J Psychiatry. 2006;163(6):954–6.

Robinson R, Lahti-Pulkkinen M, Heinonen K. Fetal programming of neuropsychiatric disorders by maternal pregnancy depression: a systematic mini-review. Paediatr Res. 2019;85:134–45.

Smith CJ, Payne WM. Epidemiology of studies of effects on lithium salts are confounded by the inability to control for other potentially teratogenic factors. Human Exp Toxicol. 2024;43:1–16.

Stein A, Pearson RM, Goodman SH, Rapa E, Rahman A, McCallum M, Howard LM, Pariante CM. Effects of perinatal mental disorders on the fetus and child. Lancet. 2014;384(9956):1800–19.

Stevenson K. Fetal programming and epigenetics. Curr Opin Endocr Metab Res. 2020;12:1–6.

Suarez EA, Bateman BT, Hernandez-Diaz S. Association of antidepressant use during pregnancy with risk of neurodevelopmental disorders in children. JAMA Int Med. 2022;182(11):1149–60.

Viguera A. Polypharmacy for perinatal mood and anxiety disorders. Lancet Psychiatry. 2024;11(8):575–7.

Viguera AC, Whitfield T, Baldessarini RJ, Newport DJ, Stowe Z, et al. Risk of recurrence in women with bipolar disorder during pregnancy: prospective study of mood stabilizer discontinuation. Amer J Psychiatry. 2007;164(12):1817–24.

Wang S, Ding C, Du C, Zhu Z, Zhang D, Yi O. Associations between maternal prenatal depression and neonatal behavior and brain function–evidence from the functional near-infrared spectroscopy. Psychoneuroendocrinology. 2022;146:105896.

WHO. Guideline: protecting, promoting and supporting breastfeeding in facilities providing maternity and newborn services. Geneva: World Health Organization; 2017.

Wisner KL. The last therapeutic orphan: the pregnant woman. Am J Psychiatry. 2012;169(6):554–6.

The Role of Paternal Mental Health During the Perinatal Period: From Preconception to Postpartum

5

Giulia Francesconi, Rosa Volgare, Umberto Volpe, and Laura Orsolini

5.1 Introduction

Paternal health and lifestyle behaviors are critically unrepresented in reproductive health discussions. Despite being formally acknowledged as a vital component of reproductive health, paternal involvement in clinical practice and assessment is often overlooked (Montagnoli et al. 2021). Paternal traits and behaviors may influence offspring's physical and mental health through both direct genetic inheritance and epigenetic modifications, as well as through indirect mechanisms that overly affect the maternal environment. Direct effects include epigenetic changes in sperm caused by lifestyle choices such as diet and smoking, which can alter gene expression patterns and affect offspring's phenotypes across generations (Donkin and Barrès 2018; Sharp et al. 2019) impacting on the behavioral and cognitive characteristics (Yeshurun and Hannan 2019). Indirect paternal effects influence the maternal environment through behaviors such as smoking, alcohol consumption, and stress, which can harm both the mother and the child or affect maternal behaviors that are important for the child's health (Scheffers-van Schayck et al. 2019; Braun et al. 2020). These modifications can affect offspring phenotypes, including susceptibility to chronic diseases such as obesity and diabetes (Fleming et al. 2018).

Recently, increasing attention has been given to paternal mental health. Evidence from several human studies suggested that preconception paternal mental health may be associated with adverse health outcomes in their offspring through both genetic and non-genetic mechanisms (Coleman et al. 2020). Depression in fathers before conception is linked to late preterm births, excessive infant crying, and potential changes in newborn's brain structure, such as accelerated white matter

G. Francesconi · R. Volgare · U. Volpe · L. Orsolini (✉)
Unit of Clinical Psychiatry, Department of Experimental and Clinical Medicine (DIMSC), Polytechnic University of Marche, Ancona, Italy
e-mail: l.orsolini@staff.univpm.it

F. Uguz, L. Orsolini (eds.), *Perinatal Psychopharmacology*,
https://doi.org/10.1007/978-3-031-99720-4_5

development (van den Berg et al. 2009; Karlsson et al. 2020; Spry et al. 2020). A recent study revealed that men diagnosed with depression before pregnancy had offspring with increased attention-deficit/hyperactivity disorder (ADHD) and autism spectrum disorder (ASD) risks (Chen et al. 2020). It is possible that preconceptional paternal depression persisted to the postnatal stage to affect children via altered parenting styles with fewer positive activities, such as reading, singing, and hugging, and a higher level of conflict in the father-child relationships making it difficult to satisfy the child's attachment in their early years and potentially affecting the development of a psychopathology later in childhood or adulthood. Family factors, such as maternal depression and couple conflicts, could also mediate the association between paternal postnatal depression and child outcomes (Tan et al. 2023). The underlying biological mechanisms are still unclear. Special attention should also be paid to the use of psychoactive drugs, with selective serotonin reuptake inhibitors (SSRIs) and valproic acid among the most studied substances, that have been hypothesized to be associated with the occurrence of neurodevelopmental disorders in children born from fathers who used these substances in the preconception period (Evans-Hoeker et al. 2018; Yang et al. 2018; Montagnoli et al. 2021).

5.2 Paternal Mental Health

Fathers have become increasingly more involved in parenting due to mothers' growing active roles in the workforce, cultural changes regarding masculinity and fatherhood, and greater equality in gender roles. While maternal mental health issues such as depression, stress, and anxiety are well-documented contributors to adverse child outcomes (Barona et al. 2017; Cook et al. 2018; Tuovinen et al. 2018; Vehmeijer et al. 2019), the impact of paternal mental health remains less clear (Sweeney and MacBeth 2016; Gentile and Fusco 2017; Cui et al. 2020; Challacombe et al. 2023). Several studies indicated that preconception paternal mental health may significantly impact offspring's mental, cognitive, and behavioral health through genetic and non-genetic mechanisms (Yeshurun and Hannan 2019; Coleman et al. 2020). Preconception paternal mental health, including depression and anxiety, seemed to correlate with offspring risks for mental health conditions such as ADHD, ASD, and emotional disturbances. These effects could be due to altered parenting styles (e.g., fewer positive interactions, and increased conflicts) due to psychiatric pathologies (Chen et al. 2020; Tan et al. 2023). Maternal mental health appears to correlate with paternal mental health. Paulson and Bazemore (2010) reported a correlation between paternal and maternal depression during the prenatal and postnatal periods, suggesting that paternal depression could influence maternal depression, which could adversely affect fetal and infant development through a spillover effect. Additionally, females mated with stressed males exhibit altered maternal care, further impacting offspring health, suggesting a bidirectional influence on child outcomes (Chen et al. 2020; Zutshi et al. 2021; Tan et al. 2023). Paternal mental health is also important when considering fertility. Depression has been diagnosed in up to 49% of male partners suffering from infertility, while female partners of depressed men are less likely to conceive. Although human and animal studies have demonstrated the association between father's mental health and an increased risk of adverse health outcomes in their offspring, the underlying biological mechanisms are unclear. Further research is therefore needed, although recently paternal mental health has become an emerging area of research interest, with a special focus on depression.

5.2.1 Paternal Mental Health: Depressive Disorders

Approximately 10% of fathers have symptoms that meet the criteria for depressive episodes of varying severity in the perinatal period (Fisher 2016) which is approximately half the rate of maternal postpartum depression (14–18%) (Liu et al. 2022). Perinatal paternal depression (PPD) can begin as early as the first trimester of pregnancy to 1 year after the birth of the child, though it most commonly emerges around 4 weeks postpartum (DSM-5-TR) (APA 2013). Several paternal factors may increase the risk of depression during the peripartum period. These include unemployment, legal problems, addiction, neurotic personality traits, financial strain, an unplanned pregnancy, and distress related to the imminent birth. Additionally, a lack of social support, avoidant coping strategies, low self-esteem, exposure to negative life events, poor sleep quality, and perceived stress can further contribute to this risk (Wang et al. 2021). Among these, maternal depression emerged as the most significant factor influencing paternal peripartum depression, with severe depression in the partner appearing to increase the father's risk of major depressive disorder (MDD) up to 50% (Wee et al. 2011). Similarly, a positive family and/or personal history of depression appears to influence the occurrence of depression (Goodman 2004). Several studies confirmed that marital dissatisfaction is a robust risk factor for paternal perinatal depression. There is also some evidence suggesting that infant factors, such as difficult temperament and feeding challenges, may play a role in increasing the risk of paternal depression, though research in this area is less extensive. The mechanisms determining the onset of perinatal depression in fathers are currently not completely defined. Certainly, the disruption of the circadian rhythm and sleep deprivation for childcare represent potential determinants. The nightly activities and care needs of the child can negatively impact fathers' productivity in their work, which is typically uninterrupted. This dynamic makes it challenging for fathers to adjust to their new role, often leading to increased frustration (Sokół-Szawłowska 2020).

Depression in men may manifest differently compared to the female counterpart. Clinical studies reported that men usually display increased irritability, impulsivity, persistent sadness, anxiety, dysphoria, low self-esteem, stiffness of affect, feelings of isolation, social withdrawal, disrupted eating patterns, insomnia, tendency to abuse substances (sometimes as part of autotherapy), self-harm ideation, and, in some cases, suicidal thoughts (Addis 2008; Da Costa et al. 2019; Bruno et al. 2020). The different clinical picture can make diagnosis difficult as well as man's tendency to downplay his mental state. It is important to consider that when comparing men and women, men are less likely to report their experiences of depression in the same way that women do and they also less likely seek treatment, mainly due to poor social support, inability to express feelings of sadness/depression for the fear to be judged and/or for internal stigma (Carlberg et al. 2018). As a result, paternal perinatal depression has been underreported, underrecognized, underdiagnosed, and undertreated.

The most common assessment screening tool is the Edinburgh Postnatal Depression Scale (EPDS) (Kozinszky and Dudas 2015). Other tools available to assess paternal depression are represented by the Gotland Male Depression Scale (GMDS) (Sigurdsson et al. 2015), the Masculine Depression Scale (Magovcevic and Addis 2008), the Male Depression Risk Scale (Herreen et al. 2022), and the Beck Depression Inventory-II (BDI-II). Diagnosis is needed since depressive symptomatology may significantly alter the father-infant relationship modifying the child's development and response to stress, with studies showing an association between a father's depressed mood and negative temperament in the child, a higher emotional dysregulation (Ramchandani et al. 2008), and a higher occurrence of both internalizing (sadness, anxiety, or physical symptoms like stomachaches) and externalizing (aggression, oppositional behavior, property destruction, or misbehavior like stealing) problems (Cross et al. 2024). Furthermore, it has also been demonstrated an association between a father's depressed mood and the emergence of reduced social skills, and higher rates of psychiatric disorders in children, particularly at school age (Gentile and Fusco 2017). There is also evidence that fathers' depression during their offspring's childhood can be associated with offspring's mental health problems, most frequently anxiety and depression, during the transition to adulthood (Fisher 2016). Furthermore, depressed fathers display a worse quality in the interaction with their children. They are less prone to play face-to-face with the child, impairing the child's communication skills. Depressed fathers more likely manifest their violence toward family members compared to healthy fathers and tend to be less engaged in offering a cognitive stimulation for their children (Sweeney et al. 2016; Sundstom et al. 2017; Sokół-Szawłowska 2020; Cross et al. 2024).

Moreover, one should argue that depression is often accompanied by poor nutrition, substance use, stress, and lack of exercise, which may also lead to alterations in sperm that can, in turn, adversely affect offspring (Yeshurun et al. 2019; Hoek et al. 2020). Conversely, the involvement of a non-depressed father may protect against some of the offspring risks associated with maternal depression (Melrose 2010).

Relatedly, paternal depression puts the mother at increased risk for depression as well, indirectly contributing to a further increased childhood risk for psychopathology. This can result in a higher prevalence of psychopathological symptoms during preschool years and an increase in psychiatric diagnoses by the time they reach school age (Cross et al. 2024). Interestingly, some findings contradict these associations. Higher paternal depressive symptoms during the prenatal period were associated with fewer child behavioral difficulties, particularly lower externalizing symptoms like conduct and hyperactivity problems. Interestingly, indeed, greater paternal depression and anxiety symptoms measured during childhood seemed to correlate with higher child Intelligence Quotient (IQ) (Jones et al. 2023). Therefore, one should argue that there are complex and nuanced relationships between paternal mental health and child development, mostly still not fully investigated and understood, which suggests a careful approach and the need for more longitudinal studies to fully understand these dynamics. Finally, a recent study showed evidence of an association between preconception parental mental health disorders and preterm birth, with persistent common mental disorder symptoms across adolescence and young adulthood showing the greatest impact. Little evidence of an association between paternal antenatal mental health disorders and small for gestational age was found. The underlying process has not yet been identified (Spry et al. 2020).

5.2.2 Paternal Mental Health: Anxiety Disorders

Anxiety appears to be more prevalent than depression among new fathers. A systematic review conducted by Leach et al. (2016) found that anxiety seemed to affect around 4–16% of fathers during the prenatal period and around 2–18% in the postnatal period. Paternal anxiety is highly comorbid with depression, and it may include a variable set of symptoms including worries, fear, physical complaints, and cognitive symptoms. Fathers are at risk for increased anxiety levels during pregnancy, postpartum, and throughout child development, with levels comparable to mothers. Risk factors include having children with chronic illnesses, low-birthweight infants, or co-parents with mental health issues, as well as low social support and poor marital quality (Luoma et al. 2013; Cimino et al. 2015). Paternal anxiety correlates with child internalizing and externalizing behaviors and other psychiatric conditions, highlighting a clear longitudinal connection between paternal anxiety and adverse child outcomes. Anxious fathers often exhibit overprotective, overinvolved parenting styles, which can model and reinforce anxiety in children. These behaviors, even occurring in infancy, may hinder children's development of independence and increase their risk of psychopathology (Breaux et al. 2014; Möller et al. 2015; Fisher 2016). A recent study showed that fathers' prenatal anxiety symptoms are associated with lower dehydroepiandrosterone (DHEA) levels and higher rates of internalizing symptoms in children. In conclusion, these findings highlight the often overlooked importance of paternal factors during pregnancy in child development, suggesting that prenatal paternal anxiety symptoms may be associated with the child's neuroendocrine function and, in turn, with internalizing symptoms that occur at least until middle childhood (Jones et al. 2024).

5.2.3 Paternal Mental Health: Bipolar Disorders

Bipolar disorder in fathers, characterized by episodes of mania, hypomania, and depression, impacts interparental and parent-child relationships and, ultimately, the child's emotional health. Research mainly found higher rates of manic, hypomanic, and mixed episodes in fathers during the postpartum period, compared to the general population (Pinheiro et al. 2011). Children of fathers with bipolar disorder face a significantly increased risk of bipolar and other mood, anxiety, and externalizing disorders. While bipolar disorder affects parenting behaviors and self-efficacy, gender-specific impacts on fathers' parenting styles remain under-investigated. Maladaptive parenting style associated with bipolar disorder seems to be linked with the emergence of children's internalizing and externalizing problems, despite more studies being needed to clarify this relationship (Fisher 2016).

5.2.4 Paternal Mental Health: Posttraumatic Stress Disorders

Research on posttraumatic stress disorder (PTSD) in fathers found that traumatic experiences, such as witnessing a difficult birth, dealing with a child's serious illness, or exposure to natural disasters and war, can lead to intrusive memories, avoidance, negative mood, and heightened arousal. These symptoms impair paternal functioning and parenting, negatively affecting children's mental health (Nicholls and Ayers 2007). Fathers who develop PTSD from childbirth trauma may struggle with bonding and interparental relationships, affecting infant outcomes (Ribi et al. 2007). Fathers with PTSD often exhibit externalizing parenting behaviors, such as irritability and detachment, contributing to their children's anxiety, depression, and behavioral problems. One study showed that the child's gender and age may be determinants of the type of behavioral problems resulting from paternal PTSD: pre-adolescent girls had somatic complaints and aggression, while adolescent girls showed more depressive symptoms; pre-adolescent boys were more anxious, while adolescent boys had somatic complaints and hyperactivity. Overall, paternal PTSD, regardless of its cause, significantly hinders functional parenting and poses a risk to children's emotional and behavioral health (Fisher 2016).

5.2.5 Paternal Mental Health: Obsessive-Compulsive Disorders

Obsessive-compulsive disorder (OCD) in fathers is one of the least explored paternal mental health conditions. This disorder is characterized by intrusive and recurrent thoughts or images (obsessions) and/or ritualistic and repetitive behaviors that relieve anxiety (compulsions), causing significant distress and being difficult to control. Currently, there is no data available on the prevalence of OCD in fathers, but it seems to be linked to maladaptive parenting styles. A study conducted by Yoshida et al. found that fathers with OCD or depression with severe obsessive traits tended to be significantly more overprotective of their children than fathers without obsessive traits or with mild obsessive traits (Yoshida et al. 2005). However, the available evidence is insufficient to determine with certainty the impact of paternal OCD on parenting behavior and children's mental health (Fisher 2016).

5.2.6 Paternal Mental Health: Substance Use Disorders

Alcohol and other substances, such as tobacco, cannabis, alcohol, and recreational drugs, have been extensively demonstrated to exert teratogenic effects when consumed prenatally by the mother, contributing to developmental delays, physical anomalies, and growth defects in offspring. Paternal substance use seems to significantly affect fertility, pregnancy outcomes, and offspring health through genetic and epigenetic mechanisms or via social, psychological, or behavioral influences on the maternal environment (Abel 2004; Thomas et al. 2023).

Paternal smoking is a modifiable risk factor that significantly influences pregnancy and infant health. It is important to consider that paternal smoking has a direct effect on fetal development through secondhand smoke. While no studies report a direct association between paternal smoking and small for gestational age or decreased birth weight of the offspring, it is known that paternal smoking, even light smoking, increases the risk of heart defects. The father's smoking habit is also associated with an increased risk of overweight and obesity (odds ratio [OR] = 1.41, 95% confidence interval [CI] = 1.17–1.85), the development of childhood leukemia, and appears to negatively impact offspring lung function. It has also been linked to higher rates of ADHD in offspring (Carter et al. 2023).

Regular cannabis use during adolescence, a critical period for testicular development, has been linked to reduced sperm concentration, lower total sperm count, significant testicular atrophy, impaired reproductive hormones, and male infertility (Durairajanayagam 2018; Montagnoli et al. 2021). Cannabis use before conception has also been associated with increased pregnancy loss, decreased birth weight in children, and behavioral and neurodevelopmental problems in offspring. These effects are thought to result from changes in cholinergic synaptic function and related behavioral outcomes (Slotkin et al. 2020).

Opioids appeared to impair male fertility by altering reproductive hormones and spermatogenesis. Their use is associated with reduced testicular volume and erectile dysfunction. Additionally, cocaine and opioid addiction in fathers has been linked to low birth weight, early mortality, and ADHD in children (Fang et al. 2018; Montagnoli et al. 2021). Paternal morphine exposure has been shown to increase behavioral vulnerability to addiction in male offspring through long-lasting neural adaptations in reward pathways (Toussaint et al. 2022).

Paternal alcohol consumption also affects fertility and pregnancy outcomes (Finelli et al. 2021). Alcohol consumption impairs the quality of spermatozoa by reducing their number, motility, and morphology. These effects have been observed even after 1 month of abstinence, suggesting that alcohol-induced changes in spermatozoa may last for weeks or months (Roach et al. 2024). In addition, preconception paternal alcohol consumption alters the hormone balance, essential for reproduction (Bedi et al. 2022; American Addiction Centre 2025). The effects of paternal alcohol use extend beyond the embryonic stage, negatively impacting pregnancy outcomes and the health of offspring. Paternal alcohol use has been linked to higher rates of miscarriage, stillbirth, and low birth weight. Additionally, paternal alcohol use disorder (AUD) has been associated with increased risks of congenital anomalies and infant mortality (Klonoff-Cohen et al. 2003). Children of fathers who drank heavily before conception have also been found to exhibit higher rates of behavioral and mental health problems, mostly represented by ADHD, hyperactivity, anxiety, depression, and sleep disorders (Easey and Sharp 2021; Lo et al. 2024; Jansen et al. 2024). These effects often manifest early in life, with risks peaking at ages 2, 4, and 6. Interestingly, girls appear to show higher rates of emotional reactivity and cognitive challenges compared to boys who are more likely to display somatic complaints and rule-breaking behaviors (Luan et al. 2022). The association between fathers' alcohol consumption and an increased risk of neurodevelopmental disorders is also significant. A recent study by May et al. (2023) suggested that paternal alcohol use may increase the risk of fetal alcohol spectrum disorders (FASD)—a condition characterized by cognitive difficulties (problems with learning, memory, attention, and problem-solving skills), behavioral disorders (impulsivity, hyperactivity, and difficulty with self-regulation), problems in interpersonal interactions, and physical abnormalities (distinctive facial features, growth delays, and organ anomalies) (Berlina 2024). May et al. (2023) found that fathers of children with FASD are more likely to have a history of heavy drinking. On average, these fathers consume 9.2 drinks per occasion, compared to 4.8 drinks in control groups, and exhibit significantly higher rates of AUD. Although the mechanisms remain unclear, this association raises the possibility that paternal alcohol use may influence FASD risk through genetic or environmental factors, or by affecting family dynamics and maternal health. A recent Swedish study (Khemiri et al. 2023) explored the impact of paternal AUD on the offspring's risk of intellectual disability (ID), a neurodevelopmental disorder with altered cognitive, social, and physical development (DSM 2013). The exact mechanisms remain unclear, but probably the paternal alcohol use near conception may induce genetic mutations or epigenetic changes, contributing to ID risk. Moreover, the relationship between paternal alcohol consumption and child outcomes appears to be dose-dependent: the more a father drinks, the greater the risks for his children (Luan et al. 2022).

5.3 The Impact of Paternal Psychopharmacotherapy

Most studies evaluating the safety of parental drug exposure during pregnancy and conception primarily focus on maternal exposure. However, recent publications have also highlighted the potential impact of paternal drug exposure on pregnancy outcomes. Antipsychotics, anxiolytics, hypnotics, sedatives, and antidepressants are frequently prescribed to fathers (Wensink et al. 2021) with some studies showing an association between the use of some of these medications and the occurrence of negative changes in sperm quality, as well as an increased risk of fetal mortality and impaired fetal growth (Baumgartner et al. 2001; Safarinejad 2008; Engeland et al. 2013; Akasheh et al. 2014). In a prospective study by Wensink et al. (2022), rates of preterm births were slightly higher in the drug-exposed groups (>6%) than in the unexposed group (5%). Birth defects were generally similar between the two groups (3.3–3.9% exposed vs 3.3% unexposed). The only drug group that showed a slightly increased risk of malformations (most frequently in the urinary tract) was diazepines, oxazepines, thiazepines, and oxepines (such as antipsychotics), which showed a moderately elevated adjusted OR of 1.22 but not statistically significant. However, there is no clear link between the drug and the malformation. The trend of increased risk for diazepines, oxazepines, thiazepines, and oxepines could be due to the underlying disease rather than the drug. It is not currently known whether paternal use of these drugs during sperm development is associated with the risk of birth defects. Further research is needed, with the current study primarily focusing on SSRIs and valproic acid.

5.3.1 The Impact of Paternal Psychopharmacotherapy: Selective Reuptake Inhibitors (SRI)

The use of selective serotonin reuptake inhibitors (SSRIs) has grown since their introduction in the 1980s (Kendrick 2021). Studies suggested that paternal use of these medications may harm male fertility and fetal development. Some studies also reported that SSRIs seemed to be associated with lower semen concentration, reduced total sperm count, decreased sperm motility, altered sperm morphology, and increased sperm DNA fragmentation (Yland et al. 2021). However, other research has concluded that SSRIs do not directly impair semen parameters, although a significant difference in sperm morphology has been observed with escitalopram use (Pham et al. 2022). Two Scandinavian cohort studies (Engeland et al. 2013; Wensink et al. 2022) have investigated the effects of preconception paternal SSRI use on major congenital malformations and preterm birth finding no increased risk of major congenital malformations, but reporting a higher risk of preterm delivery. A study conducted by Garvik et al. (2024) examined the relationship between paternal SSRI use within 3 months before conception and adverse health outcomes in offspring, including birth outcomes and early life events during the first year of life. The study did not find any statistically significant increased risk for low Apgar scores, being small for gestational age (SGA), or major congenital malformations. However, citalopram and escitalopram were associated with a statistically significant 1.15-fold increased risk of preterm birth. Regarding adverse early life events, no clinically significant risks were associated with paternal SSRI use overall, though citalopram was linked to a 1.12-fold increased risk of hospitalizations during the first year of life. Some studies focused on the possible association between paternal use of SSRIs and ASD or ADHD in offspring, despite conflicting data. A study by Viktorin et al. (2018) compared the incidence of ASD in children born to fathers undergoing antidepressant treatment during the time of conception (from 4 weeks before conception to 4 weeks after), children born to fathers who started antidepressant treatment during pregnancy, and children born to untreated fathers. No association was observed between the use of antidepressants during conception and ASD or ID. Children whose fathers started antidepressant treatment during pregnancy had a higher risk of ID (OR = 1.66; 95%CI = 1.06 to 2.59). A study based on Danish national registers found that compared to unexposed children, exposed children had a 1.62-fold higher risk of ASD (95% CI 1.33–1.96), particularly for fathers who had used SSRIs in the year before conception (Yang et al. 2017). However, the slight increase in risk may be attributable to paternal baseline psychiatric indications related to SSRI use or other confounders. Yang et al. (2018) found that exposure to SSRIs 1 year before conception showed a hazard ratio of ADHD of 1.35, while paternal SSRI use only in the last 3 months before conception had an adjusted HR of 1.31, compared to non-exposed peers. However, the slight increase in ADHD risk might be linked to the underlying conditions for which SSRIs were prescribed.

5.3.2 The Impact of Paternal Psychopharmacotherapy: Valproic Acid

Epilepsy is a prevalent neurological disorder among males of reproductive age (Christensen et al. 2023). Valproate, a commonly prescribed antiseizure medication (ASM), is frequently used to manage epilepsy in this population (Marson et al. 2021). In 2014, the European Medicines Agency (EMA) issued contraindications for the use of valproate during pregnancy and restricted its use in female patients of childbearing age due to teratogenic risks (EMA 2014). The potential risks associated with paternal exposure at conception remain unclear (Bromley et al. 2023). Nevertheless, in November 2023, the U.K. Medicines and Healthcare Products Regulatory Agency (MHRA) expanded these restrictions to include male patients, stating that valproate should not be prescribed to patients younger than 55 years of age unless no alternative treatments are available (MHRA 2023). In January 2024, the EMA recommended that valproate treatment for male patients should only be initiated and supervised by specialists. These specialists should inform patients of the potential risks, discuss the use of effective contraceptives for both the patient and their partner, and conduct regular reviews to reassess the need for treatment, particularly if the patient is planning a pregnancy (EMA 2024). These restrictions are based on a retrospective observational study initiated by the EMA which suggested a possible increased risk of neurodevelopmental disorders (such as ASD) and both major and minor congenital malformations in children conceived by men who had taken valproate in the 3 months preceding conception (EMA 2023). However, the EMA was unable to establish a direct causal link to valproate. Recent studies (Sundelin et al. 2016; Brikell et al. 2018; Garey et al. 2024) reported an increased risk of ASD and ADHD in children of parents with epilepsy, without, however, mentioning any anticonvulsant therapy used. Moreover, recent literature, although limited in data, has not demonstrated an increased risk of developmental disorders associated with paternal exposure to valproate. These results were consistent across various analyses, including comparisons with the general population, dose-response assessments, sibling comparisons, and analyses limited to fathers with epilepsy. (Tomson et al. 2020; Honybun et al. 2024; Christensen et al. 2024). According to the literature, paternal valproate exposure may potentially impact male germ cells (Sakai et al. 2023). Overall, current literature about the safety of other psychotropic drugs in fathers is still limited. Therefore, further research is needed to draw definitive conclusions about the safety of other psychotropic medications.

5.4 Management Strategies

The prevalence of mental health issues among parents is difficult to estimate due to underreporting and varying recording practices. However, estimates suggest that between 15% and 23% of children live with a parent who has a mental illness (Pierce et al. 2020). Dealing with families facing complex issues such as mental health problems presents challenges. The separation between adult mental health services and child-focused services, as well as between these services and child protection, often hinders the integration of care. Fragmented services can exacerbate reliance on healthcare resources and deepen mental health issues in children, particularly when parental mental health problems are present (Cooper et al. 2016). It is important to educate fathers through multimodal prenatal education about paternal perinatal depression in the form of in-office posters, verbal dialogue, and a handout (Guillemette et al. 2023). Early diagnosis through screening tests is crucial. Once the diagnosis is made, it is important to begin appropriate treatment including both pharmacological and nonpharmacological treatments.

The effectiveness of cognitive behavioral therapy (CBT) in treating depression and anxiety is well established, with benefits that often extend beyond the end of treatment. In some cases, CBT may even be more effective than antidepressant medications. Nontraditional methods, such as internet discussion forums, e-therapy, therapy tailored to align with masculine gender role norms, or group-based workshops (particularly if the group is exclusively male), show considerable promise (O'Brien et al. 2017). CBT-based group interventions with the family may improve parenting effectiveness and children's coping skills to reduce stress related to parental depression, also proved successful for both parents' and children's mental health (Compas et al. 2009).

Recognizing the success of home visiting programs aimed at supporting mothers during the perinatal period, Hamil et al. (2021) developed the Fathers and Babies (FAB) intervention to engage fathers. The FAB program consists of 12 sessions, featuring digital components and running concurrently with the Mothers and Babies (MB) intervention in participating families. It uniquely focuses on how fathers can enhance both their own mental health and that of their partners. Feedback from initial focus groups and survey responses indicated that the pilot program was well-received, feasible, and acceptable, with promising signs of effectiveness. In a similar vein, Kavanagh et al. (2021) developed a digital intervention designed for both new mothers and fathers. The app features various modules covering topics such as baby care, role transitions, self-care, and supporting partners. While there were no significant differences in depression and quality of life ratings between the intervention and control groups, participants in the intervention group did report greater improvements in parenting self-efficacy scores. Another form of therapy is Parent–Child Interaction Therapy (PCIT), which seems to be effective in reducing both children's internalizing and externalizing symptoms. Additionally, it leads to decreases in parental depressive symptoms and overall parenting stress (McCabe et al. 2022). Psychopharmacological therapy should not be demonized, as the literature shows that the available data is limited and often conflicting. It is therefore essential to assess the risk-benefit ratio on a case-by-case basis. Regardless of the treatment modality, targeting both parent depression and parenting skills in conjunction appears to be critical to improvements in child mental health outcomes (Cross et al. 2024).

5.5 Conclusions

This chapter has highlighted the importance of paternal mental health, an area that is often overlooked but plays a crucial role in the emotional, cognitive, and behavioral development of children, underscoring the urgency of broadening the focus of research and clinical practices, which have historically focused almost exclusively on the maternal figure. The evidence gathered shows that conditions such as depression, anxiety, bipolar disorder, OCD, AUD, and SUD not only impact the quality of the father-child relationship but can also have lasting repercussions on children's physical and mental health. Moreover, implications of paternal mental health on family dynamics are equally relevant, including interdependence with maternal mental health. Research should include an inductive investigation of fathers' psychological, socio-environmental, and biological experiences, rather than simply replicating studies on mothers. Parental role differences, based on biological sex and cultural expectations, specifically influence parenting experiences, the risk, and the clinical manifestation of mental health problems. It is important to overcome barriers to accurate diagnosis of male depression and to analyze both parents' experiences in parallel to understand the etiology and interaction of paternal and maternal mental health and long-term associations with child health. The integration of early diagnostic approaches, innovative psychotherapeutic interventions, and educational programs for fathers-to-be could help improve the psychological well-being of the family.

Therefore, it seems essential to include the fathers in perinatal depression screening, also involving less common parenting structures, such as single fathers or same-sex couples, to understand the unique experiences and risks that may affect their children. In addition, it has emerged that the use of psychotropic drugs by fathers requires careful evaluation to balance therapeutic benefits with potential risks to offspring. However, further research is needed to clarify the underlying mechanisms and develop evidence-based guidelines capable of equally involving both parents in the perinatal care journey. With a more inclusive and balanced approach, the scientific and health community can help reduce gender disparities in perinatal health and promote a healthier family environment conducive to the optimal development of the next generation.

References

Abel E. Paternal contribution to fetal alcohol syndrome. Addict Biol. 2004;9(2):127–36. https://doi.org/10.1080/13556210410001716980.

Addis ME. Gender and depression in men. Clin Psychol Sci Pract. 2008;15:153. https://doi.org/10.1111/j.1468-2850.2008.00125.x.

Akasheh G, Sirati L, Noshad Kamran AR, et al. Comparison of the effect of sertraline with behavioral therapy on semen parameters in men with primary premature ejaculation. Urology. 2014;83:800–4. https://doi.org/10.1016/j.urology.2013.12.004.

American Addiction Center. Stacy Mosel LMSW. Alcohol Addiction & Abuse: Signs, Symptoms, and Treatment. American Addiction Center; 2025.

American Psychiatric Association. Diagnostic and statistical manual of mental disorders (DSM). 5th ed. American Psychiatric Association; 2013.

Barona M, Taborelli E, Corfield F, Pawlby S, Easter A, Schmidt U, Treasure J, Micali N. Neurobehavioural and cognitive development in infants born to mothers with eating disorders. J Child Psychol Psychiatry. 2017;58(8):931–8. https://doi.org/10.1111/jcpp.12736.

Baumgartner A, Schmid TE, Schuetz CG, Adler ID. Detection of aneuploidy in rodent and human sperm by multicolor fish after chronic exposure to diazepam. Mutat Res. 2001;490:11–9. https://doi.org/10.1016/S1383-5718(00)00141-8.

Bedi YS, Wang H, Thomas KN, Basel A, Prunier J, Robert C, Golding MC. Alcohol induced increases in sperm histone H3 lysine 4 trimethylation correlate with increased placental CTCF occupancy and altered developmental programming. Sci Rep. 2022;12(1):8839. https://doi.org/10.1038/s41598-022-12188-3.

Berlina WB. Understanding fetal alcohol spectrum disorders: a guide for expecting parents, caregivers, and families. SAMHSA, 2024.

Braun M, Klingelhöfer D, Oremek GM, Quarcoo D, Groneberg DA. Influence of second-hand smoke and prenatal tobacco smoke exposure on biomarkers, genetics and physiological processes in children-an overview in research insights of the last few years. Int J Environ Res Public Health. 2020;17(9):3212. https://doi.org/10.3390/ijerph17093212.

Breaux RP, Harvey EA, Lugo-Candelas CI. The role of parent psychopathology in the development of preschool children with behavior problems. J Clin Child Adolesc Psychol. 2014;43(5):777–90. https://doi.org/10.1080/15374416.2013.836451.

Brikell I, Ghirardi L, D'Onofrio BM, Dunn DW, Almqvist C, Dalsgaard S, Kuja-Halkola R, Larsson H. Familial liability to epilepsy and attention-deficit/hyperactivity disorder: a Nationwide cohort study. Biol Psychiatry. 2018;83(2):173–80. https://doi.org/10.1016/j.biopsych.2017.08.006.

Bromley R, Adab N, Bluett-Duncan M, Clayton-Smith J, Christensen J, Edwards K, Greenhalgh J, Hill RA, Jackson CF, Khanom S, McGinty RN, Tudur Smith C, Pulman J, Marson AG. Monotherapy treatment of epilepsy in pregnancy: congenital malformation outcomes in the child. Cochrane Database Syst Rev. 2023;8(8):CD010224. https://doi.org/10.1002/14651858.CD010224.pub3.

Bruno A, Celebre L, Mento C, Rizzo A, Silvestri MC, De Stefano R, Zoccali RA, Muscatello MRA. When fathers begin to falter: a comprehensive review on paternal perinatal depression. Int J Environ Res Public Health. 2020;17(4):1139. https://doi.org/10.3390/ijerph17041139.

Carlberg M, Edhborg M, Lindberg L. Paternal perinatal depression assessed by the Edinburgh postnatal depression scale and the Gotland male depression scale: prevalence and possible risk factors. Am J Mens Health. 2018;12(4):720–9. https://doi.org/10.1177/1557988317749071.

Carter T, Schoenaker D, Adams J, et al. Paternal preconception modifiable risk factors for adverse pregnancy and offspring outcomes: a review of contemporary evidence from observational studies. BMC Public Health. 2023;23:509. https://doi.org/10.1186/s12889-023-15335-1.

Challacombe FL, Pietikäinen JT, Kiviruusu O, Saarenpää-Heikkilä O, Paunio T, Paavonen EJ. Paternal perinatal stress is associated with children's emotional problems at 2 years. J Child Psychol Psychiatry. 2023;64(2):277–88. https://doi.org/10.1111/jcpp.13695.

Chen LC, Chen MH, Hsu JW, Huang KL, Bai JM, Chen TJ, Wang PW, Pan TL, Su TP. Association of parental depression with offspring attention deficit hyperactivity disorder and autism spectrum disorder: a nationwide birth cohort study.J. Affect Disord. 2020;277:109–14. https://doi.org/10.1016/j.jad.2020.07.059.

Christensen J, Dreier JW, Sun Y, Linehan C, Tomson T, Marson A, Forsgren L, Granbichler CA, Trinka E, Illiescu C, Malmgren K, Kjellberg J, Ibsen R, Jennum PJ, et al. Estimates of epilepsy prevalence, psychiatric co-morbidity and cost. Seizure. 2023;107:162–71. https://doi.org/10.1016/j.seizure.2022.06.010.

Christensen J, Trabjerg BB, Dreier JW. Valproate use during spermatogenesis and risk to offspring. JAMA Netw Open. 2024;7:e2414709. https://doi.org/10.1001/jamanetworkopen.2024.14709.

Cimino S, Cerniglia L, Paciello M. Mothers with depression, anxiety or eating disorders: outcomes on their children and the role of paternal psychological profiles. Child Psychiatry Hum Dev. 2015;46(2):228–36. https://doi.org/10.1007/s10578-014-0462-6.

Coleman JRI, Gaspar HA, Bryois J. The genetics of the mood disorder Spectrum: genome-wide association analyses of more than 185,000 cases and 439,000 controls. Biol Psychiatry. 2020;88(2):169–84. https://doi.org/10.1016/j.biopsych.2019.10.015.

Compas BE, Forehand R, Keller G, Champion JE, Rakow A, Reeslund KL, McKee L, Fear JM, Colletti CJ, Hardcastle E, Merchant MJ, Roberts L, Potts J, Garai E, Coffelt N, Roland E, Sterba SK, Cole DA. Randomized controlled trial of a family cognitive-behavioral preventive intervention for children of depressed parents. J Consult Clin Psychol. 2009;77(6):1007–20. https://doi.org/10.1037/a0016930.

Cook N, Ayers S, Horsch A. Maternal posttraumatic stress disorder during the perinatal period and child outcomes: a systematic review. J Affect Disord. 2018;225:18–31. https://doi.org/10.1016/j.jad.2017.07.045.

Cooper M, Evans Y, Pybis J. Interagency collaboration in children and young people's mental health: a systematic review of outcomes, facilitating factors and inhibiting factors. Child Care Health Dev. 2016;42(3):325–42. https://doi.org/10.1111/cch.12322.

Cross M, Abdul-Karim Y, Johnson A, Victor C, Rosenfeld A. Healing together: a narrative review on how psychiatric treatment for parental depression impacts children. Int J Environ Res Public Health. 2024;21(3):367. https://doi.org/10.3390/ijerph21030367.

Cui C, Li M, Yang Y, Liu C, Cao P, Wang L. The effects of paternal perinatal depression on socio-emotional and behavioral development of children: a meta-analysis of prospective studies. Psychiatry Res. 2020;284:112775. https://doi.org/10.1016/j.psychres.2020.112775.

Da Costa D, Danieli C, Abrahamowicz M, et al. A prospective study of postnatal depressive symptoms and associated risk factors in first-time fathers. J Affect Disord. 2019;249:371–7. https://doi.org/10.1016/j.jad.2019.02.033.

Donkin I, Barrès R. Sperm epigenetics and influence of environmental factors. Mol Metab. 2018;14:1–11. https://doi.org/10.1016/j.molmet.2018.02.006.

Durairajanayagam D. Lifestyle causes of male infertility. Arab J Urol. 2018;16(1):10–20. https://doi.org/10.1016/j.aju.2017.12.004.

Easey KE, Sharp GC. The impact of paternal alcohol, tobacco, caffeine use and physical activity on offspring mental health: a systematic review and meta-analysis. Reprod Health. 2021;18(1):214. https://doi.org/10.1186/s12978-021-01266-w.

Engeland A, Bjørge T, Daltveit AK, Skurtveit S, Vangen S, Vollset SE, Furu K. Effects of preconceptional paternal drug exposure on birth outcomes: cohort study of 340000 pregnancies using Norwegian population-based databases. Br J Clin Pharmacol. 2013;75(4):1134–41.

European Medicines Agencies (EMA). PRAC recommends strengthening the restrictions on the use of valproate in women and girls. Internet Document; 2014.

European Medicines Agencies (EMA). A post-authorisation safety study (PASS) to evaluate the paternal exposure to valproate and the risk of neurodevelopmental disorders including autism spectrum disorder as well as congenital abnormalities in offspring – a population-based retrospective study; 2023.

European Medicines Agencies (EMA). Potential risk of neurodevelopmental disorders in children born to men treated with valproate medicines: PRAC recommends precautionary measures; 2024.

Available at https://www.ema.europa.eu/en/news/potential-riskneurodevelopmental-disorders-children-born-men-treated-valproate-medicines-prac-recommends-precautionary-measures

Evans-Hoeker EA, Eisenberg E, Diamond MP, Legro RS, Alvero R, Coutifaris C, Casson PR, Christman GM, Hansen KR, Zhang H, Santoro N, Steiner AZ. Major depression, antidepressant use, and male and female fertility. Fertil Steril. 2018;109(5):879–87. https://doi.org/10.1016/j.fertnstert.2018.01.029.

Fang SY, Huang N, Tsay JH, Chang SH, Chen CY. Excess mortality in children born to opioid-addicted parents: a national register study in Taiwan. Drug Alcohol Depend. 2018;183:118–26. https://doi.org/10.1016/j.drugalcdep.2017.10.015.

Finelli R, Mottola F, Agarwal A. Impact of alcohol consumption on male fertility potential: a narrative review. Int J Environ Res Public Health. 2021;19(1):328. https://doi.org/10.3390/ijerph19010328.

Fisher SD. Paternal mental health: why is it relevant? Am J Lifestyle Med. 2016;11(3):200–11. https://doi.org/10.1177/1559827616629895.

Fleming T, Bavin L, Lucassen M, Stasiak K, Hopkins S, Merry S. Beyond the trial: systematic review of real-world uptake and engagement with digital self-help interventions for depression, low mood, or anxiety. J Med Internet Res. 2018;20(6):e199. https://doi.org/10.2196/jmir.9275.

Garvik OS, Jølving LR, Lund K, Friedman S, Nørgård BM. Paternal use of selective serotonin reuptake inhibitors and adverse health outcomes: a nationwide cohort study on 13,547 exposed children. Andrology. 2024;13:259.

Gentile S, Fusco ML. Untreated perinatal paternal depression: effects on offspring. Psychiatry Res. 2017;252:325–32. https://doi.org/10.1016/j.psychres.2017.02.064.

Goodman JH. Paternal postpartum depression, its relationship to maternal postpartum depression, and implications for family health. J Adv Nurs. 2004;45(1):26–35. https://doi.org/10.1046/j.1365-2648.2003.02857.x.

Guillemette TN, Monn JL, Chronister M. An evidence-based project to improve paternal postpartum depression. J Nurse Pract. 2023;19:104495. https://doi.org/10.1016/j.nurpra.2022.11.005.

Hamil J, Gier E, Garfield CF, Tandon D. The development and pilot of a technology-based intervention in the United States for father's mental health in the perinatal period. Am J Mens Health. 2021;15(5):15579883211044306. https://doi.org/10.1177/15579883211044306.

Herreen D, Rice S, Zajac I. Brief assessment of male depression in clinical care: validation of the male depression risk scale short form in a cross-sectional study of Australian men. BMJ Open. 2022;12(3):e053650. https://doi.org/10.1136/bmjopen-2021-053650.

Hoek J, Steegers-Theunissen RPM, Willemsen SP, Schoenmakers S. Paternal folate status and sperm quality, pregnancy outcomes, and epigenetics: a systematic review and meta-analysis. Mol Nutr Food Res. 2020;64(9):e1900696. https://doi.org/10.1002/mnfr.201900696.

Honybun E, Rayner G, Malpas CB, et al. Paternal exposure to antiseizure medications and offspring outcomes: a systematic review. J Neurol Neurosurg Psychiatry. 2024;96(1):15–25. https://doi.org/10.1136/jnnp-2024-334077.

Jansen E, Marceau K, Sellers R, Chen T, Garfield CF, Leve LD, Neiderhiser JM, Spotts EL, Roary M. The role of fathers in child development from preconception to postnatal influences: opportunities for the National Institutes of Health environmental influences on child health outcomes (ECHO) program. Dev Psychobiol. 2024;66(2):e22451. https://doi.org/10.1002/dev.22451.

Jones SL, Caccese C, Davis KP, Lew J, Elgbeili G, Herba CM, Barnwell J, Robert CH, Gavanski I, Horsley K, Fraser WD, Da Costa D, Séguin JR, Nguyen TV, Montreuil TC. Longitudinal associations between paternal mental health and child behavior and cognition in middle childhood. Front Psychol. 2023;14

Jones SL, De Braga V, Caccese C, Lew J, Elgbeili G, Castellanos-Ryan N, Parent S, Muckle G, Herba CM, Fraser WD, Ducharme S, Barnwell J, Trasler J, Séguin JR, Nguyen TV, Montreuil TC. Prenatal paternal anxiety symptoms predict child DHEA levels and internalizing symptoms during adrenarche. Front Behav Neurosci. 2024;17:1217846. https://doi.org/10.3389/fnbeh.2023.1217846.

Karlsson H, Merisaari H, Karlsson L, Scheinin NM, Parkkola R, Saunavaara J, Lähdesmäki T, Lehtola SJ, Keskinen M, Pelto J, Lewis JD, Tuulari JJ. Association of cumulative paternal early life stress with white matter maturation in newborns. JAMA Netw Open. 2020;3(11):e2024832.

Kavanagh DJ, Connolly J, Fisher J, Halford WK, Hamilton K, Hides L, Milgrom J, Rowe H, Scuffham PA, White KM, Wittkowski A, Appleton S, Sanders D. The baby steps web program for the well-being of new parents: randomized controlled trial. J Med Internet Res. 2021;23(11):e23659. https://doi.org/10.2196/23659.

Kendrick T. Strategies to reduce use of antidepressants. Br J Clin Pharmacol. 2021;87(1):23–33.

Khemiri L, Kuja-Halkola R, Larsson H, Butwicka A, Tideman M, D'Onofrio BM, Latvala A, Lichtenstein P. Parental substance use disorder and risk of intellectual disability in offspring in Sweden: a national register study. eClinicalMedicine. 2023;63:102170. https://doi.org/10.1016/j.eclinm.2023.102170.

Klonoff-Cohen H, Lam-Kruglick P, Gonzalez C. Effects of maternal and paternal alcohol consumption on the success rates of in vitro fertilization and gamete intrafallopian transfer. Fertil Steril. 2003;79(2):330–9. https://doi.org/10.1016/s0015-0282(02)04582-x.

Kozinszky Z, Dudas RB. Validation studies of the Edinburgh postnatal depression scale for the antenatal period. J Affect Disord. 2015;176:95–105. https://doi.org/10.1016/j.jad.2015.01.044.

Leach LS, Poyser C, Cooklin AR, Giallo R. Prevalence and course of anxiety disorders (and symptom levels) in men across the perinatal period: a systematic review. J Affect Disord. 2016;190:675–86. https://doi.org/10.1016/j.jad.2015.09.063.

Liu X, Wang S, Wang G. Prevalence and risk factors of postpartum depression in women: a systematic review and meta-analysis. J Clin Nurs. 2022;31(19–20):2665–77. https://doi.org/10.1111/jocn.16121.

Lo JO, Hedges JC, Chou WH, Tager KR, Bachli ID, Hagen OL, Murphy SK, Hanna CB, Easley CA 4th. Influence of substance use on male reproductive health and offspring outcomes. Nat Rev Urol. 2024;21(9):534–64. https://doi.org/10.1038/s41585-024-00868-w.

Luan M, Zhang X, Fang G, Liang H, Yang F, Song X, Chen Y, Yuan W, Miao M. Preconceptional paternal alcohol consumption and the risk of child behavioral problems: a prospective cohort study. Sci Rep. 2022;12(1):1508. https://doi.org/10.1038/s41598-022-05611-2.

Luoma I, Puura K, Mäntymaa M, Latva R, Salmelin R, Tamminen T. Fathers' postnatal depressive and anxiety symptoms: an exploration of links with paternal, maternal, infant and family factors. Nord J Psychiatry. 2013;67(6):407–13. https://doi.org/10.3109/08039488.2012.752034.

Magovcevic M, Addis ME. The masculine depression scale: development and psychometric evaluation. Psychol Men Masculinity. 2008;9:117. https://doi.org/10.1037/1524-9220.9.3.117.

Marson A, Burnside G, Appleton R, Smith D, Leach JP, Sills G, Tudur-Smith C, Plumpton C, Hughes DA, Williamson P, Baker GA, Balabanova S, Taylor C, Brown R, Hindley D, Howell S, Maguire M, Mohanraj R, Smith PE, et al. The SANAD II study of the effectiveness and cost-effectiveness of valproate versus levetiracetam for newly diagnosed generalised and unclassifiable epilepsy: an open-label, non-inferiority, multicentre, phase 4, randomised controlled trial. Lancet. 2021;397(10282):1375–86. https://doi.org/10.1016/S0140-6736(21)00246-4. Erratum in: Lancet. 2021 Apr 24;397(10284):1544. doi: 10.1016/S0140-6736(21)00886-2. Erratum in: Lancet. 2021 May 15;397(10287):1808. doi: 10.1016/S0140-6736(21)01011-4. PMID: 33838758; PMCID: PMC8047813

May PA, Hasken JM, de Vries MM, Marais AS, Abdul-Rahman O, Robinson LK, Adam MP, Manning MA, Kalberg WO, Buckley D, Seedat S, Parry CDH, Hoyme HE. Maternal and paternal risk factors for fetal alcohol spectrum disorders: alcohol and other drug use as proximal influences. Alcohol Clin Exp Res (Hoboken). 2023;47(11):2090–109. https://doi.org/10.1111/acer.15193.

McCabe K, Zerr A, Cook M, Ringlee L, Yeh M. The relation between parent mental health and child internalizing symptoms in parent–child interaction therapy. J Child Fam Stud. 2022;31:2065. https://doi.org/10.1007/s10826-022-02254-9.

Melrose S. Paternal postpartum depression: how can nurses begin to help? Contemp Nurse. 2010;34(2):199–210. https://doi.org/10.5172/conu.2010.34.2.199.

MHRA. Valproate: review of safety data and expert advice on management of risks. public assessment report; 2023. Available at https://assets.publishing.service.gov.uk/media/65660310312f400013e5d508/Valproate-report-review-and-expert-advice.pdf

Möller EL, Majdandžić M, Bögels SM. Parental anxiety, parenting behavior, and infant anxiety: differential associations for fathers and mothers. J Child Fam Stud. 2015;24(9):2626–37. https://doi.org/10.1007/s10826-014-0075-9.

Montagnoli C, Ruggeri S, Cinelli G, Tozzi AE, Bovo C, Bortolus R, Zanconato G. Anything new about paternal contribution to reproductive outcomes? A review of the evidence. World J Mens Health. 2021;39(4):626–44. https://doi.org/10.5534/wjmh.200147.

Nicholls K, Ayers S. Childbirth-related post-traumatic stress disorder in couples: a qualitative study. Br J Health Psychol. 2007;12(Pt 4):491–509. https://doi.org/10.1348/135910706X120627.

O'Brien AP, McNeil KA, Fletcher R, Conrad A, Wilson AJ, Jones D, Chan SW. New fathers' perinatal depression and anxiety-treatment options: an integrative review. Am J Mens Health. 2017;11(4):863–76. https://doi.org/10.1177/1557988316669047.

Paulson JF, Bazemore SD. Prenatal and postpartum depression in fathers and its association with maternal depression: a meta-analysis. JAMA. 2010;303(19):1961–9. https://doi.org/10.1001/jama.2010.605.

Pham MN, Siebert AL, Faw CA, Dubin JM, Hudnall MT, Lai JD, Wren JM, Bennett NE, Brannigan RE, Halpern JA. Selective serotonin reuptake inhibitor (SSRI) use is not associated with impaired semen parameters. Urology. 2022 Jun;164:140–4.

Pierce M, Hope H, Ford T, Hatch S, Hotopf M, John A, Kontopantelis E, Webb R, Wessely S, McManus S, Abel KM. Mental health before and during the COVID-19 pandemic: a longitudinal probability sample survey of the UK population. Lancet Psychiatry. 2020;7(10):883–92. https://doi.org/10.1016/S2215-0366(20)30308-4.

Pinheiro KA, Coelho FM, Quevedo Lde Á, Jansen K, Souza Lde M, Oses JP, Horta BL, da Silva RA, Pinheiro RT. Paternal postpartum mood: bipolar episodes? Braz J Psychiatry. 2011;33(3):283–6. https://doi.org/10.1590/s1516-44462011000300012.

Ramchandani PG, Stein A, O'Connor TG, Heron J, Murray L, Evans J. Depression in men in the postnatal period and later child psychopathology: a population cohort study. J Am Acad Child Adolesc Psychiatry. 2008;47(4):390–8. https://doi.org/10.1097/CHI.0b013e31816429c2.

Ribi K, Vollrath ME, Sennhauser FH, Gnehm HE, Landolt MA. Prediction of posttraumatic stress in fathers of children with chronic diseases or unintentional injuries: a six-months follow-up study. Child Adolesc Psychiatry Ment Health. 2007;1(1):16. https://doi.org/10.1186/1753-2000-1-16.

Roach AN, Bhadsavle SS, Higgins SL, Derrico DD, Basel A, Thomas KN, Golding MC. Alterations in sperm RNAs persist after alcohol cessation and correlate with epididymal mitochondrial dysfunction. Andrology. 2024;12(5):1012–23. https://doi.org/10.1111/andr.13566.

Safarinejad MR. Sperm DNA damage and semen quality impairment after treatment with selective serotonin reuptake inhibitors were detected using semen analysis and sperm chromatin structure assay. J Urol. 2008;180:2124–8. https://doi.org/10.1016/j.juro.2008.07.034.

Sakai K, Hara K, Tanemura K. Testicular histone hyperacetylation in mice by valproic acid administration affects the next generation by changes in sperm DNA methylation. PLoS One. 2023;18(3):e0282898. https://doi.org/10.1371/journal.pone.0282898.

Scheffers-van Schayck T, Tuithof M, Otten R, Engels R, Kleinjan M. Smoking behavior of women before, during, and after pregnancy: indicators of smoking, quitting, and relapse. Eur Addict Res. 2019;25(3):132–44. https://doi.org/10.1159/000498988.

Sharp GC, Schellhas L, Richardson SS, Lawlor DA. Time to cut the cord: recognizing and addressing the imbalance of DOHaD research towards the study of maternal pregnancy exposures. J Dev Orig Health Dis. 2019;10(5):509–12. https://doi.org/10.1017/S2040174419000072.

Sigurdsson B, Palsson SP, Aevarsson O, Olafsdottir M, Johannsson M. Validity of Gotland male depression scale for male depression in a community study: the Sudurnesjamenn study. J Affect Disord. 2015;173:81–9. https://doi.org/10.1016/j.jad.2014.10.065.

Slotkin TA, Skavicus S, Levin ED, Seidler FJ. Paternal Δ9-tetrahydrocannabinol exposure prior to mating elicits deficits in cholinergic synaptic function in the offspring. Toxicol Sci. 2020;174(2):210–7. https://doi.org/10.1093/toxsci/kfaa004.

Sokół-Szawłowska M. Paternal perinatal depression: cases. Przypadki depresji okołoporodowej u ojców. Psychiatr Pol. 2020;54(6):1123–35. https://doi.org/10.12740/PP/110610.

Spry EA, Wilson CA, Middleton M, Moreno-Betancur M, Doyle LW, Howard LM, Hannan AJ, Wlodek ME, Cheong JL, Hines LA, Coffey C, Brown S, Olsson CA, Patton GC. Parental mental health before and during pregnancy and offspring birth outcomes: a 20-year preconception cohort of maternal and paternal exposure. eClinicalMedicine. 2020;27:100564.

Sundelin HE, Larsson H, Lichtenstein P, Almqvist C, Hultman CM, Tomson T, Ludvigsson JF. Autism and epilepsy: a population-based nationwide cohort study. Neurology. 2016;87(2):192–7. https://doi.org/10.1212/WNL.0000000000002836.

Sundstom Poromaa I, Comasco E, Georgakis MK, Skalkidou A. Sex differences in depression during pregnancy and the postpartum period. J Neurosci Res. 2017;95(1–2):719–30. https://doi.org/10.1002/jnr.23859.

Sweeney S, MacBeth A. The effects of paternal depression on child and adolescent outcomes: a systematic review. J Affect Disord. 2016;205:44–59. https://doi.org/10.1016/j.jad.2016.05.073.

Tan X, Luo J, Ding X, Li H. Preconception paternal mental disorders and child health: mechanisms and interventions. Neurosci Biobehav Rev. 2023;144:104976. https://doi.org/10.1016/j.neubiorev.2022.104976.

Thomas KN, Derrico DD, Golding MC. Paternal alcohol exposure and dental-facial anomalies in offspring. Reply. J Clin Invest. 2023;133(19):e174216. https://doi.org/10.1172/JCI174216.

Tomson T, Muraca G, Razaz N. Paternal exposure to antiepileptic drugs and offspring outcomes: a nationwide population-based cohort study in Sweden. J Neurol Neurosurg Psychiatry. 2020;91(9):907–13. https://doi.org/10.1136/jnnp-2020-323028.

Toussaint AB, Foster W, Jones JM, Kaufmann S, Wachira M, Hughes R, Bongiovanni AR, Famularo ST, Dunham BP, Schwark R, Karbalaei R, Dressler C, Bavley CC, Fried NT, Wimmer ME, Abdus-Saboor I. Chronic paternal morphine exposure increases sensitivity to morphine-derived pain relief in male progeny. Sci Adv. 2022;8(7):eabk2425. https://doi.org/10.1126/sciadv.abk2425.

Tuovinen S, Lahti-Pulkkinen M, Girchenko P, Lipsanen J, Lahti J, Heinonen K, Reynolds RM, Hämäläinen E, Kajantie E, Laivuori H, Pesonen AK, Villa PM, Räikkönen K. Maternal depressive symptoms during and after pregnancy and child developmental milestones. Depress Anxiety. 2018;35(8):732–41. https://doi.org/10.1002/da.22756.

van den Berg MP, van der Ende J, Crijnen AAM, Jaddoe VWV, Moll HA, Mackenbach JP, Hofman A, Hengeveld MW, Tiemeier H, Verhulst FC. Paternal depressive symptoms during pregnancy are related to excessive infant crying. Pediatrics. 2009;124(1):e96–e103. https://doi.org/10.1542/peds.2008-3100.

Vehmeijer FOL, Guxens M, Duijts L, El Marroun H. Maternal psychological distress during pregnancy and childhood health outcomes: a narrative review. J Dev Orig Health Dis. 2019;10(3):274–85. https://doi.org/10.1017/S2040174418000557.

Viktorin A, Levine SZ, Altemus M, Reichenberg A, Sandin S. Paternal use of antidepressants and offspring outcomes in Sweden: nationwide prospective cohort study. BMJ. 2018;361:k2233.

Wang D, Li YL, Qiu D, Xiao SY. Factors influencing paternal postpartum depression: a systematic review and meta-analysis. J Affect Disord. 2021;293:51–63. https://doi.org/10.1016/j.jad.2021.05.088.

Wee KY, Skouteris H, Pier C, Richardson B, Milgrom J. Correlates of ante- and postnatal depression in fathers: a systematic review. J Affect Disord. 2011;130(3):358–77. https://doi.org/10.1016/j.jad.2010.06.019.

Wensink MJ, Rizzi S, Jensen TK, et al. Paternal prescription medication before conception: a retrospective cohort study of all births in Denmark 1997-2017. Scand J Public Health. 2021;49:884–90. https://doi.org/10.1177/1403494820987468.

Wensink M, Lu Y, Tian L, Jensen TK, Skakkebæk NE, Lindahl-Jacobsen R, Eisenberg M. Nervous system drugs taken by future fathers and birth defects in offspring: a prospective registry-based cohort study. BMJ Open. 2022;12(3):e053946.

Yang F, Chen J, Miao MH, Yuan W, Li L, Liang H, Ehrenstein V, Li J. Risk of autism spectrum disorder in offspring following paternal use of selective serotonin reuptake inhibitors before conception: a population-based cohort study. BMJ Open. 2017;7(12):e016368.

Yang F, Liang H, Chen J, Miao M, Yuan W, Nørgaard M, Li J. Prenatal paternal selective serotonin reuptake inhibitors use and risk of ADHD in offspring. Pediatrics. 2018;141(1):e20171081. https://doi.org/10.1542/peds.2017-1081.

Yeshurun S, Hannan AJ. Transgenerational epigenetic influences of paternal environmental exposures on brain function and predisposition to psychiatric disorders. Mol Psychiatry. 2019;24(4):536–48. https://doi.org/10.1038/s41380-018-0039-z.

Yland JJ, Eisenberg ML, Hatch EE, Rothman KJ, McKinnon CJ, Nillni YI, Sommer GJ, Wang TR, Wise LA. A north American prospective study of depression, psychotropic medication use, and semen quality. Fertil Steril. 2021;116(3):833–42.

Yoshida T, Taga C, Matsumoto Y, Fukui K. Paternal overprotection in obsessive-compulsive disorder and depression with obsessive traits. Psychiatry Clin Neurosci. 2005;59(5):533–8. https://doi.org/10.1111/j.1440-1819.2005.01410.x.

Zutshi I, Gupta S, Zanoletti O, Sandi C, Poirier GL. Early life adoption shows rearing environment supersedes transgenerational effects of paternal stress on aggressive temperament in the offspring. Transl Psychiatry. 2021;11(1):533. https://doi.org/10.1038/s41398-021-01659-2.

Part II

Safety of Psychotropic Drugs During Pregnancy and Lactation

Antidepressants in Pregnancy

6

Esra Yazıcı and Özlem Akçay Ciner

6.1 Introduction

Pregnancy can be a time of joy and anticipation, but it also brings significant emotional and physical changes that may increase the risk of developing depression and anxiety disorders. Women's depression is prevalent, especially around childbearing years, affecting 10–23% of women aged 18 or older. Symptoms often include sleeplessness, hopelessness, and low energy (Jahan et al. 2021).

The prevalence of prenatal anxiety disorders exhibits variability across different studies and evaluations. Anxiety associated with pregnancy is prevalent; 54% of women indicate experiencing anxiety during at least one trimester. As per recent investigations, anxiety levels are projected to be 6.6–15% lower during the second trimester when juxtaposed with the initial and third trimesters, which appear to present heightened anxiety levels. Indeed, it has been observed that women encounter anxiety in a non-linear trajectory, with the first and third trimesters of pregnancy identified as particularly high-risk periods (Karnwal and Sharmila 2024).

An exhaustive analysis of the 26 scholarly articles indicated that a total of 4303 individuals tested positive for depressive disorders within a cohort of 28,248 expectant mothers, resulting in a prevalence rate of 15%. After the elimination of confounding variables, the sample size was recalibrated to 25,771, with 4223 individuals identified as exhibiting depressive symptoms, thus yielding a revised prevalence rate of 16.4%. Furthermore, the investigation disclosed that antepartum depression (AD) is most frequently encountered during the final trimester of gestation and least prevalent during the second trimester (Okagbue et al. 2019).

E. Yazıcı (✉)
Faculty of Medicine, Department of Psychiatry, Sakarya University, Sakarya, Türkiye

Ö. A. Ciner
Düzce State Hospital, Düzce, Türkiye

F. Uguz, L. Orsolini (eds.), *Perinatal Psychopharmacology*,
https://doi.org/10.1007/978-3-031-99720-4_6

Socioeconomic factors, such as low income and lack of family support, along with obstetric factors like unplanned pregnancies, are significant risk factors for these mental health issues (Nagandla et al. 2017; Adina et al. 2022). The literature highlights the importance of early screening and intervention to manage these conditions effectively, as they can have adverse effects on both maternal and fetal health (Karnwal and Sharmila 2024; Okagbue et al. 2019). Overall, while depression is most pronounced in the first trimester, anxiety and stress tend to escalate as pregnancy advances, highlighting the need for continuous mental health support throughout the pregnancy (Karnwal and Sharmila 2024).

Mental disorders during pregnancy challenges can affect not only the well-being of the mother but also the developing fetus, potentially leading to complications in both pregnancy and postpartum recovery. Addressing these mental health issues is crucial, as early intervention and support can help mitigate risks and promote a healthier environment for both the mother and child. Women may need to use antidepressants during pregnancy due to the significant risks associated with untreated depression, which can adversely affect both maternal and fetal health (Desaunay et al. 2023; Yazici et al. 2015).

Antidepressant prescriptions decrease from 70% before pregnancy to 27% during pregnancy, partly due to concerns over drug effects on the fetus and inadequate post-diagnosis prescription refills (Jahan et al. 2021). On the other hand, rates of antidepressant use during pregnancy vary significantly across different regions, with estimates indicating that approximately 2–3% of pregnant women in Nordic countries and up to 10% in the United States utilize these medications (Olivier et al. 2013). A comprehensive study in Denmark revealed that 2.4% of pregnancies involved at least one antidepressant prescription, with a notable increase from 0.4% in 1997 to 4.6% in 2011, followed by a decline to 3.1% in 2016 (Sun et al. 2019). In a cohort analysis across the UK, Norway, and Sweden, including 2,528,916 singleton births, 120,209 (4.8%) of deliveries were exposed to maternal antidepressant use (Martin et al. 2024). The rising trend in antidepressant prescriptions during pregnancy highlights the complex interplay between managing maternal mental health and potential risks to fetal outcomes, necessitating further research to understand the implications of these medications (Urato 2015) (Fabiano et al. 2025).

The use of antidepressants during pregnancy presents a complex balance of risks and benefits that must be carefully considered. On the one hand, untreated maternal depression is associated with significant adverse outcomes, including increased risks of suicidal ideation, miscarriage, neonatal growth problems, and postpartum depression, which can affect both maternal and fetal health (Gallitelli et al. 2024; Lam 2023). On the other hand, the use of antidepressants, particularly selective serotonin reuptake inhibitors (SSRIs) and other classes like duloxetine, mirtazapine, and atomoxetine, has been linked to risks such as preterm birth, low birth weight, congenital malformations, and low Apgar scores (Desaunay et al. 2023; Martin et al. 2024). However, the absolute risks of these outcomes remain relatively low, and the severity of maternal depression may confound these associations.

Some studies suggest that antidepressant use does not significantly increase the risk of preterm birth, one of the complications generally linked to antidepressant use during pregnancy, when accounting for the severity of depression (Amit et al. 2024). Moreover, the continuation of antidepressants during pregnancy may prevent relapse of depression, which is crucial for maternal mental health (Knopf 2023). There existed a robust body of evidence suggesting that the continuation of antidepressant medication throughout the course of pregnancy was not linked to an elevated risk of autism, attention-deficit/hyperactivity disorder (ADHD), or intellectual disability when compared to the cessation of such medications prior to conception in both our primary and ancillary analyses. Conversely, the evidence was notably less robust concerning the comparative analyses of the initiation versus non-initiation of antidepressant treatment during pregnancy, with the inherent lack of precision due to a reduced sample size and broader confidence intervals constituting a significant limitation (Heuvelman et al. 2023). Importantly, the decision to use antidepressants during pregnancy should be individualized, involving a multidisciplinary team to weigh the potential risks against the benefits of treating maternal depression (Gallitelli et al. 2024; Yazici et al. 2015). Personalized treatment plans and careful monitoring can help mitigate risks while addressing the mental health needs of pregnant women (Dama and Van Lieshout 2023).

In this chapter, we will concentrate on the pharmacology of antidepressants during pregnancy, examining the nuances of medications and their probable consequences.

6.2 Risks of Maternal Stress, Anxiety, and Depression

Maternal mortality review committees ascertain that over 80% of all pregnancy-associated fatalities in the United States are avertable. Within the spectrum of avertable fatalities, mental health disorders necessitate specific scrutiny as they have been identified as the predominant underlying factor (Combellick et al. 2024). Untreated depression is shown to be a strong predictor of postpartum depression (Yazici et al. 2015). A study by Nesrin Jahan reviewed 20 cohort studies of antenatally depressed women are more likely to experience severe peripartum complications such as heavy bleeding, vaginal tears, placental abnormalities, and convulsions. Additionally postpartum problems like fever, urinary/fecal incontinence, and failure to use a bed net during pregnancy are more prevalent among women with prenatal depression. Furthermore, there was a strong association between antenatal depression and an increased likelihood of cesarean section (CS) delivery, driven by higher anxiety levels and fear of labor among depressed women. The study concluded that psychological distress from depression can hinder uterine contractions, leading to prolonged labor, stalled progress, and fetal distress, raising the chances of undergoing a cesarean section. Additionally, it's reported that mothers with severe depression are at a significantly higher risk of complications like preeclampsia, preterm birth, fetal demise, and intrauterine growth restriction compared to non-depressed mothers (Jahan et al. 2021). In a study by Ogunyemi et al., anxiety/depression cases (6.3%) were analyzed against unaffected pregnancies (93.7%) using logistic regression. A higher likelihood of being Non-Hispanic White, using substances, being unmarried, relying on public insurance, and experiencing medical complications was observed. Untreated anxiety/depression correlated with adverse maternal outcomes including labor induction (aOR = 2.02) and postpartum hemorrhage (aOR = 2.57), while treated cases saw increased blood transfusions (aOR = 4.81) but decreased cesarean deliveries (aOR = 0.59). Neonatal outcomes for treated cases included risks for small for gestational age (aOR = 3.04) and neonatal seizures (aOR = 12.3), while untreated cases faced hypoxia (aOR = 2.83) and encephalopathy (aOR = 18.3). The use of multiple psychotropic medications elevated risks for neonatal adaptation syndrome and hypoglycemia. In conclusion, untreated cases led to more maternal adverse outcomes, whereas treated cases presented with greater neonatal complications compared to unaffected pregnancies (Ogunyemi et al. 2018). Maternal depression has long-term outcomes, increased susceptibility to mental health issues in the child, difficulties in social relationships, and a higher likelihood of behavioral problems as they grow older, as well as fetal and delivery effects (Nagandla et al. 2017).

Maternal depression during pregnancy has significant negative effects on both mothers and their infants. A prospective investigation conducted by Haq et al. assessed women exhibiting antenatal depression in accordance with Edinburgh Postnatal Depression Scale (EPDS) scores in a longitudinal manner. The incidence of preterm delivery was markedly elevated in the study cohort, with 40% of births categorized as preterm and 23.4% classified as early preterm, in contrast to the figures of 19.1% and 12.4% observed in the control group, respectively. In a similar vein, the depression group demonstrated lower birth weights alongside diminished 1-minute (20%) and 5-minute Apgar scores. The multivariate regression analysis indicated a statistically significant and independent association between maternal depression and the occurrence of preterm delivery (aOR: 3.27, 95% CI: 1.23–9.47) (Haq et al. 2024). Another cohort study evaluated 68 mother-baby dyads and found that maternal depressive symptoms can adversely affect child neurodevelopment, particularly in emotional processing, as evidenced by altered brain connectivity (Vartiainen et al. 2024). Furthermore, antenatal depression has been linked to lower cognitive and motor development in infants at 12 months, highlighting the importance of mental health screening during pregnancy (Roy et al. 2022).

The prevalence of depressive symptoms can also lead to long-term maternal health issues, including postpartum depression, emphasizing the need for integrated mental health care in maternal health services (Di Vincenzo et al. 2023). Effective interventions that address maternal mental health during pregnancy can significantly improve outcomes for both mothers and their infants, fostering healthier family dynamics and promoting overall well-being (Rohanachandra 2021) by providing essential support systems that not only alleviate maternal stress but also enhance the emotional and cognitive development of children, ultimately contributing to a more resilient future generation (Roy et al. 2022).

These empirical findings highlight the paramount importance of maternal mental health not solely in relation to pregnancy outcomes but also concerning the enduring development and overall well-being of offspring, thereby necessitating the establishment of comprehensive support frameworks for expectant mothers.

Furthermore, the effective management of depressive and anxiety disorders, along with the prevention of relapses of such conditions during gestation, emerges as a pivotal concern for both maternal and child mental health, as well as for public health at large.

6.3 Impact of Pregnancy on the Pharmacokinetics and Pharmacodynamics of Antidepressants

Understanding how pregnancy alters the pharmacokinetics and pharmacodynamics of antidepressants is essential for optimizing treatment strategies, as these changes can affect drug absorption, distribution, metabolism, and excretion in expectant mothers. This knowledge is vital for clinicians to tailor antidepressant therapies effectively, ensuring both maternal mental health and fetal safety throughout the course of pregnancy. Research has shown that certain antidepressants may behave differently during pregnancy, necessitating careful monitoring and potential dosage adjustments to maintain therapeutic efficacy while minimizing risks.

Pregnancy leads physiological changes, such as increased blood volume, altered hormone levels, and enhanced renal and hepatic function and these changes can modify drug absorption, distribution, metabolism, and excretion, impacting the efficacy and safety of antidepressants, leading to individualized management of treatments (Dodeja et al. 2025; Eke 2022). Specifically, the activity of cytochrome P450 enzymes, crucial for drug metabolism, is altered; for instance, CYP2D6 activity increases, leading to decreased serum concentrations of drugs like paroxetine and fluoxetine, while CYP2C19 activity decreases, affecting drugs like sertraline (Svensson et al. 2020; Poweleit et al. 2022). These changes can result in subtherapeutic drug levels or an increased risk of adverse effects if not properly managed (Yue et al. 2023; Schoretsanitis et al. 2020). The variability in pharmacokinetics is further complicated by genetic polymorphisms in CYP enzymes, which can influence individual responses to antidepressants during the pregnancy period (Cafaro et al. 2022). Despite the widespread use of SSRIs as first-line treatments for depression and anxiety disorders in pregnant women, there is still a lack of comprehensive pharmacokinetic data, leading to challenges in establishing evidence-based dosing guidelines (Avram et al. 2016). Studies have shown that dose-adjusted plasma concentrations of certain antidepressants, such as trimipramine and nortriptyline, decrease significantly in the third trimester, while others like escitalopram and venlafaxine show negligible changes (Schoretsanitis et al. 2020). The presence of the feto-placental unit adds another layer of complexity as well as gestational age, fetal growth, and positions, as drugs can cross the placental barrier, potentially affecting fetal development (Velasquez et al. 2016). Therefore, therapeutic drug monitoring and individualized treatment plans are crucial to optimize antidepressant therapy during pregnancy, ensuring maternal mental health while minimizing risks to the fetus (Campbell et al. 2016). Further research is needed to better understand these pharmacokinetic changes and to develop guidelines for safe and effective antidepressant use in pregnant populations (Schoretsanitis et al. 2020; Svensson et al.

2020). Understanding the implications of these findings is essential for healthcare providers, as it highlights the need for ongoing assessment and adjustment of medication regimens throughout pregnancy to maintain both maternal well-being and fetal safety.

6.4 Conception and Antidepressants

Fertility constitutes a significant topic of contemporary discourse and has been demonstrated to be influenced by depressive disorders as well as pharmacological interventions for depression. Antidepressants, particularly SSRIs, have been shown to affect conception and fertility in both men and women, though the effects vary. In men, SSRIs can decrease sperm count and viability, and disrupt sperm morphology, which can impair fertility (Milosavljević et al. 2022; Santos et al. 2025). For women, certain SSRIs like paroxetine and escitalopram may negatively impact fertility by affecting fallopian tube motility, although their use in women undergoing in vitro fertilization (IVF) does not seem to adversely affect outcomes (Milosavljević et al. 2022). Depression itself, independent of antidepressant use, is associated with reduced fertility and increased time to pregnancy, as well as a higher risk of infertility in both men and women (Liao et al. 2024). The decision to use antidepressants during conception is complex due to fertility; additionally, the medication during conception means medication during the first trimester of pregnancy generally. So the decision needs weighing its potential risks to fetal development, such as congenital malformations and developmental issues, although these risks are not conclusively proven and may be confounded by the severity of maternal depression (Cristina 2023; Rotem-Kohavi et al. 2021; Yang et al. 2024; Sujan 2022). Despite these concerns, untreated depression poses significant risks to both maternal and fetal health, including preterm labor and low birth weight, which highlights the importance of managing depression effectively during the reproductive period (Zeszutek 2021). Therefore, while antidepressants can affect conception, the decision to use them should carefully weigh the benefits of treating depression against potential risks to fertility and pregnancy outcomes.

6.5 Risk Associated with Antidepressant Use During Pregnancy

Antidepressant use during pregnancy is not only related to the type of antidepressant. Also age of mother, socioeconomic status, and pre-existing health conditions can play crucial roles in determining the overall impact on both maternal and fetal well-being (Desaunay et al. 2023). Comorbid clinical conditions as gestational diabetes, hypertension, and obesity may further complicate the management of depression during pregnancy, necessitating a tailored approach to treatment that considers both mental health and physical health outcomes for the mother and child.

6.5.1 Fetal and Neonatal Outcomes

6.5.1.1 Congenital Malformations

The relationship between antidepressant use during pregnancy and the risk of congenital malformations is complex and varies depending on the type of antidepressant and the specific malformation considered. Studies indicate that SSRIs, such as sertraline, are associated with an increased risk of congenital heart defects (CHDs), including only septal heart malformations, not other major malformations and although the severity of these malformations is generally not extreme (Kolding et al. 2023; Shen et al. 2017). Several studies have explored this association with mixed results. A study conducted with Mendelian randomization found no significant overall association between antidepressant use and congenital malformations, although specific associations were suggested, such as between fluoxetine and nervous system malformations, and SSRIs with respiratory system malformations (Yang et al. 2024). A population-based cohort study in Hong Kong reported no robust association between first-trimester antidepressant exposure and major congenital malformations, but noted increased risks for cardiac and respiratory anomalies, particularly with SSRIs and multiple antidepressant classes (Chan et al. 2024). In a population-based study, Chan et al. analyzed data from 465,069 women in Hong Kong who delivered their first singleton child between 2003 and 2018, focusing on the effects of first-trimester antidepressant use on the risk of congenital malformations. The study found no overall association between major malformations and antidepressant use, with a weighted odds ratio of 0.88, but identified increased risks for specific anomalies, such as cardiac (wOR, 1.82) and respiratory anomalies (wOR, 4.11). The research highlighted that while exposure to SSRIs and multiple antidepressant classes was linked to respiratory and cardiac anomalies, respectively, these associations were not consistently confirmed across sensitivity analyses, indicating a need for further research to clarify the safety of individual antidepressants regarding specific malformations (Chan et al. 2024).

Similarly, a meta-analysis of cohort studies by Lou et al. (2022), which included data from eight different studies that examined the outcomes of infants born to mothers who were exposed to serotonin-norepinephrine reuptake inhibitors (SNRIs) during early pregnancy, found that SNRIs are not significantly associated with an increased risk of overall congenital malformations, but there is a noted increase in cardiac malformations, although this risk is not statistically significant when compared to SSRIs or no exposure with clinical indication (Lou et al. 2022).

Another meta-analysis found that SSRIs and SNRIs were associated with increased odds of congenital heart defects, with specific SSRIs like paroxetine and fluoxetine showing significant associations. In the aforementioned study, a total of 20 distinct investigations were recognized, which collectively encompassed 5,337,223 instances of pregnancies. The odds ratio associated with maternal administration of any antidepressant during the initial trimester of gestation, in relation to the occurrence of congenital heart defects, as determined by random effects meta-analysis, was calculated to be 1.28 (95% confidence interval [CI] 1.17–1.41). Reported significant odds ratios included 1.69 (95% CI 1.37–2.10) for serotonin-norepinephrine reuptake inhibitors (SNRIs) and 1.25 (95% CI 1.15–1.37) for SSRIs, respectively. Conversely, a non-statistically significant odds ratio of 1.02 (95% CI 0.82–1.25) was observed for tricyclic antidepressants. Examination of individual SSRIs yielded significant odds ratios of 1.57 (95% CI 1.25–1.97), 1.36 (95% CI 1.08–1.72), and 1.29 (95% CI 1.14–1.45) for paroxetine, fluoxetine, and sertraline, respectively. Furthermore, the norepinephrine-dopamine reuptake inhibitor bupropion also demonstrated a significant odds ratio of 1.23 (95% CI 1.01–1.49) (Courtney De Vries et al. 2021b). A European register-based study supported the teratogenic effect of SSRIs for certain anomalies, including specific congenital heart defects but cannot exclude confounding by indication or associated factors (Wemakor et al. 2015). However, a systematic review and meta-analysis concluded that while antidepressants were not associated with an increased risk of overall congenital malformations, there was a statistically significant, albeit marginal, increased risk for cardiovascular malformations, particularly with paroxetine (Grigoriadis et al. 2013). These findings suggest that while there is no consensus on a broad teratogenic effect of antidepressants, certain drugs, particularly SSRIs, may pose specific risks, warranting careful consideration of the benefits and risks of antidepressant use during pregnancy. Further research is needed to clarify these associations and the underlying mechanisms (Chan et al. 2024; De Vries et al. 2021b; Grigoriadis et al. 2013; Lou et al. 2022; Wemakor et al. 2015; Yang et al. 2024).

Furthermore, a prospective cohort study in Central China encompassing 5,337,223 pregnancies reported that maternal antidepressant use before and during early pregnancy is associated with a higher risk of CHDs. The odds ratio for maternal use of any antidepressant during the first trimester of pregnancy and the presence of congenital heart defects from the random effects meta-analysis was 1.28 (95% confidence interval [CI] 1.17–1.41), with specific phenotypes such as transposition of the great arteries and ventricular septal defects being more prevalent (Sun et al. 2022). Several studies have shown that sertraline is associated with septal heart malformations, although the risk of more severe heart malformations is not significantly increased. This association may be influenced by confounding factors, such as the underlying depression itself, and should not deter necessary treatment for maternal depression (Kolding et al. 2023). Additionally, research using animal models, such as zebrafish, suggests that serotonin signaling disruption, particularly involving the 5-HT2B receptor, may play a role in cardiac development, further implicating SSRIs in potential cardiac malformations (Kent et al. 2022).

Despite these findings, the overall risk of congenital malformations with SSRIs, including sertraline, remains relatively low, and the benefits of treating maternal depression often outweigh the risks (Desaunay et al. 2023; Nunes et al. 2021). While some studies suggest an increased risk of CHD with antidepressant use before and during early pregnancy, the evidence is not conclusive, and the risk varies depending on the specific antidepressant and timing of exposure (Sun et al. 2022). Therefore, a careful risk-benefit analysis is crucial when considering antidepressant therapy during pregnancy, and ongoing research is needed to better understand the mechanisms and mitigate potential risks associated with these medications (Desaunay et al. 2023; Lou et al. 2022).

Effective communication between healthcare providers and expectant mothers is essential to ensure that mental health concerns are addressed, allowing for informed decisions regarding treatment options while prioritizing both maternal well-being and fetal safety.

6.5.1.2 Preterm Birth

The relationship between antidepressant use during pregnancy and the risk of preterm birth (PTB) is complex and multifaceted, with studies presenting varying results. Several studies indicate that antidepressant use, particularly SSRIs, is associated with an increased risk of PTB. For instance, a systematic review and meta-analysis found that maternal antidepressant use is linked to a significantly increased risk of PTB, especially in women with depression, with SSRIs showing a similar trend (Chang et al. 2020). Another study highlighted that late SSRI exposure during pregnancy is associated with a higher risk of PTB and low birth weight, suggesting that the timing of exposure is crucial and late exposure is more risky (OR = 1.5 to nonexposed group) (Hwang et al. 2023). However, other research suggests that the risk of PTB is more closely related to maternal depression itself rather than antidepressant use. This cohort study analyzed the effects of antidepressant use and maternal depression on the risk of PTB using data from 216,070 deliveries in the UK between January 1996 and February 2019. The study found that exposure to antidepressants, specifically SSRIs, during the first 22 weeks of gestation did not significantly increase the risk of preterm birth (PTB) compared to unexposed patients (HR 1.08, CI [0.98,1.18], $P = 0.11$). Additionally, a history of depression was associated with an increased risk of PTB among untreated patients (HR 1.10, CI [1.04,1.15], $P < 0.01$). Overall, antidepressant treatment does not increase the risk of PTB in pregnant women with depression (Amit et al. 2024). Similarly, another study concluded that antidepressant use alone was not associated with increased odds of spontaneous PTB, although opioid use was (Padilla-Azain et al. 2024). Furthermore, a large cohort study across multiple countries analyzed electronic health record data from over 2.5 million singleton births across the UK, Norway, and Sweden to investigate the impact of maternal antidepressant use during pregnancy on various birth outcomes, including stillbirth, preterm delivery, and low Apgar scores. It was found that maternal antidepressant use during pregnancy is associated with an increased risk of preterm delivery, with an adjusted odds ratio (aOR) of 1.26 (95% CI 1.23 to 1.30), but the absolute risks remained low, and confounding factors such as the severity of depression could not be entirely ruled out (Martin et al. 2023). The decision to use antidepressants during pregnancy should therefore be carefully weighed against the risks of untreated maternal depression, as untreated depression itself is a known risk factor for adverse birth outcomes (Chen et al. 2021; Febrianti 2024). Overall, while there is evidence suggesting an association between antidepressant use and PTB, the potential confounding effects of underlying maternal depression and other factors must be considered in clinical decision-making.

6.5.1.3 Low Birth Weight

Several studies indicate that antidepressant use during pregnancy is associated with an increased risk of low birth weight (LBW) in infants. For instance, a meta-analysis found that children whose mothers used antidepressants during pregnancy had a higher risk of LBW compared to those born to untreated depressed women (Xing et al. 2020) Similarly, another study reported that antidepressant exposure was associated with adverse outcomes at birth, including lower gestational age and preterm birth, although it did not find a direct association with LBW when compared to untreated depression (Fitton et al. 2020). However, the evidence is not entirely consistent. Nevertheless, the data is not completely uniform. Some research indicates that the detected correlations could be influenced by the existing maternal depression instead of the use of antidepressants themselves. For instance, a comprehensive review that evaluated 20 meta-analyses regarding the neonatal outcomes of antidepressants taken during pregnancy pointed out that the likelihood of negative neonatal outcomes, such as low birth weight, may be more linked to maternal depression than to the exposure to antidepressants (Uguz 2021). Additionally, a study focusing on SSRIs found no significant increase in the risk of LBW when comparing exposed and unexposed groups, suggesting that the medication itself might not be the primary factor (Amit et al. 2024).

At this point, it's important to understand the difference between clinical significance and statistical significance. For instance, in the case of LBW that we are currently examining, it has been found that women who continue to use antidepressants during pregnancy have a statistically significantly lower infant birth weight. According to the data from the study, the difference between the two groups is 71.9 grams (Wartko et al. 2021).

Overall, while there is wide evidence linking antidepressant use during pregnancy to LBW; the role of maternal depression as a confounding factor complicates the interpretation of these findings. Further research is needed to disentangle the effects of antidepressants from those of untreated maternal depression to provide clearer guidance for clinical decision-making during pregnancy.

6.5.1.4 Stillbirth

The risk of stillbirth associated with antidepressant use during pregnancy has been a subject of extensive research, with varying conclusions across studies. A systematic review and meta-analysis indicated a small increased risk of stillbirth with antidepressant use during pregnancy, with a summary effect estimate of 1.19, although this finding was likely influenced by confounding factors and the low quality of included studies (Martin et al. 2023). A large cohort study using data from the UK, Norway, and Sweden found that maternal antidepressant use was associated with increased odds of stillbirth (adjusted odds ratio [aOR] 1.16), but the absolute risk remained low, and the association was attenuated when restricted to women with depression or anxiety (Martin et al. 2024). In contrast, a population-based cohort study from Nordic countries found no significant association between SSRI use during pregnancy and stillbirth after adjusting for maternal characteristics and previous psychiatric hospitalization (Stephansson et al. 2013). Similarly, another study using the Danish Fertility Database reported no association between SSRI use and stillbirth across different trimesters of pregnancy (Jimenez-Solem et al. 2013). A systematic review and disproportionality analysis in the WHO Safety Database suggested an increased risk of fetal death, including stillbirth, with antidepressant exposure, particularly SSRIs during the first trimester, but highlighted the need for further research to address potential indication bias (Desaunay et al. 2024). Overall, while some studies suggest a modest association between antidepressant use and stillbirth, the evidence is inconsistent, and confounding factors such as the severity of maternal psychiatric conditions and familial environment may play a significant role. Therefore, the decision to use antidepressants during pregnancy should be individualized, weighing the potential risks against the benefits of treating maternal mental health conditions (Desaunay et al. 2023; Yazıcı and Şahin 2023).

6.5.1.5 Low APGAR Scores

The prevalence of low Apgar scores among newborns whose mothers used antidepressants during pregnancy is notably higher compared to those unexposed. A study analyzing data from the UK, Norway, and Sweden found that maternal antidepressant use was associated with increased odds of a low Apgar score, defined as less than 7 at 5 min post-delivery, with an adjusted odds ratio (aOR) of 1.83 (95% CI 1.75 to 1.91) (Martin et al. 2024). This association was consistent even when accounting for familial and environmental confounding factors, as indicated by a modest association with paternal antidepressant use (Martin et al. 2024). Another study focusing on SSRIs reported that infants exposed to SSRIs in late pregnancy had a higher incidence of delayed neonatal adaptation, which includes low Apgar scores, with a relative risk of 2.52 (95% CI 2.36 to 2.70) compared to unexposed infants (Cornet et al. 2024). Furthermore, a systematic review and meta-analysis confirmed increased risks for low Apgar scores among infants exposed to serotonin-reuptake inhibitors (SRIs) during pregnancy, although the clinical significance of these findings remains debated due to data quality issues (Kautzky et al. 2022). These findings collectively suggest that prenatal exposure to antidepressants, particularly SSRIs and SRIs, is associated with an increased risk of low Apgar scores, although the absolute risk remains relatively low. The studies emphasize the importance of weighing the benefits of treating maternal depression against potential neonatal risks, advocating for the lowest effective dose of antidepressants during pregnancy (Cornet et al. 2024; Kautzky et al. 2022; Martin et al. 2024).

6.5.1.6 Persistent Pulmonary Hypertension of the Neonate (PPHN)

The prevalence of persistent pulmonary hypertension of the neonate (PPHN) in infants exposed to maternal antidepressants during pregnancy is a significant concern, with studies indicating an increased risk associated with SSRIs and other antidepressants. For instance, one study found that 2.7% of infants exposed to SSRIs experienced delayed neonatal adaptation, which includes PPHN as a severe outcome (Cornet et al. 2024). Additionally, a comprehensive analysis of 2,528,916 births revealed that maternal antidepressant use was linked to adverse outcomes, including a higher likelihood of low Apgar scores and stillbirths, although the absolute risks remained low (Martin et al. 2024). Risk factors for PPHN include the type and dosage of antidepressants, as well as maternal health conditions such as pulmonary hypertension, which affects approximately 0.04% of pregnant women and is associated with significantly higher rates of adverse cardiovascular events and maternal mortality (Maligireddy et al. 2024). In research conducted by Garm et al. (2024), a total of 33,776 newborns were examined. Discontinuation of antidepressants during pregnancy was linked to a significantly lower risk of hospitalization in comparison to ongoing exposure to Citalopram throughout the pregnancy. Additionally, halting monotherapy was associated with a significant reduction in the risk of PPHN compared to continued exposure to Citalopram (Gram et al. 2024). In that study, the basis of the decision to continue or discontinue antidepressant medication is not known. Certain female patients might cease pharmacological treatment upon observing alleviation of symptoms, whereas others may persist in their regimen as a preventive measure against recurrence. The clinical significance of the findings and potential influences of confounding variables must be assessed during the decision-making process (Vigod et al. 2024).

6.5.1.7 Neonatal Adaptation Syndrome

Neonatal adaptation syndrome (NAS) is a complex condition that can arise in newborns exposed to certain medications during pregnancy, including antidepressants. It is often referred to as neonatal abstinence syndrome, a condition observed in newborns following in utero exposure to antidepressants, particularly SSRIs and SNRIs. The syndrome is characterized by a range of withdrawal symptoms such as irritability, jitteriness, lethargy, and feeding difficulties, which can vary in severity from mild to severe. Studies have shown that antidepressants like venlafaxine, a common SNRI, can lead to NAS symptoms such as hypothermia and lethargy in neonates, necessitating medical intervention (Oswald et al. 2024). The prevalence and severity of NAS in infants exposed to SSRIs and SNRIs are not routinely screened, which can lead to underdiagnosis and lack of treatment (Arulandoo and Kugathasan 2023). Disproportionality analyses using databases like VigiBase have identified significant reporting odds ratios for neonatal withdrawal syndrome associated with various antidepressants, indicating a moderate signal of risk across different classes, including SSRIs and tricyclic antidepressants (TCAs) (Gastaldon et al. 2023a, b). In a study which compared the Neonatal Abstinence Score (NAS) in neonates exposed to antidepressants in utero with those who were not exposed, a total of 221 women were recruited, with 83 in the exposed group and 138 in the control group. The results indicated that 3% of infants in the exposed group showed severe abstinence symptoms, while 28% exhibited mild abstinence symptoms, compared to 7% in the control group. Additionally, the study found that 10% of infants prenatally exposed to antidepressants experienced neonatal hypoglycemia, in contrast to only 1% in the control group. The findings highlight the importance of informing obstetric and neonatal teams about the mother's medication, as infants may require a review by neonatology after delivery due to potential withdrawal symptoms (Murad 2022). Maternal CYP polymorphisms were investigated to understand variability in NAS symptoms, but no significant association was found, suggesting other factors may contribute to the syndrome's manifestation (Shea et al. 2021). Meta-analyses have identified specific withdrawal signs such as hypoglycemia, tremors, and respiratory distress in neonates exposed to SSRIs and venlafaxine, highlighting the need for careful management of antidepressant use during pregnancy (Wang and Cosci 2021). Comparisons with second-generation antipsychotics (SGAs) show similar rates of poor neonatal adaptation syndrome (PNAS), suggesting a common underlying mechanism for NAS across different psychotropic medications (Viguera et al. 2023). Despite the observed risks, the clinical relevance of these findings remains debated due to variability in study quality and outcomes, claiming the need for more systematic research to guide clinical practice. Prospective cohort studies have confirmed that while severe NAS is relatively rare, mild symptoms are common, and healthcare providers improve multiprofessional counseling in the many women dealing with MDD, perinatal anxiety and stress during pregnancy and the peripartum, and should be prepared to manage these cases effectively (Kautzky et al. 2022). Overall, the evidence suggests that while NAS associated with antidepressant exposure is generally mild and self-limiting, it requires awareness and appropriate management to ensure optimal neonatal outcomes.

6.5.2 Long-Term Outcome of Antidepressant Use During Pregnancy

6.5.2.1 Emotional and Psychiatric Disorders

The effects of maternal antidepressant use during pregnancy on emotional and psychiatric disorders in children are complex and multifaceted, as evidenced by the studies of Bliddal and Koc, among others. Bliddal et al. conducted a comprehensive Danish register study that followed over a million children and found that those exposed to SSRIs in utero had a higher incidence of depressive, anxiety, or adjustment disorders, with an earlier onset compared to unexposed children. However, the study also highlighted that these associations might be influenced by the severity of maternal illness and other confounding factors, as similar risks were observed with paternal SSRI use and maternal use post-pregnancy (Bliddal et al. 2023). Koc et al.'s study, on the other hand, focused on the brain morphologic trajectory and found that prenatal SSRI exposure was associated with changes in brain regions involved in emotional regulation, such as the amygdala and fusiform gyrus, although these changes did not persist into early adolescence (Koc et al. 2023). Other studies, such as those by Lee et al. in a cohort of Taiwan National Health Insurance system between 2004 and 2016 antidepressant-exposed pregnancies and antidepressant-unexposed group (n = 2,245,689) and Suarez et al. in a cohort of 145,702 antidepressant-exposed and 3,032,745 unexposed pregnancies, suggest that while there is an association between prenatal antidepressant exposure and neurodevelopmental disorders like ASD and ADHD, these associations are likely confounded by maternal mental health conditions and genetic factors rather than the medication itself (Lee et al. 2024; Suarez et al. 2022). Furthermore, a systematic review by Rommel et al. indicated that while there are associations with affective disorders, many observed outcomes are driven by the underlying maternal disorder rather than the antidepressant exposure per se (Rommel et al. 2020). Overall, while there is evidence of increased risks of emotional and psychiatric disorders in children exposed to antidepressants in utero, these risks are often intertwined with maternal mental health and other confounding factors, necessitating careful consideration in clinical decision-making.

6.5.2.2 Neurodevelopmental Disorders

The impact of antidepressant use during pregnancy on neurodevelopmental outcomes in children has been extensively studied, with a focus on specific antidepressant types and neurodevelopmental disorders such as autism spectrum disorder (ASD) and attention-deficit/hyperactivity disorder (ADHD). Several studies suggest that while there is an observed association between prenatal antidepressant exposure and increased risks of ASD and ADHD, these associations are often confounded by maternal depression and other genetic and environmental factors rather than the antidepressant use itself. For instance, a study in Taiwan found increased risks of ASD and ADHD with prenatal antidepressant exposure, but these risks were not significant when comparing exposed children to their unexposed siblings, indicating that the association might be due to maternal depression rather than the medication (Lee et al. 2024). Similarly, research in the UK using various causal inference methods found little evidence of a substantial association between continued antidepressant use during pregnancy and neurodevelopmental disorders, although there was some inconsistent evidence regarding the initiation of antidepressants and autism (Heuvelman et al. 2023). A large cohort study in the United States also found no significant association between antidepressant use and neurodevelopmental disorders after adjusting for confounders, suggesting that antidepressant exposure may be a marker for the need for early screening rather than a direct cause of these disorders (Suarez et al. 2022). Furthermore, studies examining specific antidepressants, such as SSRIs, indicate that while SSRIs like fluoxetine and paroxetine may affect neuronal development in vitro, these effects are not necessarily observed in vivo, and the adverse outcomes are more likely linked to maternal depression (Hosseini et al. 2024). In a study of public-school children in Denmark, children (age 7–17) whose mothers used antidepressants during pregnancy had a statistically significant 2-point lower mathematics test score compared to those whose mothers did not. The small magnitude of this difference raises questions about its clinical relevance, necessitating consideration of the benefits of treating maternal depression during pregnancy (Christensen et al. 2021). Overall, the literature suggests that while prenatal antidepressant exposure is associated with some neurodevelopmental deficits, these are largely attenuated or eliminated when accounting for maternal depression and other confounding factors, indicating that antidepressants may not be the direct cause of these outcomes (Andrade 2022). Therefore, the decision to use antidepressants during pregnancy should be carefully considered, weighing the benefits of treating maternal depression against potential risks, with a focus on shared decision-making between the patient and healthcare provider.

6.5.2.3 Cognitive and Motor Development

The impact of maternal antidepressant use during pregnancy on the cognitive and motor development of children is a complex issue with mixed findings across various studies. Research indicates that prenatal exposure to SSRIs like fluoxetine, citalopram, and paroxetine can affect neurodevelopment, although the exact mechanisms and outcomes remain debated. For instance, in vitro studies have shown that fluoxetine and paroxetine can reduce neurite outgrowth and dysregulate genes associated with neuronal development, suggesting potential adverse effects on neural development independent of serotonin transporter activity (Hosseini et al. 2024). Animal studies further support these findings, with maternal fluoxetine exposure impairing synaptic transmission and plasticity in the medial prefrontal cortex of offspring, particularly affecting female mice, which exhibited deteriorated cognitive performance and altered serotonergic neuron structure (Bobula et al. 2024). However, human cohort studies present a more nuanced picture. A 3-D study examined 1489 mother-child pairs, with 61 (4.1%) reporting prenatal antidepressant use. Prenatal exposure correlated negatively with motor development (B = −0.91, 95% CI −1.73, −0.09 for fine motor; B = −0.89, 95% CI −1.81, 0.02 for gross motor), but not with cognitive (B = −0.53, 95% CI −1.82, 0.72) or language (B = 4.13, 95% CI −3.72, 11.89) development. The findings indicate a negative correlation between prenatal antidepressant exposure and motor development at age two, with a minimal effect size of approximately one Bayley Scales of Infant and Toddler Development (BSID-III) point lower on average, even after controlling for maternal distress (Tanguay et al. 2023). Longitudinal studies have also observed changes in brain morphology, such as reduced gray matter and altered amygdala development, in children exposed to SSRIs, although these changes may not persist into adolescence (Knopf 2023; Koc et al. 2023). There is a lack of data about newer antidepressants and their association with neurodevelopment; a study suggests that newer antidepressants like vortioxetine may have some slight adverse effects on neurodevelopment (Ergun et al. 2024). Overall, while there is evidence of potential risks associated with prenatal antidepressant exposure, the findings are inconsistent, and the role of maternal mental health and genetic factors is significant, necessitating further research to clarify these associations.

6.5.3 Maternal Outcomes

The use of antidepressants during pregnancy, delivery, and postpartum can have several side effects on the mother, although these must be weighed against the risks of untreated depression. SSRIs are the most commonly prescribed antidepressants during pregnancy, and their use has been associated with a modestly increased risk of adverse events such as postpartum hemorrhage, miscarriage, preterm birth, and cesarean delivery (Ushkalova and Ushkalova 2023; Smithson and Mitchell 2015). On the other hand, untreated maternal depression poses significant risks, including preeclampsia, poor prenatal care, and increased likelihood of postpartum depression, which can adversely affect maternal-infant bonding and child development

(Dubovicky et al. 2017; Zeszutek 2021). For example, a study evaluated the maternal and neonatal outcomes of 281 pregnant women with depressive disorders, comparing those treated with pharmacotherapy to those who were untreated, against a control group of 200 healthy pregnant women. Results indicated that untreated women experienced higher rates of cesarean sections, preterm deliveries, and lower neonatal weights and APGAR scores, while treated women had a reduced rate of cesarean sections but still exhibited lower APGAR scores. The findings suggest that pharmacological treatment during pregnancy is associated with better outcomes for both mothers and newborns, emphasizing the importance of managing depressive disorders to mitigate complications. The study concludes that untreated depressive disorders lead to poorer pregnancy outcomes compared to those who receive appropriate psychotropic treatment (Parpinel et al. 2022).

6.5.3.1 Postpartum Hemorrhage

The relationship between postpartum hemorrhage (PPH) and antidepressant use, particularly SSRIs, has been a subject of investigation due to the potential for increased bleeding risk associated with these medications. Several studies have identified a correlation between the use of antidepressants during late pregnancy and an elevated risk of PPH. For instance, a systematic review highlighted that antidepressant use in late pregnancy especially for exposures occurring within 30 days of delivery, compared with unexposed deliveries. is associated with an increased risk of PPH, although the causal link remains debated (Bobo et al. 2024). This association is further supported by findings that SSRIs can impair platelet aggregation, thereby increasing the risk of hemorrhage (Salkeld et al. 2008). A cohort study utilizing Medicaid data indicated that PPH prevalence was 2.8% among women with mood/anxiety disorders unexposed to antidepressants, 4.0% among current serotonin reuptake inhibitor users, and 3.8% among current non-serotonin reuptake inhibitor users, revealing a 1.47-fold increased risk of PPH for those exposed to SSRIs near delivery compared to non-exposed individuals, with comparable risks noted for non-serotonin reuptake inhibitors (Palmsten et al. 2013). Such studies necessitate replication while controlling for confounding variables such as obesity, age, and comorbidities. The pharmacological mechanism underlying this increased risk is thought to involve the inhibition of serotonin uptake into platelets, which is crucial for platelet aggregation and vasoconstriction, thus potentially prolonging bleeding times (Heerdink 2013).

6.5.3.2 Eclampsia, Hypertension

The prevalence of eclampsia and hypertension among mothers who used antidepressants during pregnancy is a significant concern, as highlighted by multiple studies. Antidepressant use, particularly SNRIs, has been associated with an increased risk of hypertensive disorders of pregnancy (HDP), including gestational hypertension and preeclampsia. For instance, a study using the EFEMERIS database found that women exposed to SNRIs had a significantly higher risk of HDP compared to those exposed to SSRIs and unexposed women, with adjusted odds ratios indicating a notable increase in risk (Benevent et al. 2023). Similarly, another study reported that SNRI use was independently associated with a higher risk of developing HDP, use of SNRIs (adjusted risk ratio = 9.10, 95% confidence interval = [3.82, 21.67]) and unmedicated depression (adjusted risk ratio = 3.11, 95% confidence interval = [1.32, 7.35]) suggesting a strong link between SNRI use and hypertensive complications during pregnancy (Galbally et al. 2023). Furthermore, a systematic review indicated that antidepressant use during pregnancy, particularly SSRIs and SNRIs, was associated with a moderately increased risk of gestational hypertension and preeclampsia, although the data were not conclusive due to methodological limitations (Uguz 2017). Additionally, a retrospective cohort study found that women who continued antidepressant use beyond 20 weeks of gestation had an increased risk of gestational hypertension, with significant associations observed for SSRIs and prolonged use (Zakiyah et al. 2018). These findings are corroborated by another study that highlighted the increased risk of preeclampsia among women who used antidepressants, especially if the medication was continued after the 16th week of gestation (Bernard et al. 2019). Overall, while the exact prevalence rates of eclampsia and hypertension among antidepressant users during pregnancy are not uniformly reported, the evidence suggests a heightened risk of hypertensive disorders, necessitating careful monitoring and consideration of antidepressant use during pregnancy.

6.6 Review of Risks of Medications

6.6.1 SSRIs

SSRIs are the most commonly prescribed antidepressants during pregnancy due to their extensive study and relatively favorable safety profile, particularly sertraline, which is noted for its low placental transfer and minimal presence in breast milk, making it a preferred choice for nursing mothers (Ushkalova and Ushkalova 2023). However, SSRIs are associated with several adverse outcomes, including preterm birth, low birth weight, and neonatal adaptation issues, such as low Apgar scores and increased neonatal intensive care unit admissions (Cornet et al. 2024; Febrianti 2024; Martin et al. 2024). These risks are not unique to SSRIs, as other antidepressants like duloxetine and mirtazapine also show associations with congenital malformations and similar neonatal outcomes (Febrianti 2024). The potential for delayed neonatal adaptation is particularly noted with SSRIs, with a dose-dependent relationship observed, especially with escitalopram and fluoxetine (Cornet et al. 2024). Long-term outcomes for children exposed to SSRIs in utero include altered brain development trajectories, particularly in regions associated with emotional regulation, although some changes, such as those in the amygdala, may not persist into adolescence (Knopf 2023; Koc et al. 2023). Additionally, prenatal SSRI exposure has been linked to an increased risk of emotional disorders in offspring, although this may be confounded by the severity of maternal depression (Bliddal et al. 2023). Confounding factors, such as maternal depression, can significantly affect the observed associations between SSRI exposure and birth defects. Maternal depression itself is linked to adverse pregnancy outcomes, including preterm birth, low birth weight, and fetal growth restriction, which complicates the isolation of effects solely attributable to antidepressant exposure (Febrianti 2024). The severity of maternal depression, which often necessitates antidepressant use, may independently contribute to these adverse outcomes, suggesting that observed associations might be confounded by the underlying condition rather than the medication itself (Bliddal et al. 2023; Martin et al. 2024). For instance, studies have shown that when restricting analyses to women with depression or anxiety, the association between antidepressant exposure and adverse outcomes like stillbirth attenuates, indicating that the severity of the underlying condition could be a confounding factor (Martin et al. 2024). Additionally, genetic predispositions related to maternal depression, as explored through polygenic scores, suggest that genetic liability may also play a role in these associations, although this relationship is not straightforward (Rommel et al. 2024). Furthermore, the timing of antidepressant exposure during pregnancy, such as early versus late exposure, can influence outcomes like preterm birth and low birth weight, which may reflect confounding by the progression and management of maternal depression (Hwang et al. 2023). The potential for confounding by indication is also highlighted in studies that show associations between paternal antidepressant use and adverse outcomes, suggesting that familial or environmental factors could contribute to the observed risks (Martin et al. 2024) (Bliddal et al. 2023). Overall, while sertraline and other SSRIs have been associated with specific congenital malformations, such as septal heart defects, these associations may be influenced by systematic errors and confounding factors, including the severity of maternal depression and genetic predispositions, necessitating careful consideration in clinical decision-making (Kolding et al. 2023).

6.6.1.1 Sertraline

Sertraline, a commonly prescribed SSRI during pregnancy, presents unique side effects compared to other SSRIs, particularly concerning fetal cardiac health. Studies have shown that sertraline is associated with an increased risk of septal heart malformations, such as atrial and ventricular septal defects, although it is not linked to more severe cardiac malformations (Kolding et al. 2023; Shen et al. 2017). This association may be influenced by confounding factors, but it remains a consideration for pregnant women undergoing treatment for depression. Additionally, sertraline exposure during pregnancy has been linked to congenital cardiovascular disorders, with data from the FDA Adverse Event Reporting System highlighting heart disease congenital and patent ductus arteriosus as common outcomes Beyond cardiac concerns, sertraline has been implicated in other adverse pregnancy outcomes, such as low birth weight, preterm birth, and intrauterine growth restriction, likely due to its impact on serotonin homeostasis and placental blood perfusion. Maternal SSRI usage elevates serotonin levels in both mother and fetus. This elevation may induce vasoconstriction in uterine and placental vessels, thereby diminishing blood flow to the uterus, placenta, and fetus, potentially affecting placental functionality and fetal growth (Domingues et al. 2023).

Animal studies further suggest that sertraline can be teratogenic, causing skeletal abnormalities and cleft palate in mice, although these findings are not directly translatable to humans (Cabrera et al. 2020). Moreover, sertraline use during the peripartum period has been associated with increased pup mortality and altered calcium metabolism in animal models, indicating potential risks to both the mother and offspring (Sheftel et al. 2020). Despite these risks, sertraline is often preferred over other SSRIs like paroxetine, which has a stronger association with fetal cardiovascular defects (Desaunay et al. 2023). Overall, while sertraline is a viable option for managing depression during pregnancy, its use requires careful consideration of potential fetal risks, particularly concerning cardiac and developmental outcomes.

6.6.1.2 Paroxetine

Paroxetine, an SSRI, exhibits unique side effects compared to other SSRIs, particularly when used during pregnancy. One of the most significant concerns associated with paroxetine is its potential to increase the risk of cardiac malformations in infants when used during the first trimester. Studies have shown that paroxetine exposure is linked to a higher incidence of major congenital malformations, including cardiac defects such as bulbus cordis anomalies, anomalies of cardiac septal closure, atrial septal defects, and right ventricular outflow tract defects (Bérard et al. 2016).

Paroxetine exposure during pregnancy has been associated with an increased risk of birth defects, particularly cardiac malformations. Several studies and meta-analyses have consistently reported this association. For instance, a systematic review and meta-analysis found that first-trimester exposure to paroxetine was linked to an increased risk of major congenital malformations, including cardiac defects, with a pooled odds ratio (OR) of 1.23 for any major malformations and 1.28 for major cardiac malformations. In a study by Yan Gao et al., 29 cohort studies involving over 9 million births were analyzed. SSRIs were linked to a heightened risk of major congenital anomalies (MCAs, RR 1.11, 95% CI 1.03 to 1.19) and congenital heart defects (CHD, RR 1.24, 95% CI 1.11 to 1.37). No significant risk increase was found in women with psychiatric diagnoses (MCAs, RR 1.04, 95% CI 0.95 to 1.13; CHD, RR 1.06, 95% CI 0.90 to 1.26). Significant associations were noted with maternal citalopram (MCAs, RR 1.20, 95% CI 1.09 to 1.31; CHD, RR 1.24, 95% CI 1.02 to 1.51), fluoxetine (MCAs, RR 1.17, 95% CI 1.07 to 1.28; CHD, RR 1.30, 95% CI 1.12 to 1.53), and paroxetine (MCAs, RR 1.18, 95% CI 1.05 to 1.32; CHD, RR 1.17, 95% CI 0.97 to 1.41), with analyses in psychiatric populations yielding no statistically significant results (Gao et al. 2018).

In addition to congenital malformations, research findings have indicated that exposure to paroxetine is correlated with particular cardiac anomalies, including bulbus cordis anomalies and defects in cardiac septal closure, with an odds ratio (OR) of 1.42, as well as atrial septal defects, which exhibit an OR of 2.38 (Bérard et al. 2016). Similarly, a meta-analysis reported significant odds ratios for paroxetine, indicating an increased risk of congenital heart defects, with an OR of 1.57 (Courtney De Vries et al. 2021a). The FDA issued a warning in 2005 about the increased risk of cardiac malformations with paroxetine. According to subsequent meta-analyses and systematic reviews; compared to other SSRIs, paroxetine has been consistently associated with a higher risk of these specific cardiac anomalies, although the absolute risk remains relatively small (Alwan et al. 2016; Gao et al. 2018; Wemakor et al. 2015). Additionally, paroxetine, like other SSRIs, is associated with other adverse pregnancy outcomes such as preterm birth, low birth weight, and potential neurodevelopmental disorders in children (Domingues et al. 2023). However, the risk of cardiac malformations appears to be more pronounced with paroxetine than with other SSRIs, such as fluoxetine or sertraline, which have been linked to different types of congenital anomalies (Gao et al. 2018; Wemakor et al. 2015). The decision to use paroxetine during pregnancy should involve a careful consideration of the risks and benefits, taking into account the potential for untreated maternal depression to also adversely affect pregnancy outcomes. Therefore, healthcare providers often recommend alternative treatments or additional prenatal monitoring for women who require antidepressant therapy during pregnancy.

6.6.1.3 Fluoxetine

Fluoxetine, a widely prescribed SSRI, exhibits unique side effects compared to other SSRIs, particularly when used during pregnancy. One notable concern is its impact on fetal development. Thus, in a population-based case-malformed control study conducted in 12 EUROCAT CA registries covering 2.1 million births, fluoxetine exposure has been associated with congenital anomalies, including cardiac defects such as Tetralogy of Fallot and Ebstein's anomaly, as well as non-cardiac anomalies like ano-rectal atresia and renal dysplasia (Wemakor et al. 2015). Such risks haven't been replicated in new studies and confounding factors are limiting the study's results but additionally, fluoxetine has been linked to neurodevelopmental disorders, including an increased risk of autism spectrum disorders in offspring, potentially due to serotonergic dysregulation during critical periods of brain development (Maloney et al. 2017). Furthermore, fluoxetine exposure during pregnancy can impair synaptic transmission and plasticity in the offspring's medial prefrontal cortex, leading to cognitive and affective disorders, with a distinct sex-dependent sensitivity observed in female offspring (Bobula et al. 2024). In terms of physical development, fluoxetine has been shown to compromise bone health in neonates, resulting in reduced bone mineral density and shorter femurs (Weaver et al. 2019).

Research indicates that SSRIs, including fluoxetine, are associated with delayed neonatal adaptation, which manifests as low Apgar scores, the need for resuscitation at birth, or admission to neonatal intensive care units for respiratory support. This risk is dose-dependent and particularly pronounced with fluoxetine and escitalopram, suggesting a causal relationship between SSRI exposure and neonatal adaptation issues (Cornet et al. 2024). Additionally, prenatal SSRI exposure has been linked to changes in brain morphology, such as reduced cerebral gray matter and altered amygdala volume, although some of these changes may not persist into adolescence (Koc et al. 2023). The increase in maternal and fetal serotonin levels due to SSRI use can lead to vasoconstriction in the uterine and placental vascular beds, potentially reducing blood perfusion and impacting fetal development, resulting in outcomes like low birthweight and preterm birth (Domingues et al. 2023).

Specifically, fluoxetine has been shown to reduce placentome growth and gestation length, leading to decreased birthweight and neonatal acidemia in animal models, which suggests intrauterine growth restriction (Domingues et al. 2022). Furthermore, SSRI exposure is associated with increased risks of preterm birth and neonatal respiratory distress, with these risks escalating with higher doses (Bandoli et al. 2020). Placental histopathology studies have also found that SSRI use correlates with fetal vascular malperfusion lesions, which are linked to adverse neonatal outcomes (Levy et al. 2020). Despite these risks, the teratogenic potential of SSRIs is considered low, and the decision to use these medications during pregnancy should be individualized, balancing the benefits of treating maternal depression against potential neonatal risks. Overall, while SSRIs, including fluoxetine, are commonly prescribed during pregnancy, their use requires careful consideration of the potential impacts on fetal and neonatal health.

6.6.1.4 Escitalopram and Citalopram

Escitalopram, an SSRI, presents specific risks during pregnancy that may differ from other SSRIs in terms of fetal exposure and neonatal outcomes. Studies have shown that SSRI use, including escitalopram, is associated with delayed neonatal adaptation, which encompasses symptoms such as low Apgar scores, respiratory distress, and the need for neonatal intensive care unit (NICU) admission. Escitalopram, along with fluoxetine, has been identified as having a higher risk for these outcomes compared to other SSRIs, suggesting a type and dose-dependent relationship with delayed neonatal adaptation (Cornet et al. 2024). Additionally, escitalopram exposure during pregnancy has been linked to increased rates of neonatal adaptation syndrome and NICU admissions, with these risks being particularly pronounced when exposure occurs in the third trimester (Marks et al. 2020). While SSRIs in general are associated with adverse neonatal outcomes such as preterm birth and low birth weight, the specific risks associated with escitalopram may be more pronounced due to its pharmacokinetic properties and placental transfer rates (Febrianti 2024; Hwang et al. 2023). Furthermore, the potential for fetal death, including stillbirth, has been associated with SSRI exposure, although escitalopram is not specifically highlighted in this context, indicating a need for further research to delineate its unique risks (Desaunay et al. 2024). Despite these concerns, it is crucial to balance the risks of escitalopram use against the potential consequences of untreated maternal depression, which can also lead to adverse outcomes such as preterm birth and low birth weight (Zeszutek 2021). Overall, while escitalopram shares some common risks with other SSRIs, its association with delayed neonatal adaptation and NICU admissions suggests it may pose distinct challenges in managing depression during pregnancy.

6.6.1.5 Fluvoxamine

Fetal exposure to fluvoxamine, an SSRI, has been studied to assess its impact on neonatal outcomes. Research indicates that fluvoxamine, like other SSRIs, can cross the placental barrier, potentially affecting fetal development. In animal studies, neonatal administration of fluvoxamine in rats led to increased lethality, reduced body weight, and delayed motor reflex maturation, suggesting that early exposure can alter the serotoninergic system and delay physical and motor development (Glazova et al. 2014). In human studies, fluvoxamine exposure during pregnancy has been associated with poor neonatal adaptation (PNA), a condition characterized by symptoms such as respiratory distress, jitteriness, and feeding difficulties, which occur in approximately 20–30% of infants exposed to SSRIs in utero (Kieviet et al. 2015). However, a prospective study comparing fluvoxamine-exposed pregnancies to those exposed to other SSRIs and non-teratogenic agents found no significant increase in major congenital malformations or adverse neonatal outcomes, such as miscarriage or prematurity, suggesting that fluvoxamine does not pose a higher teratogenic risk than other SSRIs (Einarson et al. 2009; Sivojelezova 2004). Additionally, while some studies have reported increased risks of delayed neonatal adaptation with SSRI exposure, these findings are often dose-dependent and vary with the type of SSRI used, with fluvoxamine not being specifically highlighted as having a higher risk compared to others like escitalopram and fluoxetine (Cornet et al. 2024). Overall, while fluvoxamine exposure during pregnancy is associated with certain risks, these are generally consistent with those observed for other SSRIs, and careful consideration of the benefits and risks is essential when prescribing fluvoxamine to pregnant women.

6.6.2 SNRIs

The comparative efficacy of SNRIs during pregnancy, particularly concerning fetal, neonatal, and maternal outcomes, reveals a complex risk-benefit profile when compared to other antidepressant classes such SSRIs. SNRIs have been associated with an increased risk of hypertensive disorders of pregnancy (HDP), including gestational hypertension and preeclampsia, with studies indicating a significantly higher risk compared to SSRIs and unexposed groups. In recent research conducted by Benevent et al., out of a total of 156,133 pregnancies, a cohort of 143,391 was incorporated into the study population, which comprised 210 (0.1%) individuals in the SNRI category, 1316 (0.9%) individuals in the SSRI category, and 141,865 (98.9%) individuals in the unexposed category. Following the adjustment for the severity of depression and additional mental health conditions, the incidence of hypertensive disorders of pregnancy (HDP) was markedly elevated among women who were exposed to SNRIs (n = 20; 9.5%) in comparison to those who were exposed to SSRIs (n = 72; 5.5%; adjusted odds ratio [aOR] [95% CI] = 2.32 [1.28–4.20]) and to women who were not exposed (n = 6224; 4.4%; aOR [95% CI] = 1.89 [1.13–3.18]) (Benevent et al. 2023). In terms of fetal and neonatal outcomes, both SNRIs and SSRIs have been linked to transient neonatal behavioral changes, such as poor neonatal adaptation and an increased rate of persistent pulmonary hypertension of the newborn (PPHN), although the absolute risk remains low (Nörby et al. 2016; Ornoy and Koren 2019). The potential for congenital malformations, particularly cardiac anomalies, has been noted, albeit with a small increased risk, and these risks are similar across different antidepressant classes (Goracci et al. 2015; Ornoy and

Koren 2017). Furthermore, untreated maternal depression itself poses significant risks, including adverse effects on child development and increased maternal morbidity, which necessitates a careful evaluation of the risks associated with discontinuing antidepressant treatment during pregnancy (Desaunay et al. 2023). The decision to use SNRIs or other antidepressants during pregnancy should therefore be guided by a thorough assessment of the maternal benefits against the potential fetal and neonatal risks, with a focus on maintaining the minimal effective dose to mitigate adverse outcomes. Overall, while SNRIs present certain risks, particularly concerning maternal hypertension, the broader context of maternal mental health and the potential consequences of untreated depression must be considered in clinical decision-making.

6.6.2.1 Duloxetine

Duloxetine, an SNRI, is one of the antidepressants used during pregnancy. Studies have shown that duloxetine exposure is associated with an increased risk of preterm birth, although the risk of being born small for gestational age is not significantly elevated compared to other antidepressants like SSRIs and venlafaxine (Ankarfeldt et al. 2023; Huybrechts et al. 2020). Additionally, duloxetine has been linked to congenital malformations, although the evidence is not consistent across all studies, and the risk is not significantly higher than that associated with other antidepressants (Febrianti 2024). A cohort study utilizing data from Sweden and Denmark encompassed over 2 million births, with 1512 instances of duloxetine exposure and compared with duloxetine-nonexposed groups, which yielded an odds ratio (OR) of 0.98 (95% confidence interval [CI] 0.74 to 1.30, $p = 0.909$) concerning major malformations, an OR of 1.09 (95% CI 0.82 to 1.45, $p = 0.570$) for minor malformations, and an OR of 1.18 (95% CI 0.43 to 3.19, $p = 0.749$) relating to stillbirths. In terms of the individual subtypes of malformations, certain findings reached statistical significance; however, these were accompanied by considerable statistical uncertainty attributable to the exceedingly limited number of occurrences. The principal limitations of a study stemmed from the unavailability of data regarding the indication for duloxetine, as well as the lack of a direct assessment of depression severity, which could not be incorporated as covariates (Ankarfeldt et al. 2021a, b). Notably, duloxetine-exposed infants have higher rates of neonatal intensive care unit (NICU) admissions and adaptation syndromes compared to those exposed to other antidepressants, such as escitalopram (Marks et al. 2020). Furthermore, duloxetine exposure during pregnancy has been associated with an increased risk of postpartum hemorrhage and a potential, albeit small, increased risk of cardiac malformations (Huybrechts et al. 2020). While duloxetine does not appear to significantly increase the risk of spontaneous or elective abortions compared to SSRIs, it does show a higher risk of elective abortions when compared to non-exposed groups but confounders still need to be clarified (Ankarfeldt et al. 2021a, b). These findings highlight the importance of carefully weighing the benefits of treating maternal depression with duloxetine against the potential risks to the fetus and neonate, considering the specific adverse outcomes associated with this medication compared to other antidepressants.

6.6.2.2 Venlafaxine

Comparative studies investigating fetal exposure risks of venlafaxine versus other antidepressants have yielded varied results, highlighting both potential risks and the need for further research. Venlafaxine, an SNRI, has been associated with increased risks of fetal cardiac anomalies in animal studies, suggesting alterations in serotonin signaling as a potential mechanism (Laurent et al. 2016). However, human studies present a more nuanced picture. Venlafaxine has been associated with a higher incidence of specific birth defects, such as anencephaly and craniorachischisis, with adjusted odds ratios indicating significant risk even after accounting for underlying maternal conditions (Anderson et al. 2020). Furthermore, venlafaxine exposure has been associated with respiratory defects in human studies, highlighting its potential impact on fetal development (Bérard et al. 2017, 2019).

Lassen et al. conducted a systematic analysis encompassing eight cohort studies that elucidate the outcomes associated with in utero exposure to venlafaxine or duloxetine during the first trimester. The aggregated data pertaining to venlafaxine included 3186 exposed infants and 107 instances of major malformations, culminating in a relative risk estimate and a 95% confidence interval of 1.12 (0.92–1.35). In contrast, the relevant data for duloxetine comprised 668 infants and 16 major malformations, yielding a relative risk estimate and a 95% confidence interval of 0.80 (0.46–1.29). The findings indicate that first-trimester in utero exposure to venlafaxine is not correlated with an elevated risk of major congenital malformations. Although the volume of data concerning duloxetine is considerably smaller, it does not imply a clinically significant increase in risk (Lassen et al. 2016). Similarly, a large Nordic cohort study found no substantial increase in overall cardiac birth defects among infants exposed to venlafaxine or SSRIs, although there was a noted increase in specific defects like septal and right ventricular outflow tract defects, which were not supported by sibling-controlled analyses, suggesting potential confounding factors rather than a direct teratogenic effect (Furu et al. 2015) Compared to other antidepressants, venlafaxine-exposed infants also showed higher rates of transient tachypnea of the newborn (TTN) (Marks et al. 2020). The WHO Safety Database analysis also identified venlafaxine among antidepressants associated with fetal death, particularly when exposure occurs during the first trimester, indicating a need for cautious use during early pregnancy (Desaunay et al. 2024). Despite these findings, the literature suggests that the benefits of treating maternal depression with antidepressants, including venlafaxine, may outweigh potential risks, especially considering the adverse effects of untreated maternal depression on fetal development.

Maternal hypertensive disorders during pregnancy, such as gestational hypertension and pre-eclampsia, have been associated with adverse fetal outcomes, and the use of antidepressants, including venlafaxine, may further complicate these risks. Venlafaxine, an SNRI, has been linked to an increased risk of hypertensive disorders of pregnancy (HDP) compared to SSRIs and non-exposure to antidepressants, with adjusted odds ratios indicating a significantly higher risk of HDP in women treated with SNRIs (Benevent et al. 2023). This increased risk of HDP is concerning given that hypertensive disorders are associated with adverse neonatal outcomes such as preterm birth and small-for-gestational-age infants (Gallitelli et al. 2024).

Overall, while venlafaxine does not appear to significantly increase the risk of major congenital malformations compared to other antidepressants, the evidence suggests that venlafaxine may pose specific risks during pregnancy, particularly concerning cardiac and respiratory outcomes, the potential for specific cardiac defects and the impact of confounding factors necessitate careful consideration and further research to clarify these associations (Furu et al. 2015; Lassen et al. 2016).

6.6.3 TCAs

The comparative analysis of tricyclic antidepressants (TCAs) versus other antidepressants during pregnancy reveals nuanced outcomes for fetal, neonatal, maternal, and long-term effects. A systematic review analyzed a total of 16 studies encompassing 4,564,798 pregnancy outcomes. The mixed-methods meta-analysis revealed an odds ratio of 1.22 (95% CI: 1.11 to 1.33) for maternal antidepressant use and congenital heart defects. Class-specific analyses indicated an odds ratio of 1.50 (95% CI: 1.19 to 1.89) for first-trimester SNRI use and congenital heart defects, while SSRIs showed a significant odds ratio of 1.22 (95% CI: 1.12 to 1.33); no increased odds ratio was observed for TCAs. Individual antidepressants demonstrated significant odds ratios of 1.53 (95% CI: 1.25 to 1.88) for paroxetine, 1.28 (95% CI: 1.01 to 1.62) for fluoxetine, 1.28 (95% CI: 1.14 to 1.45) for sertraline, and 1.23 (95% CI: 1.01 to 1.50) for bupropion (De Vries et al. 2020). However, the use of antidepressants, including TCAs, during pregnancy is associated with increased risks of preterm birth, low birth weight, and neonatal adaptation syndromes, although these risks are often confounded by the underlying maternal psychiatric conditions (Marks et al. 2020; Martin et al. 2024; Uguz 2021). Specifically, maternal antidepressant use is linked to adverse neonatal outcomes such as preterm delivery and low Apgar scores, with TCAs like amitriptyline showing fewer associations with these outcomes compared to other antidepressants (Martin et al. 2024).

Long-term outcomes for children exposed to antidepressants in utero, including TCAs, suggest associations with affective disorders but not consistently with neurodevelopmental or other psychiatric disorders, indicating that many observed effects may be attributed to the underlying maternal condition rather than the medication itself (Rommel et al. 2020). Furthermore, while antidepressant use is associated with increased risks of adverse outcomes, these risks are often comparable to those in untreated depression, suggesting that the decision to continue medication should be individualized (Mitchell and Goodman 2018). Overall, while TCAs may present a lower risk for certain congenital anomalies compared to SSRIs and SNRIs, the broader implications of antidepressant use during pregnancy necessitate careful consideration of both maternal and fetal health outcomes.

6.6.4 Atypical/Other Antidepressants

6.6.4.1 Vortioxetine

The available literature does not provide evidence of a cohort study specifically focused on vortioxetine use during pregnancy. However, there are case studies and series that offer some insights into the effects of vortioxetine during pregnancy. A case study from Japan highlighted that vortioxetine exposure during pregnancy could lead to severe neonatal asphyxia, although the drug's transfer into breast milk was minimal, suggesting limited neonatal exposure and no adverse developmental effects in the infant (Kiribayashi et al. 2024). In animal studies, prenatal and lactational exposure to vortioxetine resulted in increased motor activity and anxiety in offspring, indicating potential neurodevelopmental risks, although emotional learning and memory were unaffected (Ergun et al. 2024). Another study from the Israeli Teratology Information Service documented outcomes of 19 pregnancies with first-trimester exposure to vortioxetine, resulting in 12 live births without malformations, alongside some adverse outcomes like miscarriages and stillbirths, though these were not conclusively linked to vortioxetine alone. However, the limited data on vortioxetine, especially from small sample sizes, necessitates further research to fully understand its safety profile during pregnancy (Shweiki and Diav-Citrin 2021).

Vortioxetine's adverse effects, such as gastrointestinal issues and mood-related symptoms, are similar to those of SSRIs, but it also has unique unlisted adverse reactions like hyperprolactinemia and edema (Ekhart et al. 2022; Verma and Kumar 2021). Overall, while vortioxetine shares some risks with SSRIs, its unique pharmacological profile and adverse effects warrant careful consideration and further investigation to ensure maternal and neonatal safety (Gastaldon et al. 2023a, b).

6.6.4.2 Bupropion

Bupropion, a norepinephrine-dopamine reuptake inhibitor, presents distinct risks during pregnancy compared to other antidepressants, particularly concerning fetal exposure and neonatal outcomes. Unlike SSRIs and SNRIs, which are commonly associated with PNAS and withdrawal symptoms, bupropion does not show a significant association with neonatal withdrawal syndrome, as evidenced by a pharmacovigilance study that found no disproportionate reporting for bupropion compared to other antidepressants (Gastaldon et al. 2023a, b). However, there are concerns regarding bupropion's potential to increase the risk of cardiac malformations, as suggested by data from a bupropion pregnancy registry (The Medical Letter 2024).

A retrospective cohort study which assessed 2741 pregnant women and focused on five specific antidepressants (bupropion, citalopram, escitalopram, fluoxetine, sertraline) reported that women continuously prescribed antidepressants throughout pregnancy had lower NICU admissions if they lacked third trimester exposure to bupropion (aOR 0.43, 95% CI 0.21–0.90) or escitalopram (aOR 0.49, 95% CI 0.28–0.85). Those previously on escitalopram without third-trimester exposure exhibited decreased odds of adaptation syndrome (aOR 0.19, 95% CI 0.07–0.48). No significant differences were observed in other outcomes for women on different antidepressants or for those with no early pregnancy drug exposure versus continuous exposure (Tharp et al. 2022). Furthermore, when bupropion is used in combination with serotonergic drugs, there is a potential risk of serotonin syndrome, which can lead to severe neonatal outcomes such as encephalopathy and abnormal movements, highlighting the importance of monitoring maternal medication lists during pregnancy (Brajcich et al. 2021). Overall, while bupropion may have a lower risk of certain neonatal adaptation issues compared to SSRIs and SNRIs, its potential association with cardiac malformations and the risks associated with polypharmacy necessitate careful consideration and monitoring during pregnancy.

6.6.4.3 Mirtazapine

The use of mirtazapine during pregnancy presents several considerations regarding fetal safety and pregnancy outcomes. A nationwide cohort study in Denmark found no significant association between mirtazapine exposure and major congenital malformations, spontaneous abortion, stillbirth, or neonatal death, suggesting that mirtazapine may not increase these risks compared to unexposed pregnancies (Ostenfeld et al. 2022). A study reviewed 41 observational studies over the data of 2343 mirtazapine exposed pregnancies and concluded that mirtazapine may share some risks common to antidepressants, such as congenital malformations; the evidence is not consistent across all studies (Ostenfeld et al. 2025). Additionally, mirtazapine's impact on the offspring's brain function and behavior has been studied in animal models, where it was found to have anxiolytic effects and influence neuroplasticity, potentially mitigating some negative effects of maternal stress and depression (Dubiel-Hoppanova et al. 2025). Unlike SSRIs, which have been associated with increased risks of neonatal seizures and other adaptation syndromes, mirtazapine does not appear to significantly increase the risk of neonatal seizures or adaptation syndromes, as indicated by studies comparing various antidepressants (Martin et al. 2024; Uguz 2019). Furthermore, mirtazapine was not associated with increased risks of preterm delivery or low Apgar scores, which are concerns with other antidepressants (Martin et al. 2024).

Overall, Mirtazapine has emerged as a promising treatment for hyperemesis gravidarum (HG), particularly in cases resistant to conventional therapies. Studies and case reports indicate that mirtazapine can significantly reduce symptoms of HG scores and improve overall maternal health outcomes (Galletta et al. 2022).

6.7 Statistical Significance Versus Clinical Significance

The distinction between clinical significance and statistical significance in the context of antidepressant use during pregnancy is crucial for understanding the implications of research findings. Statistical significance refers to the likelihood that a result is not due to chance, often determined by p-values or confidence intervals. For instance, studies have shown that antidepressant use during pregnancy is statistically associated with increased risks of preterm birth and congenital malformations, with specific hazard ratios and confidence intervals indicating these associations are unlikely to be due to random variation (Martin et al. 2024). However, clinical significance considers whether these statistically significant findings have meaningful implications for patient care. As another example in a study, from the Danish national registers involving 21,785 children born to 13,941 mothers by Rommel et al., the impact of intrauterine exposure to antidepressants on birth outcomes, specifically gestational age and birthweight, while considering genetic liability to maternal major depression was investigated. The antidepressant continuation group had significantly reduced mean gestational ages (adjusted β ranges: 1.7–4.5 days, $p < 0.001$–0.008) and lower mean birthweights (adjusted β ranges: 58.6–165.4 g, $p = 0.001$–0.008) than the discontinuation and unexposed groups. The difference between groups was 1.7–4.5 days as gestational age and 58.6–165.4 grams as weight (Rommel et al. 2024).

Thus, while statistical significance provides a foundation for understanding potential risks, clinical significance guides practical decision-making in managing depression during pregnancy.

6.8 Conclusion

Table 6.1 shows expert recommendations based on scientific evidence and clinical experience). This chapter can be summarized as follows:

Importance of Mental Health Maternal mental health during pregnancy is a critical factor for both maternal and fetal well-being, and managing depression and anxiety should be prioritized to prevent long-term complications.

Table 6.1 Expert recommendations based on scientific evidence and clinical experience

Prioritize managing maternal depression and anxiety during pregnancy to enhance both maternal and fetal well-being
Stay updated with clinical guidelines and research to ascertain the safest use of SSRIs and other antidepressants during pregnancy, especially concerning congenital malformations.
Tailor antidepressant treatment plans to the specific trimester of pregnancy to mitigate associated risks
Adjust antidepressant dosages carefully during pregnancy to account for physiological changes that affect drug metabolism
Emphasize the benefits of treating maternal depression, such as preventing relapse and promoting better overall maternal health
Assess both statistical and clinical significance when considering the use of antidepressants to ensure the benefits outweigh potential risks
Develop individualized treatment plans that consider the severity of the mother's depression and the safety of the fetus
Involve a multidisciplinary team, including obstetricians, psychiatrists, and pediatricians, in the management of pregnancies exposed to antidepressants
Remain vigilant about potential neonatal risks from antidepressant use, such as adaptation issues and long-term developmental challenges
Emphasize shared decision-making between the patient and healthcare providers to ensure that treatment decisions align with the patient's values and preferences

Risks of Untreated Depression Untreated depression during pregnancy can lead to significant risks, including preterm birth, low birth weight, fetal growth restriction, miscarriage, macrosomia, preeclampsia, poor prenatal care, and long-term developmental challenges in the child, such as cognitive, behavioral, and emotional disorders, attention-deficit/hyperactivity disorder, and delayed socioemotional and linguistic development.

SSRIs and Birth Defects SSRIs are associated with an increased risk of congenital malformations, particularly cardiac defects, which necessitates further research to determine safe usage during pregnancy.

Neonatal Risks The use of SSRIs and other antidepressants during pregnancy can lead to potential risks, including congenital malformations, preterm birth, low birth weight, neonatal adaptation issues, and long-term developmental challenges in the child, such as cognitive, behavioral, and emotional disorders, while untreated maternal depression itself poses additional risks like miscarriage, fetal growth restriction, and developmental delays.

Role of Timing in Exposure The timing of antidepressant exposure during pregnancy (first, second, or third trimester) plays a notable role in determining the associated risks, highlighting the need for tailored treatment plans.

Pharmacokinetic Changes in Pregnancy Pregnancy-induced physiological changes, including altered metabolism and hormone levels, affect how antidepressants are absorbed and metabolized, requiring careful dose adjustments.

Benefits of Treating Maternal Depression The benefits of treating maternal depression during pregnancy, such as preventing relapse and promoting better overall health, outweigh the risks of medication when managed properly.

Confounding Factors in Research The relationship between antidepressant use and adverse outcomes is often confounded by maternal depression itself, making it challenging to isolate the effects of medications from the impact of untreated depression.

Statistical Significance Versus Clinical Significance Statistically significant associations with outcomes like preterm birth and congenital malformations do not always translate into clinically significant impacts, as the actual risks to maternal and fetal health may be small and context-dependent. Therefore, healthcare providers must consider both statistical and clinical significance when making treatment decisions, ensuring that the benefits of medication outweigh the potential risks to both the mother and child.

Careful Medication Management The decision to use antidepressants during pregnancy must be carefully considered, taking into account both the benefits of treating maternal depression and the potential risks to fetal-maternal health.

Individualized Treatment Plans There is no one-size-fits-all approach to antidepressant use during pregnancy. Each treatment plan should be personalized, considering the severity of maternal depression, the type of antidepressant, and fetal safety.

Multidisciplinary Approach The management of a pregnancy with exposure to antidepressants should involve a multidisciplinary team, including obstetricians, psychiatrists, and pediatricians, to ensure the best outcomes for both the mother and child.

Need for Ongoing Research Continued research is essential to refine our understanding of the risks and benefits of antidepressant use during pregnancy, ensuring that healthcare providers can make informed decisions based on the latest evidence.

References

Adina J, Morawska A, Mitchell AE, Haslam D, Ayuku D. Depression and anxiety in second and third trimesters among pregnant women in Kenya: a hospital-based prevalence study. J Affect Disord Rep. 2022;10:100447.

Alwan S, Friedman JM, Chambers C. Safety of selective serotonin reuptake inhibitors in pregnancy: a review of current evidence. CNS Drugs. 2016;30(6):499–515. https://doi.org/10.1007/s40263-016-0338-3.

Amit G, Yanover C, Bivas-Benita M, Girshovitz I, Helbitz T, Sudry T, et al. Antidepressant use during pregnancy and the risk of preterm birth – a cohort study. NPJ Women's Health. 2024;2(1):5. https://doi.org/10.1038/s44294-024-00008-0.

Anderson KN, Lind JN, Simeone RM, Bobo WV, Mitchell AA, Riehle-Colarusso T, et al. Maternal use of specific antidepressant medications during early pregnancy and the risk of selected birth defects. JAMA Psychiatry. 2020;77(12):1246–55.

Andrade C. Gestational exposure to antidepressant drugs and neurodevelopment: an examination of language, mathematics, intelligence, and other cognitive outcomes. J Clin Psychiatry. 2022;83(1) https://doi.org/10.4088/JCP.22f14388.

Ankarfeldt MZ, Petersen J, Andersen JT, Fernandes MFS, Li H, Motsko SP, et al. Duloxetine exposure during pregnancy and the risk of spontaneous and elective abortion: a Danish Nationwide observational study. Drugs Real World Outcomes. 2021a;8(3):289–99. https://doi.org/10.1007/s40801-021-00252-9.

Ankarfeldt MZ, Petersen J, Andersen JT, Li H, Motsko SP, Fast T, et al. Exposure to duloxetine during pregnancy and risk of congenital malformations and stillbirth: a nationwide cohort study in Denmark and Sweden. PLoS Med. 2021b;18(11):e1003851.

Ankarfeldt MZ, Petersen J, Andersen JT, Fernandes MFS, Li H, Motsko SP, et al. Duloxetine exposure during pregnancy and the risk of offspring being born small for gestational age or prematurely: a Nationwide Danish and Swedish safety study. Drugs Real World Outcomes. 2023;10(1):69–81. https://doi.org/10.1007/s40801-022-00334-2.

Arulandoo A, Kugathasan S. Determining the severity of neonatal abstinence syndrome among newborns exposed to selective serotonin reuptake inhibitors and serotonin and norepinephrine reuptake inhibitors in utero: a protocol for a systematic review and meta-analysis. URNCST J. 2023;7:1–6.

Avram M, Stika C, Rasmussen-Torvik L, Ciolino J, Pinheiro E, George A Jr, Wisner K. Rationale and design for an investigation to optimize selective serotonin reuptake inhibitor treatment for pregnant women with depression. Clin Pharm Ther. 2016;100(1):31–3.

Bandoli G, Chambers CD, Wells A, Palmsten K. Prenatal antidepressant use and risk of adverse neonatal outcomes. Pediatrics. 2020;146(1)

Benevent J, Araujo M, Karki S, Delarue-Hurault C, Waser J, Lacroix I, et al. Risk of hypertensive disorders of pregnancy in women treated with serotonin-norepinephrine reuptake inhibitors: a comparative study using the EFEMERIS database. J Clin Psychiatry. 2023;84(4):47872.

Bérard A, Iessa N, Chaabane S, Muanda FT, Boukhris T, Zhao JP. The risk of major cardiac malformations associated with paroxetine use during the first trimester of pregnancy: a systematic review and meta-analysis. Br J Clin Pharmacol. 2016;81(4):589–604.

Bérard A, Sheehy O, Zhao JP, Vinet É, Bernatsky S, Abrahamowicz M. SSRI and SNRI use during pregnancy and the risk of persistent pulmonary hypertension of the newborn. Br J Clin Pharmacol. 2017;83(5):1126–33.

Bérard A, Levin M, Sadler T, Healy D. Selective serotonin reuptake inhibitor use during pregnancy and major malformations: the importance of serotonin for embryonic development and the effect of serotonin inhibition on the occurrence of malformations. Bioelectricity. 2019;1(1):18–29.

Bernard N, Forest J-C, Tarabulsy GM, Bujold E, Bouvier D, Giguère Y. Use of antidepressants and anxiolytics in early pregnancy and the risk of preeclampsia and gestational hypertension: a prospective study. BMC Pregnancy Childbirth. 2019;19:1–9.

Bliddal M, Wesselhoeft R, Strandberg-Larsen K, Ernst MT, Weissman MM, Gingrich JA, et al. Prenatal antidepressant exposure and emotional disorders until age 22: a danish register study. Child Adolesc Psychiatry Ment Health. 2023;17(1):73. https://doi.org/10.1186/s13034-023-00624-9.

Bobo WV, Moore KM, Betcher HK, Larish AM, Stoppel CM, VandeVoort JL, et al. The Association of Antidepressants in late pregnancy with postpartum hemorrhage: systematic review of controlled observational studies. J Child Adolesc Psychopharmacol. 2024;34(10):428–46. https://doi.org/10.1089/cap.2024.0085.

Bobula B, Bąk J, Kania A, Siwiec M, Kiełbiński M, Tokarski K, et al. Maternal fluoxetine impairs synaptic transmission and plasticity in the medial prefrontal cortex and alters the structure and function of dorsal raphe nucleus neurons in offspring mice. Pharmacol Biochem Behav. 2024;244:173849. https://doi.org/10.1016/j.pbb.2024.173849.

Brajcich MR, Palau MA, Messer RD, Murphy ME, Marks J. Why the maternal medication list matters: neonatal toxicity from combined serotonergic exposures. Pediatrics. 2021;147(2) https://doi.org/10.1542/peds.2019-2250.

Cabrera RM, Linda Lin Y, Law E, Kim J, Wlodarczyk BJ. The teratogenic effects of sertraline in mice. Birth Defects Res. 2020;112(13):1014–24. https://doi.org/10.1002/bdr2.1660.

Cafaro R, Giorgetti F, Giacovelli L, Vanzetto S, Cerolini L, Colombo A, Dell'Osso B. Analyses of pharmacokinetic, Pharmacogenetic and psychometrics correlates of antidepressants use during pregnancy and the post-partum period. Eur Psychiatry. 2022;65(S1):S234.

Campbell SC, Salisbury LM, Roberts JK, Kamyar M, Fredrickson J, Costantine MM, Sherwin CM. Therapeutic drug monitoring in pregnancy. In: Clinical challenges in therapeutic drug monitoring. Elsevier; 2016. p. 185–211.

Chan JKN, Lee KCK, Wong CSM, Chang WC. Prenatal antidepressant use and risk of congenital malformations: a population-based cohort study. Psychiatry Res. 2024;339:116038.

Chang Q, Ma X-Y, Xu X-R, Su H, Wu Q-J, Zhao Y-H. Antidepressant use in depressed women during pregnancy and the risk of preterm birth: a systematic review and meta-analysis of 23 cohort studies. Front Pharmacol. 2020;11:659.

Chen LF, Lin CE, Chung CH, Lai CH, Chien WC. Association between the use of antidepressants and the risk of preterm birth among pregnant women with depression: a retrospective cohort study in Taiwan. J Investig Med. 2021;69(5):999–1007. https://doi.org/10.1136/jim-2020-001683.

Christensen J, Trabjerg BB, Sun Y, Dreier JW. Association of Maternal Antidepressant Prescription during Pregnancy with Standardized Test Scores of Danish school-aged children. JAMA. 2021;326(17):1725–35. https://doi.org/10.1001/jama.2021.17380.

Combellick JL, Esmaeili A, Johnson AM, Haskell SG, Phibbs CS, Manzo L, Miller LJ. Perinatal mental health and pregnancy-associated mortality: opportunities for change. Arch Womens Ment Health. 2024;27(3):417–24. https://doi.org/10.1007/s00737-023-01404-2.

Cornet M-C, Wu YW, Forquer H, Avalos LA, Sriram A, Scheffler AW, et al. Maternal treatment with selective serotonin reuptake inhibitors during pregnancy and delayed neonatal adaptation: a population-based cohort study. Arch Dis Child Fetal Neonatal Ed. 2024;109(3):294–300.

Cristina D. Woman and pregnancy: focus on depression and psychopharmacological therapy. Int J Basic Clin Pharm. 2023;12(2):284–90.

Dama MH, Van Lieshout RJ. Perinatal depression: a guide to detection and management in primary care. J Am Board Family Med. 2023;36(6):1071–86.

De Vries C, Gadzhanova S, Sykes MJ, Ward M, Roughead E. A systematic review and meta-analysis considering the SSRI, SNRI and TCA classes of antidepressants and the risk for congenital heart defects; 2020. *medRxiv*, 2020.2002. 2024.20027532.

De Vries C, Gadzhanova S, Sykes MJ, Ward M, Roughead E. A systematic review and meta-analysis considering the risk for congenital heart defects of antidepressant classes and individual antidepressants. Drug Saf. 2021a;44(3):291–312. https://doi.org/10.1007/s40264-020-01027-x.

De Vries C, Gadzhanova S, Sykes MJ, Ward M, Roughead E. A systematic review and meta-analysis considering the risk for congenital heart defects of antidepressant classes and individual antidepressants. Drug Saf. 2021b;44:291–312.

Desaunay P, Eude L-G, Dreyfus M, Alexandre C, Fedrizzi S, Alexandre J, et al. Benefits and risks of antidepressant drugs during pregnancy: a systematic review of meta-analyses. Pediatr Drugs. 2023;25(3):247–65.

Desaunay P, Eslier M, Alexandre J, Dreyfus M, Chrétien B, Guenolé F. Antidepressants and fetal death: a systematic review and disproportionality analysis in the WHO safety database (VigiBase®). Psychiatry Res. 2024;339:116048.

Di Vincenzo M, Ferrandino M, Sollo V, Landolfi L, Mancuso E, Di Cerbo A, et al. Antenatal depression, obstetric outcomes, and post-partum depression: results from a longitudinal, real-world study. Eur Psychiatry. 2023;66(S1):S501–2.

Dodeja P, Chaphekar N, Caritis SN, Venkataramanan R. Optimizing drug therapy during pregnancy: a spotlight on population pharmacokinetic modeling. Expert Opin Drug Metab Toxicol. 2025;21(2):143–60. https://doi.org/10.1080/17425255.2024.2420195.

Domingues RR, Beard AD, Connelly MK, Wiltbank MC, Hernandez LL. Fluoxetine-induced perinatal morbidity in a sheep model. Front Med. 2022;9:955560.

Domingues RR, Wiltbank MC, Hernandez LL. Maternal serotonin: implications for the use of selective serotonin reuptake inhibitors during gestation. Biol Reprod. 2023;109(1):17–28. https://doi.org/10.1093/biolre/ioad046.

Dubiel-Hoppanova L et al. Pregestational stress representing a maternal depression model and prenatally applied antidepressant mirtazapine modulate hippocampal excitability in the offspring; 2025.

Dubovicky M, Belovicova K, Csatlosova K, Bogi E. Risks of using SSRI/SNRI antidepressants during pregnancy and lactation. Interdiscip Toxicol. 2017;10(1):30–4. https://doi.org/10.1515/intox-2017-0004.

Einarson A, Choi J, Einarson TR, Koren G. Incidence of major malformations in infants following antidepressant exposure in pregnancy: results of a large prospective cohort study. Can J Psychiatr. 2009;54(4):242–6. https://doi.org/10.1177/070674370905400405.

Eke AC. An update on the physiologic changes during pregnancy and their impact on drug pharmacokinetics and pharmacogenomics. J Basic Clin Physiol Pharmacol. 2022;33(5):581–98. https://doi.org/10.1515/jbcpp-2021-0312.

Ekhart C, van Hunsel F, van Puijenbroek E, Chandler R, Meldau E-L, Taavola H, Norén GN. Post-marketing safety profile of vortioxetine using a cluster analysis and a disproportionality analysis of global adverse event reports. Drug Saf. 2022;45(2):145–53.

Ergun B, et al. Effects of prenatal and lactational vortioxetine exposure on emotional states, motor activities and cognitive performances of offspring. Psychiatry Behav Sci. 2024;14(3)

Fabiano N, Wong S, Gupta A, Tran J, Bhambra N, Min KK, et al. Safety of psychotropic medications in pregnancy: an umbrella review. Mol Psychiatry. 2025;30(1):327–35. https://doi.org/10.1038/s41380-024-02697-0.

Febrianti Y. Antidepressant use in pregnancy and the risk of neonatal outcomes: a scoping review. Jurnal Ilmiah Farmasi. 2024;20(1):90–102.

Fitton C, Steiner M, Aucott L, Pell J, Mackay D, Fleming M, McLay J. In utero exposure to antidepressant medication and neonatal and child outcomes: a systematic review. Acta Psychiatr Scand. 2020;141(1):21–33.

Furu K, Kieler H, Haglund B, Engeland A, Selmer R, Stephansson O, et al. Selective serotonin reuptake inhibitors and venlafaxine in early pregnancy and risk of birth defects: population based cohort study and sibling design. BMJ. 2015;350:h1798. https://doi.org/10.1136/bmj.h1798.

Galbally M, Watson SJ, Spigset O. Depression and antidepressant treatment in the development of hypertensive disorders of pregnancy: results from a prospective cohort study. Aust N Z J Psychiatry. 2023;57(4):520–7.

Galletta MAK, Tess VLC, Pasotti IM, Pelegrini LF, Ribeiro Rocha NK, Testa CB, Francisco RPV. Use of mirtazapine and olanzapine in the treatment of refractory hyperemesis gravidarum: a case report and systematic review. Case Rep Obstet Gynecol. 2022;2022(1):7324627.

Gallitelli V, Franco R, Guidi S, Puri L, Parasiliti M, Vidiri A, et al. Depression treatment in pregnancy: is it safe, or is it not? Int J Environ Res Public Health. 2024;21(4) https://doi.org/10.3390/ijerph21040404.

Gao S-Y, Wu Q-J, Sun C, Zhang T-N, Shen Z-Q, Liu C-X, et al. Selective serotonin reuptake inhibitor use during early pregnancy and congenital malformations: a systematic review and meta-analysis of cohort studies of more than 9 million births. BMC Med. 2018;16(1):205. https://doi.org/10.1186/s12916-018-1193-5.

Gastaldon C, Arzenton E, Raschi E, Spigset O, Papola D, Ostuzzi G, et al. Neonatal withdrawal syndrome following in utero exposure to antidepressants: a disproportionality analysis of VigiBase, the WHO spontaneous reporting database. Psychol Med. 2023a;53(12):5645–53.

Gastaldon C, Arzenton E, Raschi E, Spigset O, Papola D, Ostuzzi G, et al. Pharmacovigilance analysis of the Vigibase on neonatal withdrawal syndrome following in utero exposure to antidepressants. Eur Psychiatry. 2023b;66(Suppl 1):S96.

Glazova NY, Merchieva S, Volodina M, Sebentsova E, Manchenko D, Kudrun V, Levitskaya N. Effects of neonatal fluvoxamine administration on the physical development and activity of the serotoninergic system in white rats. Acta Nat. 2014;6(3):98–105.

Goracci A, Valdagno M, Maltinti E, Sillari S, Fagiolini A. Antidepressant use in pregnancy: a critical review of the risk and benefits. Riv Psichiatr. 2015;50(3):118–26. https://doi.org/10.1708/1910.20792.

Gram MA, Laksafoss A, Hviid A. Antidepressant exposure patterns during pregnancy and risk of adverse newborn outcomes. Psychiatry Res. 2024;342:116274. https://doi.org/10.1016/j.psychres.2024.116274.

Grigoriadis S, VonderPorten EH, Mamisashvili L, Roerecke M, Rehm J, Dennis C-L, et al. Antidepressant exposure during pregnancy and congenital malformations: is there an association? A systematic review and meta-analysis of the best evidence. J Clin Psychiatry. 2013;74(4):903.

Haq MIU, Fatima S, Amjad N, Sheikh JR. Impact of maternal depression on pregnancy and neonatal outcomes: a prospective analysis: maternal stress and neonatal outcomes. Pak J Health Sci. 2024:02–7.

Heerdink ER. Antidepressants and postpartum haemorrhage. Br Med J. 2013;347:f5194. https://doi.org/10.1136/bmj.f5194.

Heuvelman H et al. Antidepressants in pregnancy: applying causal epidemiological methods to understand service-use outcomes in women and long-term neurodevelopmental outcomes in exposed children; 2023.

Hosseini K, Cediel-Ulloa A, Al-Sabri MH, Forsby A, Fredriksson R. Assessing the neurodevelopmental impact of fluoxetine, citalopram, and paroxetine on neural stem cell-derived neurons. Pharmaceuticals. 2024;17(10):1392.

Huybrechts KF, Bateman BT, Pawar A, Bessette LG, Mogun H, Levin R, et al. Maternal and fetal outcomes following exposure to duloxetine in pregnancy: cohort study. BMJ. 2020;368

Hwang YM et al. Timing of selective serotonin reuptake inhibitor use and risk for preterm birth and related adverse events; 2023. *medRxiv*, 2023.2003. 2003.23286717.

Jahan N, Went TR, Sultan W, Sapkota A, Khurshid H, Qureshi IA, Alfonso M. Untreated depression during pregnancy and its effect on pregnancy outcomes: a systematic review. Cureus. 2021;13(8):e17251. https://doi.org/10.7759/cureus.17251.

Jimenez-Solem E, Andersen JT, Petersen M, Broedbaek K, Lander AR, Afzal S, et al. SSRI use during pregnancy and risk of stillbirth and neonatal mortality. Am J Psychiatry. 2013;170(3):299–304.

Karnwal R, Sharmila K. Perspective view of stress, anxiety, and depression among pregnant women: a review. J Ecophysiol Occup Health. 2024:7–19.

Kautzky A, Slamanig R, Unger A, Höflich A. Neonatal outcome and adaption after in utero exposure to antidepressants: a systematic review and meta-analysis. Acta Psychiatr Scand. 2022;145(1):6–28.

Kent ME, Hu B, Eggleston TM, Squires RS, Zimmerman KA, Weiss RM, et al. Hypersensitivity of zebrafish htr2b mutant embryos to sertraline indicates a role for serotonin signaling in cardiac development. J Cardiovasc Pharmacol. 2022;80(2):261–9.

Kieviet N, Duijn M, Dolman K, Honig A. Poor neonatal adaptation after in utero exposure to fluvoxamine. J Obstet Gynaecol. 2015;35(2):201–2.

Kiribayashi M, Suda T, Takahashi M, Ishikawa M, Watanabe R, Ishioka K, et al. Vortioxetine exposure during pregnancy and lactation: a Japanese case study of neonatal implications and quantitative Milk and plasma analyses. Breastfeed Med. 2024;19(8):659–62.

Knopf A. Pregnant women may benefit from continued use of antidepressants. Brown Univ Child Adolesc Psychopharm Update. 2023;25(6):5.

Koc D, Tiemeier H, Stricker BH, Muetzel RL, Hillegers M, El Marroun H. Prenatal antidepressant exposure and offspring brain morphologic trajectory. JAMA Psychiatry. 2023;80(12):1208–17. https://doi.org/10.1001/jamapsychiatry.2023.3161.

Kolding L, Henriksen JN, Pedersen LH. Fetal cardiac safety of sertraline use during pregnancy. Expert Opin Drug Saf. 2023;22(8):653–7.

Lam YF. Antidepressant use patterns in pregnancy. Brown Univ Psychopharm Update. 2023;34(8):2–3.

Lassen D, Ennis ZN, Damkier P. First-trimester pregnancy exposure to venlafaxine or duloxetine and risk of major congenital malformations: a systematic review. Basic Clin Pharmacol Toxicol. 2016;118(1):32–6. https://doi.org/10.1111/bcpt.12497.

Laurent L, Huang C, Ernest SR, Berard A, Vaillancourt C, Hales BF. In utero exposure to venlafaxine, a serotonin–norepinephrine reuptake inhibitor, increases cardiac anomalies and alters placental and heart serotonin signaling in the rat. Birth Defects Res A Clin Mol Teratol. 2016;106(12):1044–55.

Lee M-J, Chen Y-L, Wu S-I, Huang C-W, Dewey ME, Chen VC-H. Association between maternal antidepressant use during pregnancy and the risk of autism spectrum disorder and attention deficit hyperactivity disorder in offspring. Eur Child Adolesc Psychiatry. 2024;33:1–11.

Levy M, Kovo M, Miremberg H, Anchel N, Herman HG, Bar J, et al. Maternal use of selective serotonin reuptake inhibitors (SSRI) during pregnancy – neonatal outcomes in correlation with placental histopathology. J Perinatol. 2020;40(7):1017–24.

Liao T, Gao Y, Yang X, Tang Y, Wang B, Yang Q, et al. Preconception depression reduces fertility: a couple-based prospective preconception cohort. Hum Reprod Open. 2024;2024(3):hoae032.

Lou Z-Q, Zhou Y-Y, Zhang X, Jiang H-Y. Exposure to selective noradrenalin reuptake inhibitors during the first trimester of pregnancy and risk of congenital malformations: a meta-analysis of cohort studies. Psychiatry Res. 2022;316:114756.

Maligireddy A, Jabri A, Zghouzi M, Rojulpote C, VanAken G, Janga C, et al. Maternal and fetal outcomes in pulmonary hypertension during pregnancy: a contemporary Nationwide analysis. Am J Cardiol. 2024;221:113–9. https://doi.org/10.1016/j.amjcard.2024.04.016.

Maloney SE et al. Maternal SSRI treatment during offspring development results in long-term behavioral, cellular, and neuroimaging disruptions2017. *bioRxiv*, 205708.

Marks C, Quinney S, Haas D. Comparing newborn outcomes after prenatal exposure to individual antidepressants. Proc IMPRS. 2020;3(1)

Martin FZ, Smith S, Rai D, Forbes H. Antidepressant use during pregnancy and risk of stillbirth: a systematic review and meta-analysis. Reprod Female Child Health. 2023;2(3):177–87.

Martin FZ et al. Antidepressant use during pregnancy and birth outcomes: analysis of electronic health data from the UK, Norway, and Sweden; 2024. *medRxiv*.

Milosavljević JZ, Milosavljević MN, Arsenijević PS, Milentijević MN, Stefanović SM. The effects of selective serotonin reuptake inhibitors on male and female fertility: a brief literature review. Int J Psychiatry Clin Pract. 2022;26(1):43–9. https://doi.org/10.1080/13651501.2021.1872647.

Mitchell J, Goodman J. Comparative effects of antidepressant medications and untreated major depression on pregnancy outcomes: a systematic review. Arch Womens Ment Health. 2018;21(5):505–16. https://doi.org/10.1007/s00737-018-0844-z.

Murad F. A prospective cohort study to assess neonatal adaptation in neonates exposed to psychotropic medications in utero. Br J Psych Open. 2022;8(S1):S62.

Nagandla K, Nalliah S, Yin LK, Majeed ZA, Ismail M, Zubaidah S, et al. Prevalence and associated risk factors of depression, anxiety and stress in pregnancy. Int J Reprod Contracept Obstet Gynecol. 2017;5(7):2380–8. https://doi.org/10.18203/2320-1770.ijrcog20162132.

Nörby U, Forsberg L, Wide K, Sjörs G, Winbladh B, Källén K. Neonatal morbidity after maternal use of antidepressant drugs during pregnancy. Pediatrics. 2016;138(5)

Nunes TP, Nunes LP, Silva ANA, Pirovani BO, Morábito MJSD, de Morais LA, et al. Effects adverse of treatment with selective inhibitors of serotonin recaptation on the fetus and neonatals of mothers with gestational depression: a critical review. Res Soc Dev. 2021;10(4):e11210413937. https://doi.org/10.33448/rsd-v10i4.13937.

Ogunyemi D, Jovanovski A, Liu J, Friedman P, Sugiyama N, Creps J, Madan I. The contribution of untreated and treated anxiety and depression to prenatal, intrapartum, and neonatal outcomes. AJP Rep. 2018;08(03):e146–57. https://doi.org/10.1055/s-0038-1661379.

Okagbue HI, Adamu PI, Bishop SA, Oguntunde PE, Opanuga AA, Akhmetshin EM. Systematic review of prevalence of antepartum depression during the trimesters of pregnancy. Open Access Maced J Med Sci. 2019;7(9):1555–60. https://doi.org/10.3889/oamjms.2019.270.

Olivier JD, Åkerud H, Kaihola H, Pawluski JL, Skalkidou A, Högberg U, Sundström Poromaa I. The effects of maternal depression and maternal selective serotonin reuptake inhibitor exposure on offspring. Front Cell Neurosci. 2013;7 https://doi.org/10.3389/fncel.2013.00073.

Ornoy A, Koren G. Selective serotonin reuptake inhibitors during pregnancy: do we have now more definite answers related to prenatal exposure? Birth Defects Res. 2017;109(12):898–908. https://doi.org/10.1002/bdr2.1078.

Ornoy A, Koren G. SSRIs and SNRIs (SRI) in pregnancy: effects on the course of pregnancy and the offspring: how far are we from having all the answers? Int J Mol Sci. 2019;20(10):2370.

Ostenfeld A, Petersen TS, Pedersen LH, Westergaard HB, Løkkegaard ECL, Andersen JT. Mirtazapine exposure in pregnancy and fetal safety: a nationwide cohort study. Acta Psychiatr Scand. 2022;145(6):557–67. https://doi.org/10.1111/acps.13431.

Ostenfeld A, Lyngholm S, Christensen SE, Petersen TS, Andersen JT, Westergaard HB, et al. Mirtazapine in pregnancy and lactation: a systematic review of adverse outcomes. Acta Psychiatr Scand. 2025;151(1):6–32. https://doi.org/10.1111/acps.13749.

Oswald M, El-Chaar G, Canter M. Hypothermia as a presenting sign of venlafaxine-induced neonatal abstinence syndrome in 2 neonates. J Pediatr Pharm Ther. 2024;29(6):654–9.

Padilla-Azain MC, Osmundson SS, Bosworth O, Wiese A, Pham A, Leech AA, et al. Opioid analgesic and antidepressant use during pregnancy and the risk of spontaneous preterm birth: a nested case–control study. Paediatr Perinat Epidemiol. 2024;

Palmsten K, Hernández-Díaz S, Huybrechts KF, Williams PL, Michels KB, Achtyes ED, et al. Use of antidepressants near delivery and risk of postpartum hemorrhage: cohort study of low income women in the United States. Br Med J. 2013;347:f4877. https://doi.org/10.1136/bmj.f4877.

Parpinel G, Rosso G, Galante A, Germano C, Aragno E, Girlando F, et al. Effect of depressive disorders and their pharmacological treatment during pregnancy on maternal and neonatal outcome. J Clin Med. 2022;11(6):1486.

Poweleit EA, Cinibulk MA, Novotny SA, Wagner-Schuman M, Ramsey LB, Strawn JR. Selective serotonin reuptake inhibitor pharmacokinetics during pregnancy: clinical and research implications. Front Pharmacol. 2022;13:833217.

Rohanachandra YM. Depression in mothers and mental health in their children: impact, risk factors, and interventions. In: The neuroscience of depression. Elsevier; 2021. p. 45–55.

Rommel A-S, Bergink V, Liu X, Munk-Olsen T, Molenaar NM. Long-term effects of intrauterine exposure to antidepressants on physical, neurodevelopmental, and psychiatric outcomes: a systematic review. J Clin Psychiatry. 2020;81(3):10661.

Rommel A-S, Semark BD, Liu X, Madsen KB, Agerbo E, Munk-Olsen T, et al. Prenatal antidepressant exposure and the risk of decreased gestational age and lower birthweight: a polygenic score approach to investigate confounding by indication. Acta Psychiatr Scand. 2024;150(5):344–54. https://doi.org/10.1111/acps.13636.

Rotem-Kohavi N, Goodman SH, Wazana A, Oberlander TF. The other side of prenatal depression: developmental outcomes associated with antidepressant medication therapy. Prenatal Stress and Child Development; 2021, p. 565–593.

Roy R, Chakraborty M, Bhattacharya K, Roychoudhury T, Mukherjee S. Impact of perinatal maternal depression on child development. Indian J Psychiatry. 2022;64(3):284–8.

Salkeld E, Ferris LE, Juurlink DN. The risk of postpartum hemorrhage with selective serotonin reuptake inhibitors and other antidepressants. J Clin Psychopharmacol. 2008;28(2):230.

Santos RA, Sousa AP, Almeida-Santos T, Ramalho-Santos J, Tavares RS. In vitro effects of antidepressants on human sperm function. Asian J Androl. 2025;27(1):30–6.

Schoretsanitis G, Spigset O, Stingl JC, Deligiannidis KM, Paulzen M, Westin AA. The impact of pregnancy on the pharmacokinetics of antidepressants: a systematic critical review and meta-analysis. Expert Opin Drug Metab Toxicol. 2020;16(5):431–40.

Shea AK, Wang DY, Snelgrove JW, Dalfen A, Hewko S, Murphy KE. Do maternal pharmacogenetics impact the neonatal abstinence syndrome following in utero exposure to antidepressant medications? J Obstet Gynaecol Can. 2021;43(6):726–32. https://doi.org/10.1016/j.jogc.2020.09.026.

Sheftel C, Sartori LC, Manuel R, Fricke H, Bell A, Mulvenna E, Hernandez LL. MON-001 peripartum sertraline (Zoloft®) increases pup mortality immediately postpartum. J Endocr Soc. 2020;4(Supplement_1) https://doi.org/10.1210/jendso/bvaa046.1840.

Shen Z-Q, Gao S-Y, Li SX, Zhang T-N, Liu C-X, Lv H-C, et al. Sertraline use in the first trimester and risk of congenital anomalies: a systemic review and meta-analysis of cohort studies. Br J Clin Pharmacol. 2017;83(4):909–22. https://doi.org/10.1111/bcp.13161.

Shweiki S, Diav-Citrin O. Pregnancy outcome after first trimester exposure to vortioxetine: a case series. Birth Defects Res. 2021;113(6):511–5.

Sivojelezova A. Fluvoxamine (LUVOX™) use in pregnancy. Clin Pharm Ther. 2004;75(2):P25. https://doi.org/10.1016/j.clpt.2003.11.094.

Smithson J, Mitchell PB. Chapter 2 – Antidepressants. In: Ray SD, editor. Side effects of drugs annual, vol. 37. Elsevier; 2015. p. 15–31.

Stephansson O, Kieler H, Haglund B, Artama M, Engeland A, Furu K, et al. Selective serotonin reuptake inhibitors during pregnancy and risk of stillbirth and infant mortality. JAMA. 2013;309(1):48–54.

Suarez EA, Bateman BT, Hernández-Díaz S, Straub L, Wisner KL, Gray KJ, et al. Association of antidepressant use during pregnancy with risk of neurodevelopmental disorders in children. JAMA Intern Med. 2022;182(11):1149–60.

Sujan AC. What do we know about in-utero antidepressant exposure, and are these medications safe to use during pregnancy? Acta Psychiatr Scand. 2022;145:541–3.

Sun Y, Dreier JW, Liu X, Glejsted Ingstrup K, Mægbæk ML, Munk-Olsen T, Christensen J. Trend of antidepressants before, during, and after pregnancy across two decades – a population-based study. Brain and behavior. 2019;9(11):e01441.

Sun M, Zhang S, Li Y, Chen L, Diao J, Li J, et al. Effect of maternal antidepressant use during the pre-pregnancy/early pregnancy period on congenital heart disease: a prospective cohort study in Central China. Front Cardiovasc Med. 2022;9:916882.

Svensson M, Reimers A, Reis M. Pharmacokinetics of antidepressants during pregnancy. Lakartidningen. 2020;117:FYLY.

Tanguay N, Abdelouahab N, Simard M-N, Séguin JR, Marc I, Herba CM, et al. Antidepressants use during pregnancy and child psychomotor, cognitive and language development at 2 years of age – results from the 3D cohort study. Front Pharmacol. 2023;14:1252251.

Tharp MA, Silvola RM, Marks C, Teal E, Quinney SK, Haas DM. Does lack of exposure to individual antidepressants at different points during pregnancy associate with reduced risk of adverse newborn outcomes? BMC Pregnancy Childbirth. 2022;22(1):926. https://doi.org/10.1186/s12884-022-05287-6.

The Medical Letter. Addendum: bupropion safety in pregnancy. Med Lett Drugs Ther. 2024;66(1699):56. https://doi.org/10.58347/tml.2024.1699c.

Uguz F. Is there any association between use of antidepressants and preeclampsia or gestational hypertension?: a systematic review of current studies. J Clin Psychopharmacol. 2017;37(1):72–7.

Uguz F. The use of antidepressant medications during pregnancy and the risk of neonatal seizures: a systematic review. J Clin Psychopharmacol. 2019;39(5):479–84.

Uguz F. Neonatal and childhood outcomes in offspring of pregnant women using antidepressant medications: a critical review of current meta-analyses. J Clin Pharmacol. 2021;61(2):146–58. https://doi.org/10.1002/jcph.1724.

Urato AC. Are the SSRI antidepressants safe in pregnancy? Understanding the debate. Int J Risk Safety Med. 2015;27(2):93–9.

Ushkalova E, Ushkalova A. Comparative analysis of the use of selective serotonin reuptake inhibitors during pregnancy and the postpartum period. Safety of sertraline. Neuro Npsy Psyc. 2023;15(5):94–101.

Vartiainen E et al. Pre-and postnatal maternal depressive symptoms associate with local connectivity of the left amygdala in 5-year-olds; 2024. *bioRxiv*, 2024.2006. 2021.600007.

Velasquez JC, Goeden N, Herod SM, Bonnin A. Maternal pharmacokinetics and fetal disposition of (±)-citalopram during mouse pregnancy. ACS Chem Neurosci. 2016;7(3):327–38.

Verma A, Kumar A. Risks associated with vortioxetine in the established therapeutic indication. Curr Neuropharmacol. 2021;19(5):711–7.

Vigod SN, Frey BN, Clark CT, Grigoriadis S, Barker LC, Brown HK, et al. Clinical practice guideline for the Management of Perinatal Mood, anxiety, and related disorders: guide de pratique 2024 du Canadian network for mood and anxiety treatments pour le traitement des troubles de l'humeur, des troubles anxieux et des troubles connexes périnatals. Can J Psychiatry. 2024;70:07067437241303031. https://doi.org/10.1177/07067437241303031.

Viguera AC, McElheny SA, Caplin PS, Kobylski LA, Rossa ET, Young AV, et al. Risk of poor neonatal adaptation syndrome among infants exposed to second-generation atypical antipsychotics compared to antidepressants: results from the National Pregnancy Registry for psychiatric medications. J Clin Psychiatry. 2023;84(1) https://doi.org/10.4088/JCP.22m14492.

Wang J, Cosci F. Neonatal withdrawal syndrome following late in utero exposure to selective serotonin reuptake inhibitors: a systematic review and meta-analysis of observational studies. Psychother Psychosom. 2021;90(5):299–307. https://doi.org/10.1159/000516031.

Wartko PD, Weiss NS, Enquobahrie DA, Chan KG, Stephenson-Famy A, Mueller BA, Dublin S. Association of antidepressant continuation in pregnancy and infant birth weight. J Clin Psychopharmacol. 2021;41(4):403–13.

Weaver SR, Xie C, Charles JF, Hernandez LL. In utero and lactational exposure to the selective serotonin reuptake inhibitor fluoxetine compromises pup bones at weaning. Sci Rep. 2019;9(1):238. https://doi.org/10.1038/s41598-018-36497-8.

Wemakor A, Casson K, Garne E, Bakker M, Addor M-C, Arriola L, et al. Selective serotonin reuptake inhibitor antidepressant use in first trimester pregnancy and risk of specific congenital anomalies: a European register-based study. Eur J Epidemiol. 2015;30(11):1187–98. https://doi.org/10.1007/s10654-015-0065-y.

Xing D, Wu R, Chen L, Wang T. Maternal use of antidepressants during pregnancy and risks for adverse perinatal outcomes: a meta-analysis. J Psychosom Res. 2020;137:110231. https://doi.org/10.1016/j.jpsychores.2020.110231.

Yang K, Qin X, Wang H, Zhou W. Exploring genetic causal relationship between antidepressants use and congenital malformations. Reprod Toxicol. 2024;130:108736.

Yazıcı E, Şahin S. Psychiatric disorders during pregnancy and postpartum period: a guide for perinatal interview. Eur J Med. 2023;55(1):S61.

Yazici E, Kirkan TS, Aslan PA, Aydin N, Yazici AB. Untreated depression in the first trimester of pregnancy leads to postpartum depression: high rates from a natural follow-up study. Neuropsychiatr Dis Treat. 2015;11:405–11.

Yue M, Kus L, Katta S, Su I, Li L, Haas DM, Quinney SK. Pharmacokinetics of antidepressants in pregnancy. J Clin Pharmacol. 2023;63:S137–58.

Zakiyah N, Ter Heijne LF, Bos JH, Hak E, Postma MJ, Schuiling-Veninga CC. Antidepressant use during pregnancy and the risk of developing gestational hypertension: a retrospective cohort study. BMC Pregnancy Childbirth. 2018;18:1–11.

Zeszutek S. Antidepressant use in pregnancy. In: Side effects of drugs annual, vol. 43. Elsevier; 2021. p. 503–12.

Antidepressants During Lactation

7

Pierre Desaunay, Camille Blouet, Mélanie Alexandre, and Fabian Guénolé

7.1 Introduction

Breastfeeding, especially when sustained, has significant benefits for both infants and mothers, such as reduced infant morbidity and mortality, development of intelligence, and lower maternal risk of breast cancer (Victora et al. 2016). In light of these benefits, the World Health Organization (WHO) and the American Academy of Pediatrics (AAP) recommend exclusive breastfeeding for the first 6 months, then children should begin eating safe and adequate complementary foods while continuing to breastfeed for up to 2 years of age (Eidelman et al. 2012; WHO, UNICEF, USAID, and AED 2008). Antidepressant drugs (ADs), with an international prevalence estimated at 4.1% during pregnancy and rising to 5.8% postpartum (Molenaar et al. 2020), have been associated with potential adverse reactions in both mother and newborn.

Perinatal anxiety and depression disorders, as well as AD use, may limit breastfeeding initiation, duration, and exclusivity (Butler et al. 2021; Hoff et al. 2019). In nursing mothers, serotonin is the main local (i.e., intramammary) regulator of lactation (while prolactin is the main systemic regulator). Homeostatic control of milk volume within the alveolar spaces of the mammary gland involves a feedback

P. Desaunay
Centre Hospitalier Universitaire de Caen Normandie, Service de psychiatrie de l'enfant et de l'adolescent, Caen, France

C. Blouet · F. Guénolé (✉)
Centre Hospitalier Universitaire de Caen Normandie, Service de psychiatrie de l'enfant et de l'adolescent, Caen, France

Pôle de formation et recherche en santé, Faculté de médecine, Université de Caen Normandie, Caen, France

M. Alexandre
Centre Hospitalier Universitaire de Caen Normandie, Service de pédiatrie, Caen, France

F. Uguz, L. Orsolini (eds.), *Perinatal Psychopharmacology*, https://doi.org/10.1007/978-3-031-99720-4_7

system mediated by serotonin signaling (Stull et al. 2007). Additionally, serotonin induces the release of parathyroid hormone-related protein, which induces mobilizing calcium through bone resorption for milk synthesis (Marshall et al. 2014). Consequently, evidence suggests that ADs, which modulate serotonin activity, may delay alveolar secretory activation, thereby delaying the onset of lactation (Marshall et al. 2010).

Nursing infants exposed to ADs via breast milk face potential risks of various adverse reactions, including drowsiness, restlessness, irritability, and, in some cases, poor feeding and insufficient weight gain. Pathophysiology may include central nervous excitation and autonomic dysfunction (Arbitman et al. 2024). The safety of ADs use during breastfeeding depends to a large extent on their excretion into breast milk, which is commonly estimated using the milk/plasma (M/P) ratio (i.e., the ratio of milk drug concentration to maternal plasma drug concentration). An M/P ratio below 1.0 indicates low transfer into breast milk. The relative infant dose (RID, i.e., the percentage of the weight- and time-adjusted infant dose relative to the weight- and time-adjusted maternal dose) is considered a more accurate indicator of safety (Begg et al. 2002; Gentile et al. 2007). Psychotropic drugs with an RID below 10% are generally deemed safe for breastfeeding (Sachs et al. 2013), though some authors advocate for a more stringent threshold of 5% (Larsen et al. 2015). The reported maximum RID, along with infant plasma AD levels, prevalence of reported adverse reactions, and reported serious ones, constitute safety parameters, all of which are incorporated into an evidence-based "safety scoring system" for the use of psychotropic drugs during lactation (Uguz 2021).

The objective of this chapter is to review recent safety data on the use of ADs during breastfeeding, considering outcomes for both nursing mothers and their infants. For mothers, the focus includes breastfeeding initiation and duration associated with AD use. For infants, the review evaluates safety data for individual ADs and provides updated safety scores.

7.2 Safety of Antidepressants for Nursing Mothers

7.2.1 Studies on Breastfeeding Initiation and Duration

Three large studies have assessed breastfeeding initiation and duration associated with AD use started during pregnancy or postpartum. All adjusted for several risk factors known to reduce breastfeeding (including maternal age, parity, smoking, socioeconomic status).

The largest study was conducted in Norway and involved a total of 80,882 mother-infant dyads (Grzeskowiak et al. 2022). The rate of breastfeeding initiation was particularly high (i.e., 99.2%) in mothers without psychiatric disorders or ADs use. Mothers with AD use from late pregnancy, compared with mothers with anxiety or depression disorders without AD use, showed a slight decrease in breastfeeding initiation (i.e., 92.3% vs. 98.6%, aRR = 0.93 [0.90–0.97]). However, there were no more likely to discontinue breastfeeding abruptly or to experience breastfeeding-related complications (including sore nipples and mastitis) during the first month postpartum, nor to stop breastfeeding within 6 months. By contrast, mothers who started ADs postnatal were at greater risk of abrupt breastfeeding discontinuation (aRR = 2.64 [2.07–3.73]) and breastfeeding problems (aRR = 1.37 [1.14–1.64]) during the first month postpartum. There were also at greater risk of breastfeeding cessation until 6 months postpartum (aRR = 0.49 [0.42–0.56]), mainly for predominant breastfeeding (aRR = 0.37 [0.22–0.61]).

The second larger study was conducted in Wales and involved 38,725 mother-infant dyads (Jordan et al. 2019). The breastfeeding rate among mothers without depression or AD use was low, estimated at 34.31% at 6–8 weeks postpartum. Results adjusted for risk factors including depression showed a reduction in breastfeeding initiation associated with SSRI use during the second or third trimester (aOR = 0.66 [0.56–0.77]), particularly with SSRIs used at high dose (aOR = 0.59 [0.44–0.78]). Mothers were at higher risk of discontinuing breastfeeding 6–8 weeks postpartum, whether they had used ADs during the first trimester of pregnancy only (any AD: aOR = 0.70 [0.57–0.85]; any SSRI: aOR = 0.64 [0.54–0.74]), or during the second or third trimesters (any AD: aOR = 0.81 [0.67–0.98]; any SSRI: aOR = 0.77 [0.62–0.95]), particularly at high dose (any SSRI: aOR = 0.45 [0.23–0.86]).

The third larger study was conducted in Australia and involved 32,662 mother-infant dyads (Leggett et al. 2017). The rate of breastfeeding at discharge from maternity hospital was particularly high (i.e., 88.9%) in mothers without psychiatric disorders or ADs use. When neonates were born at term, mothers with AD use until the second and third trimesters of pregnancy were less likely to be breastfeeding their infants at discharge compared with mothers with psychiatric disorders not using ADs (aOR = 0.73 [0.55–0.98]). With preterm newborns or admitted to the neonatal intensive care unit (NICU), no significant differences in breastfeeding rates at discharge were observed between mothers with AD use, mothers with psychiatric disorders not using ADs, and mothers without psychiatric disorders or AD use. A smallest study also conducted in Australia reported no significant difference on breastfeeding duration across depressed mothers with AD use, depressed mothers without AD use, and undepressed mothers (Galbally et al. 2019).

7.2.2 Discussion

A consistent decrease in breastfeeding initiation was shown in mothers using ADs during at least the third trimester of pregnancy, compared to control mothers, after adjusting for various risk factors including psychiatric ones (Grzeskowiak et al. 2022; Jordan et al. 2019; Leggett et al. 2017). An increased risk of abrupt breastfeeding discontinuation was also shown in mothers starting ADs postnatally (Grzeskowiak et al. 2022). These results may involve biological, psychological, or environmental factors. First, serotonin acts as a homeostatic regulator of lactation (Stull et al. 2007), and serotonergic ADs may delay alveolar secretary activation, thereby interfering with the establishment of breastfeeding (Marshall et al. 2010).

Second, depressed mothers, compared with undepressed ones, are more likely to experience difficulties in initiating breastfeeding, including high physical difficulties and significant pain (Brown et al. 2016). In addition, breastfeeding mothers with AD use have more severe depressive symptoms and functional impairment compared with those not receiving ADs (Battle et al. 2008; Molenaar et al. 2018), and they also demonstrate less efficient coping strategies for initiating and continuing breastfeeding (Da Silva Tanganhito et al. 2020). Third, AD use during late pregnancy is associated with poor neonatal adaptation symptoms including poor sucking and feeding, irritability, motor and tone symptoms, which may also hinder initiation of breastfeeding (Gastaldon et al. 2023). Finally, variable and sometimes conflicting safety advices regarding AD use during breastfeeding, difficulties in apprehending the potential risks, societal pressures on breastfeeding mothers, and inconsistent knowledge among healthcare professionals about the safety of AD use while breastfeeding may influence mother's decisions to breastfeed negatively (Battle et al. 2013; McClatchey et al. 2018; Uguz et al. 2020). However, the fact that no significant differences in breastfeeding rates at discharge were observed after premature birth or NICU admission across mothers with late pregnancy AD use, mothers without psychiatric disorders or AD use, and mothers without psychiatric disorders or AD use, suggest that under circumstances in which mothers with AD use can benefit from further breastfeeding support from healthcare providers, their breastfeeding initiation rates may become similar to those of mothers without psychiatric disorders or AD use (Leggett et al. 2017).

There was a variable reduction in breastfeeding duration. Studies conducted in Australia and Norway—countries with notably high breastfeeding rates among high-income nations (Vaz et al. 2021)—reported no increased risk of breastfeeding discontinuation during the first and 6 months postpartum, nor reduced breastfeeding mean duration, associated with AD use from pregnancy (Galbally et al. 2019; Grzeskowiak et al. 2022). In contrast, a study from Wales—a country with one of the lowest breastfeeding rates among high-income nations (Vaz et al. 2021)—identified an increased risk of breastfeeding discontinuation at 6–8 weeks postpartum associated with AD use initiated during pregnancy (Jordan et al. 2019). As for breastfeeding initiation, these results suggest that in environments supportive of breastfeeding, AD use may not significantly impact breastfeeding duration.

7.3 Safety of Antidepressants for Breastfed Infants

7.3.1 The Safety Scoring System

The safety scoring system (Uguz 2021) evaluated six safety parameters for AD use during breastfeeding: (1) reported total sample size (i.e., the total number of breastfed infants exposed to ADs, scored 0 to 2); (2) reported maximum relative infant dose RID (i.e., reported maximum weight- and time- adjusted infant dose relative to the weight- and time- adjusted maternal dose; scored 0 to 2); (3) reported sample size for relative infant dose (i.e., number of breastfed infants with reported RID values; scored 0 to 1); (4) infant plasma drug levels (i.e., proportion of breastfed infants with undetectable AD in plasma; scored 0 to 1); (5) prevalence of reported any adverse reaction (i.e., prevalence in the total sample size; scored 0 to 2); and (6) reported serious adverse reactions (i.e., report or no report of severe adverse drug reaction; scored 0 to 1). The total score ranged from 0 to 10 (≤ 3, very low safety profile; 3.1 to 5, low safety profile; 5.1 to 7.0, moderate safety profile; 7.1 to 8.5, good safety profile; 8.6 to 10.0, very good safety profile).

7.3.2 Methods

For each AD assessed, the data were drawn from two primary sources: (1) all studies referenced in LactMed®, specifically those detailing "drug levels" and "effects in breastfeeding infants", and (2) all studies included in the most recent and comprehensive review of AD use during breastfeeding (Eleftheriou et al. 2024). Included studies were case reports, case series, cohort studies, case-control studies, letters to editors, reviews, and meta-analyses published up to November 20th, 2024, and reporting pharmacological or clinical safety data on infants exposed to ADs through breastmilk.

Antidepressants evaluated covered the 21 ADs most routinely prescribed worldwide from the N06A category of the Anatomical Therapeutic Chemical classification system (Cipriani et al. 2018; Furukawa et al. 2016; Nahler 2009), as well as recently developed neurosteroid drugs for postpartum depression (Patterson et al. 2024). These included (1) all second-generation ADs approved by the regulatory agencies in the USA, Europe, or Japan (i.e., agomelatine, bupropion, citalopram, desvenlafaxine, duloxetine, escitalopram, fluoxetine, fluvoxamine, levomilnacipran, milnacipran, mirtazapine, nefazodone, paroxetine, reboxetine, sertraline, trazodone, venlafaxine, vilazodone, and vortioxetine); (2) tricyclic antidepressants (TCAs) from the WHO Model List of Essential Medicines (i.e., amitriptyline, clomipramine); (3) brexanolone and zuranolone.

Screening, data extraction, and scoring were conducted independently by two investigators (CB and PD). Any discrepancies were resolved by discussion and consensus.

7.3.3 Safety Scores

7.3.3.1 Selective Serotonin Reuptake Inhibitors (SSRIs)

Citalopram Its safety profile was moderate, due to a high reported maximum reported RID >10% (Pogliani et al. 2019) and detected drug in more than half of infant plasma. Adverse reactions were rare, and all minor. The total score was lower than in the initial version, due to recent data showing a high transfer of citalopram into milk in breastfed newborns (Pogliani et al. 2019), and detectable citalopram in most of infant's plasma in the largest study that assessed this AD during breastfeeding (Den Besten-Bertholee et al. 2024). In addition, a recent combined analysis identified a high M/P ratio (mean 2.05, range 0.78–7.23) (Schoretsanitis et al. 2021).

Escitalopram This AD is the stereoisomer of citalopram. Its safety profile was low. Although the maximum reported RID was <10% (Weisskopf et al. 2017) and the reported total sample was larger than the initial version, there was a higher proportion of reported adverse reactions - mostly minor ones - resulting in a lower total score. A case of necrotizing enterocolitis, a serious reaction, was reported in a newborn (Potts et al. 2007). In addition, escitalopram had the highest M/P ratio among SSRIs in a recent combined analysis (mean 2.19, range 1.68–3.00) (Schoretsanitis et al. 2021).

Fluoxetine This AD has long half-life compared with other SSRIs. Its safety profile was moderate, similarly to the initial version. This result was due to a high reported RID >10% (Pogliani et al. 2019), and detected fluoxetine and norfluoxetine (its active metabolite) in the serum of most breastfed infants. Adverse events were all minor.

Fluvoxamine The safety profile was moderate, similarly to the initial version. The safety of prescribing this AD during breastfeeding has been poorly documented. Available data indicate a low maximum RID (Kristensen et al. 2002), and limited adverse events in breastfed infants. A recent combined analysis identified a moderate M/P ratio (mean 0.98, range 0.29–1.57) (Schoretsanitis et al. 2021).

Paroxetine The safety profile was good, thanks to numerous data, a low maximum RID (Pogliani et al. 2019), and low detectable drug in the infant's plasma. The total score was lower than in the initial version, due to higher rate of reported adverse events in breastfed infants. However, as neonatal adaptation symptoms may be serious following in utero exposure to paroxetine (Desaunay et al. 2022), a misinterpretation of neonatal symptoms related to transplacental transfer and transfer via breast milk of paroxetine can be discussed in neonates (Costei et al. 2002). A case of severe hyponatremia in an 18-month-old breastfeed infant was reported (Abdul Aziz et al. 2004). A recent combined analysis identified a low M/P ratio (mean 0.63, range 0.05–2.37) (Schoretsanitis et al. 2021).

Sertraline The safety profile was good, thanks to numerous data, a low RID (Pogliani et al. 2019), and low detectable drug in most of the infant's plasma. Another study with meta-analysis showed that levels of sertraline and its active metabolite, desmethylsertraline, were below the limit of detection in most of the infant serums (87.4% and 70%, respectively) (Pinheiro et al. 2015). However, a recent combined analysis found a M/P ratio > 1 (mean 1.62, range 0.22–3.00) (Schoretsanitis et al. 2021). There was no report of severe adverse reaction in breastfed infants. The total score was lower than in the initial version, due to a slightly higher rate of reported adverse reactions. Indeed, a recent prospective study conducted in a pharmacy specialized in breastfeeding reported minor adverse reactions in 13 of 28 breastfed infants; a selection bias was discussed (Morze et al. 2024).

7.3.3.2 Serotonin and Norepinephrine Reuptake Inhibitors (SNRIs)

Desvenlafaxine This AD is an active metabolite of venlafaxine. Its safety profile was very low, due to a high maximum reported RID >10% (Rampono et al. 2011) and insufficient data, although no adverse reaction was reported in any of the infants described. The total drug exposure of breastfed infants has been estimated approximately half that of breastfed infants exposed to venlafaxine via breastmilk transfer (Rampono et al. 2011), and a combined analysis found a high M/P ratio (mean 1.86, range 1.40–2.47) (Schoretsanitis et al. 2021).

Duloxetine The safety profile was low. Although the maximum RID was low (Briggs et al. 2009), there were limited data regarding potential adverse reactions. A recent combined analysis identified a low M/P ratio (0.40, range 0.12–1.29) (Schoretsanitis et al. 2021).

Milnacipran The safety profile was very low, mainly due to a lack of safety data. However, the maximum RID was low (Forest Pharmaceuticals 2012 n.d.).

Venlafaxine The safety profile was low, due to a high maximum reported RID >10% (Newport et al. 2009), detectable drug in the plasma of most breastfed infants. The total score was lower than in the initial version, due to a higher rate of reported adverse reactions, and the description of two severe adverse reactions, i.e., poor weight gain and feeding interrupted by distress and easy fatigability (Tran et al. 2016), and apparent toxicity (Eleftheriou et al. 2022). In addition, a recent combined analysis identified a high M/P ratio (mean 2.59, range 0.85–4.85) (Schoretsanitis et al. 2021).

7.3.3.3 Tricyclic Antidepressants (TCAs)

Amitriptyline The safety profile was low, mainly due to a lack of safety data. However, the maximum RID was low (Bader and Newman 1980). A case of severe sedation and poor feeding was reported (Uguz 2017). The mean M/P ratio in a recent combined analysis was moderate (mean 0.95, range 0.56–1.42) (Schoretsanitis et al. 2021).

Clomipramine The safety profile was moderate, with a low maximum RID (Schimmell et al. 1991), and no adverse reaction was reported in breastfed infant. The mean M/P ratio in a recent combined analysis was moderate (mean 1.08, range 0.89–1.26) (Schoretsanitis et al. 2021).

7.3.3.4 Other Antidepressant Drugs

Agomelatine The safety profile was very low, due to scarcity of safety information, and no available data on RID. No short- or long-term adverse reactions were noted in all but one breastfed infants exposed through breastmilk in a small cohort; one baby showed drowsiness, then developmental concerns of speech and low muscle tone at 9 months of age during follow-up (Kwok et al. 2023).

Bupropion The safety profile was low, similar to the initial version. Although safety data are numerous, the reported maximum RID was high >10% (Davis et al. 2009), and a high proportion of adverse reactions is reported in breastfeeding infants. Two cases of seizure were described in 6-month-old breastfed infants (Chaudron and Schoenecker 2004; Neuman et al. 2014). In addition, a combined analysis found a high M/P ratio (mean 1.95, range 0.63–5.79) (Schoretsanitis et al. 2021).

Milnacipran The safety profile was low, due to scarcity of safety information. However, the maximum reported RID was low.

Mirtazapine The safety profile was good, thanks to numerous safety data, a low maximum reported RID (Kristensen et al. 2007), and no adverse reactions—including severe ones—reported in breastfed infants. The total score was higher than in the initial version, due to new data showing a favorable safety profile during breastfeeding. A combined analysis found a moderate M/P ratio (mean 1.08, range 0.56–1.51) (Schoretsanitis et al. 2021).

Nefazodone The safety profile was very low, due to a lack of safety data, and a severe adverse reaction reported in a 9-week-old breastfed infant, with drowsiness, lethargy, poor feeding, and low temperature (Yapp et al. 2000). However, the maximum reported RID was low (Dodd et al. 1999).

Reboxetine The safety profile was very low, due to a lack of safety data. However, the maximum reported RID was low (Hackett et al. 2006), and there was no severe adverse reaction reported. In addition, a combined analysis found a low M/P ratio (mean 0.06, range 0.05–0.08) (Schoretsanitis et al. 2021).

Trazodone The safety profile was low due to a lack of safety data. However, the maximum reported RID was low (Verbeeck et al. 1986), and there was no severe adverse reaction reported. In addition, a combined analysis found a low M/P ratio (mean 0.14 ± 0.04) (Schoretsanitis et al. 2021).

Vortioxetine The safety profile was low due to a lack of safety data. However, the maximum reported RID was low (Marshall et al. 2021).

7.3.3.5 Neurosteroids Antidepressants

Brexanolone and *zuranolone*. These ADs had low safety profile, due to a lack of safety data. However, the maximum reported RID was low (Deligiannidis et al. 2024; Wald et al. 2022).

7.3.4 Discussion

SSRIs are the most commonly prescribed ADs during pregnancy and postpartum (Molenaar et al. 2020), and showed the best safety profile during breastfeeding among all ADs assessed. Among SSRIs, sertraline and paroxetine showed good safety profiles, with sertraline obtaining the highest safety score of all ADs evaluated. Sertraline and paroxetine are preferred ADs in breastfeeding women in most international guidelines (Larsen et al. 2015; MacQueen et al. 2016; McAllister-Williams et al. 2017; Portet et al. 2024; Sie et al. 2012; Sriraman et al. 2015). Considering that sertraline is also a preferred AD during pregnancy in many international guidelines (Molenaar et al. 2018), it should be preferred in pregnant women planning to breastfeed. In contrast, paroxetine has been associated with higher risks of birth defects and poor neonatal adaptation symptoms compared to other SSRIs (Brumbaugh et al. 2023; Desaunay et al. 2023; Gastaldon et al. 2023; Haddad et al. 2005), and is non-preferred AD during pregnancy in most international guidelines (Molenaar et al. 2018). Therefore, it should preferably be initiated in the postnatal period in breastfeeding mothers.

Citalopram, fluoxetine, and fluvoxamine had moderate safety profiles. Citalopram is a preferred AD during pregnancy according to some international guidelines (Molenaar et al. 2018). However, high reported RID (Pogliani et al. 2019) and M/P ratio (Schoretsanitis et al. 2021) suggest it could pass significantly into breastmilk. Long half-life of fluoxetine and its active metabolite suggest a risk of drug accumulation in breastfed infants, although adverse reactions reported were rare and minor. Some authors and guidelines advise caution in the use of citalopram and fluoxetine during breastfeeding (McDonagh et al. 2014; Orsolini and Bellantuono 2015; Sachs et al. 2013; VA/DoD 2010), while other guideline identify citalopram as a preferred AD during breastfeeding (MacQueen et al. 2016).

Escitalopram was the only SSRI with a low safety profile during breastfeeding. Escitalopram showed the highest rate of adverse reactions in breastfed infants among SSRIs, though most were minor. Guidelines are conflicting regarding escitalopram, with some discouraging its use during breastfeeding (Larsen et al. 2015), while others classify it as a preferred AD (Eleftheriou et al. 2024; MacQueen et al. 2016). Despite its frequent prescription during pregnancy (Petersen et al. 2021), its safety profile has been poorly examined in the context of breastfeeding.

Among SNRIs, venlafaxine has been the most widely evaluated during breastfeeding. Newborns exposed in utero to venlafaxine may be at higher risk of birth defects and poor neonatal adaptation symptoms compared to those exposed to other ADs (Anderson et al. 2020; Desaunay et al. 2022; Gastaldon et al. 2023; Holland and Brown 2017), which is to consider if initiating this AD in a pregnant woman planning to breastfeed. One guideline suggests that venlafaxine should be used with caution in breastfeeding mothers (Sachs et al. 2013). Both venlafaxine and desvenlafaxine have high RIDs and are detectable in most of breastfed infant's serum; however, reported adverse reactions remain low. Duloxetine and milnacipran had low and very low safety profiles, respectively, mainly due to insufficient data despite low reported RIDs.

Tricyclic ADs are generally not prescribed as first-line treatments for major depressive disorders due to their unfavorable safety profiles. Newborns exposed in utero to TCAs may be at higher risk of poor neonatal adaptation symptoms compared to those exposed to other ADs (Desaunay et al. 2022; Gastaldon et al. 2023; Misri and Sivertz 1991). However, available data suggest that the maximum RID of TCAs is low, and these drugs are rarely detected in the plasma of breastfed infants.

Among other ADs from the N06A category, mirtazapine was the only one to achieve a high safety score. Mirtazapine excretion into milk would be very low, and no adverse reactions have been reported in breastfed infants. Bupropion, while widely used as a smoking cessation aid during pregnancy (Robijn et al. 2024), has been associated with a high rate of adverse reactions in breastfed infants, including severe. Other ADs in this category scored low or very low, despite RIDs below 10%, due to limited safety data.

For neurosteroid ADs, there is insufficient data on breastfeeding, which is a concern (Rosen-Carole and Ito 2021). Brexanolone and zuranolone all have RIDs below 10% (ranging from 0.74% to 1.3%). Lactmed reports suggest that brexanolone and zuranolone are unlikely to cause adverse reactions in breastfed infants.

7.4 General Discussion

First, studies in breastfeeding mothers show that under circumstances where mothers benefit from a supportive environment toward breastfeeding, initiation and duration of breastfeeding may improve. Mothers using ADs from pregnancy did not show reduced breastfeeding rates at hospital discharge after preterm birth or NICU admission, where healthcare providers could offer additional breastfeeding support (Leggett et al. 2017). Furthermore, studies conducted in high-income countries with known high breastfeeding rates reported no reduction in breastfeeding duration among mothers using ADs from pregnancy (Galbally et al. 2019; Grzeskowiak et al.

2022). Therefore, pregnant women or nursing mothers using ADs may benefit from breastfeeding support that could be more specific (e.g., trained staff, early and individualized support, advice on AD safety during breastfeeding…), to help them reach better breastfeeding outcomes.

Second, this review with safety score update highlights that all ADs assessed can be prescribed to breastfeeding mothers, although the safety profiles of these drugs vary. Table 7.1 summarizes this document's recommendations concerning AD use during breastfeeding. Both sertraline and paroxetine ranked high, which aligns with international guidelines recommending them as preferred ADs during breastfeeding (Molenaar et al. 2018; Portet et al. 2024). However, other ADs ranked from high to very low, with many guidelines providing no or contradictory information. For such cases, North American and European guidelines indicate that AD prescription involves an individualized risk-benefit assessment (AAP and ACOG 2015; Kittel-Schneider et al. 2022; Sriraman et al. 2015). The Academy of Breastfeeding Medicine suggests that a previously effective AD should be first-line represcribed to a breastfeeding mother, and that an effective AD during pregnancy should be continued during breastfeeding (Sriraman et al. 2015). Similarly, the American Academy of Pediatrics and American College of Obstetricians and Gynecologists recommend to not switch an effective AD to another AD because of breastfeeding, but to continue the AD with close monitoring of the infant's growth and neurodevelopment (AAP and ACOG 2015). In addition, the risk-benefit assessment should consider the substantial benefits of breastfeeding for both mother and child, including on mental maternal health (Henshaw 2023; Kendall-Tackett et al. 2011).

Third, although AD transfer to infants via breastmilk is lower than transplacental transfer during pregnancy (Schoretsanitis et al. 2021), the potential adverse reactions of AD exposure in breastfed children have been studied far less extensively compared to the numerous studies conducted during pregnancy, raising concerns. However, data from the U.S. Food and Drug Administration (FDA) Adverse Event Reporting System (FAERS) indicate that nervous system drugs account for half of the adverse drug reactions reported in breastfed infants (Yalçın et al. 2024). The overall methodological quality of lactation studies on ADs has been deemed insufficient (Den Besten-Bertholee et al. 2019). Most of the included studies in this chapter were small cohorts or case report studies, which may induce selection bias or reporting biases. Some researchers advocate for the establishment of population-based databases to monitor neurodevelopment in children exposed to ADs via breastfeeding (Nallani et al. 2023). In response to these gaps, the FDA has issued draft guidance encouraging pharmaceutical companies to conduct clinical lactation studies on ADs (FDA 2019).

Table 7.1 Expert recommendations based on scientific evidence and clinical experience

Antidepressant class and drug	Maximum reported RID	Adverse reactions in infants	Safety scores A 0–2	B 0–2	C 0–1	D 0–1	E 0–2	F 0–1	Total 0–10	Safety profile	LactMed® main recommendations	Comments on usage during breastfeeding
Selective serotonin reuptake inhibitors												
Citalopram	18.4%	9%	2.5	0.5	1	0.5	1	1	6.5	Moderate	Reported cases of minor side effects (drowsiness, fussiness). If citalopram is required by the mother, it is not a reason to discontinue breastfeeding. Continue citalopram if started during pregnancy or if other ADs have been ineffective; otherwise, prefer ADs with lower excretion into breastmilk (especially with newborns or preterm infants). Monitor the infant for excess drowsiness, restlessness, irritability, poor feeding, and poor weight gain (especially in younger, exclusively breastfed infants, or psychotropic drugs combined)	Possible
Escitalopram	9%	22%	2	1	1	0.5	0.5	0	5	Low	Reported case of necrotizing enterocolitis, case of seizure-like event, and cases of minor behavioral problems. If escitalopram is required by the mother, it is not a reason to discontinue breastfeeding. Monitor the infant for excess drowsiness, restlessness, agitation, poor feeding, and poor weight gain (especially in younger, exclusively breastfed infants, or psychotropic drugs combined)	Possible with caution

Fluoxetine	20%	12%	3	0.5	1	0.5	1	0	6	Moderate	High amount of drug in breastmilk. Reported cases as colic, fussiness, and drowsiness in some infants. If fluoxetine is required by the mother, it is not a reason to discontinue breastfeeding. Continue fluoxetine if started during pregnancy or if other ADs have been ineffective; otherwise, prefer ADs with lower excretion into breastmilk (especially with newborns or preterm infants). Monitor the infant for colic, agitation, irritability, poor feeding, poor weight gain	Possible
Fluvoxamine	1.38%	5%	1.5	2	0.5	1	1	1	7	Moderate	Limited information. Reported case of diarrhea, vomiting, and stimulation. Maternal fluvoxamine up to 300 mg daily would cause any adverse effects. If the mother requires fluvoxamine, it is not a reason to discontinue breastfeeding. Monitor the infant for diarrhea, vomiting, decreased sleep, and agitation	Possible

(continued)

Table 7.1 (continued)

Antidepressant class and drug	Maximum reported RID	Adverse reactions in infants	Safety scores A 0–2	B 0–2	C 0–1	D 0–1	E 0–2	F 0–1	Total 0–10	Safety profile	LactMed® main recommendations	Comments on usage during breastfeeding
Paroxetine	3.2%	9%	3	1.5	1	1	1	0	7.5	Good	Low levels of paroxetine in breastmilk, small amounts ingested by the infant, mostly not detected in the infant's serum. Occasional mild side effects reported (especially after in utero exposure during the third trimester of pregnancy). A preferred AD during breastfeeding. Monitor the infant for agitation, irritability, poor feeding, and poor weight gain	Acceptable
Sertraline	2.4%	8%	3	1.5	1	1	1	1	8.5	Good	Low levels of sertraline in breastmilk, small amounts ingested by the infant, usually not detected in the infant's serum (although active metabolite often detected in low levels). Rare symptoms, similar to neonatal abstinence, in preterm infants. A preferred AD during breastfeeding	Acceptable
Serotonin and norepinephrine reuptake inhibitors												
Desvenlafaxine	10.8%	63%	1	0.5	0.5	0	0	1	3	Very low	Total drug exposure of breastfed infants is approximately half that of breastfed infants exposed to venlafaxine via breastmilk transfer. Monitor breastfed infants for excessive sedation and adequate weight gain if this drug is used during lactation, especially newborns or preterm infants	Not recommended

Duloxetine	0.82%	33%	1	2	0.5	0.5	0	0.5	4.5	Low	Little published information; however, the dose in milk is low and serum levels are low. If the mother requires duloxetine, it is not a reason to discontinue breastfeeding. A better studied drug may be preferred, especially while nursing a newborns or preterm infant. Monitor breastfed infants for drowsiness, adequate feeding, weight gain and developmental milestones (especially in younger, exclusively breastfed infants, or psychotropic drugs combined)	Possible with caution
Milnacipran	5%	ND	1	1.5	0.5	0	0	0	3	Very low	Amounts of milnacipran in breastmilk are low and would not be expected to cause any adverse effects in breastfed infants. Until more data become available, milnacipran should be used with caution during breastfeeding (especially in newborn or preterm infant)	Not recommended

(continued)

Table 7.1 (continued)

Antidepressant class and drug	Maximum reported RID	Adverse reactions in infants	Safety scores A 0–2	B 0–2	C 0–1	D 0–1	E 0–2	F 0–1	Total 0–10	Safety profile	LactMed® main recommendations	Comments on usage during breastfeeding
Venlafaxine	13.3%	9.4%	2	0.5	1	0.5	1	0	5	Low	Metabolite of venlafaxine can be found in the plasma of most breastfed infants; however, concurrent side effects have rarely been reported. Monitor breastfed infants for excessive sedation and adequate weight, especially in newborns or preterm infants, or even measure serum levels of desvenlafaxine (O-desmethylvenlafaxine), to rule out toxicity if there is a concern. Bruxism has been reported in one infant	Possible with caution
TCAs												
Amitriptyline	1.8%	5.2%	1.5	2	0	1	1	0	5.5	Low	Low levels of amitriptyline and its metabolites in breastmilk. Limited data found no adverse effects on infant growth and development. Amitriptyline use during breastfeeding would usually not be expected to cause any adverse effects in breastfed infants, especially if the infant is older than 2 months. Rare sedation has been reported in a neonate. Other agents with fewer active metabolites may be preferred when large doses are required or while nursing a newborn or preterm infant	Possible with caution
Clomipramine	2.2%	0%	1.5	1.5	0	1	2	1	7	Moderate	Limited evidence indicates that use of clomipramine during breastfeeding is acceptable	Possible

Other antidepressant drugs												
Agomelatine	ND	5.8%	1.5	0	0	0	1	0	2.5	Very low	Little published information; possible drowsiness and developmental concerns in one infant, but no problems in 16 other breastfed infants. Infant exposure and adverse effects can be avoided if breastfeeding is held for 4 hours after a dose	Not recommended
Bupropion	10.6%	23.7%	2	0.5	0.5	1	0.5	0	4.5	Low	Limited information. Maternal bupropion doses of up to 300 mg daily produce low levels in breastmilk and would not be expected to cause any adverse effects. Reported case of a possible seizure. If bupropion is required by a nursing mother, it is not a reason to discontinue breastfeeding. However, another drug may be preferred (especially with newborns or preterm infants). For bupropion co-prescribed with an SSRI, monitor for vomiting, diarrhea, jitteriness, sedation, or even measure serum levels to rule out toxicity if there is a concern	Possible with caution

(continued)

Table 7.1 (continued)

Antidepressant class and drug	Maximum reported RID	Adverse reactions in infants	Safety scores A 0–2	B 0–2	C 0–1	D 0–1	E 0–2	F 0–1	Total 0–10	Safety profile	LactMed® main recommendations	Comments on usage during breastfeeding
Levomilnacipran	ND	ND									No information. However, the racemic form of milnacipran has low levels in breastmilk and would not be expected to cause any adverse effects. Until more data become available, levomilnacipran should be used with caution during breastfeeding (especially in newborns and preterm infants). Monitor for agitation, irritability, poor feeding, and poor weight gain	Possible with caution
Milnacipran	5%	ND	1	1.5	0.5	0	0	0	3	Low	Low amounts in milk; milnacipran would not be expected to cause any adverse effects in breastfed infants. Until more data become available, milnacipran should be used with caution during breastfeeding (especially in newborns and preterm infants)	Possible with caution
Mirtazapine	2.8%	0%	2	1.5	0.5	1	2	1	8	Good	Limited information; maternal doses of up to 120 mg daily produce low levels in milk and would not be expected to cause any adverse effects, especially if the infant is older than 2 months. If mirtazapine is required by the mother, it is not a reason to discontinue breastfeeding. Monitor exclusively breastfed infants for behavioral side effects and adequate growth	Acceptable

Nefazodone	6.2%	ND	0.5	1	0	0	0	0	1.5	Very low	Limited information; usual doses of nefazodone produce low but variable levels in milk that would not be expected to cause adverse effects, especially if the infant is older than 2 months. Reported adverse effects in a preterm infant. If nefazodone is required by the mother of an older infant, it is not a reason to discontinue breastfeeding. Until more data become available, other drugs may be preferred (especially with newborns or preterm infants)	Not recommended
Reboxetine	2.5%	ND	1	1.5	0	0.5	0.5	0.5	3	Very low	Limited information; doses of up to 10 mg daily produce low levels in milk and appear to not result in any adverse effects in breastfed infants. Until more data are available, reboxetine should be used with careful monitoring during breastfeeding	Not recommended
Trazodone	0.65%	ND	1	2	0.5	0	0.5	0.5	4.5	Low	Limited information; levels in milk are low and would not be expected to cause any adverse effects, especially if the infant is older than 2 months or when doses of 100 mg or less are used at bedtime for sleep	Possible with caution

(continued)

Table 7.1 (continued)

Antidepressant class and drug	Maximum reported RID	Adverse reactions in infants	Safety scores A 0–2	B 0–2	C 0–1	D 0–1	E 0–2	F 0–1	Total 0–10	Safety profile	LactMed® main recommendations	Comments on usage during breastfeeding
Vilazodone	ND	ND									*No information.* An alternate drug may be preferred, especially while nursing newborns or preterm infants	Not recommended
Vortioxetine	1.7%	ND	0.5	2	0	0	0.5	0.5	3.5	Low	Amounts of vortioxetine in milk are low. If vortioxetine is required by the mother, it is not a reason to discontinue breastfeeding. Until more data are available, vortioxetine should be used with careful infant monitoring during breastfeeding	Possible with caution
Neurosteroid agents												
Brexanolone	1.3%	ND	1	2	0.5	0	0	0	3.5	Low	Low amounts in milk and low oral bioavailability; brexanolone would not be expected to cause any adverse effects in breastfed infants. If brexanolone is required by the mother, it is not a reason to discontinue breastfeeding. Because excessive sedation or sudden loss of consciousness can occur during brexanolone infusion, patients should provide a separate caregiver for any child who is present during the infusion	Possible with caution

Zuranolone	0.74%	ND	1	2	0.5	0	0	0	3.5	Low	Low amounts in milk; zuranolone would not be expected to cause any adverse effects in breastfed infants. If zuranolone is required by the mother, it is not a reason to discontinue breastfeeding. Monitor infants for excessive sedation (especially with higher dosages and in newborns and preterm infants)	Possible with caution

ND no data, *RID* relative infant dose

7.5 Conclusion

Pregnant and postpartum women using ADs should benefit from additional support to achieve optimal breastfeeding initiation and duration. All ADs evaluated in this review can be prescribed to nursing mothers, with sertraline and paroxetine recommended as first-line options and others to be considered on a case-by-case basis. Regardless of the AD used, breastfed infants should be monitored closely, including for weight gain and neurodevelopment. Finally, larger, methodologically robust safety studies are required to better understand the implications of AD use during breastfeeding.

Bibliography

AAP, & ACOG. Breastfeeding handbook for physicians. 3rd ed; 2015.

Abdul Aziz A, Agab A, Kalis N. Severe paroxetine induced hyponatremia in a breast fed infant; 2004.

Anderson KN, Lind JN, Simeone RM, Bobo WV, Mitchell AA, Riehle-colarusso T, et al. Maternal use of specific antidepressant medications during early pregnancy and the risk of selected birth defects. JAMA Psychiatry. 2020;77(12):1246–55. https://doi.org/10.1001/jamapsychiatry.2020.2453.

Arbitman L, Chen S, Kim B, Lee M, Zou P, Doughty B, et al. Assessment of infant exposure to antidepressants through breastfeeding: a literature review of currently available approaches. Pharmaceutics. 2024;16(7):847. https://doi.org/10.3390/pharmaceutics16070847.

Bader TF, Newman K. Amitriptyline in human breast milk and the nursing infant's serum. Am J Psychiatry. 1980;137(7):855–6. https://doi.org/10.1176/ajp.137.7.855.

Battle CL, Zlotnick C, Pearlstein T, Miller IW, Howard M, Salisbury A, Stroud L. Depression and breastfeeding: which postpartum patients take antidepressant medications? Depress Anxiety. 2008;25(10):888–91. https://doi.org/10.1002/da.20299.

Battle CL, Salisbury AL, Schofield CA, Ortiz-Hernandez S. Perinatal antidepressant use: understanding women's preferences and concerns. J Psychiatr Pract. 2013;19(6):443–53. https://doi.org/10.1097/01.pra.0000438183.74359.46.

Begg EJ, Duffull SB, Hackett LP, Ilett KF. Studying drugs in human milk: time to unify the approach. J Hum Lact. 2002;18(4):323–32. https://doi.org/10.1177/089033402237904.

Briggs GG, Ambrose PJ, Llett KF, Hackett LP, Nageotte MP, Padilla G. Use of duloxetine in pregnancy and lactation. Ann Pharmacother. 2009;43(11):1898–902. https://doi.org/10.1345/aph.1M317.

Brown A, Rance J, Bennett P. Understanding the relationship between breastfeeding and postnatal depression: the role of pain and physical difficulties. J Adv Nurs. 2016;72(2):273–82. https://doi.org/10.1111/jan.12832.

Brumbaugh JE, Ball CT, Crook JE, Stoppel CJ, Carey WA, Bobo WV. Poor neonatal adaptation after antidepressant exposure during the third trimester in a geographically defined cohort. MCP:IQ&O. 2023;7(2):127–39. https://doi.org/10.1016/j.mayocpiqo.2023.02.002.

Butler MS, Young SL, Tuthill EL. Perinatal depressive symptoms and breastfeeding behaviors: a systematic literature review and biosocial research agenda. J Affect Disord. 2021;283:441–71. https://doi.org/10.1016/j.jad.2020.11.080.

Chaudron LH, Schoenecker CJ. Bupropion and breastfeeding: a case of a possible infant seizure. J Clin Psychiatry. 2004;65(6):881–2. https://doi.org/10.4088/JCP.v65n0622f.

Cipriani A, Furukawa TA, Salanti G, Chaimani A, Atkinson LZ, Ogawa Y, et al. Comparative efficacy and acceptability of 21 antidepressant drugs for the acute treatment of adults with major depressive disorder: a systematic review and network meta-analysis. Focus. 2018;16(4):420–9. https://doi.org/10.1176/appi.focus.16407.

Costei AM, Kozer E, Ho T, Ito S, Koren G. Perinatal outcome following third trimester exposure to paroxetine. Arch Pediatr Adolesc Med. 2002;156(11):1129. https://doi.org/10.1001/archpedi.156.11.1129.

Da Silva Tanganhito D, Bick D, Chang Y-S. Breastfeeding experiences and perspectives among women with postnatal depression: a qualitative evidence synthesis. Women Birth. 2020;33(3):231–9. https://doi.org/10.1016/j.wombi.2019.05.012.

Davis MF, Miller HS, Nolan PE. Bupropion levels in breast milk for 4 mother-infant pairs. J Clin Psychiatry. 2009;70(2):297–8. https://doi.org/10.4088/JCP.07l03133.

Deligiannidis KM, Bullock A, Nandy I, Dunbar J, Lasser R, Witte M, et al. Zuranolone concentrations in the breast milk of healthy, lactating individuals. J Clin Psychopharmacol. 2024;44:337. https://doi.org/10.1097/JCP.0000000000001873.

Den Besten-Bertholee D, Van Der Meer DH, Ter Horst PGJ. Quality of lactation studies investigating antidepressants. Breastfeed Med. 2019;14(6):359–65. https://doi.org/10.1089/bfm.2019.0021.

Den Besten-Bertholee D, Touw DJ, Damer EA, Mian P, Ter Horst PGJ. Sertraline, citalopram and paroxetine in lactation: passage into breastmilk and infant exposure. Front Pharmacol. 2024;15(May):1–7. https://doi.org/10.3389/fphar.2024.1414677.

Desaunay P, Dolladille C, Chrétien B, Eude L-G, Fedrizzi S, Alexandre C, et al. Neonatal Hypotonia following in utero exposure to antidepressant drugs. J Pediatr. 2022;245:222. https://doi.org/10.1016/j.jpeds.2022.02.028.

Desaunay P, Eude L-G, Dreyfus M, Alexandre C, Fedrizzi S, Alexandre J, et al. Benefits and risks of antidepressant drugs during pregnancy: a systematic review of meta-analyses. Pediatr Drugs. 2023;0123456789:247. https://doi.org/10.1007/s40272-023-00561-2.

Dodd S, Buist A, Burrows GD, Maguire KP, Norman TR. Determination of nefazodone and its pharmacologically active metabolites in human blood plasma and breast milk by high-performance liquid chromatography. J Chromatogr B Biomed Sci Appl. 1999;730(2):249–55. https://doi.org/10.1016/S0378-4347(99)00225-X.

Eidelman AI, Schanler RJ, Johnston M, Landers S, Noble L, Szucs K, Viehmann L. Breastfeeding and the use of human milk. Pediatrics. 2012;129(3):e827–41. https://doi.org/10.1542/peds.2011-3552.

Eleftheriou G, Butera R, Gallo M, Giampreti A, Faraoni L, Contessa MG, Bacis G. Breastfeeding during venlafaxine therapy: a case report of neonatal toxicity. Clin Toxicol. 2022;60:58.

Eleftheriou G, Zandonella Callegher R, Butera R, De Santis M, Cavaliere AF, Vecchio S, et al. Consensus panel recommendations for the pharmacological management of breastfeeding women with postpartum depression. Int J Environ Res Public Health. 2024;21(5):551. https://doi.org/10.3390/ijerph21050551.

FDA. Clinical lactation studies: considerations for study design guidance for industry. In Draft guidance; 2019. Retrieved from https://www.fda.gov/Drugs/GuidanceComplianceRegulatoryInformation/Guidances/default.htm

Forest Pharmaceuticals. An open-label, single-dose pharmacokinetic study in healthy, lactating women. Study MLN-PK-22 2012; n.d..

Furukawa TA, Salanti G, Atkinson LZ, Leucht S, Ruhe HG, Turner EH, et al. Comparative efficacy and acceptability of first-generation and second-generation antidepressants in the acute treatment of major depression: protocol for a network meta-analysis. BMJ Open. 2016;6(7):e010919. https://doi.org/10.1136/bmjopen-2015-010919.

Galbally M, Watson SJ, Ball H, Lewis AJ. Breastfeeding, antidepressants, and depression in the mercy pregnancy and emotional well-being study. J Hum Lact. 2019;35(1):127–36. https://doi.org/10.1177/0890334418758658.

Gastaldon C, Arzenton E, Raschi E, Spigset O, Papola D, Ostuzzi G, et al. Neonatal withdrawal syndrome following in utero exposure to antidepressants: a disproportionality analysis of VigiBase, the WHO spontaneous reporting database. Psychol Med. 2023;53(12):5645–53. https://doi.org/10.1017/S0033291722002859.

Gentile S, Rossi A, Bellantuono C. SSRIs during breastfeeding: spotlight on milk-to-plasma ratio. Arch Womens Ment Health. 2007;10(2):39–51. https://doi.org/10.1007/s00737-007-0173-0.

Grzeskowiak LE, Saha MR, Nordeng H, Ystrom E, Amir LH. Perinatal antidepressant use and breastfeeding outcomes: findings from the Norwegian mother, father and child cohort study. Acta Obstet Gynecol Scand. 2022;101(3):344–54. https://doi.org/10.1111/aogs.14324.

Hackett LP, Ilett KF, Rampono J, Kristensen JH, Kohan R. Transfer of reboxetine into breast-milk, its plasma concentrations and lack of adverse effects in the breastfed infant. Eur J Clin Pharmacol. 2006;62(8):633–8. https://doi.org/10.1007/s00228-006-0140-0.

Haddad PM, Pal BR, Clarke P, Wieck A, Sridhiran S. Neonatal symptoms following maternal paroxetine treatment: serotonin toxicity or paroxetine discontinuation syndrome? J Psychopharmacol. 2005;19(5):554–7. https://doi.org/10.1177/0269881105056554.

Henshaw EJ. Breastfeeding and postpartum depression: a review of relationships and potential mechanisms. Curr Psychiatry Rep. 2023;25(12):803–8. https://doi.org/10.1007/s11920-023-01471-3.

Hoff CE, Movva N, Rosen Vollmar AK, Pérez-Escamilla R. Impact of maternal anxiety on breastfeeding outcomes: a systematic review. Adv Nutr. 2019;10(5):816–26. https://doi.org/10.1093/advances/nmy132.

Holland J, Brown R. Neonatal venlafaxine discontinuation syndrome: a mini-review. Eur J Paediatr Neurol. 2017;21(2):264–8. https://doi.org/10.1016/j.ejpn.2016.11.003.

Jordan S, Davies GI, Thayer DS, Tucker D, Humphreys I. Antidepressant prescriptions, discontinuation, depression and perinatal outcomes, including breastfeeding: a population cohort analysis. PLoS One. 2019;14(11):e0225133. https://doi.org/10.1371/journal.pone.0225133.

Kendall-Tackett K, Cong Z, Hale TW. The effect of feeding method on sleep duration, maternal well-being, and postpartum depression. Clin Lactation. 2011;2(2):22–6. https://doi.org/10.1891/215805311807011593.

Kittel-Schneider S, Felice E, Buhagiar R, Lambregtse-van den Berg M, Wilson CA, Banjac Baljak V, et al. Treatment of Peripartum depression with antidepressants and other psychotropic medications: a synthesis of clinical practice guidelines in Europe. Int J Environ Res Public Health. 2022;19(4):1973. https://doi.org/10.3390/ijerph19041973.

Kristensen JH, Hackett LP, Kohan R, Paech M, Ilett KF. The amount of fluvoxamine in milk is unlikely to be a cause of adverse effects in breastfed infants. J Hum Lact. 2002;18(2):139–43. https://doi.org/10.1177/089033440201800205.

Kristensen JH, Ilett KF, Rampono J, Kohan R, Hackett LP. Transfer of the antidepressant mirtazapine into breast milk. Br J Clin Pharmacol. 2007;63(3):322–7. https://doi.org/10.1111/j.1365-2125.2006.02773.x.

Kwok S, Cupitt D, Kennedy D. Breastfeeding exposure to agomelatine – preliminary findings from an Australian observational cohort study. Neurotoxicol Teratol. 2023;98:107222. https://doi.org/10.1016/j.ntt.2023.107222.

Larsen ER, Damkier P, Pedersen LH, Fenger-Gron J, Mikkelsen RL, Nielsen RE, et al. Use of psychotropic drugs during pregnancy and breast-feeding. Acta Psychiatr Scand. 2015;132:1–28. https://doi.org/10.1111/acps.12479.

Leggett C, Costi L, Morrison JL, Clifton VL, Grzeskowiak LE. Antidepressant use in late gestation and breastfeeding rates at discharge from hospital. J Hum Lact. 2017;33(4):701–9. https://doi.org/10.1177/0890334416678209.

MacQueen GM, Frey BN, Ismail Z, Jaworska N, Steiner M, Lieshout RJV, et al. Canadian network for mood and anxiety treatments (CANMAT) 2016 clinical guidelines for the management of adults with major depressive disorder: section 6. Special populations: youth, women, and the elderly. Can J Psychiatr. 2016;61(9):588–603. https://doi.org/10.1177/0706743716659276.

Marshall AM, Nommsen-Rivers LA, Hernandez LL, Dewey KG, Chantry CJ, Gregerson KA, Horseman ND. Serotonin transport and metabolism in the mammary gland modulates secretory activation and involution. J Clin Endocrinol Metab. 2010;95(2):837–46. https://doi.org/10.1210/jc.2009-1575.

Marshall AM, Hernandez LL, Horseman ND. Serotonin and serotonin transport in the regulation of lactation. J Mammary Gland Biol Neoplasia. 2014;19(1):139–46. https://doi.org/10.1007/s10911-013-9304-6.

Marshall K, Datta P, Rewers-Felkins K, Krutsch K, Baker T, Hale TW. Transfer of the serotonin modulator Vortioxetine into human milk: a case series. Breastfeed Med. 2021;16(10):843–5. https://doi.org/10.1089/bfm.2021.0074.

McAllister-Williams RH, Baldwin DS, Cantwell R, Easter A, Gilvarry E, Glover V, et al. British Association for Psychopharmacology consensus guidance on the use of psychotropic medication preconception, in pregnancy and postpartum 2017. J Psychopharmacol. 2017;31(5):519–52. https://doi.org/10.1177/0269881117699361.

McClatchey AK, Shield A, Cheong LH, Ferguson SL, Cooper GM, Kyle GJ. Why does the need for medication become a barrier to breastfeeding? A narrative review. Women Birth. 2018;31(5):362–6. https://doi.org/10.1016/j.wombi.2017.12.004.

McDonagh MS, Matthews A, Phillipi C, Romm J, Peterson K, Thakurta S, Guise JM. Depression drug treatment outcomes in pregnancy and the postpartum period: a systematic review and meta-analysis. Obstet Gynecol. 2014;124(3):526–34. https://doi.org/10.1097/AOG.0000000000000410.

Misri S, Sivertz K. Tricyclic drugs in pregnancy and lactation: a preliminary report. Int J Psychiatry Med. 1991;21(2):157–71. https://doi.org/10.2190/JDTX-BYC3-K3VP-LWAH.

Molenaar NM, Kamperman AM, Boyce P, Bergink V. Guidelines on treatment of perinatal depression with antidepressants: an international review. Aust N Z J Psychiatry. 2018;52(4):320–7. https://doi.org/10.1177/0004867418762057.

Molenaar NM, Bais B, Lambregtse-van den Berg MP, Mulder CL, Howell EA, Fox NS, et al. The international prevalence of antidepressant use before, during, and after pregnancy: a systematic review and meta-analysis of timing, type of prescriptions and geographical variability. J Affect Disord. 2020;264:82–9. https://doi.org/10.1016/j.jad.2019.12.014.

Morze K, Szałek E, Waszyk-Nowaczyk M. Drug-related problems among breastfeeding patients treated for depressive spectrum disorders. Front Pharmacol. 2024;15 https://doi.org/10.3389/fphar.2024.1440681.

Nahler G. Anatomical therapeutic chemical classification system (ATC). In: Dictionary of pharmaceutical medicine; 2009. p. 8. https://doi.org/10.1007/978-3-211-89836-9_64.

Nallani SC, Baisden K, Dinatale M, Basham L, Kwatra D, Yao L. Clinical lactation studies of neuropsychiatric medications: clinical pharmacology and labeling considerations. J Clin Pharmacol. 2023;63(S1):S159. https://doi.org/10.1002/jcph.2251.

Neuman G, Colantonio D, Delaney S, Szynkaruk M, Ito S. Bupropion and Escitalopram during lactation. Ann Pharmacother. 2014;48(7):928–31. https://doi.org/10.1177/1060028014529548.

Newport DJ, Ritchie JC, Knight BT, Glover BA, Zach EB, Stowe ZN. Venlafaxine in human breast milk and nursing infant plasma. J Clin Psychiatry. 2009;70(9):1304–10. https://doi.org/10.4088/JCP.08m05001.

Orsolini L, Bellantuono C. Serotonin reuptake inhibitors and breastfeeding: a systematic review. Hum Psychopharmacol Clin Exp. 2015;30(1):4–20. https://doi.org/10.1002/hup.2451.

Patterson R, Balan I, Morrow AL, Meltzer-Brody S. Novel neurosteroid therapeutics for postpartum depression: perspectives on clinical trials, program development, active research, and future directions. Neuropsychopharmacology. 2024;49(1):67–72. https://doi.org/10.1038/s41386-023-01721-1.

Petersen JM, Esposito DB, Werler MM. Selective serotonin reuptake inhibitor use patterns among commercially insured US pregnancies (2005–2014). Arch Womens Ment Health. 2021;24(1):155–64. https://doi.org/10.1007/s00737-020-01027-x.

Pinheiro E, Bogen DL, Hoxha D, Ciolino JD, Wisner KL. Sertraline and breastfeeding: review and meta-analysis. Arch Womens Ment Health. 2015;18(2):139–46. https://doi.org/10.1007/s00737-015-0499-y.

Pogliani L, Baldelli S, Cattaneo D, Pileri P, Clementi E, Cetin I, Zuccotti G. Selective serotonin reuptake inhibitors' passage into human milk of lactating women. J Matern Fetal Neonatal Med. 2019;32(18):3020–5. https://doi.org/10.1080/14767058.2018.1455180.

Portet F, Palmaro A, Ortala B, Lefloch P, Dupouy J, Ouanhnon L. Management of major depressive disorders in pregnant or breastfeeding women in primary care: a systematic meta-review. La Presse Médicale Open. 2024;5(May 2023):100049. https://doi.org/10.1016/j.lpmope.2024.100049.

Potts AL, Young KL, Carter BS, Shenai JP. Necrotizing enterocolitis associated with in utero and breast milk exposure to the selective serotonin reuptake inhibitor, escitalopram. J Perinatol. 2007;27(2):120–2. https://doi.org/10.1038/sj.jp.7211640.

Rampono J, Teoh S, Hackett LP, Kohan R, Ilett KF. Estimation of desvenlafaxine transfer into milk and infant exposure during its use in lactating women with postnatal depression. Arch Womens Ment Health. 2011;14(1):49–53. https://doi.org/10.1007/s00737-010-0188-9.

Robijn AL, Tran DT, Cohen JM, Donald S, Cesta CE, Furu K, et al. Smoking cessation pharmacotherapy use in pregnancy. JAMA Netw Open. 2024;7(6):e2419245. https://doi.org/10.1001/jamanetworkopen.2024.19245.

Rosen-Carole C, Ito S. Using Brexanolone for postpartum depression must account for lactation. Matern Child Health J. 2021;25(7):1007–9. https://doi.org/10.1007/s10995-021-03144-0.

Sachs HC, Frattarelli DAC, Galinkin JL, Green TP, Johnson T, Neville K, et al. The transfer of drugs and therapeutics into human breast milk: an update on selected topics. Pediatrics. 2013;132(3):e796–809. https://doi.org/10.1542/peds.2013-1985.

Schimmell MS, Katz EZ, Shaag Y, Pastuszak A, Koren G. Toxic neonatal effects following maternal clomipramine therapy. J Toxicol Clin Toxicol. 1991;29(4):479–84. https://doi.org/10.3109/15563659109025744.

Schoretsanitis G, Westin AA, Stingl JC, Deligiannidis KM, Paulzen M, Spigset O. Antidepressant transfer into amniotic fluid, umbilical cord blood; breast milk: A systematic review; combined analysis. Prog Neuro-Psychopharmacol Biol Psychiatry. 2021;107(August 2020):110228. https://doi.org/10.1016/j.pnpbp.2020.110228.

Sie SD, Wennink JMB, van Driel JJ, te Winkel AGW, Boer K, Casteelen G, van Weissenbruch MM. Maternal use of SSRIs, SNRIs and NaSSAs: practical recommendations during pregnancy and lactation. Arch Dis Child Fetal Neonatal Ed. 2012;97(6):F472–6. https://doi.org/10.1136/archdischild-2011-214239.

Sriraman NK, Melvin K, Meltzer-Brody S, Marinelli KA, Bunik M, Noble L, et al. ABM clinical protocol #18: use of antidepressants in breastfeeding mothers. Breastfeed Med. 2015;10(6):290–9. https://doi.org/10.1089/bfm.2015.29002.

Stull MA, Pai V, Vomachka AJ, Marshall AM, Jacob GA, Horseman ND. Mammary gland homeostasis employs serotonergic regulation of epithelial tight junctions. Proc Natl Acad Sci. 2007;104(42):16708–13. https://doi.org/10.1073/pnas.0708136104.

Tran MM, Fancourt N, Ging JM, Tantsis EM, Nelson T, Sharma R. Failure to thrive potentially secondary to maternal venlafaxine use. Australas Psychiatry. 2016;24(1):98–9. https://doi.org/10.1177/1039856215618528.

Uguz F. Poor feeding and severe sedation in a newborn nursed by a mother on a low dose of amitriptyline. Breastfeed Med. 2017;12(1):67–8. https://doi.org/10.1089/bfm.2016.0174.

Uguz F. A new safety scoring system for the use of psychotropic drugs during lactation. Am J Ther. 2021;28(1):e118–26. https://doi.org/10.1097/MJT.0000000000000909.

Uguz F, Kirkas A, Aksoy ZK, Yunden S. Use of psychotropic medication during lactation in postpartum psychiatric patients: results from an 8-year clinical sample. Breastfeed Med. 2020;15(8):535–7. https://doi.org/10.1089/bfm.2020.0111.

VA/DoD. Management of Bipolar Disorder Working Group. VA/DoD clinical practice guideline for management of bipolar disorder in adults, . Washington, DC; 2010

Vaz JS, Maia MFS, Neves PAR, Santos TM, Vidaletti LP, Victora C. Monitoring breastfeeding indicators in high-income countries: levels, trends and challenges. Matern Child Nutr. 2021;17(3):e13137. https://doi.org/10.1111/mcn.13137.

Verbeeck R, Ross S, McKenna E. Excretion of trazodone in breast milk. Br J Clin Pharmacol. 1986;22(3):367–70. https://doi.org/10.1111/j.1365-2125.1986.tb02903.x.

Victora CG, Bahl R, Barros AJD, França GVA, Horton S, Krasevec J, et al. Breastfeeding in the 21st century: epidemiology, mechanisms, and lifelong effect. Lancet. 2016;387(10017):475–90. https://doi.org/10.1016/S0140-6736(15)01024-7.

Wald J, Henningsson A, Hanze E, Hoffmann E, Li H, Colquhoun H, Deligiannidis KM. Allopregnanolone concentrations in breast milk and plasma from healthy volunteers receiving Brexanolone injection, with population pharmacokinetic modeling of potential relative infant dose. Clin Pharmacokinet. 2022;61(9):1307–19. https://doi.org/10.1007/s40262-022-01155-w.

Weisskopf E, Panchaud A, Nguyen KA, Grosjean D, Hascoët J-M, Csajka C, et al. Simultaneous determination of selective serotonin reuptake inhibitors and their main metabolites in human breast milk by liquid chromatography-electrospray mass spectrometry. J Chromatogr B. 2017;1057:101–9. https://doi.org/10.1016/j.jchromb.2017.04.039.

WHO, UNICEF, USAID, & AED. Indicators for assessing infant and young child feeding practices. Geneva: World Health Organization; 2008.

Yalçın HT, Yalçın N, Ceulemans M, Allegaert K. Drug safety during breastfeeding: a comparative analysis of FDA adverse event reports and LactMed®. Pharmaceuticals. 2024;17(12):1654. https://doi.org/10.3390/ph17121654.

Yapp P, Ilett KF, Kristensen JH, Hackett LP, Paech MJ, Rampono J. Drowsiness and poor feeding in a breast-fed infant: association with Nefazodone and its metabolites. Ann Pharmacother. 2000;34(11):1269–72. https://doi.org/10.1345/aph.10120.

8 Antipsychotics in Pregnancy

Carolyn Breadon and Jayashri Kulkarni

8.1 Introduction

The changing patterns of antipsychotic medication use over the past 20 years have resulted in a dramatic shift in the typical profile of the pregnant woman taking these medications. Several decades ago, the use of first-generation antipsychotic medication was restricted largely to the treatment of women suffering schizophrenia and schizophrenia spectrum disorders. In more recent times the use of second-generation antipsychotic medications has exploded, especially in North America, to treat patients with mood disorders (including bipolar disorders and major depressive disorders), anxiety spectrum disorders (including PTSD and OCD), ADHD, tic disorders, personality disorders, and intellectual disability and developmental spectrum disorders.

Additionally, the use of first-generation antipsychotics in the past may have had the effect of reducing women's fertility through elevated prolactin, effectively arresting the cycle of ovulation. Second-generation antipsychotics do not have this tendency to the same degree, though case reports and clinical experience suggest that individual women may be sensitive to this effect even when taking medications not traditionally considered to be highly active at D2-receptors, such as olanzapine and quetiapine. Hence women taking antipsychotic medication are more numerous, more fertile, and suffer a greater variety of underlying conditions which result in their use of antipsychotic medications in the contemporary era. These women could be encountered in any area of psychiatric practice.

Teratogenic risks of medications are traditionally considered to be at their highest in the first trimester of pregnancy, when women are often not aware that they are pregnant. This means that the care of every woman of childbearing age should

C. Breadon · J. Kulkarni (✉)
Monash Alfred Psychiatry Research Centre, Monash University, Melbourne, VIC, Australia
e-mail: jayashri.kulkarni@monash.edu

F. Uguz, L. Orsolini (eds.), *Perinatal Psychopharmacology*,
https://doi.org/10.1007/978-3-031-99720-4_8

incorporate a consideration of the risks of medication prescribed to a potential unborn child, and psychiatrists must be aware of these risks and communicate them clearly to their patients.

Once a woman is aware she is pregnant her next consideration is a decision about the continuation of pregnancy. For this phase of care a woman must be aware of the risks both to herself in continuing to take a medication throughout pregnancy which may affect her physical health and her experience of delivery, and the risks to her child of congenital defects, adverse events at birth, or of later neurodevelopmental delay.

Again, it is the role of her psychiatrist to inform her of the risks of treatment to her and her baby, balanced against the risks of untreated illness including relapse in pregnancy or the postpartum. Women taking antipsychotic medications in pregnancy may be more vulnerable to metabolic effects including high rates of weight gain and gestational diabetes, particularly those taking second-generation antipsychotics. Both weight gain and gestational diabetes have implications for delivery and neonatal outcomes.

Increasing evidence suggests that most antipsychotic medications do not confer a greatly increased risk of congenital malformations. However, babies may experience neonatal respiratory difficulties and medication withdrawal symptoms at delivery, suggesting that a neonatal ICU or special care nursery should be available. Available data on neurocognitive development of babies exposed to antipsychotics in pregnancy seems to suggest that at 1 year there are no developmental distinctions between these babies and their peers.

Emerging evidence relating to risks of neurodevelopmental delay, autism spectrum disorder and attention deficit-hyperactivity disorder in babies of women treated with antipsychotic medications seems to indicate that babies born to women with a broad range of mental health disorders may be at higher risk of developing these conditions, and that treatment with antipsychotic medication in pregnancy probably does not further elevate these risks.

This chapter aims to provide a concise up-to-date summary of the known risks associated with antipsychotic medication treatment in pregnancy, to aid clinicians in providing best practice care to their patient (and by extension, to their patient's family).

8.2 The True Cost of Relapse in Pregnancy and the Postpartum

Women who are prescribed antipsychotic medications face a decision point when they discover they are pregnant. Anecdotally, many women cease all medications at this point. Recent evidence suggests that this is also true for women taking antipsychotic medications (Petersen et al. 2014). However, this decision can have serious consequences for the mother and also for her unborn or newborn child. Elsewhere, researchers have examined the dollar cost of a relapse of psychosis (Hong et al. 2009). This can't begin to encompass the multiple problems associated with a relapse of psychosis for the individual and society more broadly in terms of financial, interpersonal, occupational, and psychological costs. These costs are magnified and other risks are added in the context of pregnancy and childbirth. In clinical experience, treating a pregnant woman with psychosis in a general psychiatric inpatient unit provokes anxiety and distress for everyone involved in the woman's care, including the woman herself and her family. The risks are evident: fragmented antenatal care, poor attention to nutrition, itinerancy or homelessness, with all the risks to physical safety and health that these situations entail, including the need to commence higher doses of medication in hospital to establish, rather than maintain, a stable mental state.

It has been well established that women are at greater risk of relapse of mood disorders in pregnancy and in the postpartum, when this can manifest as postpartum psychosis. Women with a history of bipolar disorder who are untreated in pregnancy face a very high risk of relapse (Bergink et al. 2012). In the postpartum this relapse carries the added risks of suicide and infanticide (Wisner et al. 2002), alongside the more subtle risks to attachment security and bonding which could occur through separation of mother and baby (Howard 2000) or through the difficulties associated with bonding and psychosis (Howard 2000).

Women living with schizophrenia are perhaps uniquely vulnerable when faced with the challenges of parenting (Hipwell et al. 1996), especially when allied with other factors related to mental illness such as poor social support and economic disadvantage (Göpfert et al. 1996). Howard et al. (2004a) lists the potential pitfalls for these women as follows: "Psychotic symptoms may affect the mother-infant relationship through involvement of the child in delusions, hallucinations or passivity experiences, by making the mother unavailable, or through the absence of desirable behaviours resulting in an impoverished environment for the child." These authors examined outcomes for unwell women with psychosis admitted to mother and baby units in the UK, and advocated for early treatment of psychosis in averting parenting orders and family separation (Howard et al. 2004a).

8.3 Evaluating the True Risks to Women and Their Babies from Treatment with Antipsychotic Medication in Pregnancy

The challenge in correctly identifying the true risk to a woman and her baby from treatment lies in unravelling the risks conferred by a medication from the risks associated with having a serious mental illness. A woman living with schizophrenia or bipolar disorder may have genetic vulnerabilities shared by her child, and may also have multiple vulnerabilities and disadvantages arising from the financial, social, and occupational costs of living with a major mental illness. Taylor et al. (2015) succinctly summarised the current state of research into confounding factors, writing "..the prevalence of these modifiable risk factors in these women is unclear as most studies have used clinical data from specialist services with limited generalisability, or have small clinical samples with limited statistical power to investigate differences between the groups, or have used administrative data of population cohorts with little detail on clinical characteristics." In reality, the field of perinatal research is very limited in data sources by the ethical considerations of research in pregnancy and postpartum, and in the ethical and logistical risks attendant on mother and baby from more traditional "gold standard" research (i.e., randomised controlled trial models). This means it is incumbent on perinatal researchers to analyse observational data sets with sophistication, and consider the outcomes they find in the context of the inherent risks associated with such data. Major potential biases in these studies are confounding by indication, confounding by severity, and residual confounding.

Attempts have been made to systematise the evaluation of the quality of observational studies to improve their utility. The Cochrane Review suggests the use of the ROBINS-I scale and as an alternative, the Newcastle-Ottawa Scale. The ROBINS-I focuses on evaluating risk of bias in estimates of the effectiveness or safety of an intervention from studies that did not use randomisation to allocate interventions. Hence, the ROBINS-I is specifically useful for observational studies using data that is collected in the course of usual clinical care. An update for observational studies, the ROBINS-E, has been published in 2024. Increasingly, recent systematic reviews and meta-analyses have been using either of these scales to guide their choice of appropriate studies for review (Tang et al. 2023).

8.3.1 Risks of Adverse Outcomes in Pregnancy Relating to a Diagnosis of Schizophrenia: Confounding by Indication

Jablensky et al. (2005) examined the underlying risk relating to a diagnosis of major mental illness such as schizophrenia or affective psychosis on pregnancy-related, obstetric or neonatal outcomes in a population of women in Western Australia in the 1980s. They found that women with schizophrenia were significantly more likely to experience obstetric complications, and their babies to experience neonatal complications, than a comparison group without a psychiatric diagnosis. All women with a psychiatric diagnosis (included in this sample women diagnosed with schizophrenia, affective psychosis, and unipolar depression) were significantly more likely to have a severe obstetric complication. Specifically, women with schizophrenia and bipolar disorder were significantly more likely to record placental abnormalities (placental abruption in women with schizophrenia, placenta praevia in women with bipolar disorder) and antepartum haemorrhage in women with bipolar disorder. Women with schizophrenia were significantly more likely to experience foetal distress in labour and their babies to require naloxone treatment at delivery.

In a clever analysis, this team attempted to account for the differential effect of maternal mental illness and treatment by comparing cohorts of women whose first delivery occurred before, and after, their first psychiatric diagnosis. This showed a significant difference in cohorts. Women whose babies were born after their first diagnosis of mental illness (who were thus more likely to be provided treatment prior to and during pregnancy) were significantly more likely to experience obstetric complications. Women whose illness was diagnosed after their baby's birth had similar risk profiles to the general population. This pattern remained when analysing cohorts of women with schizophrenia, and with affective psychosis. The exception to this pattern was the risk of three specific obstetric complications, which remained significantly higher in the cohort of women with schizophrenia regardless of when they were diagnosed: placental abruption, low birth weight for age, and cardiovascular birth defects. This difference could be accounted for by the influence of medication treatment in pregnancy on obstetric and neonatal outcomes, or alternatively relate to severity of illness, which is often greater with early onset of disease.

Gentile (2010) cited various studies to support the risks associated with major mental illness in pregnancy, including placental anomalies, eclampsia, antepartum haemorrhage, premature delivery, low birth weight and APGAR scores, shorter length at delivery, foetal distress, stillbirth, perinatal mortality, and congenital anomalies (Schneid-Kofman et al. 2008; Jablensky et al. 2005; Niemi et al. 2005). This author specifically noted the correlation drawn between schizophrenia and major neurological malformations, preterm delivery, low birth weight, and small for gestational age babies.

Confounding by indication and severity was further examined by King-Hele et al. (2009) by looking specifically at markers of severity of disease (in this case, hospitalisation for psychiatric illness) and comparing the rates of adverse neonatal outcomes including stillbirth and neonatal death with these incidences in the general population. This group found a doubling in the relative risk of stillbirth due to mental health disorders in pregnancy, and an even higher risk in those with alcohol and drug-related disorders (RR = 2.3, CI 1.2–4.2). Amongst women hospitalised with affective disorders, rates of congenital malformations were also much higher than in the general population (RR =2.4, CI 1.1–5.1). Specifically examining women with schizophrenia and related disorders, there was a high risk of neonatal death due to fatal congenital malformations (RR = 2.2, CI 1.1–4.1). The authors discussed other potential contributors to these increased risks aside from the severity of illness, including associated lifestyle factors that themselves contribute to the rates of adverse outcomes. Kulkarni et al. (2014) have also addressed this issue, using various assessments including the Positive and Negative Syndrome Scale and the Edinburgh Postnatal Depression Scale in pregnancy and postpartum, as well as the number of psychiatric hospitalisations as a proxy for illness severity in this group.

Harris et al. (2019) also considered the consequences for women and their babies of psychiatric relapse in pregnancy. This group followed 98 pregnancies to women with a diagnosis of schizophrenia between 2006 and 2017, noting that women with a psychiatric hospitalisation in pregnancy were more likely to use alcohol or illicit substances in pregnancy and more likely to have child protective services involvement, including child removal. However, this group did not have an increased rate of adverse obstetric or neonatal outcomes recorded compared with their peers who were not admitted to hospital in pregnancy: both groups had high rates of antenatal complications, at 63.8–6.5%, including pre-eclampsia and antepartum haemorrhage, and high rates of obstetric and neonatal adverse outcomes including preterm birth (6.9–15%), low (8.6–12.8%), and high (10.3–8.6%) birth weight babies, low 1- (65.8–67.2%) and 5- (81.6–84.5%) minute APGAR scores, congenital malformations (10.5–12.1%), and special care nursery admissions (48.3–61.5%). These outcomes suggest that there is a shared heightened vulnerability for women with schizophrenia in pregnancy and childbirth regardless of relapse of mental illness in pregnancy. This implies that increased medical support and physical health monitoring of both baby and mother are indicated even when a woman's mental health is well managed throughout.

Reis and Kallen (2008) addressed the problem of confounding by indication by investigating birth outcomes for all women taking antipsychotics, including those taking dixyramine and prochlorperazine, commonly used for hyperemesis gravidarum. Thus these women were compared with women taking antipsychotic medications, both first and second generation, for their mental health. Notably, the women taking dixyramine and prochlorperazine did not demonstrate an increase in rates of congenital malformations.

Habermann et al. (2013) formed a contrasting view: as there does not appear to be a significant increase in rates of malformations in women taking either antipsychotic type, the underlying disease is unlikely to have an effect on the risk of congenital birth defects. Citing Sacker et al. (1996) and Bennedsen et al. (1999), these authors write: "Because malformation rates in our study do not suggest a substantial teratogenic risk for second generation antipsychotics and first-generation antipsychotics, and mental illness is not supposed to possess a protective effect on malformation rates, we do not expect an undetected major influence of the disease on the risk of congenital birth defects."

8.3.2 Confounding Through Social Change: The Risk of Long-Term Cohort Studies

Long-term studies that enrol women over the course of more than a decade risk cultural or historical factors intruding into their data. Increasing rates of obesity in the general population over time in England (Newham et al. 2008) or Canada (Sadowski et al. 2013), for example, could affect rates of gestational hypertension or diabetes in the sample taken a decade apart. Similarly, societal change in prescribing patterns, noted by many authors (Kulkarni et al. 2015), could confuse results for large-scale studies which don't specify the type of treatment for a given mental illness. At the start of the 1990s it might have been a typical antipsychotic; by the end of the millennium, it was overwhelmingly more likely to be an atypical.

8.3.3 Risks of Adverse Outcomes in Pregnancy Relating to Lifestyle Factors

Many studies have reflected this reality for women living with a mental illness. Women taking antipsychotics in pregnancy have been found to be more likely to smoke during pregnancy (Sadowski et al. 2013; Kulkarni et al. 2014; Boden et al. 2012a, b; Frayne et al. 2019; Simoila et al. 2020) and to drink alcohol or use illicit drugs (Habermann et al. 2013; Boden et al. 2012a, b; Frayne et al. 2019; Simoila et al. 2020). These women are also often older in their first pregnancy (Hizkiyahu et al. 2009; Reis and Kallen 2008; Simoila et al. 2020) and more likely to be overweight (Boden et al. 2012a, b; Reis and Kallen 2008; Hizkiyahu et al. 2009; Frayne et al. 2019; Simoila et al. 2020) with a lower educational attainment, higher rates of unemployment (Reis and Kallen 2008), and a higher rate of unplanned pregnancy (Miller and Finnerty 1996). These women were more likely to be single or not cohabiting with their partner (Boden et al. 2012a, b; Simoila et al. 2020). Many of the exposed cohort in the study by Habermann et al. (2013) were nulliparous, consistent with other discussions on the effect of illness on fertility and decision-making around childbirth (Jablensky et al. 2005; Laursen and Munk-Olsen 2010). Women seen in Kulkarni's et al. (2014) prospective cohort had low attendance rates at antenatal clinics. Other studies have noted low rates of folate, prenatal vitamin and thyroid hormone use in pregnancy in women with mental illness (Reis and Kallen 2008). Low rates of folate intake in at-risk populations with mental illness have been conjectured to contribute to higher rates of congenital birth defects in this group (Habermann et al. 2013).

In addition to the genetic risks already discussed, Jablensky et al. (2005) also note that risk factors for placental complications could occur in greater numbers in the cohort of pregnant women with mental illnesses; these authors specifically note factors such as older age (>35) and smoking, which could independently increase the risk of this outcome.

Habermann et al. (2013) are the only authors to specifically screen for the use of folate as a confounder when comparing cohorts of women taking second-generation antipsychotics, first-generation antipsychotics, and a matched comparison group. It was notable in this study that the rate of use of folate in pregnancy was markedly lower in both groups taking antipsychotics in pregnancy (85.7% and 85.2%) when compared to women not taking antipsychotics (95.5%), raising the possibility that there are other factors aside from increased rates of smoking, alcohol use and illicit substance use which may also increase the risk of congenital malformations in babies exposed to antipsychotic medication.

Similarly to Habermann et al. (2013), Sadowski et al. (2013) found a lower rate of prenatal vitamin use in the group exposed to second-generation antipsychotics, at 87.6% compared with 99.2% ($p < 0.001$). Sadowski et al. (2013) also found that the exposed women were much more likely to smoke, and much less likely to breastfeed (both differences were statistically significant in this sample).

Taylor et al. (2015) conducted one of the few studies to include domestic abuse as a factor in infant outcomes (low birth weight, small for gestational age, or premature birth), however these authors did not find a statistically significant difference in this measure in women with psychotic or mood disorders as compared with the general population in South London. Statistically significant differences between the two groups with serious mental illness included ethnicity (Black African women were more likely to be diagnosed with a non-affective psychosis), smoking in pregnancy ($p < 0.05$), substance use in pregnancy ($p < 0.05$), age (women with non-affective psychoses were younger), level of recent acute psychiatric illness and single status. There was a high rate of ceasing or switching medications in both groups (40.4%). Both groups were substantially disadvantaged when compared with the general population, were substantially impaired in their general level of function (as measured by the HONOS), and experienced higher rates of domestic violence in pregnancy.

Nilsson et al. (2002, 2008) have examined the issue of confounding factors in assessing risk associated with antipsychotics from several angles. In 2002 this group demonstrated that increased risk for a woman with schizophrenia of having a baby of low birth weight was reduced from 80% to 30% when confounders such as smoking, low educational attainment, and single status were considered. However, as the authors noted, a 30% increase in risk remained. In their subsequent (2008) study, this group found that a diagnosis of schizophrenia made during an inpatient psychiatric admission for either mother or father conferred an increased risk of more than twice for infant death. This association remained after controlling for covariates including age, parity, education, cohabitation, and smoking. Considering the genetic factors in this association, the group then investigated whether the risk of infant death was higher amongst siblings of those with schizophrenia, but this was not the case. Very sadly, the researchers found an even higher risk of post-neonatal death (OR 3.5) than neonatal death (OR 1.8) amongst the children of mothers with schizophrenia. These researchers also found a higher rate of low birth weight babies and small for gestational age babies amongst children of fathers with schizophrenia, thus eliminating the moderating effect of antipsychotics in utero. Despite these findings, the authors felt that residual factors aside from genetics were likely to confer the bulk of risk for babies of parents with schizophrenia.

In a similar spirit, Ellman et al. (2007) examined high-risk pregnancies in Finland, discovering that the babies of women with schizophrenia were at much higher risk of adverse outcomes including eclampsia, premature delivery, gestational hypertension, reduced birth weight (by 173 g), and reduced APGAR at 1 minute (by less than 1) than other babies, but that these women's siblings' babies were not at similarly elevated risk. These researchers found that maternal smoking was likely to be the factor which mediated low birth weight in babies of women with schizophrenia, though other adverse outcomes remained unexplained. The authors hypothesised that increased maternal age, maternal stress, or other health risk behaviours such as poor nutrition, reduced vitamin use, limited prenatal care or substance abuse were the cause of adverse outcomes in the babies of women with schizophrenia, as their siblings did not show any of the patterns of elevated risk that these women did in pregnancy or the postpartum.

8.3.4 Polypharmacy in Pregnancy: The Rule Rather Than the Exception in Women with Mental Illness, and a Potential Confounding Factor Conferring Additional Risk

Most studies (Newport et al. 2007; Kulkarni et al. 2014; Sadowski et al. 2013; Huybrechts et al. 2017; Petersen et al. 2016a, b; Newham et al. 2008; Habermann et al. 2013; Reis and Kallen 2008; Boden et al. 2012a, b) found that women taking antipsychotics in pregnancy were also taking multiple other psychiatric medications, often including anti-depressants, anti-convulsants, lithium, benzodiazepines, anxiolytics/sedatives, and opioids. Of those taking second-generation antipsychotics, 53.1% were also taking another psychotropic medication, as were 67.6% of those taking first-generation antipsychotics in the cohort examined by Habermann et al. (2013). The cohorts followed by Newham et al. (2008) were similarly exposed to multiple agents including venlafaxine, nitrazepam, lithium, zopiclone, paroxetine, amitriptyline, sodium valproate, carbamazepine, and cigarettes. The cohort examined by Sadowski et al. (2013) overwhelmingly took more than one psychotropic, with polytherapy reported by 72% of women. Of these, 44% took 2 medications, 17% took 3 medications, and 11% took 4 or more. The most commonly used medications were antidepressants, benzodiazepines, and anticonvulsants. In common with other authors, Reis and Kallen (2008) found that women taking antipsychotics for mental illness were much more likely to take other psychotropics, including anticonvulsants, benzodiazepines, sedatives, hypnotics, and antidepressants of all types.

Taylor et al. (2015) found a high degree of polypharmacy in patients with both affective and psychotic illnesses; 44.8% in affective disorders vs. 38.9% in non-affective disorders. Of women taking more than one psychotropic, 21.1% of women with a non-affective psychosis were taking 2 agents, and 5.6% of women with non-affective psychosis were taking more than 2 agents in the first trimester of pregnancy. Of women with affective disorders taking psychotropics in pregnancy, 22.5% were taking 2 agents, and 8% were taking more than 2 agents in the first trimester.

Several studies discussed the uncertainty involved in various methods of ascertaining true rates of treatment; self-report, or rates of filled prescriptions being two examples for which there must exist a degree of error. Newport took the further step of assessing cord blood at delivery to determine the percentage of placental passage of antipsychotic medications, correlating this with obstetric outcomes.

Risks associated with some psychotropics (benzodiazepines, anticonvulsants, lithium) are well characterised; risks associated with others (antidepressants) continue to be refined according to newer information. All of these add to the risk to which the pregnant woman and the developing foetus is exposed.

8.3.5 How to Identify the Confounders Which Have a True Effect on Adverse Outcomes?

The challenge in choosing confounding factors lies in correctly identifying these. Lin et al. (2010) attempted to correct for confounders by excluding all women with a history of mental illness other than schizophrenia or bipolar disorder from their study, though it is unclear whether they also excluded women with schizoaffective disorder. They then excluded all women with partners who had a history of mental illness, as they felt this might also have an impact on the parameters studied: low birth weight, preterm birth, and small for gestational age infants. These researchers subsequently adjusted for gender and parity, maternal age, education, marital status, gestational hypertension or diabetes, father's age and education, and family income, but not for smoking, alcohol intake, illicit drug use, or body mass index (as noted by the authors). Lin et al. (2010) also noted in their discussion that they did not assess smoking status, likely to be a major factor in preterm birth and low birth weight in women with a mental illness who have higher rates of smoking than the general population. However, these authors did note MacCabe et al. (2007), who found that the relationship between bipolar disorder and low birth weight persisted even after adjusting for smoking.

However, despite our best efforts, confounding factors may exist which are highly likely to affect results but which remain masked or as yet unknown. Vigod et al. (2015) attempted to address this problem by using high-dimensional propensity scoring (HDPS) in a carefully matched cohort from the general population not using atypical antipsychotic medications in Ontario. This study matched women through their patterns of use of healthcare services, which much more closely mirrored the patterns of women taking antipsychotic medication. Fascinatingly, the maternal outcomes assessed (gestational diabetes, gestational hypertension, pre-eclampsia, eclampsia, and thromboembolism) did not appear to be significantly more common in the studied population, when using HDPS matched comparison groups. Notably, even with the use of HDPS techniques, the matched cohort did not mirror the treatment group in all details, specifically in relation to polypharmacy. To manage this discrepancy the authors subsequently adjusted for prescribed SSRI, non-SSRI, mood stabiliser, and/or benzodiazepine prescribing during index pregnancy.

8.4 Issues Relating to Fertility for Women with Major Mental Illnesses

8.4.1 Fertility and Stress

It is established through animal and human-based research that both mood and anxiety states can negatively affect fertility (McGrath et al. 1999; Haukka et al. 2003; Howard et al. 2002; Svensson et al. 2007; Bhatia et al. 2004). Specifically, stress, anxiety, negative life events, and the experience of depression can all have a negative effect on fertility as measured by cycle-to-cycle rates of conception. It could be theorised that women taking antipsychotic medication may also fall into this category, as women with a diagnosis of schizophrenia or bipolar disorder are subject to the stress and negative life events related to the experience of a major mental illness.

8.4.2 Fertility and Major Mental Illness: Schizophrenia and Bipolar Disorder

It is also apparent that fertility may be reduced in women who suffer from schizophrenia and bipolar disorder related not primarily to their medication treatment, but to their underlying illness. Multiple studies have observed lower fertility rates in those suffering from psychotic disorders (Power et al. 2013; Bundy et al. 2011; Simoila et al. 2018). Simoila et al. (2018) found that of a cohort of women diagnosed with schizophrenia born between 1965 and 1980, 50% of cases (5214 women) had never given birth, compared with 12% of controls. Laursen and Munk-Olsen (2010) have demonstrated a similar trend in those suffering bipolar disorder, though those with schizophrenia were the most severely affected by low fertility rates in this study. These Danish researchers and others (Jablensky et al. 2005) have considered fertility to be a proxy measure for physical and mental well-being, and thus a socioeconomic marker relating to the adversity experienced by those with mental illness. However, other researchers (Lee and Lin 2012; Lin et al. 2010) have attempted to tease out the clustering of adverse fertility indicators associated with major mental illness including poor diet, lack of exercise and obesity, and have found that the increased risk of adverse pregnancy outcomes in bipolar disorder has remained. These researchers considered the possibility of an underlying genetic vulnerability in these women relating to the illness itself, rather than to the surrounding social consequences.

McKenna et al. (2005) commented on the reproductive risks, including reduced fertility (Haukka et al. 2003; Howard et al. 2002), that women with psychotic illnesses face. These include unplanned pregnancies which may be unwanted (Miller and Finnerty 1996), resulting in a higher rate of terminations (Miller and Finnerty 1998), as well as a variety of other risks to the foetus such as higher rates of drug and alcohol use in pregnancy, reduced knowledge about contraception, and increased rates of unplanned sex (McNeil et al. 1984). Kulkarni et al. (2014) noted a rate of 7% of conceptions aided through IVF in their cohort of women with mental illness, approximately double the population rates of IVF pregnancy in Australia at that time.

English (Hope et al. 2020) and Scottish (MacBeth et al. 2023) researchers have continued to find reduced fertility rates in women with non-affective psychosis, with profound differences in the Scottish population for women with psychosis of RR 0.28, CI 0.24–2.32. These results derived from 2007 to 2013 suggest that women with major mental health challenges continue to suffer low fertility despite recent widespread availability of atypical antipsychotic medications.

Hope et al. (2020) considered both live births and terminated pregnancies, and also considered women with major mental illness who took both first and second-generation antipsychotics in their study. Interestingly, this study found that women with affective psychosis had an increase in pregnancy rate over the study period (1992–2017) whereas women with non-affective psychosis did not. Another interesting finding was that women who were treated with any antipsychotic, regardless of type, were less likely to conceive. The rate of pregnancy "almost doubled" in the first 6 months after ceasing any antipsychotic medication. All women with major mental illness were less likely to carry a baby to term than those without this diagnosis. At the time of writing, these studies (Simoila et al. 2018; Hope et al. 2020; MacBeth et al. 2023) comprise three amongst very few studies to track recent pregnancy and birth rates in women with major mental illness. Their findings suggest that the fertility of women with major mental illness is impacted by both their illness and their treatment in ways which are as yet poorly understood.

8.4.3 Fertility and Antipsychotic Medications

Treatment with antipsychotic medication has traditionally been found to have a negative effect on fertility (Ajmal et al. 2014). Historically, this has been linked to the elevated prolactin level found in women taking first-generation antipsychotic medications (Haddad and Wieck 2004). More recently, risperidone seems to be the medication amongst the second-generation antipsychotics which causes the greatest rise in prolactin, and hence suppresses ovulation (Montgomery et al. 2004). Otherwise, the reduced effect of other novel antipsychotic medications on prolactin has been cited as a major reason why fertility rates in women with major mental illnesses appear to have risen in the early twenty-first century (Vigod et al. 2012).

8.5 Obesity and Second-Generation Antipsychotics in Pregnancy

8.5.1 Obesity and Mental Illness

Molyneaux et al. (2014) examined two studies which considered the connection between obesity and serious mental illness. The first, Ban et al. (2012), noted a trend towards increased rates of bipolar disorder, schizophrenia, or other psychotic illnesses in pregnant women with obesity, though this was not significant. Boden et al. (2012a, b) noted a similar correlation, finding odds of bipolar disorder significantly higher for both obese and overweight pregnant women in comparison with pregnant women of normal weight.

A more recent international meta-analysis (Afzal et al. 2021) found rates of obesity for both men and women with major mental illness to be higher than for the general population, RR 3.04, CI 2.42–3.82, and that women with schizophrenia were more likely to suffer obesity than men RR 1.46, CI 1.23–1.72). There was no sex difference found when considering bipolar disorder.

8.5.2 Second-Generation Antipsychotic Medications and Obesity in Women with a Mental Illness

Recent research would suggest that women with mental illness are especially vulnerable to antipsychotic-induced weight gain (Kraal et al. 2017). These views were anticipated over a decade ago by Seeman (2009). In support of this conclusion Seeman cited Koga (2003), who found that the odds ratio for weight gain in women treated with antipsychotic medications for extended periods was significantly higher than for men, and Andersen et al. (2005), who found that predictors for weight gain on psychotropics included female gender.

Freeman et al. (2017), using the Massachusetts General Hospital National Pregnancy Registry for Atypical Antipsychotics, found that women were significantly more likely to have a high BMI prior to pregnancy if they were exposed to atypical antipsychotic medication than otherwise, but that both groups gained a similar amount of weight in pregnancy. This amount was more than is recommended, suggesting that women with a mental illness may be more vulnerable to pregnancy-associated weight gain.

8.5.3 Second-Generation Antipsychotic Medications, Obesity, and Pregnancy

The risk of overweight and obesity for those taking second-generation antipsychotic medication is well known (Allaire et al. 2016; Rojo et al. 2015). Studies in women taking antipsychotic medication in pregnancy demonstrate that a heightened risk also applies in this subgroup. In one UK study (Petersen et al. 2016a, b), 16.5% of women taking second-generation antipsychotics prior to pregnancy (but who ceased before the first trimester) were obese in pregnancy. Rates of obesity increased to 22% in those who continued to take second-generation antipsychotics throughout pregnancy. These elevated rates were strikingly absent in the cohort taking first-generation antipsychotics either prior to or throughout pregnancy; in this group, rates of obesity ranged between 10.6 and 10.8%, comparable with rates for those who had never been exposed to antipsychotics, at 7.3%. These results are echoed by Habermann et al. (2013), who also found a higher median BMI in women taking second-generation antipsychotics (24.2) than those taking first-generation antipsychotics (23.7) or those unexposed (21.8).

Sadowski et al. (2013) noted that women taking second-generation antipsychotics in pregnancy were significantly more likely to be of higher weight than their peers, with mean pre-pregnancy weight of those exposed to second-generation antipsychotics at 74.3 kg and those unexposed at 64.6 kg, $p < 0.001$. Interestingly, there was very little difference in maternal pregnancy weight gain between the two groups. In their 2005 study, McKenna et al. (2008) showed that women exposed to antipsychotics in pregnancy had a higher mean BMI by a large margin, falling within the obese range. 52% of exposed women had a BMI of >27, in comparison with 29% of the unexposed group. This difference was significant ($p < 0.008$). Exposed women also gained more weight in pregnancy than their comparators, though this difference was not statistically significant. In contrast to other authors who have considered clozapine or olanzapine to be the most "obesogenic" (Boden et al. 2012a, b), quetiapine appeared to be the medication taken by the women with the highest BMI amongst the exposed group. Importantly, quetiapine appears to be the most frequently prescribed antipsychotic medication in recent times (Park et al. 2017).

8.5.4 Obesity in Pregnancy and Risks to the Mother

Molyneaux et al. (2014) commented on increased risks for women with obesity in pregnancy, including pre-eclampsia, gestational diabetes, and foetal death, citing Sebire et al. (2001). There is substantial consensus on risks associated with pre-pregnancy and pregnancy rates of obesity for gestational diabetes (Torloni et al.

2009), gestational hypertension and pre-eclampsia (Wang et al. 2013), instrumental and caesarean section delivery (Dzakpasu et al. 2014), and wound infection (Stamilio et al. 2014).

8.5.5 Obesity, Second-Generation Antipsychotics and Mental Illness in Pregnancy: Risks to the Baby

In her editorial, Seeman (2009) commented specifically on the risks associated with obesity in pregnancy, including to the foetus: increased risk of neural tube defects, heart defects, anorectal atresia, hypospadias, limb reduction defects, diaphragmatic hernia, and omphalocoele. This author cited theories as to the increase in rates of these anomalies in the context of obesity, including the possibility of undiagnosed diabetes in the obese mother, and suggested that the use of weight-inducing antipsychotics in pregnancy could lead to adverse outcomes from this mechanism alone, regardless of any direct teratogenic risk.

Gentile (2010) noted the propensity for second-generation antipsychotics to induce obesity, especially in long-term treatment and in women of childbearing potential. He saw the risk of congenital malformations associated with pre-pregnancy obesity itself as an independent risk factor, suggesting that it may relate to undiagnosed diabetes (citing Waller et al. 2007). In his discussion, Gentile also considered the longer-term risks too large for gestational age babies, including later-life obesity, cardiovascular disease, and diabetes (again, citing Waller et al).

Koren et al. (2002) drew a link between obesity in pregnancy and the risk of neural tube defects, specifically in the context of the use of atypical antipsychotic medications, citing Werler et al. (1996) and Shaw et al. (1996). This group observed folate intake of men (of whom 38% were obese) and women (of whom 63% were obese) with schizophrenia, compared with general population rates of obesity in Canada of 25% and 20% respectively. This study established that levels of folate in the diets of people with schizophrenia are below those of the general population (23.2 nmol/L vs. 35.8 nmol/L). Koren's group suggested that both obesity and low folate intake present a risk for women with schizophrenia, who are also more likely to have unplanned pregnancies. Thus, their babies are at risk from multiple factors in relation to congenital defects.

This research has broadened into an exploration of the longer-term implications of pregnancy-related weight gain in recent years (Kramer et al. 2024). Recent papers have linked weight gained in pregnancy to later life cardiovascular risk for the mother (Lee et al. 2015), as well as obesity and cardiovascular risks for infants exposed to obesity in the intrauterine environment (Eriksson et al. 2014).

8.6 Gestational Diabetes

8.6.1 Gestational Diabetes in Women with Mental Illness

Hizkiyahu et al. (2009) found their cohort of women with schizophrenia had higher rates of gestational diabetes than their peers. Simoila et al. (2020) followed a large group of women diagnosed with schizophrenia who had significantly more abnormal glucose tolerance tests than their matched controls ($p < 0.001$).

Petersen et al. (2016a, b) found a strong association between obesity and gestational diabetes in women with mental illness, with an adjusted risk ratio of 5.49 (95% CI 2.67–11.2). Vigod et al. (2014) examined a cohort of women with schizophrenia, and found these women had a higher rate of diabetes prior to pregnancy than an otherwise matched control group (3.9% vs. 1.2%). Subsequently adjusted odds ratio showed no significantly increased risk of gestational diabetes when women with pre-existing diabetes were excluded (OR = 1.13 95% CI 0.90–1.44). This may reflect that women with a pre-existing diagnosis of schizophrenia have already commenced antipsychotic medication treatment prior to pregnancy, and their risk for development of diabetes has already risen. It is worth noting as previously that the same Canadian cohort, when compared with high-dimensional propensity-scored matched comparison groups, did not have elevated rates of gestational diabetes, gestational hypertension, pre-eclampsia, eclampsia, or thromboembolism.

Boden et al. (2012a, b) followed a group of women diagnosed with bipolar disorder who demonstrated a non-significantly increased risk for gestational diabetes; this tendency became more marked in the group receiving treatment. This study did not distinguish between mood stabilisers, considering lithium, antipsychotics, carbamazepine, lamotrigine, and valproate in the same category when evaluating the risk of adverse maternal outcomes.

8.6.2 Gestational Diabetes and Antipsychotic Medication Treatment: Prior to and During Pregnancy

In the 2013 study by Sadowski et al., women exposed to second-generation antipsychotics in pregnancy were not significantly more likely to develop gestational diabetes than the control group. Note that this cohort was also exposed to multiple other psychotropics (though anticonvulsants were excluded). After excluding women with pre-existing diabetes, the study by Bellet et al. (2015) found 4.7% of exposed women developed gestational diabetes compared with 4.1% of the unexposed group. Hence, there was no significant increase in risk associated with the use of aripiprazole.

The second group studied by Boden et al. (2012a, b) (women taking antipsychotics in pregnancy, of whom about half had a diagnosed psychotic disorder) was more than twice as likely to have gestational diabetes as the general population. After adjustment for confounders including birth order, maternal age, country of origin, cohabitation, smoking, and height, these differences remained but were reduced in degree and lost significance in the group only taking olanzapine or clozapine (these were considered the most "obesogenic" by researchers).

Using the Massachusetts Birth Registry for Atypical Antipsychotics, Panchaud et al. (2017) examined outcomes for gestational diabetes. They followed 303 women, compared with 149 controls not exposed to medications, not closely matched for demographics or diagnosis, with none of the reference group suffering a psychotic illness. Both groups had high rates of exposure to other psychotropics

(72% in the exposed vs. 65% of the unexposed cohort), including SSRIs in 31% and anticonvulsants in 42% of the exposed cohort. Interestingly, in the context of other studies discussed, this group did not find an increase in the risk for gestational diabetes in raw or adjusted terms (contrasted with Boden et al. 2012a, b; Petersen et al. 2016a, b; Reis and Kallen 2008). These authors found that a more compelling predictor of gestational diabetes was pre-pregnancy weight, consistent with Molyneaux et al. (2014), Sebire et al. (2001), and Torloni et al. (2009). Panchaud et al. (2017) did find a modest dose effect of medication in increasing the risk of gestational diabetes, but found that this increased risk was also mediated by higher BMI. By contrast, Yeong et al. (2014), examining women with a very similar profile through the Australian National Register of Antipsychotic Medications in Pregnancy, found extremely high rates of gestational diabetes in this population, at 22.1% compared with an expected population rate of 5.5%.

In recent years there has been a proliferation of new research (Park et al. 2018; Galbally et al. 2020; Heinonen et al. 2022) and systematic reviews (Uguz 2019; Kucukgoncu et al. 2020; Wang et al. 2021a, b) which continue to emphasise the links between antipsychotic medication treatment in pregnancy and gestational diabetes. Of the novel antipsychotic medications, olanzapine and quetiapine were associated with significant adjusted relative risk of gestational diabetes in women who continued to take antipsychotics in pregnancy (Park et al. 2018). Galbally et al. (2020) found that women taking risperidone, clozapine, and quetiapine were at significantly higher risk for gestational diabetes. Heinonen et al. (2022) similarly grouped olanzapine, quetiapine, and clozapine together as "high-risk" novel antipsychotics for gestational diabetes, finding adjusted relative risk compared to women treated before/after pregnancy (so, real-world comparator groups) of aRR 1.6 (CI 1.2–2.1).

Uguz (2019) cautioned against the uncritical acceptance of a causal association between the use of antipsychotics in pregnancy and gestational diabetes based on a comparison of treated women with never-treated controls, noting in addition the many methodological issues in relation to existing data: the use of administrative datasets providing limited clinical information (including dose and specific medications), polypharmacy impacting outcomes in several studies, missing data, and limited accounting for confounding by indication, especially considering that schizophrenia and bipolar disorder are associated with higher rates of type II diabetes, which is also associated with gestational diabetes.

In their meta-analysis, Kucukgoncu et al. (2019) found, unsurprisingly, that unadjusted RR of gestational diabetes in women taking any antipsychotic medication compared with never-treated women was 1.63 (CI 1.20–2.22), and adjusted RR was 1.3 (CI 1.023–1.66). Again, this is not a terribly clinically useful result, as the question facing women and their treating clinicians who need to decide on medication treatment in pregnancy is not, What is the difference between this patient and others in the general population who do not suffer mental illness? It is, rather, What are the risks that this woman, facing a relapse of her major mental illness in pregnancy, must contemplate? Hence the authors subsequently moved to compare treated women with women who had ceased antipsychotic use in pregnancy. This outcome was non-significant (RR 0.78, CI 0.281–2.164), an important result. Many of the prior criticisms by Uguz remain relevant, however, in interrogating this data; Kucukgoncu et al. commented that diagnosis in the studies selected for meta-analysis was at times not specified and at times ranged broadly, and given the higher risk for patients with major mental illness, the outcomes might not relate specifically to this highly vulnerable group. Additionally, the authors noted that very limited clinical data was available for many studies, including pre-pregnancy obesity, age at pregnancy, or other relevant risk factors for gestational diabetes, thus making the connection between antipsychotic treatment and gestational diabetes less clear. The authors mentioned that their analysis could not provide for differentiation between different classes of drug or specific drugs, which are known to have diverse modes of action and weight-gain risk profiles. These authors also commented on recent research indicating that a diagnosis of major mental illness itself appears to confer greater risk of abnormal glucose metabolism, citing Pillinger et al. (2017), Perry et al. (2016), and their own prior work in this area (Kucukgoncu et al. 2019).

The third systematic review and meta-analysis, Wang et al. (2021a, b), included six studies already discussed in this paper in detail, using the Newcastle Ottawa Scale to determine quality for inclusion: Boden et al. (2012a, b), Panchaud et al. (2017), Park et al. (2018), Petersen et al. (2016a, b), Reis and Kallen (2008), and Vigod et al. (2015). Pooled meta-analysis of this data showed adjusted RR of 1.24, CI 1.08–1.42. Noting that this analysis did not distinguish between FGA and SGA antipsychotic groups, the authors then provided a meta-analysis of the two studies which focused on SGAs (Panchaud et al. 2017; Park et al. 2018), finding non-significant pooled aRR of 1.12 (CI 0.79–1.60), and of the remaining 4 studies which looked at both groups, finding pooled aRR of any antipsychotic use at 1.30 (CI 1.06–1.60). However, the authors also noted in a post-hoc sensitivity analysis that the oldest study in the group (Reis and Kallen 2008) had a substantial impact on outcomes, at 17.76%; the removal of this study from the pool left a non-significant result: RR 1.19, CI 0.92–1.55. Whilst these authors concluded that exposure to antipsychotic medications in pregnancy is associated with increased risk of gestational diabetes, they also commented on the limited clinical utility of these findings, noting that the pooled outcomes provided do not differentiate between drug classes or specific drugs, also noting heterogeneity in the trimester exposure to medications and dosage, both of which may impact on outcomes for gestational diabetes.

Consistent with research on other sedating antipsychotics, clozapine appears to confer an increased risk of gestational diabetes (OR 2.44, CI 1.14–4.24 in Mehta and Van Lieshout (2017), citing Boden et al. (2012a, b). Mehta and Van Lieshout (2017) also cite case reports of gestational hypertension, excess weight gain and anaemia scattered through the literature over the past 35 years (Vavrusova and Konikova 1998; Gupta and Grover 2004; Barnas et al. 1994). However, women taking clozapine usually suffer more severe psychotic illnesses, and these women are already at risk of adverse outcomes in pregnancy. Unfortunately, as the frequency of these risks is so low, case reports cannot accurately differentiate the contribution of risk from illness as compared with its treatment.

8.6.3 Risks of Gestational Diabetes to the Mother

Vemuri and Rasgon (2007) report on a case of gestational diabetes which they consider could have been directly worsened by olanzapine treatment, as the woman's blood glucose levels became more abnormal after increases in dose of olanzapine, despite no significant weight gain. They comment on the implications of using a medication which may have an effect on obesity, diabetes and insulin resistance, in the context of pregnancy, which itself increases the risk of insulin resistance.

Fascinatingly, Frise et al. (2016) describe the case of a woman whose gestational diabetes they attribute in part to the commencement of olanzapine in pregnancy. This woman developed life-threatening ketoacidosis after an increase in her dose of olanzapine, a reduction in oral intake, and the commencement of metformin. They note the autopsies of several patients treated with clozapine and olanzapine who seem to have died from catastrophic ketoacidosis, and suggest that the combination of pregnancy as a hyper-insulinaemic state, with olanzapine, known in animal models to affect glucose metabolism, should be undertaken with caution.

8.6.4 Risks of Gestational Diabetes to the Baby

Seeman (2009) comments on the risks posed to babies from diabetes in pregnancy, presenting data that suggest an increase in risk of congenital malformations of OR 1.2 per unit increase in glycosylated haemoglobin (Guerin et al. 2007). This data also suggests that good, close glycaemic control is paramount in pregnancy, and provides further support for close monitoring of all parameters for women taking antipsychotics in pregnancy (per Gentile 2010).

8.7 Gestational Hypertension and Pre-eclampsia, Embolic Events in Pregnancy

8.7.1 Gestational Hypertension in Women with Mental Illness

Vigod et al. (2014) found that rates of gestational hypertension were higher in a cohort with schizophrenia (2.8% vs. 2.0%), having already excluded women with pre-existing hypertension. Amongst this group, women with schizophrenia were already at nearly twice the risk of those without this diagnosis (3.7% of women with a diagnosis of schizophrenia, vs. 1.9% in the control group).

Several subsequent studies have examined this outcome (Simoila et al. 2020; Fabre et al. 2021; Toufeili et al. 2022) amongst others. A well-conducted study, Fabre et al. (2021) matched women with schizophrenia with demographic and age-matched controls, finding increased rates of gestational hypertension at aOR 1.42 (CI 1.14–1.76). A pooled meta-analysis (Tang et al. 2023) including these studies and earlier studies already referenced in this chapter suggests a non-significant relationship between gestational hypertension and schizophrenia, $p = 0.325$.

8.7.2 Risk Factors for Gestational Hypertension

Whilst not commenting on hypertension in pregnant women specifically, Seeman (2009) notes that obesity can add to the risk of hypertension, especially in women. Simoila et al. (2020) note their cohort's increased risk of gestational hypertension in the first pregnancy, when compared with controls who did not have a diagnosis of schizophrenia.

8.7.3 The Risk of Pre-eclampsia for Women with Major Mental Illness

Similarly to the finding by Vigod et al. (2014) on hypertension, women with schizophrenia were at higher risk for pre-eclampsia in this study, with approximately double the rate of this complication in pregnancy (OR 1.93 CI 1.05–1.99). By contrast, Reis and Kallen (2008) did not find a significant increase in the risk for pre-eclampsia in their sample of women treated for mental illness with both first- and second-generation antipsychotics. Fabre et al. (2021) found that women with a diagnosis of schizophrenia were not more vulnerable to pre-eclampsia ($p = 0.32$), eclampsia ($p = 0.90$), or HELLP syndrome ($p = 0.50$). However, the meta-analysis by Tang et al. (2023) supports an increased risk of pre-eclampsia in women with major mental illness, $p = 0.021$.

8.7.4 Embolic Risk for Women with Major Mental Illness in Pregnancy

In her editorial on the differential impact of treatments for mental illness on women, Seeman (2009) comments that the risk of stroke in women with schizophrenia has been found to be much higher than for male patients (Lin et al. 2010). Supporting this assertion, Vigod et al. (2014) demonstrated in a large population-based sample that women with schizophrenia were already at higher risk for embolic events prior to pregnancy, with rates more than three times higher than that of the control group (1.7% vs. 0.5%). In pregnancy this risk remained significantly higher in women with schizophrenia, with a doubling of risk for this group compared with controls: unadjusted odds ratio of 2.20 (CI 1.36–3.55).

Vigod et al. (2020) utilised a population-based register linked with birth data to examine a cohort of Canadian women between 2006 and 2011. Unfortunately this data did not include maternal BMI, but did capture a population of women with a schizophrenia diagnosis, considering both direct and indirect mediators to adjust for relative risk of adverse outcomes. Consistent with earlier research, women with schizophrenia were significantly older, poorer, and more likely to smoke cigarettes, drink alcohol or use illicit drugs. They were also significantly more likely to have had prior preterm birth, a prior surgical termination of pregnancy, and to be diagnosed with HIV. They were more vulnerable to outcomes such as venous thromboembolism ($p = 0.002$), pre-eclampsia/eclampsia ($p < 0.0001$), and placental abruption ($p = 0.0002$). I note a significantly higher rate of thromboembolic disease found in the meta-analysis by Tang et al. (2023), reviewing recent findings by Fabre et al. (2021), Simoila et al. (2020), and Vigod et al. (2020), at $p < 0.001$.

8.7.5 Embolic Risk in Pregnancy Relating to Antipsychotic Use

Seeman (2009) further comments specifically on the effect of antipsychotics of both classes on the risk of thromboembolism. She cites studies showing a seven-fold increase of primary venous thromboembolism (Zornberg and Jick 2000) associated with the use of antipsychotic medication, and suggests that this risk must only escalate in the context of pregnancy, which is itself a period of higher risk of embolic events.

8.8 Obstetric Outcomes for Women with Mental Illness in Pregnancy

The 2014 study by Vigod et al. showed women with schizophrenia at significantly greater risk for a variety of adverse outcomes including placental abruption, septic shock, induction of labour, caesarean section, transfer to ICU, readmission to hospital within 3 months, and maternal death. In particular, Vigod et al. (2014) singles out maternal death, as despite being a very rare outcome overall, it remains five times more likely for women with schizophrenia (adjusted odds ratio 5.64, CI 1.39–23.0). However, in the same authors' 2015 re-examination of the same patient group, comparison with matched cohorts did not show any of these elevated risks in the treatment group, aside from labour induction and operative vaginal delivery.

Matevosyan (2011) took a highly structured approach to the analysis of risk conferred by the diagnosis of schizophrenia, pooling data from multiple studies to arrive at odds ratios of various outcomes for pregnant women with schizophrenia. This author found that these women were not at statistically greater risk of induction of labour or emergency caesarean section than their peers.

Women with bipolar disorder were much more likely to have instrumental deliveries than their peers, especially those who were treated with medication (OR = 1.39, 1.09–1.79, Boden et al. 2012a, b). Those treated were also much more likely to have caesarean section delivery (OR 1.56 CI 1.20–2.03), or to be induced (OR = 2.12, CI 1.68–2.67).

8.8.1 Caesarean Section Delivery in Women Taking Antipsychotics in Pregnancy

Diav-Citrin et al. (2005) found that women treated with haloperidol were more likely to have caesarean deliveries (25.5% vs. 16.3%, $p = 0.014$).

Sadowski et al. (2013) found a higher rate of planned caesarean section, at 11.5% in women exposed to second-generation antipsychotics in pregnancy, compared with 2.6% in those unexposed. Reis and Kallen's (2008) treatment cohort also had a significantly higher rate of caesarean section than those not taking antipsychotic medication for a mental health indication, or not taking medication at all. This study also found an increased risk of placental abruption and induction of labour in women treated for mental health problems, but neither of these outcomes reached significance. Vigod et al. (2020) further examined a clinical registry-linked dataset, described previously. Again, consistent with prior research, women with schizophrenia were more likely to have a caesarean section birth ($p = 0.011$).

Kulkarni et al. (2014) examined 147 women taking typical and atypical antipsychotics in pregnancy for psychotic and mood disorders. This group demonstrated high rates of caesarean section at 40%, compared with the expected population rate of 31.5%.

Interestingly, Petersen et al. (2016a, b) found that rates of caesarean section were higher in women who took antipsychotic medication in pregnancy than those who had never been exposed to this, but that the significance of this difference disappeared when adjusting for health and lifestyle factors. High rates of caesarean section were seen in women taking both typical (26.8%) and atypical (24.6%) antipsychotics in pregnancy, compared with the general population cohort (18%).

8.9 Congenital Malformations and Antipsychotic Medications

Rates of congenital malformations found in babies of women taking antipsychotic medications are only meaningful when compared with accurate rates for the general population (and even more so when compared with accurate rates in babies born to mothers diagnosed with a major mental illness who are not taking antipsychotic medications in pregnancy). Over time, reported rates for congenital malformations in the general population have varied widely in different settings around the world, from 2.0 to 5.5 (Brunner et al. 2013). A recent survey of 20% of the American population suggests that the rate of congenital malformations in this ethnically and socioeconomically diverse nation is 28.9/1000 (Egbe et al. 2015). The authors note this to be a conservative estimate as it excludes stillbirth and terminations.

Additionally, a distinction should be drawn between major malformations, with implications for survival or lifelong illness, and minor malformations, which may be mild cosmetic defects that are easily correctable. Some investigators make this distinction and others do not.

There is a broad range of data available on congenital malformations. That which applies to first-generation antipsychotics often borrows from the use of phenothiazines over the past 40+ years for nausea in pregnancy. The use of this data could be considered problematic, as it isn't assessing women treated for major mental illnesses, and doses are typically small and intermittent. Hence these data sets probably don't really examine the true risks for the population of women living with major mental illnesses, whether bipolar disorder or schizophrenia. However, some authors have defended this practice, arguing that it eliminates confounding by indication; that if schizophrenia itself confers an increased risk of malformations, then using data from women who don't have this diagnosis will eliminate this confounder.

8.9.1 Managing Confounding by Indication: What Is the Risk of Congenital Malformations Associated with Underlying Mental Illness in Pregnancy?

Reis and Kallen (2008) found an increase in the rates of congenital malformations in women taking antipsychotic medication for their mental health, compared with women taking antipsychotic medication for hyperemesis. When these numbers were adjusted to consider only major malformations, this difference became statistically significant. These authors excluded preauricular tags, tongue tie, patent ductus arteriosus at preterm birth, single umbilical artery, undescended testis, unstable hip, and naevus. These authors also excluded babies with chromosomal abnormalities.

In common with other authors, Reis and Kallen (2008) found that women taking antipsychotics for mental illness were significantly less likely than their peers to take multivitamins, folate, or thyroid hormone, but much more likely to take other psychotropics, including anticonvulsants, benzodiazepines, sedatives, hypnotics, and antidepressants of all types.

Other authors take a different approach to confounding by indication. Petersen et al. (2016a, b) examined data from general practice databases in the UK, comparing three groups of women: those who had taken antipsychotics prior to pregnancy, but ceased; those who took antipsychotics throughout pregnancy; and those who had never been exposed to antipsychotic medication. In this study, 3.4% of women taking antipsychotics throughout pregnancy (416 women) had babies with major congenital malformations, in comparison with 2.2% of women taking antipsychotics prior to, but not during pregnancy (670 women), and 2.1% of those women not exposed to antipsychotics (the reference cohort of 319,520). The difference between these cohorts was not statistically significant (adjusted risk ratio = 1.59 with 95% CI 0.84–3.00). This was a compelling study as it attempted to distinguish the risk associated with diagnosis from the risk associated with medication treatment in pregnancy. However, this may only have eliminated the risk for women with illnesses that were not severe enough to require medication treatment throughout pregnancy. If these less unwell women were at lesser risk of congenital malformations, this study might have missed this distinction.

A more recent study across multiple countries (Huybrechts et al. 2023) showed a pooled absolute risk of congenital malformation amongst unexposed babies was

2.7%, and that for unexposed babies of women with a mental health condition (including schizophrenia, bipolar disorder, OCD, ADHD, depression and anxiety) this risk increased to 3.7%. This suggests a strong contribution of underlying genetic, epigenetic, or other factors in babies of women with mental health disorders.

8.9.2 Schizophrenia and the Risk of Congenital Malformations, Specifically Cardiovascular Risk

Jablensky et al. (2005) provided one of the earlier large-scale population-based data sets from which to examine low-incidence events such as congenital malformations. For that reason, and for its rigour of analysis, this was a seminal paper. The drawback of this approach was that medication and other treatment for the individual, as well as other data affecting risk of teratogenesis, were not available. These authors found no significant increase in overall birth defects in women with schizophrenia compared with the reference group, though there was a trend (6.0% vs. 4.9%). When examining specific defects, however, this study found a significant increase in cardiovascular anomalies, including atrial and ventricular septal defects, patent ductus arteriosus, and aortic anomalies (adjusted odds ratio 2.50) in babies of women with schizophrenia, as well as a significant increase in minor physical abnormalities. Jablensky singles out patent ductus arteriosus, with a ten-fold increase in incidence in babies of women with schizophrenia, ventricular septal defect (with a three-fold increase in risk), and atrial septal defect, with a doubling of risk.

These authors suggest that all of these abnormalities have a strong genetic component, and hypothesise a mechanism: patent ductus arteriosus linked to abnormal expression of the prostaglandin receptor, an abnormality also found in people with schizophrenia and their relatives; ventricular septal defect linked to velocardifacial syndrome, which in turn confers a higher risk for schizophrenia; and atrial septal defect linked to chromosome 6p21.3 deletion, also related to schizophrenia risk. Vigod et al. (2014) found an increased risk for congenital anomalies (adjusted odds ratio of 1.94 with CI 1.56–2.41) for babies of women with schizophrenia, but did not include information on treatment modality. Pooling data on risk relating to a diagnosis of schizophrenia, Matevosyan (2011) found that rates of congenital defects were significantly higher in babies of mothers with schizophrenia (RR 2.1, CI 1.1–3.8), though these defects were not further characterised in this study. Hizkiyahu et al. (2009) found a significantly higher rate of congenital malformations in a cohort of women with schizophrenia than their comparators: 11.3% vs. 5.2%. Both of these rates are so high that they suggest that minor as well as major malformations may have been considered as part of this study.

8.9.3 Bipolar Disorder and the Risk of Congenital Malformations

Specifically examining women with bipolar disorder, Boden et al. (2012a, b) did look at congenital malformations in patients taking antipsychotic medications, though did not further stratify these patients into medication class. These authors found a malformation rate of 3.5% in this group, with p of 0.11; 1 each of talipes equinovarus, cleft palate, urinary system agenesis, and heart malformation.

A more recent paper (Chan et al. 2024) considered "treated" and "untreated" women with bipolar disorder and examined a range of adverse outcomes, including congenital malformations. The outcomes of this otherwise well-conducted paper were tainted by the unfortunate decision to include all "mood stabilisers", including sodium valproate, lithium, and antipsychotic medications, in a single category, possibly due to low numbers of women treated in pregnancy. As all of these medications have diverse modes of action and differing known associations with congenital malformations, this did not help to clarify the risk related to the use of antipsychotics in pregnancy and congenital malformations.

8.9.4 Typical Antipsychotic Medication and the Risk of Congenital Malformations

An older large-scale study of typical antipsychotics (Diav-Citrin et al. 2005) was an international collaboration which followed 188 women prescribed haloperidol at therapeutic doses for major mental illness (median 5 mg/day) throughout pregnancy, including in the first trimester in 78.2% of women. Most of these women, as in other studies, were also taking other medication (75%). These women were also, as in other studies, more likely to be older and to smoke than the reference group. This study found no statistical increase in the rate of major malformations in the group treated with haloperidol.

Munk et al. (2005) found increased rates of congenital abnormalities which did not reach significance in a small cohort of 69 babies exposed to first-generation antipsychotics when compared with the general population in several Danish counties.

Huybrechts et al. (2023) found a risk of congenital malformations in babies exposed to typical antipsychotics in pregnancy of 3.1% (CI 2.7–3.5%), actually lower than their unexposed comparator groups whose mothers had a history of mental health diagnosis (3.7%).

8.9.5 Typical Versus Atypical Antipsychotic Medication: Is There a Difference in Risk?

8.9.5.1 Voluntary Reporting Cohorts and Case-Control Studies of Congenital Abnormalities in Babies Exposed to Atypical Antipsychotics in Utero

I note the retrospective study by Wichman (2009) of 16 babies exposed in utero to atypical antipsychotics, compared with a tertiary hospital peer cohort. The rate of malformations was 6.25% (one baby) in this (very low powered) study, with 3 babies exhibiting heart murmurs which resolved by the end of the first year.

Brunner et al. (2013) found a congenital malformation rate of 4.4% in 610 pregnancies using voluntary reporting to Eli Lilly of pregnancy outcomes for women exposed to olanzapine. The authors suggest that the general population rate of malformations is 3–5%, and hence 4.4% falls within the expected reference range, consistent with most international surveillance authorities (Public Health Agency of Canada 2013).

McKenna et al. (2005) provide an earlier, but well-conducted study of rates of congenital malformations amongst babies exposed to atypical antipsychotics in pregnancy, comparing exposed women with unexposed age-matched peers. They found that the exposed group was overall more likely to have high rates of factors known to worsen the outcome of pregnancy, including having an unplanned pregnancy (57% vs. 23%) and not taking folate or multivitamins during pregnancy (15% vs. 2%). Interestingly, both groups reported relatively high rates of alcohol use in pregnancy (14% vs. 12%), but there was a substantial difference in smoking rates (38% vs. 13%). This study, as most others, reported a high rate of polypharmacy in women taking psychotropics, with 57% also taking an antidepressant, 34% a benzodiazepine and 17% an anticonvulsant (of whom 72% were taking valproate). These authors found a rate of major malformations in babies exposed to atypical antipsychotics of 0.9% vs. 1.5%, both lower than that found in most general population samples.

Cohen et al. (2016) reported on results from the National Pregnancy Registry for Atypical Antipsychotics at Massachusetts General Hospital, similar to the NRAMP study in Australasia, to track outcomes for women taking second-generation antipsychotic medication in pregnancy. This group published data on 214 babies exposed in pregnancy, and found there was no significant increase in risk in the exposed group (1.4%, CI 0.29–4.04). Unadjusted odds ratio found an increase in rates of 1.25 in exposed babies over those unexposed. However, after performing sensitivity analysis, these authors used propensity scoring to assess for the relative contribution of confounders they considered, using the diagnosis of bipolar disorder as a basis for comparison. Confounders considered included smoking, stimulant, illicit drug or alcohol use in the first trimester, concomitant anticonvulsant, lithium, anxiolytic, sedative, antidepressant, or typical antipsychotic use, a diagnosis of depression or anxiety, chronicity of illness, the use of prenatal vitamins, ethnicity, age, BMI, or planned pregnancy. Incorporating these factors reduced the adjusted odds ratio to close to parity. However, excluding women taking known teratogens including valproate, lithium, isotretinoin, and illicit drugs, the odds ratio returned to 1.25.

Outcomes from this register were updated in 2021 (Viguera et al. 2021) with an increased pool of 640 live births in the exposed group and 704 controls. This study showed a non-significant increased OR of 1.48, CI 0.625–3.517. The authors also noted that there was no organ-specific or other pattern in relation to the congenital malformations identified, suggesting that there was no particular mechanism that could be identified which would unify these outcomes.

8.9.5.2 Large-Scale Studies Examining Rates of Congenital Abnormalities in Women Taking Atypical Antipsychotics: Habermann et al. (2013), Huybrechts et al. (2016), Montastruc et al. (2016)

Habermann et al. (2013) found a statistical difference between the rates of congenital abnormalities in babies of women taking second-generation antipsychotics and those unexposed (OR 2.13, 95% CI 1.19–3.80), though not between babies of those taking first-generation antipsychotics and those unexposed (OR 1.75, 95% CI 0.80–3.80). This group adjusted carefully for known confounders, including maternal age, alcohol consumption, smoking, BMI, past history of malformations in pregnancy, and past history of miscarriage. Of these, only alcohol had a significant influence on the outcome and was therefore included in the final analysis. The difference in incidence remained significant after this adjustment. No specific second-generation antipsychotic was associated with statistically significant differences in rates, though these rates did vary; a rate of 3.59% was found with quetiapine (5/139) and 6.81% (3/44) with aripiprazole. No malformations were observed with amisulpride (though low numbers were examined: 13) or zotepine (2).

Habermann et al. (2013) drew a distinction between major and minor malformations, and though these authors found a slightly higher rate of minor malformations in the group of women taking first-generation antipsychotics (5.5%) than those taking second-generation antipsychotics (3.2%), this difference was not significant.

Huybrechts et al. (2016) published a large-scale dataset examining 1.3 million pregnancies, of whom 9258 took an atypical antipsychotic in the first trimester and 733 took a typical antipsychotic during the same period. In common with other research (Habermann et al. 2013; Kulkarni et al. 2014), the most commonly used atypical antipsychotic medication was quetiapine (46% of all atypical prescriptions). These authors observed that, as in other studies, women who took antipsychotic medication in pregnancy were generally older, in poorer health, and used more other medications and illicit drugs known to be associated with congenital defects than their peers. Therefore, these researchers controlled for indication and other confounders including smoking, ethnicity, age, obesity, and general physical and obstetric morbidity. Considering the large number of factors controlled for, this study used propensity scores as a method of data reduction. Absolute risk of congenital defects for those treated with atypical antipsychotics was higher at 4.5% (95% CI 40.5–48.9) than for those treated with typical antipsychotics at 3.8% (95% CI 26.6–54.7) or the baseline risk in the general population in this study of 3.3%.

Overall unadjusted cardiac risks were greater for babies of all women taking antipsychotic medications, but disappeared for those taking typical antipsychotic medications when psychiatric illness was accounted for. Huybrechts et al. (2016) noted that a large component of the increased risk for both overall and cardiovascular anomalies in babies exposed to atypical antipsychotics was accounted for by risperidone. The updated study published in 2023 (Huybrechts et al. 2023) did not confirm this preponderance of risperidone in affected babies, but did demonstrate an increase in rates of babies exposed to olanzapine developing oral cleft abnormalities.

Consistent with the outcomes for Huybrecht's group, Monstastruc et al. 2016) noted in a very large scale study examining all outcomes from the World Health Organisation Collaborating Centre for International Drug Monitoring over four decades, that only two second-generation antipsychotic medications showed a signal of increased risk of congenital malformations: risperidone and aripiprazole, specifically in relation to gastrointestinal malformations. This is a surprising finding, as major gastrointestinal abnormalities (oesophageal atresia, anorectal atresia; some authors include in this list cleft lip and palate) are not commonly noted in the literature to date in relation to novel antipsychotics. This group also found a signal for phenothiazine medications with a piperazine side chain. However, the widespread use of these medications for nausea in pregnancy throughout the past 60 years might influence the utility of this finding in relation to antipsychotic medications specifically used for mental illness. By contrast, risperidone and aripiprazole are very rarely prescribed for nausea in pregnancy. The authors were cautious not to attribute causality to this finding, but did note the necessity for further research on medication-specific risks of teratogenicity, echoing other authors such as Gentile (2010). Considering the possibility that specific medications could confer specific risks, it is worthwhile examining some of these medications in more detail.

8.9.5.3 Retrospective Reviews of Data Reporting Congenital Abnormalities

Einarsson and Boskovic (2009), of the Motherisk team at the Hospital for Sick Children in Toronto, performed a retrospective review of all studies relating to typical and atypical antipsychotics at that time. These authors discussed phenothiazines including promethazine, widely used for nausea in pregnancy, and noted that these medications do not seem to be associated with any known adverse outcomes for babies. Prochlorperazine, also widely used for nausea, was used in the first trimester in 877 pregnancies, and did not result in an increase in the rate of congenital abnormalities (Slone et al. 1977). Similarly, Briggs et al. (2008) found no increase in risk above baseline in 704 babies after first-trimester exposure to prochlorperazine. These researchers found a study in 1982 which evaluated 264 women taking chlorpromazine in pregnancy for nausea, with no increase in the rate of malformations amongst their babies (Hannah et al. 1982). Einarsson cites Diav-Citrin et al. (2005) in relation to haloperidol with no increased risk found, and Slone et al. (1977) in relation to perphenazine (no increased risk found in relation to perinatal mortality, birth weight, or intelligence at 4 years). Trifluoperazine, now rarely used in most centres, was evaluated in relation to risk of exposure in early pregnancy in a study of 480 women, for whom the incidence of birth defects was 1.1%; well within the expected incidence of the general population (Moriarty et al. 1963). For completeness' sake, Einarsson et al. (Einarsson and Boskovic 2009) include data on loxapine (3 cases of abnormalities including achondroplasia, unspecified malformations, and tremors at 15 weeks old Heel et al. 1978), and thioridazine (2 major malformations in 63 exposed newborns Briggs et al. 2008). Einarsson reports extremely limited data on flupenthixol (3 pregnancies reported without abnormalities) and fluphenazine (Briggs et al. 2008).

Though these authors did not further discuss the results, they mentioned that post-marketing data for clozapine included 523 cases of known exposure to clozapine in pregnancy, which resulted in 22 reports of malformations without any pattern of defects found. Similarly, correspondence with the manufacturers by the authors resulted in a report of 144 prospective and 98 retrospective pregnancy outcomes for women taking olanzapine with no increase in rates of malformations, but no further information regarding these. Discussion with the manufacturer of quetiapine by the authors resulted in 298 pregnancy exposures, of which there were 14 reports of congenital anomalies with no pattern of defects found. Discussion with manufacturers of ziprasidone by the authors revealed 57 known pregnancy outcomes, of which 50 showed no malformation, 5 had miscarriages, one twin pair of which one of the twins had a malformation, and one woman had a stillbirth. The frustrating aspect of these relatively large data samples is the paucity of further information on women and their babies in every category, limiting their utility for ascertaining risk.

Gentile (2010) painstakingly collated all available data, including case reports, on both typical and atypical antipsychotics at the time of writing, and found inadequate human data to guide prescribing on amisulpride, ziprazidone and sertindole. He found 3 case reports on aripiprazole. Hence he advised avoidance of all these medications in pregnancy due to limited data. He found 200 babies exposed to clozapine in utero, of whom there were 15 cases of congenital malformation reported, though these could not be further investigated in most cases. He found 419 cases of olanzapine-exposed foetuses, of whom 26 had congenital malformations, including neural tube defects in 4. Further, this study found 227 babies exposed to quetiapine, of whom 8 had congenital malformations, not further specified, and 321 babies exposed to risperidone, of whom 15 had congenital malformations. 411 babies were exposed to haloperidol in utero, of whom 14 cases of foetal abnormalities were observed, including 3 limb malformations. Gentile notes the risks of late uterine exposure associated with haloperidol, including body temperature instability. He also found over 400 cases of exposure to chlorpromazine, of which only 5 cases of malformations were described. His recommendations based on this review are discussed elsewhere.

8.9.5.4 Meta-Analyses of Data Reporting Congenital Abnormalities

Coughlin et al. (2015) attempted to provide a comprehensive analysis of available data, given the small sample sizes of most studies. This meta-analysis compiled results from 3346 babies over a variety of outcomes. Investigators noted a large degree of heterogeneity amongst trials, but no publication bias. This study found no significant difference between the rates of congenital malformations for babies exposed to either typical or atypical antipsychotics. The most common abnormality reported was a heart defect. This meta-analysis found that exposure to antipsychotic medication, typical or atypical, significantly increased the risk of heart defects with OR 2.09, CI 1.50–2.91, $p < 0.001$.

A similar approach to aggregating data was undertaken by Terrana et al. (2015), focusing on outcomes for babies of mothers taking second-generation antipsychotics in pregnancy, specifically congenital malformations. Examining all reported case-control studies, this group found an aggregate of 12 studies meeting at least level 6 on the Newcastle-Ottawa Assessment Scale. A total of 1872 subjects formed the final pool of data including 631 women taking olanzapine, 424 taking quetiapine, 314 taking risperidone, 254 taking aripiprazole, 152 taking clozapine, 37 taking ziprasidone, 17 taking amisulpride, and 7 taking zotepine. Importantly, when this data was analysed, babies of these women were significantly more likely to have congenital malformations, with OR 2.03 (1.41–2.93). A specific pattern of malformations was not found.

8.9.6 Polypharmacy: Does the Use of Multiple Medications in Pregnancy Escalate the Risk of Congenital Malformations?

Examining data from the Motherisk Program in Toronto, Sadowski et al. (2013) found that rates of major congenital malformations were higher in the cohort exposed to second-generation antipsychotics than the unexposed group, at 6.2% compared with 2.6%. However, this difference did not reach significance. All babies who had major malformations at birth were exposed to polypharmacy in utero, suggesting that there may be other factors at play in the development of congenital malformations in this group. These authors suggested that the practice of polypharmacy severely affected outcomes for babies, and advocated for the use of a minimal number of medications in pregnancy.

8.9.7 Cardiovascular Risk Revisited; the Risk Posed by Specific Classes of Antipsychotic

When considering major malformations, the striking example in the study by Habermann's group was cardiac malformations. At a rate of 2.8% in the second-generation-exposed subgroup in comparison with 1.4% in the first-generation-exposed and 0.6% in the unexposed subgroup, these authors found a significant difference between the second-generation-exposed and unexposed cohorts (OR = 3.21, 95% CI 1.34–7.67). These defects were largely atrial or ventricular septal defects. This result is complicated by the co-administration of lithium to 3 children in the second-generation-exposed cohort (the total number of children with a cardiovascular abnormality in this cohort was 12).

In reference to the finding of elevated rates of cardiac malformations in babies of women taking second-generation antipsychotics in pregnancy, Habermann et al. (2013) recommend that babies of mothers exposed to these medications in the first trimester of pregnancy should be offered a detailed ultrasound to confirm normal cardiac development.

8.9.8 Special Cases

8.9.8.1 Risperidone

Coppola et al. (2007) found 197 retrospective reports of risperidone in pregnancy, amongst which there were 12 reports of major congenital abnormality without any clear pattern of organ system involvement. Ten of these women were also taking other medications known to increase the risk of congenital abnormality. These authors concluded that the low rate of malformations reported (6.09%), together with the absence of specific organ pattern involvement, suggested that risperidone is not likely to be implicated in specific teratogenic risk.

In their large dataset analysis, Huybrechts et al. (2016) found that within the group of women taking atypical antipsychotic medication, the overall risk of malformations in those taking risperidone was significant (RR 1.26, 95% CI 1.02–1.56), and remained appreciable, though non-significant when considering cardiac defects specifically (RR 1.26, 95%CI 0.88–1.81). Interestingly, this group also examined the relationship between the dose of medications and the risk of defects. This did not appear to be a factor for any medications aside from risperidone, for which doses above 2 mg/day were related to an increased risk for cardiac malformations (RR 2.08, 95% CI 1.32–3.28). These authors are cautious about interpretation of their results, referring to the increased risk associated with risperidone use in the first trimester as a "safety signal", though they also point to a prior systematic review (Ennis and Damkier 2015) which found a similar unadjusted RR of 1.5 for risperidone and major malformations (though 95% CI was 0.9–2.2). Updated data from Huybrechts et al. (2023) included an additional 1232 risperidone-exposed pregnancies, with a propensity-score weighted SMR rate of 0.9/1000 exposed babies (or non-significant aRR 0.95 (CI 0.66–1.37).

8.9.8.2 Aripiprazole

Aripiprazole is an unusual antipsychotic with a distinct mode of action, acting as a partial agonist at D2 and 5-HT1A receptors, and as an antagonist at 5-HT2A receptors (Bellet et al. 2015). Its use merits specific discussion because of its uniqueness in mode of action (which could lead to unique teratogenic risks) and its reduced effect on weight gain when compared to other second-generation antipsychotic medications such as olanzapine or quetiapine. Hence it may be an option considered if weight gain, gestational diabetes, hypertension or other metabolic risks are a major concern for a woman considering pregnancy.

A review conducted by Cuomo et al. (2017) suggests that concerns raised by non-human teratogenesis relating to aripiprazole use have not been replicated in human subjects. These researchers mention the miscarriage signal in aripiprazole use in pregnancy reported by Sakai et al. (2017), but also mention other studies which do not seem to support an increase in the rate of congenital malformations or of miscarriage (Huybrechts et al. 2016; Habermann et al. 2013).

Bellet et al. (2015) divided congenital malformations into major and minor categories according to EUROCAT, and found that the rate of major malformations was higher in the group exposed to aripiprazole (2.8%) compared with the unexposed group (1.2%), though this difference was not statistically significant.

Interestingly, one of the babies suffering a malformation had a gastrointestinal tract abnormality (oesophageal atresia) consistent with the findings by Montastruc et al. (2016) in regard to aripiprazole in pregnancy (see previous section for more detail).

Freeman et al. (2021) found that, comparing 158 babies exposed to aripiprazole with 690 controls, aOR for major malformations was 1.35, with CI 0.43–4.20, a non-significant result.

8.9.8.3 Clozapine

The use of clozapine in pregnancy presents special challenges. Most women take clozapine for treatment-refractory symptoms of psychosis, hence switching medications or ceasing medications during pregnancy is not always feasible. Cessation of clozapine in particular can result in severe relapses of psychotic symptoms, as demonstrated by case reports (Mendhekar et al. 2003). The chaos associated with a severe relapse of psychosis could have multiple negative effects for both mother and baby. Therefore, decisions about treatment with clozapine in pregnancy need to be well informed of all potential risks to both mother and baby.

Mehta and Van Lieshout (2017) note that Novartis Pharmaceuticals has reported 523 cases of clozapine exposure in pregnancy, of whom 22 have reported malformations. At 4.2%, this lies within baseline rates for the general population. Higher rates of 8.2% have been reported by Dev and Krupp (1995) in a series of 61 babies exposed to clozapine. Boden et al. (2012a, b) report macrocephaly associated with clozapine or olanzapine in pregnancy. Kulkarni et al. (2014) report on the relatively high rate of congenital abnormalities in their group of babies exposed to clozapine in utero: of 11 babies, 2 were born with major congenital abnormalities: craniosynostosis, hypospadias and hypertelorism in one baby, and gastroschisis and horseshoe kidney in the other. Notably, there does not appear to be a pattern of organs affected by clozapine in this case series.

Nguyen et al. (2020) report on a case series of 9 women taking clozapine throughout pregnancy, none of whom had mental health relapses during their pregnancy. Of their babies, notably all those who underwent CTG monitoring (7) all had at least one non-reactive CTG. 8 required neonatal resuscitation, and 4 were transferred to the special care nursery. No babies experienced agranulocytosis, and all babies were formula fed because of concerns about induced agranulocytosis. All babies received antenatal ultrasound testing, resulting in 2 congenital abnormalities noted: pyloric stenosis in one baby and pulmonary artery stenosis and atrial septal defect in another. Both cases were managed conservatively.

8.9.8.4 Olanzapine

An unexpected signal relating to olanzapine and teratogenesis in pregnancy was found in a Finnish national register, which also included terminations for reasons of major congenital malformations (Ellfolk et al. 2021). This group found an increased risk of major congenital malformations in olanzapine-exposed babies of OR 2.12 (CI 1.19–3.76), specifically musculoskeletal malformations: OR 3.71 (CI 1.35–10.1). These authors also seemed bemused by their finding, as their overall assessment of second-generation antipsychotic use in pregnancy did not appear to support an association with congenital malformations. Authors hypothesised a potential link with genetic vulnerabilities to hyperglycaemia prevalent in the study population, suggesting that a possible mechanism might be olanzapine promoting an increase in congenital malformations through hyperglycaemia in early pregnancy.

A signal in relation to olanzapine was also found in a large multinational study incorporating American and Scandinavian populations (Huybrechts et al. 2023). This study found babies exposed to olanzapine in pregnancy were more likely to have oral cleft abnormalities, with aRR 2.14 (1.07–4.27). Again, the authors were cautious about this finding, suggesting that future studies would be helpful to confirm or disconfirm.

8.10 Elective Terminations, Spontaneous Abortion, Miscarriage, and Stillbirth

Many authors have commented on the high rate of elective terminations found in women prescribed antipsychotics in pregnancy (Huybrechts et al. 2016; Habermann et al. 2013; Coughlin et al. 2015; Diav-Citrin 2005; McKenna et al. 2005; Brunner et al. 2013). Several have speculated on the reasons for this, some citing the high rates of unplanned pregnancy in this group (McKenna et al. 2005).

A 2015 meta-analysis by Coughlin et al. confirmed this trend, with pooled odds ratio of 5.98 (CI = 2.94–12.14, $p < 0.001$). These authors considered the possibility that this high rate may be masking a concealed higher rate of congenital malformations, but noted that the indication for termination was not mentioned in the studies which reported this result. Huybrechts et al. (2016) noted that the relative risk for any congenital malformation in the context of atypical antipsychotic use increased from 1.05 to 1.09–1.14 after accounting for the increased rates of termination amongst treated and untreated women. Somewhat confusingly, a recent study (Fabre et al. 2021) considered stillbirth and medical abortions in the same category, and found an increased rate of stillbirth/medical abortion in women with schizophrenia at aOR 2.17 (1.62–2.90).

Increased termination rates appear to relate to women taking both typical and atypical medications. Diav-Citrin et al. (2005) found a higher rate of elective terminations in women exposed to haloperidol than in a control group (8.8% vs. 3.8%), $p = 0.004$. Habermann et al. (2013) found an increased rate of elective terminations of pregnancy in women taking both second-generation and first-generation antipsychotics (9.4%, 8.1%) compared with those not taking these medications (5.7%). McKenna et al. (2005) found a high rate of elective terminations amongst women exposed to atypical antipsychotics: 9.9% vs. 1.3% in the comparator group.

8.10.1 Stillbirths and Neonatal Deaths in Women with Major Mental Illness

Lee and Lin (2012) cite Howard et al. (2004a, b) in suggesting that women with a history of psychotic disorders have higher rates of stillbirths and neonatal deaths than other women. These authors also cite other earlier studies suggesting that women with schizophrenia are at increased risk of stillbirth (Nilsson et al. 2002; Rifkin et al. 1994; Bennedsen et al. 1999; Sacker et al. 1996), and cite Webb et al. (2007) in suggesting that maternal mood disorders are associated with a higher risk of fatal congenital defects.

Whereas these earlier studies seemed to link a diagnosis of major mental illness with an increased risk of stillbirth, this finding is not corroborated by more recent research. Habermann et al. (2013), Vigod et al. (2015), Reis and Kallen (2008), Diav-Citrin et al. (2005), Terrana et al. (2015), Coughlin et al. (2015), Brunner et al. (2013), and Boden et al. (2012a, b) all found rates of stillbirth or neonatal death which approximated rates found in the general population. Jablensky et al. (2005) found no significant differences between women with schizophrenia, affective psychosis, or the general population in terms of stillbirth, neonatal deaths, or deaths within the first year of life. Of note, Vigod et al. (2014) did not find a significantly elevated risk of neonatal death in a population-based sample examining obstetric outcomes for women with schizophrenia. However, in their subsequent review of research findings, the authors commented that the observed neonatal mortality rate of 1% was still twice that of the general population.

8.10.2 Miscarriage/Spontaneous Abortion/Ectopic Pregnancy/Foetal Death in Utero

In a pooled meta-analysis of women diagnosed with schizophrenia, Matevosyan (2011) found rates of miscarriage of 5.1% (RR = 2.04). The authors reported this to be a higher rate than the reference population, though this difference did not reach significance. Sadowski et al. (2013) defined miscarriage as occurring prior to 20 weeks, foetal death as occurring after 20 weeks, and found that neither occurred more frequently in women exposed to second-generation antipsychotics. Habermann et al. (2013) found no significant increase in risk of spontaneous abortion after exposure to antipsychotics either second or first generation, reporting consistency with outcomes observed by other authors (Goldstein et al. 2000; Garayt and Merieux 2009; Paulus et al. 2005). Diav-Citrin et al. (2005), Terrana et al. (2015), Coppola et al. (2007), Coughlin et al. (2015), and Brunner et al. (2013) found no significant difference between rates of miscarriage in women treated with either typical or atypical antipsychotic medications, and the general population. Two authors mentioned no difference in rates of ectopic pregnancy between women treated with antipsychotics and those unexposed (Diav-Citrin et al. 2005; Brunner et al. 2013).

8.10.3 Specific Antipsychotics: Aripiprazole and the Risk of Miscarriage

Sakai et al. (2017) examined the relative risk for miscarriage of aripiprazole specifically, in comparison with other second-generation antipsychotics including risperidone, olanzapine, and quetiapine. These researchers used a voluntary reporting database in Japan for this study. The relative risk for spontaneous miscarriage was found to be significantly greater for women taking aripiprazole than for unexposed women; this significant difference was not present for other second-generation antipsychotics: ROR 2.76 (CI 1.62–4.69). Of the 18 women reporting miscarriage with aripiprazole, 12 had a diagnosis of schizophrenia, treated with a median dose of aripiprazole 12 mg. This finding has been discussed elsewhere in the literature; Cuomo et al. (2017) mention the miscarriage signal for aripiprazole use in pregnancy reported by these Japanese researchers, but also mention other studies which do not support an increase in the rate of congenital malformations or of miscarriage for women taking aripiprazole (Huybrechts et al. 2016; Habermann et al. 2013).

By contrast with research by Sakai et al. (2017), Bellet et al. (2015) conducted a review of 86 cases of babies exposed to aripiprazole in pregnancy excluding all exposures to known teratogens, including other psychotropic medications, in the first trimester. This team drew cases from a reporting service available in France for monitoring adverse outcomes, and screened for substance use, smoking, and other lifestyle factors in the women identified. Women with pre-existing diabetes were excluded. Pregnancy outcomes included a high rate of elective termination (9.3%), consistent with other studies, and a miscarriage rate within the general population rate (again, 9.3%).

8.10.4 Clozapine and Risk of Stillbirth or Miscarriage in Pregnancy

Mendhekar et al. (2003) report on a stillbirth associated with monotherapy of clozapine 75 mg throughout pregnancy, including the first trimester. Aside from case reports, there is very little information about stillbirth, miscarriage, or ectopic pregnancy rates in babies exposed to clozapine in pregnancy.

8.11 Premature Infants/Low Birth Weight Infants

8.11.1 Schizophrenia and Premature Birth/Low Birth Weight: Another Instance of Potential Confounding by Indication

Looking primarily at diagnosis rather than treatment modality and examining women treated prior to the era of widespread use of atypical antipsychotics, Jablensky et al. (2005) noted a slight trend to preterm birth, a lower mean birth weight, reduced head circumference and reduced length in babies of women with schizophrenia. There was a suggestion in this study that babies of women with schizophrenia experienced intrauterine growth restriction after adjustment for ethnicity, maternal age, infant gender, plural birth, and marital status. This group also adjusted for the expected impact of smoking (extrapolated from other studies; this data set did not include smoking rates) and found an additional residual effect of schizophrenia diagnosis alone (or the presence of an unaccounted-for additional moderator). This study could be considered a proxy for examining treatment using first-generation antipsychotic agents, as it studied a population of women diagnosed (and presumably treated) in the 1980s.

Consistent with these earlier results, Vigod et al. (2014) found a much higher rate of preterm birth in the babies of women with schizophrenia regardless of treatment modality, with rates of 11.2% compared with 6.2% in the control group. Adjusted odds ratio was 1.75 (CI 1.46–2.08). Women with schizophrenia were also statistically more likely to deliver very preterm infants (<32 weeks). Similarly, the women in Reis and Kallen's 2008 cohort taking antipsychotics for mental health reasons were significantly more likely to have babies born before 37 weeks, with an odds ratio of 1.73 (95% CI 1.31–2.29). Matevosyan (2011) found rates of premature labour in women with schizophrenia which the author considered high (5.1% RR 1.98), but which remained well within statistical norms. This author did find a statistical increase in rates of babies with growth retardation born to mothers with schizophrenia (RR 2.16, CI 1.48–3.87). These findings were echoed by Hizkiyahu et al. (2009), who found that babies born to women with a diagnosis of schizophrenia were significantly more likely to be of low birth weight (13.4% vs. 7.8%, $p = 0.042$). Later research by Vigod et al. (2020) also found a higher rate of preterm birth (aRR 1.64 (CI 1.51–1.77) and small for gestational age babies (aRR 1.40, CI 1.20–1.64) in babies of women with schizophrenia. Similarly, Fabre et al. (2021) in their recent study found increased rates of intra-uterine growth retardation at aOR 1.37 (1.17–1.59), small for gestational age (aOR 1.34, CI 1.19–1.50) and preterm birth (aOR 1.64, CI 1.42–1.90) in babies of women with a diagnosis of schizophrenia.

8.11.2 Women with Schizophrenia and Low Birth Weight Babies Born at Term

Vigod et al. (2014) found a correlation between diagnosis of schizophrenia in the mother and small for gestational age infants, though these researchers did not stratify according to treatment. The unadjusted odds ratio for small for gestational age babies (<third centile) born to women with schizophrenia was 1.56 (95% CI 1.25–1.95). Reis and Kallen (2008) found that women taking antipsychotics for mental health reasons were also significantly more likely to have babies born at low birth weight (<2500 g): OR 1.67 (95%CI 1.21–2.29). Jablensky et al. (2005) found a significant increase in low birth weight infants born to mothers with schizophrenia, regardless of the timing of onset of their illness (whether prior to or after the birth). This approach seemed to account well for any effect associated with treatment.

Lin et al. (2010) found that women with diagnoses of bipolar disorder and schizophrenia were more likely than women without a mental illness to have babies of low birth weight, even after adjustment for sociodemographic and metabolic factors. These babies were also more likely to be small for gestational age.

8.11.3 Bipolar Disorder and Premature Birth/Low Birth Weight Infants

Lin et al. (2010) found that women with bipolar disorder were more likely than relatively demographically matched controls to have preterm babies (OR 2.08 CI 1.53–2.83). In support of this view, Lee and Lin (2012) cite MacCabe et al. (2007) in suggesting that mothers with mood disorders have elevated risk of preterm birth and small for gestational age babies. Both treated and untreated women with bipolar disorder studied by Boden et al. (2012a, b) had similarly increased rates of preterm birth, further supporting the view that perhaps this risk may not relate to medication treatment, but instead to other factors underlying the diagnosis or associated sociodemographic risks.

8.11.4 Women with Bipolar Disorder and Low Birth Weight Babies Born at Term

In the 2012 study by Boden et al., women with bipolar disorder who remained untreated were much more likely to have babies of low birth weight at delivery. Interestingly, this study examined head circumference, which alone of weight, length, and head circumference remained significant after adjustment for confounders in women with untreated bipolar disorder. These researchers suggested that maternal psychosocial stress in pregnancy in the context of untreated bipolar disorder may be the mechanism responsible, or that women with bipolar disorder were more vulnerable to adverse neonatal outcomes such as low birth weight because of associated demographic and lifestyle factors. These researchers also drew an association between small for gestational age infants and neonatal hypoglycaemia, which could be associated primarily with the condition of small-for-gestational-age itself rather than with the administration of psychotropic medications.

8.11.5 Typical Antipsychotic Medications and Prematurity/Low Birth Weight

There appears to be a consensus relating to the correlation between typical antipsychotic exposure and preterm birth in most early studies, and this is borne out in recent work as well. The study by Munk et al. (2005) suffered from low numbers in the target population, but did find a trend towards risk of preterm birth and low birth weight in women taking first-generation antipsychotics throughout pregnancy.

Diav-Citrin et al. (2005) found that gestational age at delivery was lower in a cohort of women taking haloperidol for multiple different diagnostic indications, as was median birth weight. Babies exposed to haloperidol in pregnancy were 2 times more likely to be born prior to 37 weeks. When the data were analysed for the relative strength of predictors of low birth weight, only haloperidol and smoking were significant predictors.

8.11.6 Typical Antipsychotic Medications and Low Birth Weight Babies Born at Term

Habermann et al. (2013) found that babies of women taking first-generation antipsychotics had the lowest birth weights when compared with babies of women taking second-generation antipsychotics or those unexposed, but that the difference in birth weights was not clinically significant, especially when preterm babies were excluded from this analysis: these researchers found median weight at delivery of 3.38 kg for first-generation-exposed babies compared with 3.4 kg for second-generation-exposed babies, and 3.44 kg for unexposed babies. Diav-Citrin et al. (2005) noted that their group of term infants exposed to haloperidol in utero was lighter by 165 g than the reference cohort. Overall, Newham et al. (2008) found in a small sample that babies exposed to typical antipsychotics weighed significantly less than babies exposed to atypical antipsychotics than a reference group of unexposed babies ($p < 0.05$).

8.11.7 Atypical Antipsychotics and Prematurity/Low Birth Weight

Infants exposed to second-generation antipsychotics in the study by Sadowski et al. (2013) were approximately 2.5 times more vulnerable to prematurity compared with controls (10.6% vs. 4.3%). There was also a marked difference between gestational age of neonates exposed to one second-generation antipsychotic in comparison with those exposed to polypharmacy ($p = 0.005$). Similarly, unmatched cohorts in the study by Vigod et al. (2015) showed a higher rate of preterm birth in women taking atypical antipsychotic medication in pregnancy, at 14.8% vs. 10.3%. However, there was not a significant increase in low birth weight even in the unmatched cohort in this study. Boden's group of women taking only antipsychotic medication demonstrated higher rates of preterm birth when comparing medications other than olanzapine and clozapine with unexposed groups. McKenna et al. (2005) found a trend to prematurity in women treated with atypical antipsychotics (13% vs. unexposed 8%) but this difference was not significant. 10% of exposed babies were of low birth weight, vs. 2% of comparators; this difference was significant ($p = 0.05$).

Wichman (2009), conducting a retrospective review of birthing records for a tertiary referral maternity centre, found 16 women prescribed atypical antipsychotics in pregnancy. These women predominantly had diagnoses of major depressive disorder (44%), schizoaffective disorder, or bipolar disorder, and over half were prescribed quetiapine. There is no data on concomitant medications, which are likely to have been prescribed given the diagnostic categories treated. The average age at delivery was 37 weeks and 5 days, with 18.75% of babies born prematurely. Comparison data were not available in this study to evaluate significance. Average birth weight was low, at 3188 g.

Terrana et al. (2015) conducted a meta-analysis of cohort studies examining second-generation antipsychotics. This group found that these babies were significantly more at risk of preterm birth (OR = 1.85 (1.20–2.86), though this impact was decreased under a fixed effects model (OR = 1.51, CI 1.15–1.98) and further decreased with adjustment (aOR = 1.34, CI 0.85–2.11) to lose statistical significance. This meta-analysis did not find a significant increase in the risk for small-for-gestational age or large-for-gestational age babies, respectively, though noting that the studies evaluating large for gestational age babies were not homogeneous.

Hence the data is more mixed in relation to the risk of low birth weight in babies exposed to atypical antipsychotics in pregnancy, though the trend to mild prematurity seems in most studies to remain.

8.11.8 Atypical Antipsychotics and Low Birth Weight Babies Born at Term

Sadowski et al. (2013) did not find a significant difference in the incidence of babies who were small for gestational age at delivery between women exposed to second-generation antipsychotics and those unexposed. This group also did not find any significant difference in birth weight. Examining antipsychotic medication exposure in pregnancy, Boden et al. (2012a, b) found a much higher unadjusted risk (more than double) of small for gestational age babies than the general population, regardless of the type of antipsychotic medication to which they were exposed. However, significance disappeared once maternal factors were adjusted for. McKenna et al. (2005) found 10% of exposed babies had a low birth weight, compared with 2% of unexposed babies. This difference was not statistically significant.

A meta-analysis by Coughlin et al. (2015) presented some complexity when considering birth weight. Including both typical and atypical antipsychotic medications in this analysis led to a slight reduction in the birth weight of babies born to treated mothers, but the mean difference was small: 57.9 g. This analysis showed a relationship between antipsychotic exposure of all kinds and small for gestational age infants, but not for large for gestational age infants, again not separating the effects of typical and atypical agents. This analysis noted that heterogeneity between studies existed in relation to reporting of smoking status, obesity, alcohol use, illicit drug use, socioeconomic status, confounding by indication or concomitant medication use, all of which are known to affect all parameters studied. Virtually none of the studies reported doses, which could also affect the risk to the exposed foetus. Interestingly, these authors took issue with the "typical/atypical" division commonly used in analysing antipsychotic medications, noting that both groups include a diversity of medications which can have different risks associated with their use. These authors advocated drug-specific data reporting, to help clarify the true risk presented by each medication.

The study by Bellet et al. (2015) found a significant increase in the rate of preterm birth (16.4%, OR 2.57, CI 1.06–6.27) in babies exposed to aripiprazole. There was also a significantly increased rate of foetal growth retardation in the exposed group (OR 2.97, CI 1.23–7.16). There was a slightly reduced mean weight in exposed neonates compared with their peers (3268 g compared with 3339 g).

8.11.9 Studies Comparing First- (Typical) and Second-Generation (Atypical) Antipsychotics and the Risk of Prematurity

Petersen et al. (2016a, b) found that babies of women taking typical antipsychotics in pregnancy appeared at higher risk of prematurity or low birth weight (11.8%) than those taking atypical antipsychotics in pregnancy (8.4%), and much higher risk than those never exposed to antipsychotic medication (3.9%). Habermann et al. (2013) found those exposed to first-generation antipsychotics had higher rates of premature birth (15.7%) than either women taking second-generation antipsychotics (9.2%) or those unexposed to any antipsychotic in pregnancy (8.7%), and that this difference was statistically significant (OR 1.96 first-generation antipsychotic vs. unexposed cohort, 95% CI 1.29–2.98), also citing similar results in Lin et al. (2010). One confounding variable raised by Habermann's group was the very high rate of concurrent antidepressant use in the cohort treated with first-generation antipsychotics, which could also have an effect on preterm birth.

The 2015 meta-analysis by Coughlin et al. showed a statistically significant increase in rates of preterm birth of babies exposed to both typical and atypical antipsychotics in utero, but these studies were heterogeneous. It seemed that the impact of antipsychotic exposure in pregnancy on gestational age at delivery was present, but small, leading to babies born a mean of 0.21 weeks earlier.

In passing (as their focus was on weight at term birth), Newham et al. (2008) excluded from their sample 16% of infants exposed to typical antipsychotics and 17% exposed to atypical antipsychotics, who were delivered prematurely. Of this group, 21.4% of patients taking olanzapine had preterm deliveries (compared with no patients taking haloperidol or risperidone). They compared this group with a reference group of unexposed infants, of whom 2% were premature and 5% were post-dates. This result contrasts with the study by Brunner et al. (2013) using the Eli Lilly reporting database on olanzapine, which found rates of premature birth of 9.8% in these babies compared with a population rate of 12.8%.

Kulkarni et al. (2014) did not stratify their results according to antipsychotic class, noting that a large majority of their cohort took atypical antipsychotics. Interestingly, these authors stratified by dose, and found that dose of antipsychotic (measured in risperidone equivalents) correlated inversely with prematurity. Babies born at term were exposed in the first trimester to an average of 2.6 mg risperidone equivalent dose, whereas babies born prematurely were exposed to an average of 5.0 mg, $p = 0.02$.

8.12 Second-Generation Antipsychotics and High Birth Weight Infants

8.12.1 The Influence of a Diagnosis of Mental Illness: Schizophrenia

Vigod et al. (2014) did not sub-categorise women's treatment medication, but considered all women with a diagnosis of schizophrenia together. In this cohort they found that 4.5% of babies born to women with schizophrenia were born at larger than the 97th centile, compared with 2.7% in the referent group. This comparison was adjusted for maternal age, parity, income, community size, pre-existing diabetes, hypertension, thromboembolic disease, and infant gender. The adjusted odds ratio for this was 1.53 (CI 1.17–1.99).

8.12.2 Second-Generation Antipsychotics and High Birth Weight Infants

The same group subsequently more closely examined the nexus between treatment of mental illness in pregnancy and large for gestational age babies (Vigod et al. 2015). Focusing on atypical antipsychotic use, this study showed an increase in high birth weight (>97th centile) babies born to the cohort treated with atypical antipsychotics compared with the unmatched general population. However, when matched for health service usage and demographics, this outcome was no longer significantly different in the treatment group, suggesting that lifestyle risks associated with a diagnosis of mental illness could also be responsible for the discrepancy.

Habermann et al. (2013) did not find a significant increase in birth weight of babies exposed to second-generation antipsychotics in utero in comparison with controls. Similarly, Reis and Kallen (2008), observing a cohort of women taking both first- and second—generation antipsychotics for their mental health, did not find a significant increase in rates of high birth weight.

Boden et al. (2012a, b) did not separately examine the effect of antipsychotics on birth weight. However, treatment of women with bipolar disorder with mood stabilisers including antipsychotics resulted in a non-statistically significant increase in the risk of large for gestational age infants. The authors' hypothesis, that macrocephaly might relate to specific medications (olanzapine and clozapine) seemed to be borne out in the results of the second study undertaken by this group, in women taking antipsychotic medication. The most striking finding was that this group of infants had an adjusted OR of 3.02 (1.60–5.71) for head circumference more than 2 standard deviations from the average. This was such an unusual finding that the authors assessed for the possibility that hydrocephalus might account for the difference, which it did not.

Sadowski et al. (2013) found that babies born to women taking second-generation antipsychotics in pregnancy were more likely to be large for gestational age (>90th centile), at $p < 0.05$. However, after analysing for treatment effect, this group felt that the major predictor of large for gestational age babies was pre-pregnancy weight of the mother. Notably, this does not discount the effect of second-generation antipsychotics on this outcome, but suggests that the impact may occur prior to conception.

Interestingly, in contrast to most other published data, Newport et al. (2007) performed a placental transfer study showing that only haloperidol was associated with high birth weight babies (>4000 g) in 15.4% of patients, whereas olanzapine, risperidone, and quetiapine were not correlated with this outcome. This outcome was noted in a study with low total number of 51 women.

The blockbuster study in this area is Newham et al. (2008) with results that, if replicated, have significant implications for medication choices in treating women with multiple risks for obesity in pregnancy. Newham et al. (2008) note that, aside from the putative effect of atypical antipsychotic medication, risk factors for macrosomia at delivery are maternal obesity, type I diabetes, gestational diabetes and excess pregnancy weight gain. This group focused on gestational weight at term delivery, excluding all women with a diagnosis of diabetes, those whose babies had congenital malformations, or who were taking both a typical and atypical antipsychotic medication. Large and small for gestational age were defined as below the tenth or above the 90th centile. Newham et al. (2008) found a highly significant increased rate of large for gestational age infants in the group exposed to atypical antipsychotics (20%) than in both the typical antipsychotics (2%) or the reference unexposed group (3%), $p < 0.05$. This difference was even more marked when the babies exposed to olanzapine and clozapine were compared with the reference group. Of these babies, 31% were large for gestational age. Notably, this study did not record maternal smoking or alcohol use, which they considered a limitation. These authors also considered a cohort effect on infant size over time, as rates of obesity in women have increased over that time period.

They further note that large for gestational age infants can cause their own complications at delivery for the mother including vaginal lacerations, postpartum haemorrhage, and increased risk of emergency caesarean section. Risks for the baby cited by Newham et al. (2008) include birth trauma, shoulder dystocia and foetal hypoxia, as well as risks for higher BMI and greater incidence of diabetes in later life.

8.13 Neonatal Distress and Adverse Neonatal Events

8.13.1 Definitions

There is a plurality of names for the cluster of signs and symptoms that may manifest when placental transfer of a substance and its metabolites comes to an abrupt end at delivery. Habermann et al. (2013) note the difficulty in comparing rates of neonatal distress due to the absence of an internationally agreed measure or scale for these events.

Convertino et al. (2016) hypothesise that this cluster may represent either the residual toxic effects of a substance which is no longer efficiently metabolised by infant kidneys and liver, or alternatively a withdrawal from a high blood level of a substance which is no longer available. These authors suggest that in the case of antipsychotics, some symptoms occur as a consequence of cholinergic rebound, and others relate to dopamine blockade. The multiple names for this syndrome include "neonatal abstinence syndrome", "neonatal withdrawal syndrome", "neonatal adaptation syndrome", or "neonatal behavioural syndrome" and in the case of antipsychotics, encompass a range of symptoms and signs including agitation, feeding disorders, abnormalities of tone, respiratory distress, somnolence, and tremors (Vigod et al. 2015). They can appear within hours after delivery, and some reports suggest that they can remain up to a month afterwards (Vigod et al. 2015).

8.13.2 The Influence of Diagnosis of Mental Illness on Adverse Events at Delivery

Reis and Kallen (2008) found increased rates of low APGAR scores, respiratory diagnoses and hypoglycaemia in the babies of women treated with antipsychotics for mental illness, but none of these differences reached significance. These scores were adjusted for maternal age, parity, smoking, and history of prior miscarriage. Vigod et al. (2020) also found low APGAR scores in babies of women with a diagnosis of schizophrenia, APGAR <8 at 1 min (aRR 1.49, CI 1.40–1.59) and APGAR <8 at 5 min (aRR 1.90 CI 1.68–2.16).

Babies whose mothers had either treated or untreated bipolar diagnoses (Boden et al. 2012a, b) had a diverse APGAR range, which was difficult to interpret. Babies whose mothers were not treated seemed more at risk of low APGAR though this difference did not reach significance; babies whose mothers were treated with medication did not seem to be as much at risk of low APGAR as the general population. Boden et al. (2012a, b) also examined the risk of neonatal hypoglycaemia; both treated and untreated populations were more highly at risk for this outcome, though this risk only reached significance in the untreated cohort.

Jablensky et al. (2005), focusing on risks relating to underlying maternal diagnoses of psychiatric illness, noted that there was a trend towards lower APGAR score at 5 min, respiratory depression and intubation in babies of women with schizophrenia. Matevosyan (2011) echoed this outcome, finding a statistical increase in rates of low APGAR scores at 5 min for babies of mothers with schizophrenia.

Vigod et al. (2014) found a highly elevated risk of neonatal abstinence syndrome for babies of mothers with schizophrenia (aOR = 53.7, 95%CI = 36.8–78.4). In this research, neonatal abstinence syndrome is classified separately from Respiratory Distress Syndrome, which these authors also found more commonly in babies of mothers with schizophrenia (aOR = 1.86, 95%CI = 1.23–2.81), as were seizures (aOR = 4.21, 95%CI = 2.31–7.65), intraventricular haemorrhage (aOR =2.43, 95%CI = 1.34–4.41), and persistent foetal circulation (aOR = 3.19, 95%CI = 1.43–7.14).

The fascinating coda to this alarming warning was that, on re-examining the data and matching with controls with similar patterns of healthcare utilisation (Vigod et al. 2015), these differences became less marked. When these data were also controlled for the use of psychotropics other than antipsychotic medications, in particular antidepressants, mood stabilisers,and benzodiazepines, these outcomes lost significance. Regardless, the authors argue that these women and their babies are still at much higher risk of adverse outcomes than the general population, and hence should be observed and supported much more closely. It seems, however, on the basis of this analysis, that it is not necessary to avoid the use of antipsychotics for these women, which should help maintain mental stability throughout pregnancy and beyond.

8.13.3 First-Generation Antipsychotics and Adverse Neonatal Events

There has been awareness of the possibility of withdrawal syndromes and extrapyramidal side effects from antipsychotic use in pregnancy for many years (Falterman and Richardson 1980, via Petersen et al. 2016a, b). More recently, both the United States' Food and Drug Administration and the United Kingdom's Medicines and Healthcare Products Regulatory Agency updated their advice on risks of extrapyramidal effects and withdrawal syndromes in 2011 in regard to typical antipsychotic medication use in pregnancy. Advice from the US FDA was based on 69 cases reported between 2008 and 2011. Symptoms included agitation, hypertonia, hypotonia, tremor, somnolence, respiratory distress, and feeding disorder.

Einarsson and Boskovic (2009), completing an exhaustive review of all known studies relating to antipsychotics in pregnancy, found a paper from 1971 which described neonatal withdrawal and extrapyramidal symptoms in babies exposed to higher doses of chlorpromazine, up to several weeks after birth (Farkas et al. 1971). These authors note other reports of extrapyramidal side effects after exposure to typical antipsychotics which persisted up to months after delivery (O'Connor et al. 1981), and two reports of paralytic ileus in neonates after exposure to typical antipsychotics (Falterman et al. 1980).

8.13.4 Adverse Events Associated with First- and Second-Generation Antipsychotics: Is This a Useful Distinction in Assessing Risk for Neonates?

Convertino et al. (2016) note that both first-generation and second-generation antipsychotic use in later pregnancy have been associated with increased rates of abnormal neuromotor performance, hypertonicity, and tremors. These authors mention in this context the 2011 USFDA warning, mentioned above. Convertino et al. (2016) also mentioned results from Kulkarni et al. (2014) in the Australian National Register of Antipsychotic Medications in Pregnancy (NRAMP) of rates of medical withdrawal symptoms in 15% of babies, which appeared to be dose-related and which took up to 6–8 weeks to subside. Kulkarni et al. (2014) noted that there was a trend towards exposure to higher doses of medication at 12 weeks' gestation in babies who experienced withdrawal symptoms ($p = 0.162$).

Interestingly, Convertino et al. (2016) also drew some distinctions between reported symptom profiles after withdrawal from specific medications: seizures in one case of a baby exposed to risperidone; heat regulation, hyperbilirubinaemia and feeding difficulties in another. These authors note case reports of thermoregulation difficulties, tremor, vomiting, poor feeding and decreased muscle tone in haloperidol exposure, and respiratory distress, hypotonia, poor feeding in olanzapine exposure; retinopathy and transient neonatal hypoxaemic encephalopathy in clozapine exposure. They also note a report of delayed neurological and extrapyramidal symptoms in fluphenazine exposure, presenting a month after delivery. Worsley et al. (2013) commented on outcomes for 114 babies in the NRAMP database referred to above. In this analysis, babies who were exclusively breastfed from delivery (12.2%) were less likely to have withdrawal symptoms than babies who were exclusively bottle-fed (27.5%), with OR 2.74, CI 1.02–7.32, $p = 0.04$. A full discussion of this issue is beyond the scope of this chapter, however it remains an interesting outcome when considering ways to reduce the impact of adverse events on neonates.

Sadowski et al. (2013) found higher rates of foetal distress at delivery amongst babies exposed to second-generation antipsychotics, at rates of 22.5% vs. 14.3% in those unexposed (though this did not reach statistical significance). This group also had much higher rates of Neonatal Intensive Care Unit (NICU) admission, at 25.3% vs. 9.5%, and much greater rates of signs of neonatal abstinence syndrome (which they labelled "PNA": 16.5% vs. 5.2%). These researchers considered PNA to include central nervous system, respiratory, and gastrointestinal problems.

The 2007 study by Newport et al. demonstrated APGAR at 5 min to be broadly similar across all treatment groups, with a mean between 8 and 9. Olanzapine and quetiapine were associated with higher rates of NICU admission (30.8% and 9.5% respectively), both of which are higher rates than those observed in the general population. Notably, again, olanzapine seemed to be associated with a higher rate of cardiovascular and respiratory complications, with 23.1% and 30.8% of babies experiencing these adverse outcomes at delivery.

Gentile's 2010 review found high rates of neonatal adverse events in babies of mothers taking clozapine in pregnancy, including transient floppy infant syndrome, noting that most of these women were also taking other medications. He found 63 of 419 babies exposed to olanzapine who experienced "perinatal complications", not further specified. He found neonatal complications in babies exposed to risperidone, including withdrawals and seizures, but did not further characterise these. He also found reports of neonatal adverse events relating to late-pregnancy use of chlorpromazine including extrapyramidal signs, respiratory distress, seizures, and transient neurodevelopmental delay.

8.13.5 Aripiprazole and Adverse Neonatal Events

Bellet et al. (2015) found 2 babies who experienced neonatal adverse events associated with aripiprazole exposure. The first had a withdrawal syndrome with pulmonary hypertension and respiratory distress. The second had an aspiration pneumonia in the context of premature rupture of membranes. More generally, APGAR scores were lower at both 1 and 5 min in babies exposed to aripiprazole.

8.13.6 Clozapine and Adverse Neonatal Events

Isolated case reports of reduced heart rate variability have been noted in foetuses of women taking clozapine in pregnancy (Yogev et al. 2002; Guyon et al. 2015; Nguyen et al. 2020). There have been several case reports of floppy infant syndrome in babies exposed to clozapine in utero (Di Michele et al. 1996; Karakula et al. 2004). The longer-term sequelae of this syndrome can include motor delay and other developmental difficulties (Igarashi 2004). Seizures have been reported in clozapine-exposed babies (Stoner et al. 1997; Karakula et al. 2004). The authors speculated that these could result from immature infant hepatic metabolism, or alternatively from withdrawals from the medication, given that some seizures have occurred several days after delivery. There have been several reports of shoulder dystocia, suggesting possible macrosomia at delivery (Waldman and Safferman 1993; Dickson and Hogg 1998).

Reports of agranulocytosis of babies breastfed by mothers taking clozapine (Dev and Krupp 1995) suggest that this effect could also occur as a consequence of treatment in utero. On this basis, Kulkarni et al. (2015) have suggested that weekly white cell monitoring should occur up to 6 months after delivery for babies exposed to clozapine in utero.

8.13.7 Lifestyle Factors Elevating Risk of Adverse Neonatal Events

Whereas the absolute rates of adverse neonatal events were higher in babies of women taking antipsychotics throughout pregnancy at 6% in the 2016 study by Petersen et al., it is notable that 4.7% of babies of women not taking antipsychotics in pregnancy, but who had previously been prescribed these, also experienced these outcomes. Rates of adverse neonatal events for babies of women never exposed to antipsychotics were much lower, at 2.5%. After adjustment for age, obesity, alcohol problems, smoking, illicit drug use, and antidepressant and anticonvulsant prescribing, the differences between these groups were not significant. These results raise the issue, also raised elsewhere, of the contribution of underlying illness or clustering lifestyle factors to adverse outcomes, rather than solely relating to the administration of medication itself.

8.13.8 Polypharmacy Escalates Risk of Adverse Neonatal Events

Coppola et al. (2007), considering only risperidone, noted 1 of 68 pregnancies in which the baby experienced a possible withdrawal syndrome. The mother of this child was also taking imipramine, clonazepam and alcohol through pregnancy. The baby experienced sleepiness, jitteriness, and slow sucking, but did not require transfer to a NICU or special care nursery. These authors also found 21 of 197 retrospectively reported pregnancies exposed to risperidone which reported adverse neonatal events. These included drug withdrawal in 13 (in 5 of which drug withdrawal was attributed to other drugs taken by the woman in pregnancy), movement disorder or tremor in 9, jitteriness or irritability in 8, feeding problems in 8, somnolence and lethargy in 3 and seizures in 3. 18 of the 21 were complicated by concomitant use of other drugs, illicit or prescribed, known to be associated with withdrawal syndromes. 3 of these babies were transferred to NICU for further care, 3 required oxygen, tube feeding or treatment with anticonvulsants, and 15 did not require any specific treatment.

Consistent with these findings, Sadowski et al. (2013) found that adverse neonatal events were much more common in those exposed to polypharmacy, with signs at 21.2% vs. 4% of monotherapy babies, and NICU admission at rates of 28.8% vs. 16%. When those exposed to polypharmacy were excluded, babies exposed to second-generation antipsychotics had similar rates of abstinence symptoms to those in the unexposed group. Similarly, Diav-Citrin et al. (2005) found that the rate of neonatal adverse outcomes was 5% in a cohort treated with haloperidol. Most of these babies were born to women treated with multiple psychotropic medications. The cohort examined by Kulkarni et al. (2014) also demonstrated high rates of polypharmacy, with 11% of women taking an additional antipsychotic medication, and 43% of women prescribed antipsychotics also taking an antidepressant. This study found a strikingly high rate of neonatal respiratory distress in babies exposed to these multiple medications, at 37%. The authors noted that babies also exposed to mood stabilisers were over six times more likely to experience respiratory distress. Overall, these babies were also sicker than most other cohorts examined; over 40% required transfer to a neonatal ICU or special care nursery (SCN), compared with expected community rates of 14.2%. The authors noted that higher doses of antipsychotics in pregnancy increased the risk of admission to NICU or SCN.

The 2013 study by Habermann et al. adjusted for alcohol consumption, smoking, and gestational age at birth, all of which were shown to have a significant effect on neonatal adverse events. After adjustment, exposure to second-generation antipsychotics was also significant in this regard (OR = 6.24, 95% CI = 3.51–11.10) as was exposure to first-generation antipsychotics (OR = 5.03, 95%CI = 2.21–11.44). The outcomes measured for newborns included jitteriness, somnolence, and seizures. The authors noted that co-medication with additional psychoactive medications greatly added to the risk of postnatal disorders for all babies exposed to antipsychotics in utero, raising rates from 10.8% and 10.3% respectively to 29.5% and 36.4%. Hence polypharmacy appears to dramatically escalate the risk of neonatal morbidity in these vulnerable babies. The medications most associated with neonatal symptoms included quetiapine at 25.8% and aripiprazole at 23.5%, followed by olanzapine at 15.1%. As a consequence of these very marked results, Habermann et al. (2013) recommend that babies born to women taking any antipsychotic medication in the final week of pregnancy should have their delivery planned with access to a neonatal intensive care unit.

8.14 Neurocognitive Development of the Infant: Developmental Delay, Autism Spectrum Disorder, and Attention Deficit-Hyperactivity Disorder: What Is the Evidence?

The quality and quantity of evidence in relation to conditions such as developmental delay, autism spectrum disorder (ASD), and attention deficit-hyperactivity disorder (ADHD) have improved substantially in the past few years. There is existing support for a strong genetic component to the development of ADHD and autism, which also often co-occur. Twin-twin concordance studies have shown a strong degree of heritability in particular for autism spectrum disorder of up to 90% (Tick et al. 2016), with 70% heritability for ADHD (Sciberras et al. 2017). Multiple studies have implicated a variety of genes in the later development of autism, intellectual disability and ADHD (Torrico et al. 2015; Forrest et al. 2018; Lahbib et al. 2019). In a search for environmental or other influences which could accentuate vulnerability to either condition, researchers have posited a number of factors.

Autism spectrum disorder has been associated with various environmental pollutants, such as traffic fumes (Gong et al. 2017), flame retardants (Lyall et al. 2017), or plastics (Hamra et al. 2019); in-pregnancy exposures such as use of NSAIDS (Chowdhury et al. 2023) or low levels of vitamin D in pregnancy (Windham et al. 2020), vitamin supplementation rates (DeVilbiss et al. 2017), maternal melatonin levels (Braam et al. 2018), or prenatal stress (Hecht et al. 2016), and genetic vulnerability such as intellectual disability or epilepsy (Breuillard et al. 2016), as well as other factors including birth complications (Modabbernia et al. 2016), autoimmune (Vinet et al. 2015; Spann et al. 2019; Sjölander et al. 2022) or inflammatory conditions (Dale et al. 2017; Brynge et al. 2022; Ramirez-Celis et al. 2022), infections (Guisso et al. 2018), obesity (Ahlberg et al. 2022), and even fish consumption at conception (Gao et al. 2016). Others have focused on maternal physical health conditions such as PCOS (Kosidou et al. 2016) or other metabolic disorders (Connolly et al. 2016; Qin et al. 2017), or family migration (Fairthorne et al. 2017; Abdullahi et al. 2019; Morinaga et al. 2021).

The diversity of influences and comorbid conditions (for example, co-occurring intellectual disability in children with ASD), as well as the identification of multiple loci of interest in relation to heritable ASD and ID traits, has led to a widespread view that ASD is an umbrella term which describes a number of individual phenotypes which may have distinct aetiologies, or a number of clustering contributors which separately add to the risk of ASD as a diagnosable outcome.

8.14.1 Evidence Relating to the Use of Antipsychotic Medication in Pregnancy and Risks of Developmental Delay, ASD and ADHD

Specifically in relation to the risks around the use of antipsychotic medications in pregnancy, several papers have been published in recent years which have made substantial improvements in study design and analysis on prior research. This was the case with a large Scandinavian study published in 2021 (Hálfdánarson et al. 2022), covering 2 decades and including 4 million children, of whom 15,466 were exposed to antipsychotic medication in utero. Responding perhaps to criticism of earlier studies with less sophisticated design and analysis, this study considered women with major mental illness whose pregnancies were not exposed to antipsychotic medication as a comparator group to account for confounding by indication, and then considered unexposed sibling pairs to account for unmeasured confounders such as genetic or shared environmental confounders. Primary outcomes of interest were childhood diagnoses of ADHD or ASD. Importantly for the clarity of this research, children diagnosed with a chromosomal abnormality or foetal alcohol syndrome were excluded from the analysis. The study considered both first- and second-generation antipsychotics separately, and did not include lithium or prochlorperazine in the results. Whilst any exposure in pregnancy was considered, the authors also looked at trimester timing of exposure. Covariates examined included sociodemographic status, smoking, BMI, maternal age, parity and child's sex. Country and birth year were also considered, possibly due to differences in regional diagnoses for these conditions and the changes in diagnosis of each condition over time.

Much of the prior research into ADHD and ASD risk has been affected by comparison of large datasets of children with ADHD comparing rates between exposed and unexposed groups. This of course yields an impressive hazard ratio, as it did in this case: 2.28 (CI 2.08–2.49). However, it is not a sophisticated reading of the relationship, as demonstrated in Hálfdánarson et al. (2022), who went on to perform a multivariate regression using the covariates described above, resulting in a less substantial HR of 1.10, CI 1.00–1.21. I would still consider this type of analysis to be misleading, however, as it does not consider major confounders such as maternal mental illness and other genetic and epigenetic vulnerabilities; it would be far more appropriate to compare the cohort of women taking antipsychotics to a more similar comparator group. Fortunately, this was the next step for Hálfdánarson et al., who then found HR for ADHD of 0.90 (CI 0.70–1.15) for babies of women with psychotic illnesses or bipolar disorder; 0.96 (0.82–1.12) for babies of women with other psychiatric disorders, and 1.44 (1.25–1.66) for babies of women with no diagnosed psychiatric condition. This shows, interestingly, that women with psychosis or bipolar who take medication in pregnancy are actually, if anything, less likely to have babies with ADHD than their unmedicated comparators who also suffer these conditions. Even this analysis can be criticised due to confounding by severity, prompting a further secondary analysis, which considered women who took antipsychotic medication before pregnancy (hence requiring treatment) and then ceased in pregnancy. These women were found more likely to have babies who developed ADHD, suggesting that a genetic vulnerability related to underlying mental ill-health is probably a relevant factor.

A similar relationship was found between antipsychotic exposure and ASD, for which an unadjusted HR was 2.12 (1.86–2.41) but when covariates were considered this dropped to insignificance, with HR 1.12 (CI 0.97–1.29). Aside from the relationship between antipsychotic exposure in women with no psychiatric condition recorded (HR 1.27, CI 1.00–1.60), none of the subgroups of women suffering mental illness reached significance. This group is a highly unusual one: who takes an antipsychotic in pregnancy with no mental health indication? Considering this was the only group in whom a significant result was obtained, it would be interesting to know more about the reasons for prescribing.

Sibling analysis, considering an even more closely paired comparator group, was similarly revealing: of 322 children whose siblings were not exposed to antipsychotics there was a non-significant HR of 1.14 (CI 0.79–1.64) for ADHD and for 127 children whose siblings were unexposed there was also a non-significant HR of 1.34 (CI 0.75–2.39) for ASD.

It was interesting that trimester timing of exposure did not appear to affect outcomes for this study. This is consistent with the development of the neurological system in utero, which continues throughout gestation, and also consistent with the effect of sodium valproate on neurological development, which does not appear to be tethered to a specific trimester. The authors commented on the robust association between underlying maternal psychotic and bipolar disorder and children's development of the conditions of interest. A strength of this study was the relatively long follow-up period of up to 9 years, though I note that longer-term follow-up into adulthood may be an additional benefit in future research.

A slightly earlier British study tracked neurodevelopmental and multiple other outcomes for babies in a large UK primary care dataset between 1995 and 2012 (Petersen et al. 2016a, b). Exposures of interest were antipsychotic and mood stabiliser medications, including sodium valproate and lithium taken in pregnancy. Within this cohort, 554 women were prescribed antipsychotic medication in pregnancy. A large percentage of these were also taking other psychotropics: 387 were also taking an antidepressant; 80 were also taking an antidepressant and a hypnotic; 35 were taking antidepressant, hypnotic, anxiolytic as well as an antipsychotic, and 34 were taking an anticonvulsant and antidepressant in addition to an antipsychotic. Thus of the 554 total, only 18 were solely taking an antipsychotic medication in pregnancy. From these pregnancies, 290 children exposed to antipsychotic medication were followed through to between 2 and 3 years post-birth.

This study included women taking antipsychotic medication prior to pregnancy as a comparator group, as well as the larger "healthy women" cohort from the broader dataset. Notably, even this smaller comparator group had half the incidence of obesity as the cohort of interest (10.7% vs. 20%) and a lower smoking and alcohol use rate. Women treated in pregnancy were older than either comparator cohort.

Relevant outcomes for neonates included a broad "developmental delay" category as well as behavioural problems within the scope of the study (i.e. prior to 15 months of age).

When compared with the broader cohort, babies exposed to antipsychotic medications in pregnancy were found to be no more likely to be at risk of neurodevelopmental and behavioural disorder, after adjustment for confounders. When compared with other women who had taken antipsychotic medication prior to pregnancy, these pregnancies were no more likely to result in birth of a child suffering neurodevelopmental delay or behavioural problems, even prior to adjustment for confounders. Whilst this study did not differentiate between antipsychotics, the overall lack of a signal for adverse outcomes meant adjustment was not as important a consideration.

This study noted by contrast the strong signal for sodium valproate in relation to congenital birth defects and neurodevelopmental abnormalities, consistent with existing research, and related guidelines emphasising the importance of considering childbearing potential when prescribing valproate.

Yet another administrative dataset studied similar outcomes, this time for American women and babies (Straub et al. 2022). These authors noted the expanded uses to which antipsychotic medications are put in an American context, also noting the ability of these drugs to cross the placenta. Babies were followed for up to 14 years. Interestingly, this research selected for antipsychotic prescribing in the second half of pregnancy, rather than the first, due to a view that neural synaptogenesis occurs later in pregnancy. This approach differs somewhat from other studies (e.g. Halfdanarson) which have emphasised neural tube development in the first trimester. Specific diagnoses of ADHD and ASD were evaluated, as well as neurodevelopmental disorder more broadly. 9551 + 1221 pregnancies were exposed to antipsychotics during the period 2000–2014. Given the larger sample size, this study could evaluate for specific antipsychotics as well as distinguish between classes. This study utilised high-dimensional propensity scoring to account for residual confounding. A potential signal was found for aripiprazole, which then caused the researchers to focus on this drug in a subsequent analysis.

In this study, the vast majority of prescriptions were for quetiapine, accounting for about 40% of exposures; slightly less commonly prescribed was aripiprazole (16–23%). Most women took only 1 antipsychotic in pregnancy. This study noted the older age of women taking antipsychotics in pregnancy, and that they were more likely to take illicit drugs, smoke cigarettes, and drink alcohol.

Straub et al. (2022) showed very high rates of diagnosis with neurodevelopmental abnormalities, with 37% of publicly insured children exposed to antipsychotics in the second half of pregnancy subsequently diagnosed with NDD by age 8, including 24.5% diagnosed with ADHD and 3.5% diagnosed with ASD. Rates were lower in the privately insured cohort, but still very high by international standards: 24.5% NDD, 17.5% ADHD, 3.8% ASD. However, in adjusted analysis, there was no statistical difference found between exposed and unexposed groups, aside from aripiprazole in the second half of pregnancy: pooled adjusted HR for NDD 1.35, CI 1.14–1.63; this lost significance for the two specific outcomes of ADHD (paHR 1.36, CI 0.98–1.89) and ASD (paHR 1.49, CI 0.91–2.47).

Authors considered the possibility that aripiprazole is prescribed for women with more severe illness, so compared women taking higher doses of aripiprazole in pregnancy with those taking lower doses; this did not meaningfully affect the outcomes, which remained consistent also when aripiprazole was prescribed in the first half of pregnancy. They then compared these women with those taking aripiprazole prior to pregnancy, which again did not meaningfully affect the results. The authors pointed out the slightly different mechanism of action for aripiprazole which might affect prolactin, and considered the risk for an effect on breastfeeding, which might in turn affect NDD.

A well-designed Danish study (Momen et al. 2022) utilised a population-based register to examine all births 1998–2015. Of these, authors considered women taking antipsychotics prior to pregnancy, and compared those who continued taking antipsychotics in pregnancy with those who did not. This neatly addressed concerns about confounding by indication and about lifestyle, sociodemographic and residual confounders which arise when those who do not suffer mental ill-health requiring antipsychotic medications are compared with those who do. The authors also considered paternal antipsychotic use in the hope that this may address additional genetic or environmental factors which could influence outcomes related to intrauterine exposure to antipsychotics. As a consequence of this decision, all children for whom paternal information was missing were also excluded from the dataset. The authors further excluded children with diagnosed chromosomal abnormalities. The eventual target cohort of children of women continuing to take antipsychotic medications in pregnancy was 2035, compared with 6976 pregnancies where antipsychotic medication was discontinued in pregnancy. A new user group of 857 women was included in this study, of women who had not previously taken antipsychotic medication in pregnancy who then started this medication de novo in pregnancy. Children were followed until the end of the study period or until they reached an endpoint as defined by the outcomes of the study. This study examined children up to the age of 15 years.

Comparisons were adjusted using covariates such as maternal and paternal age, severity of illness (judged by hospital admissions; women who had inpatient psychiatric admissions in the 2 years prior to birth were excluded from the analysis), socioeconomic status, smoking, and year of delivery, amongst other variables. Exposure timing in trimesters was specified. Unfortunately this dataset did not provide diagnosis codes for maternal mental health, so the indication for use of antipsychotic was unclear. These patients were subsequently added for sensitivity analysis, and there was no a significant difference in their outcomes. Some exclusions from the data seem counterintuitive, such as excluding all women who had a psychiatric admission in the 2 years prior to delivery, as this would have been a useful indicator of severity of illness, which is an important consideration and is difficult to adjust for. Additionally, women who received comorbid diagnosis of substance use disorder were excluded, as were women who took other psychotropic medications in pregnancy. Again, these are women who are frequently seen in clinical practice, and the information on their babies' outcomes is important to ascertain. Often this information is not available in other studies, and in this case could have been used as a covariate for analysis. I hope that this may be considered in this group's future research.

In comparing babies exposed to antipsychotics in pregnancy with those whose mothers had ceased taking antipsychotics in pregnancy, exposed babies went on to have 10% higher rates of psychiatric disorders overall than the comparator group, though this was not statistically significant: HR 1.10, CI 0.93–1.30. In relation to timing, interestingly second and third trimesters appeared to have a greater magnitude of effect (HR 1.42) but the difference was non-significant (CI 0.86–2.35). The authors considered duration of use of antipsychotic medication in pregnancy, and this also did not appear to increase risk: HR 1.00, CI 0.98–1.02. Paternal use of antipsychotics was overall not significant: HR 1.05 (CI 0.89–1.24).

In relation to ADHD and ASD diagnoses, point prevalence was lower in the cohorts exposed to intrauterine antipsychotic: ADHD HR 0.85 (CI 0.62–1.15), ASD HR 0.83 (CI 0.90–1.26), though the difference was non-significant. Hence other behavioural and emotional disorders, neurotic, stress-related and somatoform disorders, and psychiatric disorders more generally, all appear to have been higher in the treatment group.

This study also looked at antipsychotics differentiated by structure; this was a bit confusing and might not be immediately useful to clinicians. All antipsychotic structures, including N05AA Phenothiazines with aliphatic side-chain antipsychotic (prochlorperazine, chlorpromazine, and promethazine), antipsychotics with piperidine side chains (risperidone), thioxanthenes (flupenthixol, zuclopenthixol) appeared to have lower HRs than the control group, aside from thioxanthene derivatives (flupenthixol, zuclopenthixol): HR 1.28, CI 1.01–1.62. The authors noted the limitations of being unable to consider indication in this study, as well as dosage, due to low power in the available dataset, and advised future studies to evaluate these. They also mentioned that the reduced time of follow-up meant that adult-onset disorders may not be fully ascertained. Their discussion noted that when comparing sex of the child, there was a higher risk of neurodevelopmental abnormalities in male babies, which is a well-established finding.

A Taiwanese study (Yeh et al. 2021) utilised nationalised health register data to enrol 5669 women since 2002 with an ICD-9 diagnosis of Bipolar Disorder, of whom 426 women took a psychiatric medication prior to and during pregnancy, and only 45 were taking antipsychotic medication during pregnancy. These women were matched with women without a diagnosis of major mental illness according to age and residence. Children of these pregnancies were then followed until 2011 (so a maximum of 9 years post-partum) to elicit a diagnosis of ADHD or ASD. The authors stratified exposure into trimester, and adjusted for urban environment.

This study again reinforced the influence of underlying mental illness on ADHD and ASD outcomes, finding that all women diagnosed with bipolar disorder regardless of medication treatment were more likely to have children with ADHD (OR 1.51, CI 1.28–1.77) and ASD (OR 1.85, CI 1.20–2.85) than those who did not have a diagnosis of major mental illness. When comparing those with bipolar disorder who took medication in pregnancy with those who did not, for those taking an antipsychotic medication at any point during pregnancy the association with ADHD and ASD was not significant: OR 1.38, CI 0.56–3.41. The authors highlighted that for women taking antipsychotic medication specifically within the third trimester, the association with later onset ADHD was significant, at OR 3.83 (CI 1.12–13.12), but I would note the absolute number of these women was 35, and the CI correspondingly broad, suggesting this is not a highly reliable result.

Wang et al. (2021a, b) used a clinical data register in Hong Kong to evaluate children born between 2001 and 2015 and exposed to antipsychotic medications in utero for outcomes of ADHD and ASD. This study used sibling matching to address residual confounding, and a propensity score stratification method to manage measured confounders. To ascertain the outcome of ADHD, researchers limited their study to children who were aged at least 6 at the end of the study period, and for ASD, to children aged at least 3. Babies were excluded if they were also exposed to lithium or an antidepressant in pregnancy. Comparator groups included women with and without a psychiatric diagnosis who had never taken antipsychotics, and those who had previously taken antipsychotics but discontinued these in pregnancy. Covariates were maternal age, year at delivery, sex, parity, maternal comorbidities including epilepsy, gestational diabetes and pre-existing diabetes, and socioeconomic status. In relation to ADHD, babies exposed to antipsychotics in utero were slightly less likely than their unexposed peers to develop ADHD if their mother had previously taken antipsychotics prior to pregnancy: HR 0.99, CI 0.60–1.61. Babies whose mothers had previously taken antipsychotics but ceased them in pregnancy were more likely to develop ADHD than those whose mothers had never taken antipsychotics, as were babies of women who had never taken antipsychotics but had a mental health diagnosis compared with those whose mothers had never taken an antipsychotic and didn't have a mental health diagnosis. These two results highlight what has been shown in other studies, the risk associated with underlying mental illness, which seems to be robust in relation to the association between bipolar disorder and ADHD.

Similarly, all outcomes for ASD were non-significant aside from the association between those who had never taken antipsychotics but had a diagnosis of mental disorder, compared with those who had never taken an antipsychotic and did not have a mental health diagnosis (the broader population).

Propensity score stratified matching for sibling pairs suggested that babies exposed to antipsychotics in pregnancy were marginally less likely than their siblings to develop ADHD or ASD in childhood, though neither of these results held significance. Whilst this study examined the effect of trimester exposure, the authors did not find any trimester held a greater risk than another for the outcomes examined.

The overall impression gained from these later studies undertaken between 2016 and 2022 is that maternal mental ill-health seems to play a role in children's later development of ASD and ADHD, and treatment with antipsychotic medication in pregnancy appears not to have a substantial impact on this risk. To quantify this impression, Wang et al. (2024) undertook a meta-analysis of these studies. This meta-analysis found a slight increase in risk when pooled results were used to compare exposed cohorts with "never exposed" cohorts; RR of ADHD 1.11, CI 1.03–1.19. However, all studies also considered the impact of maternal characteristics, comparing prior exposure with current exposure: RR of ADHD 0.78 (0.63–0.96), or sibling characteristics: RR of ADHD 1.11, CI 0.78–1.60. When these more similar cohorts were compared, the relationship did not reach significance. Results were similar for ASD. All cohorts, exposed or previously exposed to antipsychotics, were far more likely to develop ADHD or ASD, suggesting that the relationship may not be mediated by the direct effect of antipsychotic medication on the baby's developing brain, but related instead to the indication for treatment in the mother. This is consistent with earlier research suggesting an association between ADHD and ASD in children of women with mental health disorders (Fairthorne et al. 2016; Vizzini et al. 2019; Nidey et al. 2021). The authors noted that, despite their use of tools which assess for bias, their analysis was limited by the limitations inherent in the studies examined:

1. The heterogeneity of diagnoses for which antipsychotics are utilised, which made it more difficult to ascertain whether there was a specific underlying diagnosis, or severity of illness, more closely associated with the development of ADHD or ASD.
2. Whether there is a dose effect, or if specific antipsychotics are more closely associated with development of ADHD/ASD.
3. Whether a longer-term follow-up may ascertain a larger number of cases.

These issues remain open for subsequent research.

8.15 Conclusion

Table 8.1 shows expert recommendations based on scientific evidence and clinical experience on this topic.

A woman with a diagnosis of major mental illness facing pregnancy also faces a host of related challenges which include the direct effect of her illness on her mental and physical health and that of her baby, and also the social and economic disadvantage that this illness confers.

There is a broad consensus on important contributing factors to adverse outcomes for women in this population: poorer general health in women suffering major mental illness including high rates of obesity and diabetes, increased rates of smoking, alcohol and illicit drug use. For pregnant women in particular, factors contributing to adverse outcomes include reduced attendance at antenatal appointments, reduced use of prenatal vitamins, folate and thyroid hormone, increased rates of unplanned and unwanted pregnancy, limited social support and increased rates of domestic abuse, poverty and disadvantage.

The study of the impact of antipsychotic medications in pregnancy is complicated by the imperative for many women to remain well in pregnancy and the postpartum. Multiple potential error sources in data derived from studies observing these women include confounding by indication; such confounders already identified include severity of illness, socioeconomic, historical or lifestyle factors, and detection bias.

Table 8.1 Expert recommendations based on scientific evidence and clinical experience

Pre-conception planning for women with major mental illness includes contraception and fertility advice and management in addition to medication safety advice in pregnancy
Women with major mental illness require both physical and mental health monitoring throughout pregnancy
Physical health issues to address with women presenting with major mental illness in pregnancy include
Support around smoking, drug and alcohol use cessation
Prenatal vitamin supplementation
Evidence-based advice around medication safety
Avoid or minimise polypharmacy and switching medications
Mental health monitoring and support includes additional support for social safety, including detecting and addressing issues of homelessness, domestic abuse, and social disadvantage or poverty
Assess for and address obesity in all women of childbearing age who present with a major mental illness
Monitor and manage obesity in pregnancy for women taking antipsychotic medications
Assess for and manage diabetes in pregnancy for women taking antipsychotic medications, including liaison with expert medical teams
Antipsychotic medication and congenital abnormalities
Whereas the data does not at this stage suggest significantly increased risk of structural abnormalities for babies exposed to antipsychotic medications in utero, the evidence base is small
Antipsychotic medication can increase the risk for premature birth, low birth weight or small for gestational age infants, or high birth weight infants
Consider intrauterine ultrasound for structural and growth abnormalities in all babies exposed to antipsychotic medication in utero. In particular, consider high-resolution ultrasound for cardiac defects at 20 weeks and at 36 weeks
A baby exposed to antipsychotic medications in utero is at increased risk of neonatal withdrawal symptoms and distress; ensure that tertiary neonatal support is available at delivery
There is at present no strong evidence supporting developmental delay or disadvantage for babies exposed to antipsychotic medication in utero

What is striking about recent research is that more sophisticated methods of analysis suggest that problems relating to the experience of disadvantage for women with a major mental illness may actually form a significant aspect of the negative outcomes measured for these women (Vigod et al. 2015). There are two further conclusions that can be drawn from this: firstly, that harms previously attributed either to the illness itself or to antipsychotic medication treatment may relate more closely to socioeconomic factors.

Secondly, if a more holistic approach to support of these women in pregnancy included efforts to avert homelessness, identify and protect against physical or emotional abuse, support the use of prenatal vitamins, and reduce incidence of smoking, alcohol and illicit drug use, a large proportion of the harms to the foetus and baby could be minimised. Hence care in pregnancy for women with a major mental illness needs to encompass far more than just careful prescribing of appropriate medications; this is only the first step in averting harm. As psychiatrists, we must advocate for best practice in using evidence-based prescribing as part of an overall care package which incorporates these other elements as well.

Emerging evidence does suggest that iatrogenic harms can accrue to the mother and her baby from psychotropic medication treatment. In the case of antipsychotic medication, the harms seem to be becoming more clearly defined. In the first instance, the risk of harms to women appears to be shifting slightly over time. Whereas the risk of reduced fertility from hyperprolactinaemia was previously highly prevalent and associated with first-generation antipsychotic medication (Ajmal et al. 2014), reproductive risks in the era of widespread use of second-generation antipsychotic medication relate more to the risks associated with obesity and diabetes in pregnancy (Newham et al. 2008).

A common thread in several recent research papers is the risk of pre-pregnancy weight gain for subsequent development of gestational diabetes. This suggests that this risk should be considered for every woman with reproductive potential suffering a major mental illness from the age of 15–50. This is especially important given the increased rates of unplanned pregnancy in this group. The cascading risks relating to obesity and gestational diabetes for both mother and baby in pregnancy include increased rates of congenital malformations and macrosomia, increased rates of instrumental delivery and emergency caesarean section, and increased rates of transfer to neonatal intensive care.

Despite these associated risks, the risk and rate of major congenital abnormalities relating directly to exposure to antipsychotic medications in pregnancy does not seem to be significantly elevated (Huybrechts et al. 2016). However, rates of neonatal distress and withdrawal symptoms are high in these babies, and seem to be higher for some antipsychotic medications than others. There is some very limited research to suggest that there is also a dose-related increase in these symptoms.

Notably, in addition to all the socioeconomic harms previously mentioned, these babies are very rarely exposed to just one medication, or just one class of medications. The dramatically elevated risk of neonatal adverse events severe enough to prompt transfer to a NICU occurs in the context of polypharmacy (Sadowski et al. 2013). This is a harm that can be greatly curtailed by sensible, sparing prescribing of only those medications (such as antipsychotics) which are required to maintain a stable mental state. The high rates of transient adverse outcomes at delivery for these babies also suggest that babies of women prescribed psychotropics in pregnancy should birth in a centre with access to neonatal resuscitation and intensive care support (Habermann et al. 2013).

There is a positive note in this discussion; that neurodevelopmental studies, limited though they are at this stage, suggest that developmental delay noted in babies exposed to antipsychotics in pregnancy is unlikely to persist to 1 year postpartum, despite high rates of psychiatric symptoms in women in the first year after delivery (Kulkarni et al. 2014). In recent years, focus has been placed on specific conditions such as autism spectrum disorders and attention deficit hyperactivity disorder. Several well-conducted studies using appropriate analytic techniques to manage the risks inherent in observational data have found, reassuringly, that treatment with antipsychotic medication in pregnancy does not appear to be associated with an increased risk of these specific conditions. However, women who have diagnoses of schizophrenia and bipolar disorder, amongst other mental health diagnoses, may have a genetic vulnerability to these conditions which they may then pass on to their children. This is clearly an avenue of ongoing future research as our understanding of these conditions matures.

In concert with a more sophisticated approach to modelling and analysis, borrowing approaches from other research fields such as health economics (high dimensional propensity scoring, for example, or machine learning techniques), several authors have called for a more sophisticated approach to research in psychotropics (Gentile 2010; Convertino et al. 2016; Habermann et al. 2013; Uguz 2019). It is probably not good enough to lump antipsychotic medications into two baskets and analyse harms associated with each; individual drugs within both novel and older antipsychotic groups have specific modes of action and associated risks which may be distinct, and whose specific harms may be masked by considering them all together. Whereas in the past few years aripiprazole was a focus of concern, now olanzapine appears to be associated with slightly more adverse outcomes for mothers and babies than previously appreciated.

The future of best practice care for women living with a major mental illness in pregnancy and the postpartum incorporates careful analysis of both large population-based data sets and granular review of symptoms and side effects in long-term follow-up studies of mother and baby pairs to inform prescribing practice. Consideration of a woman's reproductive health should be integrated into her care throughout her life, and the care of mothers and babies in the context of maternal mental illness should be a trigger to provide enhanced social, emotional, economic and psychiatric support to avert harm and improve outcomes.

References

Abdullahi I, Wong K, Mutch R, Glasson E, de Klerk N, Cherian S, Downs J, Leonard H. Risk of developmental disorders in children of immigrant mothers: a population-based data linkage evaluation. J Pediatr. 2019;204:275–84.

Afzal M, Siddiqi N, Ahmad B, Afsheen N, Aslam F, Ali A, Ayesha R, Bryant M, Holt R, Khalid H, Ishaq K. Prevalence of overweight and obesity in people with severe mental illness: systematic review and meta-analysis. Front Endocrinol. 2021;12:769309.

Ahlberg R, Garcia-Argibay M, Hirvikoski T, Boman M, Chen Q, Taylor M, Frans E, Bölte S, Larsson H. Shared familial risk factors between autism spectrum disorder and obesity – a register-based familial coaggregation cohort study. J Child Psychol Psychiatry. 2022;63(8):890–9.

Ajmal A, Joffe H, Nachtigall L. Psychotropic-induced hyperprolactinemia: a clinical review. Psychosomatics. 2014;55(1):29–36.

Allaire B, Raghavan R, Brown D. Morbid obesity and use of second generation antipsychotics among adolescents in foster care: evidence from Medicaid. Child Youth Serv Rev. 2016;67:27–31.

Andersen SW, Clemow DB, Corya SA. Long-term weight gain in patients treated with open-label olanzapine in combination with fluoxetine for major depressive disorder. J Clin Psychiatry. 2005;66:1468–76.

Ban L, Gibson J, West J, Fiaschi L, Oates M, Tata L. Impact of socioeconomic deprivation on maternal perinatal mental illnesses presenting to UK general practice. Br J Gen Pract. 2012;62:e671–8.

Barnas C, Bergant A, Hummer M, Saria A, Fleischhacker W. Clozapine concentrations in maternal and fetal plasma, amniotic fluid, and breast milk. Am J Psychiatry. 1994;151(6):945.

Bellet F, Beyens M, Bernard N, Beghin D, Elefant E, Vial T. Exposure to aripiprazole during embryogenesis: a prospective multicenter cohort study. Pharmacoepidemiol Drug Saf. 2015;24(4):368–80.

Bennedsen B, Mortensen P, Olesen A, Henriksen T. Preterm birth and intra-uterine growth retardation among children of women with schizophrenia. Br J Psychiatry. 1999;175:239–45.

Bergink V, Bouvy P, Vervoort J, Koorengevel K, Steegers E, Kushner S. Prevention of postpartum psychosis and mania in women at high risk. Am J Psychiatry. 2012;169(6):609–15.

Bhatia T, Franzos M, Wood J, Nimgaonkar V, Deshpande S. Gender and procreation among patients with schizophrenia. Schizophr Res. 2004;68:387–94.

Boden R, Lundgren M, Brandt L, Reutfors J, Andersen M, Kieler H. Risks of adverse pregnancy and birth outcomes in women treated or not treated with mood stabilisers for bipolar disorder: population based cohort study. BMJ. 2012a;345:e7085.

Boden R, Lundgren M, Brandt L, Reutfors J, Kieler H. Antipsychotics during pregnancy: relation to fetal and maternal metabolic effects. Arch Gen Psychiatry. 2012b;96:715–21.

Braam W, Ehrhart F, Maas A, Smits M, Curfs L. Low maternal melatonin level increases autism spectrum disorder risk in children. Res Dev Disabil. 2018;82:79–89.

Breuillard D, Leunen D, Chemaly N, Auclair L, Pinard JM, Kaminska A, Desguerre I, Ouss L, Nabbout R. Autism spectrum disorder phenotype and intellectual disability in females with epilepsy and PCDH-19 mutations. Epilepsy Behav. 2016;60:75–80.

Briggs G, Freeman R, Yaffe S. Drugs in pregnancy and lactation, eighth edition. Philadelphia: Lippincott, Williams and Wilkins. 2008.

Brunner E, Falk D, Jones M, Dey D, Shatapathy C. Olanzapine in pregnancy and breastfeeding: a review of data from global safety surveillance. Br Med Council Pharmacol Toxicol. 2013;2-13(14):38.

Brynge M, Gardner RM, Sjöqvist H, Lee BK, Dalman C, Karlsson H. Maternal levels of cytokines in early pregnancy and risk of autism spectrum disorders in offspring. Front Public Health. 2022;10:917563.

Bundy H, Stahl D, MacCabe J. A systematic review and meta-analysis of the fertility of patients with schizophrenia and their unaffected relatives. Acta Psychiatr Scand. 2011;123:98–106.

Chan J, Hung S, Lee K, Cheung K, Seto M, Wong C, Lin J, Chang W. Risk of adverse pregnancy, delivery and neonatal outcomes associated with bipolar disorder and prenatal use of mood stabilizers: a population-based cohort study. Psychiatry Res. 2024;339:116050.

Chowdhury M, Hardin J, Love B, Merchant A, McDermott S. Relationship of nonsteroidal anti-inflammatory drug use during pregnancy with autism spectrum disorder and intellectual disability among offspring. J Women's Health. 2023;32(3):356–65.

Cohen L, Viguera A, McInerney K, Freeman M, et al. Reproductive safety of second-generation antipsychotics: current data from the Massachusetts General Hospital National Pregnancy Registry for atypical antipsychotics. Am J Psychiatry. 2016;173(3):263–70.

Connolly N, Anixt J, Manning P, Ping-I Lin D, Marsolo KA, Bowers K. Maternal metabolic risk factors for autism spectrum disorder-an analysis of electronic medical records and linked birth data. Autism Res. 2016;9(8):829–37.

Convertino I, Sansone A, Marino A, Galiulo M, Mantarro S, Antionioli L, Fornai M, Binadizzi C, Tuccori M. Neonatal adaptation issues after maternal exposure to prescription drugs: withdrawal syndromes and residual pharmacological effects. Drug Saf. 2016;39:903–24.

Coppola D, Russo L, Kwarta R, Varughese R, Schmider J. Evaluating the postmarketing experience of risperidone use during pregnancy: pregnancy and neonatal outcomes. Drug Saf. 2007;30:247–64.

Coughlin C, Blackwell K, Bartley C, Hay M, Yonkers K, Bloch M. Obstetric and neonatal outcomes after antipsychotic medication exposure in pregnancy. Obstet Gynecol. 2015;125:1224–35.

Cuomo A, Goracci A, Fagiolini A. Aripiprazole use during pregnancy, peripartum and lactation. A systematic literature search and review to inform clinical practice. J Affect Disord. 2017;228:229–37.

Dale R, Barnett M, Kiernan M. Maternal autoimmunity: risk of neurodevelopmental and neuropsychiatric outcomes. J Neurol Neurosurg Psychiatry. 2017;88:713–4.

Dev V, Krupp P. The side effects and safety of clozapine. Rev Contempor Pharmacother. 1995;6:197–208.

DeVilbiss E, Magnusson C, Gardner R, Rai D, Newschaffer C, Lyall K, Dalman C, Lee B. Antenatal nutritional supplementation and autism spectrum disorders in the Stockholm youth cohort: population based cohort study. BMJ. 2017;359:j4273.

Di Michele V, Ramenghi L, Sabatino G. Clozapine and lorazepam administration in pregnancy. Eur Psychiatry. 1996;11(4):214.

Diav-Citrin O, Shechtman S, Ornoy S, Arnon J, Schaefer C, Garbis H, Clementi M, Ornoy A. Safety of haloperidol and penfluridol in pregnancy: a multicenter prospective controlled study. J Clin Psychiatry. 2005;66:317–22.

Dickson R, Hogg L. Pregnancy of a patient treated with clozapine. Psychiatr Serv. 1998;49(8):1081–3.

Egbe A, Uppu S, Lee S, Stroustrup A, Ho D, Srivastava S. Congenital malformations in the newborn population: a population study and analysis of the effect of sex and prematurity. Pediatr Neonatol. 2015;56(1):25–30.

Einarsson A, Boskovic R. Use and safety of antipsychotic drugs during pregnancy. J Psychiatr Pract. 2009;15:183–92.

Ellfolk M, Leinonen MK, Gissler M, Kiuru-Kuhlefelt S, Saastamoinen L, Malm H. Second-generation antipsychotic use during pregnancy and risk of congenital malformations. Eur J Clin Pharmacol. 2021;77(11):1737–45.

Ellman L, Huttunen M, Lonnqvist J, Cannon T. The effects of genetic liability for schizophrenia and maternal smoking during pregnancy on obstetric complications. Schizophr Res. 2007;93(1–3):229–36.

Ennis Z, Damkier P. Pregnancy exposure to olanzapine, quetiapine, risperidone, aripiprazole and risk of congenital malformations: a systematic review. Basic Clin Pharmacol Toxicol. 2015;116(4):315.

Eriksson J, Sandboge S, Salonen M, Kajantie E, Osmond C. Long-term consequences of maternal overweight in pregnancy on offspring later health: findings from the Helsinki birth cohort study. Ann Med. 2014;46(6):434–8.

Fabre C, Pauly V, Baumstarck K, Etchecopar-Etchart D, Orleans V, Llorca PM, Blanc J, Lancon C, Auquier P, Boyer L, Fond G. Pregnancy, delivery and neonatal complications in women with schizophrenia: a national population-based cohort study. Lancet Reg Health Eur. 2021;10:100209.

Fairthorne J, Hammond G, Bourke J, de Klerk N, Leonard H. Maternal psychiatric disorder and the risk of autism Spectrum disorder or intellectual disability in subsequent offspring. J Autism Dev Disord. 2016;46(2):523–33.

Fairthorne J, de Klerk N, Leonard H, Schieve L, Yeargin-Allsopp M. Maternal race-ethnicity, immigrant status, country of birth, and the odds of a child with autism. Child Neurol Open. 2017;4:2329048X16688125.

Falterman CG, Richardson CJ. Small left colon syndrome associated with maternal ingestion of psychotropic drugs. The Journal of pediatrics. 1980;97(2):308–10.

Farkas V, Farkas G. Teratogenic action of hyperemesis in pregnancy and of medication used to treat it. Zentralbl Gynakol. 1971;10:325–330.

Forrest M, Hill M, Kavanagh D, Tansey K, Waite A, Blake D. The psychiatric risk gene transcription factor 4 (TCF4) regulates neurodevelopmental pathways associated with schizophrenia, autism, and intellectual disability. Schizophr Bull. 2018;44(5):1100–10.

Frayne J, Nguyen T, Allen S, Hauck Y, Liira H, Vickery A. Obstetric outcomes for women with severe mental illness: 10 years of experience in a tertiary multidisciplinary antenatal clinic. Arch Gynecol Obstet. 2019;300(4):889–96.

Freeman M, Viguera A, Góez-Mogollón L, Young A, Caplin P, McElheny S, Church T, Chitayat D, Hernández-Díaz S, Cohen L. Reproductive safety of aripiprazole: data from the Massachusetts General Hospital National Pregnancy Registry for atypical antipsychotics. Arch Womens Ment Health. 2021;24(4):659–67.

Frise C, Attwood B, Watkinson P, Mackillop L. Life-threatening ketoacidosis in a pregnant woman with psychotic disorder. Obstet Med. 2016;9(1):46–9.

Galbally M, Frayne J, Watson S, Morgan V, Snellen M. The association between gestational diabetes mellitus, antipsychotics and severe mental illness in pregnancy: a multicentre study. ANZJOG. 2020;60(1):63–9.

Gao L, Cui SS, Han Y, Dai W, Su YY, Zhang X. Does periconceptional fish consumption by parents affect the incidence of autism spectrum disorder and intelligence deficiency? A case-control study in Tianjin, China. Biomed Environ Sci. 2016;29(12):885–92.

Garayt C, Merieux C. Pregnancy outcome in women exposed to atypical antipsychotics European network of teratology information service conference; 2009.

Gentile S. Antipsychotic therapy during early and late pregnancy. A systematic review. Schizophr Bull. 2010;36(3):518–33.

Goldstein D, Corbin L, Fung M. Olanzapine-exposed pregnancies and lactation: early experience. J Clin Psychopharmacol. 2000;20(4):399–403.

Gong T, Dalman C, Wicks S, Dal H, Magnusson C, Lundholm C, Almqvist C, Pershagen G. Perinatal exposure to traffic-related air pollution and autism spectrum disorders. Environ Health Perspect. 2017;125(1):119–26.

Göpfert M, Reupert A, Maybery D, Nicholson J, Seeman MV, eds. Parental psychiatric disorder: distressed parents and their families. 1st ed. Cambridge University Press; 1996.

Guerin A, Nisenbaym R, Rag J. Use of maternal GHb concentration to estimate the risk of congenital anomalies in the offspring of women with prepregnancy diabetes. Diabetes Care. 2007;30:1920–5.

Guisso D, Saadeh F, Saab D, El Deek J, Chamseddine S, Abou-El-Hassan H, Majari G, Boustany R. Association of autism with maternal infections, perinatal and other risk factors: a case-control study. J Autism Dev Disord. 2018;48(6):2010–21.

Gupta N, Grover S. Safety of clozapine in 2 successive pregnancies. Can J Psychiatr. 2004;49(12):863.

Guyon L, Auffret M, Coussemacq M, Bene J, Deruelle P, Gautier S. Alteration of the fetal heart rate pattern induced by the use of clozapine during pregnancy. Therapie. 2015;70(3):301–3.

Habermann F, Fritzsche J, Fuhlbruck F, Wacker E, Allignol A, Weber-Schoendorfer C, Meister R, Schaefer C. Atypical antipsychotic drugs and pregnancy outcome: a prospective cohort study. J Clin Psychopharmacol. 2013;33:453–62.

Haddad P, Wieck A. Antipsychotic-induced hyperprolactinaemia: mechanisms, clinical features and management. Drugs. 2004;64(20):2291–314.

Hálfdánarson Ó, Cohen J, Karlstad Ø, Cesta C, Bjørk M, Håberg S, Einarsdóttir K, Furu K, Gissler M, Hjellvik V, Kieler H, Leinonen MK, Nørgaard M, Öztürk Essen B, Ulrichsen S, Reutfors J, Zoega H. Antipsychotic use in pregnancy and risk of attention/deficit-hyperactivity disorder and autism spectrum disorder: a Nordic cohort study. Evid Based Ment Health. 2022;25(2):54–62.

Hamra G, Lyall K, Windham G, Calafat A, Sjödin A, Volk H, Croen L. Prenatal exposure to endocrine-disrupting chemicals in relation to autism spectrum disorder and intellectual disability. Epidemiology. 2019;30(3):418–26.

Hannah RS, Roth SH, Spira AW. The effects of chlorpromazine and phenobarbital on cerebellar Purkinje cells. Teratology.1982;26:21–25.

Harris E, Frayne J, Allen S, Renganathan K, Nguyen T. Psychiatric admission during pregnancy in women with schizophrenia who attended a specialist antenatal clinic. J Psychosom Obstet Gynaecol. 2019;40(3):211–6.

Haukka J, Suvisaari J, Lonnqvist J. Fertility of patients with schizophrenia, their siblings, and the general population: a cohort study from 1950 to 1959 in Finland. Am J Psychiatry. 2003;160:460–3.

Hecht P, Hudson M, Connors S, Tilley M, Liu X, Beversdorf D. Maternal serotonin transporter genotype affects risk for ASD with exposure to prenatal stress. Autism Res. 2016;9(11):1151–60.

Heel RC, Brogden RN, Speight TM, Avery GS. Loxapine: a review of its pharmacological properties and therapeutic efficacy as an antipsychotic agent. Drugs. 1978 Mar;15(3):198–217.

Hipwell AE, Kumar R. Maternal psychopathology and prediction of outcome based on mother-infant interaction ratings (BMIS). The British Journal of Psychiatry. 1996;169(5):655–61.

Hizkiyahu R, Levy A, Sheiner E. Pregnancy outcome of patients with schizophrenia. Am J Perinat. 2009;27(1):9–23.

Hong J, Windmeijer F, Novick D, Haro JM, Brown J. The cost of relapse in patients with schizophrenia in the European SOHO (Schizophrenia Outpatient Health Outcomes) study. Prog Neuropsychopharmacol Biol Psychiatry. 2009;33(5):835–41.

Hope H, Parisi R, Ashcroft D, Williams R, Coton S, Kosidou K, et al. Fertility trends of women with serious mental illness in the United Kingdom 1992–2017: a primary care cohort study using the clinical practice research datalink. J Affect Disord. 2020;269:141–7.

Howard LM. The separation of mothers and babies in the treatment of postpartum psychotic disorders in Britain 1900–1960. Archives of Women's Mental Health. 2000 ;3(1):1–5.

Howard L, Kumar C, Leese M, Thornicroft G. The general fertility rate in women with psychotic disorders. Am J Psychiatry. 2002;159:991–7.

Howard L, Goss C, Leese M, Thornicroft G. Medical outcome of pregnancy in women with psychotic disorders and their infants in the first year after birth. Br J Psychiatry. 2003;182:63–7.

Howard L, Goss G, Leese M, Appleby L, Thornicroft G. The psychosocial outcome of pregnancy in women with psychotic disorders. Schizophr Res. 2004a;71:49–60.

Howard L, Thornicroft G, Salmon M, Appleby L. Predictors of parenting outcome in women with psychotic disorders discharged from mother and baby units. Acta Psychiatr Scand. 2004b;110:347–55.

Huybrechts K, Hernandez-Diaz S, Patorno E, Desai R, Mogun H, Dejene S, Cohen J, Panchaud A, Cohen L, Bateman B. Antipsychotic use in pregnancy and the risk for congenital malformations. JAMA Psychiatry. 2016;73(9):938–46.

Huybrechts KF, Bateman BT, Desai RJ, Hernandez-Diaz S, Rough K, Mogun H, Kerzner LS, Davis JM, Stover M, Bartels D, Cottral J. Risk of neonatal drug withdrawal after intrauterine co-exposure to opioids and psychotropic medications: cohort study. bmj. 2017;358.

Huybrechts K, Straub L, Karlsson P, Pazzagli L, Furu K, Gissler M, Hernandez-Diaz S, Nørgaard M, Zoega H, Bateman B, Cesta C, Cohen J, Leinonen M, Reutfors J, Selmer R, Suarez E, Ulrichsen S, Kieler H. Association of in utero antipsychotic medication exposure with risk of congenital malformations in Nordic countries and the US. JAMA Psychiatry. 2023;80(2):156–66.

Igarashi M. Floppy infant syndrome. J Clin Neuromuscular Disorders. 2004;6(2):69–90.

Jablensky A, Morgan V, Zubrick S, Bower C, Yellachich L. Pregnancy, delivery, and neonatal complications in a population cohort of women with schizophrenia and major affective disorders. Am J Psychiatry. 2005;162:79–91.

Karakula H, Szajer K, Rpila B, Grzywa A, Chuchra M. Clozapine and pregnancy-a case history. Pharmacopsychiatry. 2004;37(6):303–4.

King-Hele S, Webb R, Mortensen P, Appleby L, Pickles A, Abel K. Risk of stillbirth and neonatal death linked with maternal mental illness: a national cohort study. Arch Dis Child Fetal Neonatal Edition. 2009;94(2):105–10.

Koga M. Clinical factors related to gains in body mass index (BMI) among patients under long-term antipsychotic treatment. Seishin Shinkeigaku Zasshi. 2003;105(4):473–88.

Koren G, Cohn T, Chitayat D, Kapur B, Remington G, Reid D, Zipursky R. Use of atypical antipsychotics during pregnancy and the risk of neural tube defects in infants. Am J Psychiatry. 2002;159(1):136–7.

Kosidou K, Dalman C, Widman L, Arver S, Lee B, Magnusson C, Gardner R. Maternal polycystic ovary syndrome and the risk of autism spectrum disorders in the offspring: a population-based nationwide study in Sweden. Mol Psychiatry. 2016;21(10):1441–8.

Kraal AZ, Ward KM, Ellingrod VL. Sex differences in antipsychotic related metabolic functioning in schizophrenia spectrum disorders. Psychopharmacology bulletin. 2017;47(2):8.

Kramer C, Ye C, Hanley A, Connelly P, Sermer M, Zinman B, Retnakaran R. Postpartum weight retention and the early evolution of cardiovascular risk over the first 5 years after pregnancy. Cardiovasc Diabetol. 2024;23(1):101.

Kucukgoncu S, Kosir U, Zhou E, Sullivan E, Srihari VH, Tek C. Glucose metabolism dysregulation at the onset of mental illness is not limited to first episode psychosis: a systematic review and meta-analysis. Early Interv Psychiatry. 2019;13(5):1021–31.

Kucukgoncu S, Guloksuz S, Celik K, Bahtiyar M, Luykx J, Rutten B, Tek C. Antipsychotic exposure in pregnancy and the risk of gestational diabetes: a systematic review and meta-analysis. Schizophr Bull. 2020;46(2):311–8.

Kulkarni J, Worsley R, Gilbert H, Gavrilidis E, Van Rheenen T, Wang W, McCauley K, Fitzgerald P. A prospective cohort study of antipsychotic medications in pregnancy: the first 147 pregnancies and 100 one year old babies. PLoS One. 2014;9(5):e94788.

Kulkarni J, Storch A, Baraniuk A, Gilbert H, Gavrilidis E, Worsley R. Antipsychotic use in pregnancy. Expert Opin Pharmacother. 2015;16(9):1335–45.

Lahbib S, Leblond C, Hamza M, Regnault B, Lemée L, Mathieu A, Jaouadi H, Mkaouar R, Youssef-Turki I, Belhadj A, Kraoua I, Bourgeron T, Abdelhak S. Homozygous 2p11.2 deletion supports the implication of ELMOD3 in hearing loss and reveals the potential association of CAPG with ASD/ID etiology. J Appl Genet. 2019;60(1):49–56.

Laursen T, Munk-Olsen T. Reproductive patterns in psychotic patients. Schizophr Res. 2010;121:234–40.

Lee H, Lin H. Maternal bipolar disorder increased low birth weight and preterm births: a nationwide population-based study. J Affect Disord. 2012;121:100–5.

Lee K, Raja E, Lee A, Bhattacharya S, Bhattacharya S, Norman J, Reynolds R. Maternal obesity during pregnancy associates with premature mortality and major cardiovascular events in later life. Hypertension. 2015;66(5):938–44.

Lin H, Chen I, Chen Y, Lee H, Wu F. Maternal schizophrenia and pregnancy outcome: does the use of antipsychotics make a difference? Schizophr Res. 2010;116:55–60.

Lyall K, Croen L, Weiss L, Kharrazi M, Traglia M, Delorenze G, Windham G. Prenatal serum concentrations of brominated flame retardants and autism spectrum disorder and intellectual disability in the early markers of autism study: a population-based case-control study in California. Environ Health Perspect. 2017;125(8):087023.

MacBeth A, McSkimming P, Bhattacharya S, Park J, Gumley A, St Clair D, Barry S. General and age-specific fertility rates in non-affective psychosis: population-based analysis of Scottish women. Soc Psychiatry Psychiatr Epidemiol. 2023;58(1):105–12.

MacCabe J, Martinsson L, Lichtenstein P, Nilsson E, Cnattingius S, Murray E, Hultman C. Adverse pregnancy outcomes in mothers with affective psychosis. Bipolar Disord. 2007;9(3):305–9.

Matevosyan N. Pregnancy and postpartum specifics in women with schizophrenia: a meta-study. Arch Gynecol Obstet. 2011;283(2):141–7.

McGrath J, Hearle J, Jenner L, Plant K, Drummond A, Barkla J. The fertility and fecundity of patients with psychoses. Acta Psychiatr Scand. 1999;99:441–6.

McKenna K, Koren G, Tetelbaum M, Wilton L, Shakir S, Diav-Citrin O, Levinson A, Zipursky R, Einarson A. Pregnancy outcome of women using atypical antipsychotic drugs: a prospective comparative study. J Clin Psychiatry. 2005;66(4):444–9.

McNeil T, Kaij L, Malmquist-Larsson A. Women with nonorganic psychosis: pregnancy's effect on mental health during pregnancy. Acta Psychiatr Scand. 1984;70:140–8.

Mehta T, Van Lieshout R. A review of the safety of clozapine during pregnancy and lactation. Arch Womens Ment Health. 2017;20(1):1–9.

Mendhekar D, Sharma J, Srivastava P, War L. Clozapine and pregnancy. J Clin Psychiatry. 2003;64(7):850.

Miller L, Finnerty M. Sexuality, pregnancy, and childrearing among women with schizophrenia spectrum disorders. Psychiatr Serv. 1996;47:502–6.

Miller L, Finnerty M. Family planning knowledge, attitudes and practices in women with schizophrenic spectrum disorders. J Psychosoc Obstet Gynaecol. 1998;19:210–7.

Modabbernia A, Mollon J, Boffetta P, Reichenberg A. Impaired gas exchange at birth and risk of intellectual disability and autism: a meta-analysis. J Autism Dev Disord. 2016;46(5):1847–59.

Molyneaux E, Poston L, Ashurst-Williams S, Howard L. Obesity and mental disorders during pregnancy and postpartum: a systematic review and meta-analysis. Obstet Gynecol. 2014;123(4):857–67.

Momen N, Robakis T, Liu X, Reichenberg A, Bergink V, Munk-Olsen T. In utero exposure to antipsychotic medication and psychiatric outcomes in the offspring. Neuropsychopharmacology. 2022;47(3):759–66.

Montastruc F, Salvo F, Arnaud M, Bead B, Pariente A. Signal of gastrointestinal congenital malformations with antipsychotics after minimising competition bias: a disproportionality analysis using data from Vigibase. Drug Saf. 2016;39(7):689–96.

Montgomery J, Winterbottom E, Jessani M, Kohegyi E, Fulmer J, Seamonds B, Josiassen R. Prevalence of hyperprolactinemia in schizophrenia: association with typical and atypical antipsychotic treatment. J Clin Psychiatry. 2004;65(11):1491–8.

Moriarty AJ, Nance MR. Trifluoperazine and pregnancy [letter]. Can Med Assoc J. 1963;88:375–6.

Morinaga M, Rai D, Hollander AC, Petros N, Dalman C, Magnusson C. Migration or ethnic minority status and risk of autism spectrum disorders and intellectual disability: systematic review. Eur J Pub Health. 2021;31(2):304–12.

Munk E, Norgaard B, Gislum M, Mortensen P, Sorensen H. Use of antipsychotic drugs during pregnancy and the risk of adverse birth outcomes: a population-based cohort study. Schizophr Bull. 2005;31:233.

Newham J, Thomas S, MacRitchie K, McElhatton P, McAllister-Williams R. Birth weight of infants after maternal exposure to typical and atypical antipsychotics: prospective comparison study. Br J Psychiatry. 2008;192:333–7.

Newport D, Calamaras M, DeVane C, Donovan J, Beach A, Winn S, Knight B, Gibson B, Viguera A, Owens M, Nemeroff C, Stowe Z. Atypical antipsychotic administration during late pregnancy: placental passage and obstetrical outcomes. Am J Psychiatry. 2007;164:1214–20.

Nguyen T, Mordecai J, Watt F, Frayne J. Obstetric and neonatal outcomes of clozapine exposure in pregnancy: a consecutive case series. Arch Womens Ment Health. 2020;23(3):441–5.

Nidey NL, Momany AM, Strathearn L, Carter KD, Wehby GL, Bao W, Xu G, Scheiber FA, Tabb K, Froehlich TE, Ryckman K. Association between perinatal depression and risk of attention deficit hyperactivity disorder among children: a retrospective cohort study. Ann Epidemiol. 2021;63:1–6.

Niemi LT, Suvisaari JM, Haukka JK, Lönnqvist JK. Childhood predictors of future psychiatric morbidity in offspring of mothers with psychotic disorder: results from the Helsinki High-Risk Study. The British Journal of Psychiatry. 2005;186(2):108–14.

Nilsson E, Lichtenstein P, Cnattingius S, Murray R, Hultman C. Women with schizophrenia: pregnancy outcome and infant death among their offspring. Schizophr Res. 2002;58(2–3):221–9.

Nilsson E, Hultman C, Cnattingius S, Olausson P, Bjork C, Lichtenstein P. Schizophrenia and offspring's risk for adverse pregnancy outcomes and infant death. Br J Psychiatry. 2008;193(4):311–5.

O'Connor M, Johnson GH, James DI. Intrauterine effects of phenothiazines. Med J Aust. 1981;1:416–17.

Panchaud A, Hernandez-Diaz S, Freeman M, Viguera A, MacDonald S, Sosinksy A, Cohen L. Use of atypical antipsychotics in pregnancy and maternal gestational diabetes. J Psychiatr Res. 2017;95:84–90.

Park Y, Huybrechts K, Cohen J, Bateman B, Desair R, Patorno E, Mogun H, Cohen L, Hernandez-Diaz S. Antipsychotic medication use among publicly insured pregnant women in the United States. Psychiatr Serv. 2017;68(11):1112–9.

Park Y, Hernandez-Diaz S, Bateman B, Cohen J, Desai R, Patorno E, Glynn R, Cohen L, Mogun H, Huybrechts K. Continuation of atypical antipsychotic medication during early pregnancy and the risk of gestational diabetes. Am J Psychiatry. 2018;175(6):564–74.

Paulus W, Shloemp S, Sterzik K. Atypical antipsychotic agents in early pregnancy. Reprod Toxicol. 2005;20:477.

Perry BI, McIntosh G, Weich S, Singh S, Rees K. The association between first-episode psychosis and abnormal glycaemic control: systematic review and meta-analysis. Lancet Psychiatry. 2016;3(11):1049–58.

Petersen I, McCrea R, Osborn D, Evans S, Pinfold V, Cowen P, Gilbert R, Nazareth I. Discontinuation of antipsychotic medication in pregnancy: a cohort study. Schizophr Res. 2014;159(1):218–25.

Petersen I, Sammon C, McCrea D, Evans S, Cowen P, Nazareth I. Risks associated with antipsychotic treatment in pregnancy: comparative cohort studies based on electronic health records. Schizophr Res. 2016a;176:349–56.

Petersen I, McCrea R, Sammon C, Osborn D, Evans S, Cowen P, Freemantle N, Nazareth I. Risks and benefits of psychotropic medication in pregnancy: cohort studies based on UK electronic primary care health records. Health Technol Assess. 2016b;20(23):1–176.

Pillinger T, Beck K, Gobjila C, Donocik JG, Jauhar S, Howes OD. Impaired glucose homeostasis in first-episode schizophrenia: a systematic review and meta-analysis. JAMA Psychiatry. 2017;74(3):261–9.

Power R, Kyaga S, Uher R, MacCabe J, Langstrom N, Landen M, McGuffin P, Lewis C, Lichtenstein P, Svensson A. Fecundity of patients with schizophrenia, autism, bipolar disorder, depression, anorexia nervosa, or substance abuse vs their unaffected siblings. JAMA Psychiatry. 2013;70(1):22–30.

Public Health Agency of Canada. Congenital anomalies in Canada 2013: a perinatal health surveillance report. Ottawa, 2013.

Ramirez-Celis A, Croen L, Yoshida C, Alexeeff S, Schauer J, Yolken R, Ashwood P, Van de Water J. Maternal autoantibody profiles as biomarkers for ASD and ASD with co-occurring intellectual disability. Mol Psychiatry. 2022;27(9):3760–7.

Reis M, Kallen B. Maternal use of antipsychotics in early pregnancy and delivery outcome. J Clin Psychopharmacol. 2008;28:279–88.

Rifkin L, Lewis S, Jones P, Toone B, Murray R. Low birth weight and schizophrenia. Br J Psychiatry. 1994;165:357–62.

Rojo L, Gaspar P, Silva H, Risco L, Arena P, Cubillos-Robles K, Jara B. Metabolic syndrome and obesity among users of second generation antipsychotics: a global challenge for modern psychopharmacology. Pharmacol Res. 2015;101:74–85.

Sacker A, Done D, Crow T. Obstetric complications in children born to parents with schizophrenia: a meta-analysis of case-control studies. Psychol Med. 1996;26:279–87.

Sadowski A, Todorow M, Brojeni P, Koren G, Nulman I. Pregnancy outcomes following maternal exposure to second-generation antipsychotics given with other psychotropic drugs: a cohort study. BMJ Open. 2013;3:e003062.

Sakai T, Ohtsu F, Mori C, Tanabe K, Goto N. Signal of miscarriage with aripiprazole: a disproportionality analysis of the Japanese adverse drug event report database. Drug Saf. 2017;40(11):1141–6.

Schneid-Kofman N, Sheiner E, Levy A. Psychiatric illness and adverse pregnancy outcome. Int J Gynaecol Obstet. 2008;101:53–6.

Sciberras E, Mulraney M, Silva D, Coghill D. Prenatal risk factors and the etiology of ADHD – review of existing evidence. Curr Psychiatry Rep. 2017;19:1.

Sebire N, Jolly M, Harris J, Wadsworth J, Joffe M, Beard R, Regan L, Robinson S. Maternal obesity and pregnancy outcome: a study of 287,213 pregnancies in London. Int J Obes Relat Metab Disord. 2001;25:1175–82.

Seeman M. Secondary effects of antipsychotics: women at greater risk than men. Schizophr Bull. 2009;35(5):937–48.

Shaw G, Velie E, Schaffer D. Risk of neural tube defect-affected pregnancies among obese women. JAMA. 1996;275(14):1093–6.

Simoila L, Isometsä E, Gissler M, Suvisaari J, Sailas E, Halmesmäki E, Lindberg N. Schizophrenia and induced abortions: a national register-based follow-up study among Finnish women born between 1965-1980 with schizophrenia or schizoaffective disorder. Schizophr Res. 2018;192:142–7.

Simoila L, Isometsä E, Gissler M, Suvisaari J, Halmesmäki E, Lindberg N. Schizophrenia and pregnancy: a national register-based follow-up study among Finnish women born between 1965 and 1980. Arch Womens Ment Health. 2020;23(1):91–100.

Sjölander A, Öberg S, Frisell T. Generalizability and effect measure modification in sibling comparison studies. Eur J Epidemiol. 2022;37(5):461–76.

Slone D, Siskind V, Heinonen O, Monson R, Kaufman D, Shapiro S. Antenatal exposure to the phenothiazines in relation to congenital malformations, perinatal mortality rate, birth weight and intelligence quotient score. Am J Obstet Gynecol. 1977;128(5):486–8.

Spann M, Timonen-Soivio L, Suominen A, Cheslack-Postava K, McKeague I, Sourander A, Brown A. Proband and familial autoimmune diseases are associated with proband diagnosis of autism spectrum disorders. J Am Acad Child Adolesc Psychiatry. 2019;58(5):496–505.

Stamilio DM, Scifres CM. Extreme obesity and postcesarean maternal complications. Obstetrics & gynecology. 2014 Aug;124(2 PART 1):227–32.

Stoner S, Sommi R, Marken P, Anya I, Vaughn J. Clozapine use in two full-term pregnancies. J Clin Psychiatry. 1997;58(8):364–5.

Straub L, Hernández-Díaz S, Bateman B, Wisner K, Gray K, Pennell P, Lester B, McDougle C, Suarez E, Zhu Y, Zakoul H, Mogun H, Huybrechts K. Association of antipsychotic drug exposure in pregnancy with risk of neurodevelopmental disorders: a national birth cohort study. JAMA Intern Med. 2022;182(5):522–33.

Svensson A, LichtensteinP SS, Hultman C. Fertility of first-degree relatives of patients with schizophrenia: a three-generation perspective. Schizophr Res. 2007;91:238–45.

Tang W, Zhou L, Zhang W, Jia Y, Hu F, Chen H. Adverse perinatal pregnancy outcomes in women with schizophrenia: a systematic review and meta-analysis. Schizophr Res. 2023;262:156–67.

Taylor C, Stewart R, Ogden J, Broadbent M, Pasupathy D, Howard L. The characteristics and health needs of pregnant women with schizophrenia compared with bipolar disorder and affective psychoses. Br Med Council Psychiatry. 2015;15:88.

Terrana N, Koren G, Pivovarov J, Etwel F, Nulman I. Pregnancy outcomes following in utero exposure to second-generation antipsychotics: a systematic review and meta-analysis. J Clin Psychopharmacol. 2015;35(5):559–65.

Tick B, Bolton P, Happé F, Rutter M, Rijsdijk F. Heritability of autism spectrum disorders: a meta-analysis of twin studies. J Child Psychol Psychiatry Allied Discip. 2016;57:585–95.

Torloni MR, Betrán AP, Horta BL, Nakamura MU, Atallah AN, Moron AF, Valente O. Prepregnancy BMI and the risk of gestational diabetes: a systematic review of the literature with meta-analysis. Obesity reviews. 2009;10(2):194–203.

Torrico B, Fernàndez-Castillo N, Hervás A, Milà M, Salgado M, Rueda I, Buitelaar J, Rommelse N, Oerlemans A, Bralten J, Freitag C, Reif A, Battaglia A, Mazzone L, Maestrini E, Cormand B, Toma C. Contribution of common and rare variants of the PTCHD1 gene to autism spectrum disorders and intellectual disability. Eur J Hum Genet. 2015;23(12):1694–701.

Toufeili A, Cohen E, Ray J, Wilton A, Brown H, Saunders N, Dennis C, Holloway A, Morrison K, Hanley G, Oberlander T, Bérard A, Tu K, Barker L, Vigod S. Complex chronic conditions among children born to women with schizophrenia. Schizophr Res. 2022;241:24–35.

Uguz F. Antipsychotic use during pregnancy and the risk of gestational diabetes mellitus: a systematic review. J Clin Psychopharmacol. 2019;39(2):162–7.

Vavrusova L, Konikova M. Clozapine administration during pregnancy. Ceska Slovenska Psychiatrie. 1998;94:282–5.

Vemuri M, Rasgon N. A case of olanzapine-induced gestational diabetes mellitus in the absence of weight gain. J Clin Psychiatry. 2007;68(12):1989.

Vigod S, Seeman M, Ray J, Anderson G, Dennis C, Grigoriadis S, Gruneir A, Kurdyak P, Rochon P. Temporal trends in general and age-specific fertility rates among women with schizophrenia (1996–2009): apopulation-based study in Ontario, Canada. Schizophr Res. 2012;139(1–3):169–75.

Vigod S, Kurdyak P, Dennis C, Gruneir A, Newman A, Seeman M, Rochon P, Anderson G, Grigoriadis S, Ray J. Maternal and newborn outcomes among women with schizophrenia: a retrospective population-based cohort study. Br J Obst Gynaecol. 2014;121(5):566–74.

Vigod S, Gomes T, Wilton A, Taylor V, Ray J. Antipsychotic drug use in pregnancy: high dimensional, propensity matched, population based cohort study. BMJ. 2015;350:h2298.

Viguera A, Freeman M, Góez-Mogollón L, Sosinsky A, McElheny S, Church T, Young A, Caplin P, Chitayat D, Hernández-Díaz S, Cohen L. Reproductive safety of second-generation antipsychotics: updated data from the Massachusetts General Hospital National Pregnancy Registry for atypical antipsychotics. J Clin Psychiatry. 2021;82(4):20m13745.

Vinet É, Pineau CA, Clarke AE, Scott S, Fombonne É, Joseph L, Platt RW, Bernatsky S. Increased risk of autism spectrum disorders in children born to women with systemic lupus erythematosus: results from a large population-based cohort. Arthritis Rheumatol. 2015;67(12):3201–8.

Vizzini L, Popovic M, Zugna D, Vitiello B, Trevisan M, Pizzi C, Rusconi F, Gagliardi L, Merletti F, Richiardi L. Maternal anxiety, depression and sleep disorders before and during pregnancy, and preschool ADHD symptoms in the NINFEA birth cohort study. Epidemiol Psychiatr Sci. 2019;28(5):521–31.

Waldman M, Safferman A. Pregnancy and clozapine. Am J Psychiatry. 1993;150(1):168–9.
Waller D, Shaw G, Rasmussen A, Hobbs C, Canfield M, Siega-Riz A, Gallaway M, Correa A. Pre-pregnancy obesity as a risk factor for structural birth defects. Arch Pediatr Adolesc Med. 2007;161:745–50.
Wang IK, Muo CH, Chang YC, Liang CC, Chang CT, Lin SY et al. Association between hypertensive disorders during pregnancy and end-stage renal disease: a population-based study. CMAJ. 2013;185:207–213.
Wang Z, Chan A, Coghill D, Ip P, Lau W, Simonoff E, Brauer R, Wei L, Wong I, Man K. Association between prenatal exposure to antipsychotics and attention-deficit/hyperactivity disorder, autism spectrum disorder, preterm birth, and small for gestational age. JAMA Intern Med. 2021a;181(10):1332–40.
Wang Z, Wong I, Man K, Alfageh B, Mongkhon P, Brauer R. The use of antipsychotic agents during pregnancy and the risk of gestational diabetes mellitus: a systematic review and meta-analysis. Psychol Med. 2021b;51(6):1028–37.
Wang Z, Yuen A, Wong K, Chan A, Coghill D, Simonoff E, Lau W, Wong I, Park S, Man K. Association between prenatal antipsychotic exposure and the risk of attention-deficit/hyperactivity disorder and autism spectrum disorder: a systematic review and meta-analysis. Neurosci Biobehav Rev. 2024;160:105635.
Werler MM, Louik C, Shapiro S, Mitchell A. Pre-pregnancy weight in relation to risk of neural tube defects. JAMA. 1996;275(14):1089–92.
Wichman CL. Atypical antipsychotic use in pregnancy: a retrospective review. Arch Womens Ment Health. 2009;12:53–7.
Windham G, Pearl M, Poon V, Berger K, Soriano J, Eyles D, Lyall K, Kharrazi M, Croen L. Maternal vitamin D levels during pregnancy in association with autism Spectrum disorders (ASD) or intellectual disability (ID) in offspring; exploring non-linear patterns and demographic sub-groups. Autism Res. 2020;13(12):2216–29.
Wisner K, Gracious B, Piontek C, Peindl K, Perel J. Postpartum disorders: phenomenology, treatment approaches, and relationship to infanticide. In: Spinelli MG, editor. Infanticide: psychosocial and legal perspectives on mothers who kill. Washington: American Psychiatric Publishing; 2002. p. 36–60.
Worsley R, Gilbert H, Gavrilidis E, Naughton B, Kulkarni J. Breastfeeding and psychotropic medication. Lancet. 2013;381:905.
Yeh T, Bai Y, Hsu J, Huang K, Tsai S, Chu H, Liang C, Chen M. Bipolar women's antepartum psychotropic exposure and offspring risk of attention-deficit/hyperactivity disorder and autism spectrum disorder. J Affect Disord. 2021;295:1407–14.
Yeong CC, Worsley R, Gilbert H, Kulkarni J. Gestational diabetes in women with mental illness. Aust N Z J Psychiatry. 2014;48(10):958.
Yogev Y, Ben-Haroush A, Kaplan B. Maternal clozapine treatment and decreased fetal heart rate variability. Int J Gynecol Obstet. 2002;79(3):259–60.
Zornberg GL, Jick H. Antipsychotic drug use and risk of first-time idiopathic venous thromboembolism: a case control study. Lancet. 2000;356:1219–23.

Suggested Reading

Abel K. Fetal antipsychotic exposure in a changing landscape: seeing the future. Br J Psychiatry. 2013;202(5):321–3.
Australian Royal. Royal Australian and New Zealand College of Psychiatrists clinical practice guidelines for the treatment of schizophrenia and related disorders. Aust N Z J Psychiatry. 2016;50(5):1–117.
Babu G, Desai G, Chandra P. Antipsychotics in pregnancy and lactation. Indian J Psychiatry. 2015;57(Suppl 2):S303–7.
Bennedsen B. Adverse pregnancy outcome in schizophrenic women: occurrence and risk factors. Schizophr Res. 1998;33:1–26.

Bennedsen B, Mortensen P, et al. Congenital malformations, stillbirths, and infant deaths among children of women with schizophrenia. Arch Gen Psychiatry. 2001;58:674–9.

Daniels J, Forssen U, Hultman C, Cnattingius S, David A, Feychting M, Sparen P. Parental psychiatric disorders associated with autism spectrum disorders in the offspring. Pediatrics. 2008;121:1357–62.

Di Florio A, Forty L, Gordon-Smith K, Heron J, Jones L, Craddock N, Jones I. Perinatal episodes across the mood disorder spectrum. JAMA Psychiatry. 2013;70:168–75.

Epstein R, Bobo W, Shelton R, Arbogast P, Morrow J, Wang W, Chandrasekar R, Cooper W. Increasing use of atypical antipsychotics and anticonvulsants during pregnancy. Pharmacoepidemiol Drug Saf. 2013;22:794–801.

Freeman M, Sosinsky A, Moustafa D, Viguera A, Cohen L. Supplement use by women during pregnancy: data from the Massachusetts General Hospital National Pregnancy Registry for Atypical Antipsychotics. Arch Womens Ment Health. 2016;19(3):437–41.

Freeman M, Sosinsky A, Goez-Mogollon L, Savella G, Moustafa D, Viguera A, Cohen L. Gestational weight gain and pre-pregnancy body mass index associated with second-generation antipsychotic drug use during pregnancy. Psychosomatics. 2018;59(2):125–34.

Galbally M, Snellen M, Power J. Antipsychotic drugs in pregnancy: a review of their maternal and fetal effects. Ther Adv Drug Saf. 2014;5(2):100–9.

Gassó P, Mas S, Molina O, Bernardo M, Lafuente A, Parellada E. Neurotoxic/neuroprotective activity of haloperidol, risperidone and paliperidone in neuroblastoma cells. Prog Neuro-Psychopharmacol Biol Psychiatry. 2012;36(1):71–7.

Gentile S. Clinical utilisation of atypical antipsychotics in pregnancy and lactation. Ann Pharmacother. 2004;38:1265–71.

Gentile S. More than half the women with a history of psychosis have a psychiatric episode in the first year after childbirth. Evidence Based Ment Health. 2005;8(2):33.

Gentile S. A safety evaluation of aripiprazole for treating schizophrenia during pregnancy and puerperium. Expert Opin Drug Saf. 2014;13(12):1733–42.

Gentile S, Fusco M. Neurodevelopmental outcomes in infants exposed in utero to antipsychotics: a systematic review of published data. CNS Spectr. 2017;22(3):273–81.

Getz K, Anderka M, Werler M, Jick S. Maternal pre-pregnancy body mass index and autism spectrum disorder among offspring: a population-based case-control study. Paediatr Perinat Epidemiol. 2016;30(5):479–87.

Gilbert H. About Helen – antipsychotic medication use during pregnancy. A case study. Aust Nurs J. 2009;16(7):20.

Goh I, Bollano E, Einarson T, Koren G. Prenatal multivitamin supplementation and rates of congenital anomalies: a meta-analysis. J Obstet Gynaecol Can. 2006;28(8):680–9.

Howard L, Seneviratne T. Management of women with psychosis during pregnancy. Prog Neurol Psychiatry. 2008;12(2):9–12.

Howard L, Oram S, Galley H, Trevillion K, Feder G. Domestic violence and perinatal mental disorders: a systematic review and meta-analysis. PLoS Med. 2013;10(5):e1001452.

Hunt N, Silverstone T. Does puerperal illness distinguish a subgroup of bipolar patients? J Affect Disord. 1995;34:101–7.

Johnson K, LaPrairie J, Brennan P, Stowe Z, Newport D. Prenatal antipsychotic exposure and neuromotor performance during infancy. Arch Gen Psychiatry. 2012;69(8):787–94.

Jokiranta E, Brown A, Heinimaa M, Cheslack-Postava K, Partanen A, Sourander A. Parental psychiatric disorders and autism spectrum disorders. Psychiatry Res. 2013;207(3):203–11.

Judd F, Komiti A, Sheehan P, Newman L, Castle D, Everall I. Adverse obstetric and neonatal outcomes for women with severe mental illness: to what extent can they be prevented? Schizophr Res. 2014;157(1–3):305–9.

Kallen B, Borg N, Reis M. The use of central nervous system active drugs during pregnancy. Pharmaceuticals (Basel). 2013;6(10):1221–86.

Koren G. Misrepresentation and miscommunication of teratogenic risk of drugs; analysis of three highly publicised international cases. Reprod Toxicol. 2001;15(1):1–3.

Koren G. What adversely affects the unborn – psychotropic drugs or maternal morbidity? J Clin Psychiatry. 2015;76(7):e904–5.

Kulkarni J, McCauley-Elsom K, Marston N, Gilbert H, Gurvich C, de Castella A, Fitzgerald P. Preliminary findings from the National Register of antipsychotic medication in pregnancy. Aust N Z J Psychiatry. 2008;42:38–44.

Larsson H, Eaton W, Madsen K, Vestergard M, Olesen A, Agerbo E, Schendel D, Thorsen P, Mortensen P. Risk factors for autism: perinatal factors, parental psychiatric history, and socioeconomic status. Am J Epidemiol. 2005;161:916–25.

Lobstein R, Koren G. Pregnancy outcome and neurodevelopment of children exposed in utero to psychoactive drugs: the Motherisk experience. J Psychiatry Neurosci. 1997;22(3):192–6.

Lopez-Yarto M, Ruiz-Mirazo E, Holloway A, Taylor V, McDonald S. Do psychiatric medications, especially antidepressants, adversely impact maternal metabolic outcomes? J Affect Disord. 2012;141:120–9.

McCauley-Elsom K, Kulkarni J. Managing psychosis in pregnancy. Aust N Z J Psychiatry. 2007;41:289–92.

McCauley-Elsom K, Gurvich C, Elsom S, Kularni J. Antipsychotics in pregnancy. J Psychiatric Ment Health Nurs. 2009;17(2):97–104.

McColl H, Dhillon M, Howard LM. A systematic review of the nutritional status of women of a childbearing age with severe mental illness. Arch Womens Ment Health. 2013;16(1):39–46.

McEvoy J, Meyer J, Goff D, Nasrallah H, Davis S, Sullivan L, Meltzer H, Hsiao J, Scott Stroup T, Lieberman J. Prevalence of the metabolic syndrome in patients with schizophrenia: baseline results from the clinical antipsychotic trials of intervention effectiveness (CATIE) schizophrenia trial and comparison with national estimates from NHANES III. Schizophr Res. 2005;80:19–32.

McKenna K, Einarson A, Levinson A, Gideon K. Significant changes in antipsychotic drug use during pregnancy. Vet Human Toxicol. 2004;46(1):44–6.

Macritchie K, Young A, McElhatton P. Birth outcome following therapeutic atypical antipsychotics exposure during pregnancy: an ongoing prospective study. Clin Toxicol. 2006;44(4):401–586.

Margulis A, Kang E, Hammad T. Patterns of prescription of antidepressants and antipsychotics across and within pregnancies in a population-based UK cohort. J Matern Child Health. 2014;18:1742–52.

Mei-Dan E, Ray J, Vigod S. Perinatal outcomes among women with bipolar disorder: a population-based cohort study. Am J Obstet Gynecol. 2015;212(3):367.e1–8.

Mendhekar D. Possible delayed speech acquisition with clozapine therapy during pregnancy and lactation. J Neuropsychiatry Clin Neurosci. 2007;19(2):196–7.

Miller L. Comprehensive care of pregnant mentally ill women. J Mental Health Adm. 1992;19:170–7.

Morgan V, Croft M, Valuri G, Zubrick S, Bower C, McNeil T, Jablensky A. Intellectual disability and other neuropsychiatric outcomes in high-risk children of mothers with schizophrenia, bipolar disorder and unipolar major depression. Br J Psychiatry. 2012;200(4):282–9.

NICE. National Institute for Health and Care Excellence; >NICE Guidance>Conditions and diseases>Fertility, pregnancy and childbirth>postnatal care; nice.org.uk

Nguyen T, Faulkner D, Frayne J, Allen S, Hauck Y, Rock D, Rampono J. Obstetric and neonatal outcomes of pregnant women with severe mental illness at a specialist antenatal clinic. Med J Aust. 2013;199(suppl):S26–9.

Nulman I, Citron S, Todorow M, Uleryk E. Neurodevelopment of children exposed to antidepressant and antipsychotic medications during pregnancy. In: Preece P, Riley E, editors. Alcohol, drugs and medication in pregnancy: the long-term outcome for the child. London: Mac Keith Press; 2011. p. 56–84.

Odegard O. Fertility of psychiatric first admissions in Norway 1936–1975. Acta Psychiatr Scand. 1980;62:212–20.

Park S, Phuong V, Lee C, Lee J, Seo M, Cho H, Fang Z, Lee B, Kim Y. Effects of antipsychotic drugs on BDNF, GSK-3β, and β-catenin expression in rats subjected to immobilization stress. Neurosci Res. 2011;71(4):335–40.

Paulus W. Is the use of aripiprazole safe during first trimester of pregnancy? Reprod Toxicol. 2013;37:87.

Peng M, Gao K, Dong Y, Ou J, Calabrese J, Wu R, Zhao J. Effects of prenatal exposure to atypical antipsychotics on postnatal development and growth of infants: a case-controlled, prospective study. Psychopharmacol (Berlin). 2013;228(4):577–84.

Pinkofsky H, Fitzgerald M, Reeves R. Psychotropic treatment during pregnancy [letter]. Am J Psychiatry. 1997;154:718–9.

Scalzo F, Ali S, Holson R. Behavioral effects of prenatal haloperidol exposure. Pharmacol Biochem Behav. 1989;34(4):727–31.

Shao P, Ou J, Peng M, Zhao J, Chen J, Wu R. Effects of clozapine and other atypical antipsychotics on infants development who were exposed to as fetus: a post-hoc analysis. PLoS One. 2015;10(4):e0123373.

Skovlund C, Morch L, Kessing L, Lidegaard O. Association of hormonal contraception with depression. JAMA Psychiatry. 2016;73(11):1154–62.

Stein A, Pearson R, Goodman S, Rapa E, Rahman A, McCallum M, Howard L, Pariante C. Effects of perinatal mental disorders on the fetus and child. Lancet. 2014;384(9956):1800–19.

Štika L, Elisová K, Honzáková H, Hrochova H, Plechatoa H, Strnadova J, Skop B, Svihovec J, Vachova M, Vinar O. Effects of drug administration in pregnancy on children's school behaviour. Pharm Weekbl Sci Edition. 1990;12(6):252–5.

Sutter-Dallay A, Bales M, Pambrun E, Glangeaud-Freudenthal N, Wisner K, Verdoux H. Impact of prenatal exposure to psychotropic drugs on neonatal outcome in infants of mothers with serious psychiatric illnesses. J Clin Psychiatry. 2015;76(7):967–73.

Toh S, Li Q, Cheetham T, Cooper W, Davis R, Dublin S, Hammad T, Li D, Pawloski P, Pinheiro S, Raebel M, Scott P, Smith D, Bobo W, Lawrence J, Dashevsky I, Haffenreffer K, Avalos L, Andrade S. Prevalence and trends in the use of antipsychotic medications during pregnancy in the US 2001-2007: a population-based study of 585,615 deliveries. Arch Womens Ment Health. 2013;16(2):149–57.

Trixler M, Gati A, Fekete S, Tenyi T. Use of antipsychotics in the management of schizophrenia during pregnancy. Drugs. 2005;65(9):1193–206.

Viguera A, Cohen L, Baldessarini R, Nonacs R. Managing bipolar disorder during pregnancy: weighing the risks and benefits. Can J Psychiatr. 2002;47(5):426–36.

Viguera A, Whitfield T, Baldessarini R, Newport D, Stowe Z, Reminick A, Zurick A, Cohen L. Risk of recurrence in women with bipolar disorder during pregnancy: prospective study of mood stabilizer discontinuation. Am J Psychiatry. 2007;16412:1817–24.

Walker A, Rosemberg M, Balaban-Gil K. Neurodevelopmental and neurobehavioral sequelae of selected substances of abuse and psychiatric medications in utero. Child Adolesc Psychiatr Clin N Am. 1999;8(4):845–67.

Wangel A, Molin J, Moghaddassi M, Ostman M. Prior psychiatric inpatient care and risk of caesarean sections: a registry study. J Psychosom Obstet Gynaecol. 2011;32(4):189–97.

Webb R, Abel K, Pickles A, Appleby L. Mortality in offspring of parents with psychotic disorders: a critical review and meta-analysis. Am J Psychiatry. 2005;162(6):1045–56.

Webb R, Pickles A, King-Hele S, Appleby L, Mortensen P, Abel K. Parental mental illness and fatal birth defects in a national birth cohort. Psychol Med. 2008;38(10):1495–503.

Wesseloo R, Kamperman A, Munk-Olsen T, Pop V, Kushner S, Bergink V. Risk of postpartum relapse in bipolar disorder and postpartum psychosis: a systematic review and meta-analysis. Am J Psychiatry. 2016;173:117–27.

Westin A, Brekke M, Molden E, Skogvoll E, Castberg I, Spigset O. Treatment with antipsychotics in pregnancy: changes in drug disposition. Clin Pharmacol Ther. 2018;103(3):477–84.

Wilsgaard T, Schirmer H, Arnesen E. Impact of body weight on blood pressure with a focus on sex differences: the Tromso study, 1986-1995. Arch Int Med. 2000;160(18):2847–53.

Worly B, Gur T. The effect of mental illness and psychotropic medication on gametes and fertility: a systematic review. J Clin Psychiatry. 2015;76(7):974–85.

Yeshayahu Y. The use of olanzapine in pregnancy and congenital cardiac and musculoskeletal abnormalities. Am J Psychiatry. 2007;164:11.

Antipsychotics During Lactation

9

Adele C. Viguera, Alexia M. Jones, Joshua Niforatos, and Carrie Swetlik

9.1 Introduction

Historically, women with serious mood and psychotic disorders have often been discouraged from breastfeeding due to limited lactation safety data for mood stabilizers and second-generation antipsychotics (SGAs.) (Viguera et al. 2010; Sachs and Committee On Drugs 2013; Viguera et al. 2002) While 83.2% of mothers in the United States initiate breastfeeding (Center for Disease Control and Prevention 2022), only approximately 49% of mothers with psychiatric disorders attempt to breastfeed (Santucci et al. 2017), with rates as low as 15% for mothers with bipolar disorder (Shao et al. 2015).

The American Academy of Pediatrics strongly advocates for exclusive breastfeeding during the first six months of life, citing well-documented nutritional, immunological, physical, neurodevelopmental, and psychological benefits for both mother and infant (Center for Disease Control and Prevention 2022; Meek et al. 2022). However, this recommendation becomes more nuanced for women

A. C. Viguera (✉)
Department of Psychiatry and Psychology, Cleveland Clinic, Cleveland, OH, USA
e-mail: viguera@ccf.org

A. M. Jones
Cleveland Clinic, Cleveland, OH, USA
e-mail: jonesa131@ccf.org

J. Niforatos
Department of Emergency Medicine, John Hopkins University – School of Medicine, Baltimore, MD, USA
e-mail: jnifora1@jhmi.edu

C. Swetlik
Department of Neurology, MetroHealth Hospital, Cleveland, OH, USA
e-mail: cswetlik@metrohealth.org

F. Uguz, L. Orsolini (eds.), *Perinatal Psychopharmacology*,
https://doi.org/10.1007/978-3-031-99720-4_9

managing psychiatric conditions whose treatment typically involves multiple psychotropic medications (Galbally et al. 2019; Viguera et al. 2022; Viguera 2024; Baldessarini et al. 2008).

The postpartum period represents a time of increased risk for either onset or relapse of mood, anxiety, and psychotic disorders (Jones and Craddock 2005; Viguera et al. 2007a, 2011; Kendell et al. 1987). Therefore, prioritizing maternal mental health and stability often represents the most prudent clinical approach when evaluating risks and benefits of treatment during the perinatal period (Viguera et al. 2007a; Miller et al. 2023; Cohen et al. 2006). Moreover, medication exposure differs significantly between prenatal exposure and exposure through breast milk (Verstegen et al. 2022).

During pregnancy, drug concentrations in the fetal bloodstream equilibrate with maternal levels, resulting in substantial exposure. In contrast, during breastfeeding infants receive only a small fraction of the mother's medication dose through breastmilk (Verstegen et al. 2022). Data also suggest that for most medications, adverse effects from breast milk exposure are rare (Sachs and Committee On Drugs 2013; Anderson et al. 2016). Consequently, there is no compelling rationale to advise against breastfeeding for postpartum mothers who require psychotropic medications (Sachs and Committee On Drugs 2013; Miller et al. 2023).

Growing evidence indicates that most psychotropic medications, with only a few exceptions, are safe for breastfeeding mothers (Klinger et al. 2013; Pacchiarotti et al. 2016; Fortinguerra et al. 2009; Larsen et al. 2015; Uguz 2016; Gentile 2008; McAllister-Williams et al. 2017). This chapter examines the lactation safety data of antipsychotic medications, with particular emphasis on second-generation antipsychotics (SGAs), and outlines a clinical decision-framework for treatment management.

9.2 Current Clinical Practices and Evolving Treatment Paradigms

9.2.1 Insights from the National Pregnancy Registry for Atypical Antipsychotics

Recent evidence from the National Pregnancy Registry for Atypical Antipsychotics (NPRAA) has provided valuable insights into real-world breastfeeding practices among women taking second-generation antipsychotics (Viguera et al. 2022). This prospective cohort study, conducted between 2008 and 2020, enrolled 2004 women with a history of psychiatric disorders aged 18–45 years, with 1394 completing postpartum follow-up (Viguera et al. 2022). The study revealed significant differences in breastfeeding patterns between women taking SGAs, most of whom were diagnosed with bipolar disorder, and those who were not. The control group consisted of mostly women treated with SSRI/SNRI for unipolar and anxiety disorders. Of women taking SGAs, 59.3% initiated breastfeeding, compared to 88.2% in the control group. By 3 months postpartum, only 23% of women on SGAs maintained breastfeeding compared to 47% in the control group of women with psychiatric disorders taking other psychotropics other than SGAs. Of the women taking SGAs, 60.4% were also on other psychotropic medications (polytherapy), compared to only 24.4% in the control group. Importantly, no serious adverse effects were reported in either the cases or controls per medical record review.

Polytherapy has historically been considered incompatible with breastfeeding (Klinger et al. 2013; Uguz 2016; Viguera et al. 2007b; Sadowski et al. 2013). Thus, the high rate of polytherapy with SGAs observed in this study is striking, and aligns with data demonstrating that multiple psychotropic medications are increasingly used during pregnancy and breastfeeding, especially for mood, anxiety, and psychotic disorders (Sadowski et al. 2013). This finding underscores the clinical reality faced by many women with psychiatric disorders who need more than one medication to maintain symptom stability (Galbally et al. 2019; Viguera 2024; Baldessarini et al. 2008). Although lactation safety data for multiple concurrent psychotropics remains sparse, these findings demonstrate that women who are successfully managed on complex medication regimens may continue breastfeeding their infants safely.

This current trend may reflect a growing awareness among mothers and clinicians that the substantial benefits of breastfeeding outweigh concerns about the uncertain risks of multiple medications during lactation. This finding may also suggest women are independently deciding to breastfeed while taking multiple medications, contrary to clinical recommendations. Similar behavior has been observed among women who were lithium monotherapy responders who chose to breastfeed, despite it being considered a contraindication by many clinicians (Viguera et al. 2007b). Researchers found that healthy, full-term infants who were closely monitored with appropriate labs (TSH, BUN/Cr) in collaboration with a pediatrician were able to successfully breastfeed while their mothers took lithium, with no serious adverse events reported (Viguera et al. 2007b). This suggests that limited data or experience with a particular medication during breastfeeding does not necessarily constitute a contraindication, but rather indicates that breastfeeding may be attempted with appropriate close monitoring and follow-up.

9.3 Pharmacological Principles of Drug Transfer into Breast Milk

Understanding medication transfer into breast milk is complex and requires consideration of multiple pharmacological principles. Drug transfer into breast milk occurs primarily via passive diffusion (Hale's Medications and Mothers' Milk 2026; Begg et al. 2002; Kelsey 2016; Hale 2004). Factors that influence the amount of drug available for secretion into breast milk include molecular weight, protein binding, lipid solubility, drug half-life, and pKa levels (Verstegen et al. 2022; Anderson et al. 2016; Hale's Medications and Mothers' Milk 2026; Begg et al. 2002; Kelsey 2016; Hale 2004). Molecular weight significantly influences medication transfer, with lower molecular weight compounds passing more readily than those with higher molecular weight. While most antipsychotics have low molecular weights allowing moderate milk transfer, quetiapine is an exception with its high molecular weight (Klinger et al. 2013). Protein binding represents another critical factor; medications with high protein binding (>90%) demonstrate limited breast milk transfer. This is particularly relevant for antipsychotics, which feature high protein binding (Klinger et al. 2013). Thus, only a small fraction of the antipsychotic in the form of free drug is available for excretion into breast milk, keeping most of the drug bound in maternal plasma and preventing transfer into breast milk (Klinger et al. 2013).

The lipid solubility of medications significantly impacts their concentration in breast milk (Verstegen et al. 2022). Lipophilic medications tend to concentrate in breast milk due to its higher fat content compared to plasma. Most psychotropics, including antipsychotics, are generally lipophilic compounds (Klinger et al. 2013). Additionally, the pH gradient between breast milk and plasma influences medication transfer. Breast milk (pH 7.2) is slightly more acidic than plasma (pH 7.4), and this pH difference can lead to ion trapping of basic medications in breast milk, potentially increasing infant exposure (Kelsey 2016). Other factors including bioavailability, volume of distribution, and the permeability of the blood-brain barrier also play a role in determining the impact of medication exposure in the infant (Kelsey 2016).

9.3.1 Metrics for Measuring Infant Exposure

There are several methods for evaluating medication exposure through breastfeeding. However, two metrics, the Milk-to-Plasma (M/P) ratio and the Relative Infant Dose (RID), have been typically used in clinical practice and are important metrics in assigning risk categories to various medications (Verstegen et al. 2022; Hale's Medications and Mothers' Milk 2026; Begg et al. 2002; Kelsey 2016). The M/P ratio, which represents the ratio of the concentration of drug in the milk to that in the maternal plasma, is commonly reported in the literature (Verstegen et al. 2022; Uguz 2016). However, its clinical utility remains limited as it only accounts for drug transfer from the mother's blood to breastmilk without accounting for actual infant exposure (Verstegen et al. 2022).

In contrast, the RID attempts to quantify infant exposure and offers a more comprehensive assessment by measuring what percentage of the mother's medication dose reaches her breastfed infant, incorporating both maternal and infant weight into its calculations (Verstegen et al. 2022; McAllister-Williams et al. 2017; Hale's Medications and Mothers' Milk 2026). The current standard considers a relative infant dose of less than 10% of the maternal dose to be safe and compatible with breastfeeding (Verstegen et al. 2022). Notably, almost all psychiatric medications fall below this safe threshold, offering reassurance to both clinicians and mothers (Hale's Medications and Mothers' Milk 2026). For the most commonly prescribed antipsychotics, quetiapine has the lowest RID (0.09–0.43%), followed by aripiprazole (0.7–1.4%), olanzapine (1.0–1.8%), and finally risperidone (2.3–4.7%) suggesting minimal infant exposure through breast milk (Viguera et al. 2007b).

While these metrics provide valuable information, they should not be the sole basis for determining medication compatibility with breastfeeding. They function primarily as *proxy* measures and do not address the true clinical concern of whether the exposure correlates with any serious adverse effects in the infant (Verstegen et al. 2022; Hale's Medications and Mothers' Milk 2026). Other important factors, not captured in these metrics, that may make infants particularly vulnerable to serious adverse reactions include prematurity, enhanced permeability of the blood-brain barrier, and compromised liver function (Payne 2021; Viguera et al. 2007b; Sadowski et al. 2013; Begg et al. 2002).

9.3.2 Medication Risk Category Classifications

Medication risk categorization systems such as the well-established Hale's Lactation Risk Categories (Hale's Medications and Mothers' Milk 2026), provide a standardized framework for evaluating medication safety during breastfeeding based on pharmacokinetic parameters. Other recently published scoring systems consider additional non-pharmacokinetic parameters such as the number of exposed infants reported in the literature and prevalence of reported adverse events in calculating a safety score (Uguz 2021). These various category risk systems provide useful guidance and reduce complex information into a simplified rating score which is certainly user-friendly for clinicians. However, they do not take into consideration other important individual variables which are essential for nuanced clinical decision making—such as infant age and health condition, maternal illness severity, and risks of untreated condition—are not fully captured in these standardized frameworks. Furthermore, inconsistency between these different systems can create confusion, as the same medication may receive different risk categorizations depending on which framework is consulted. Given these constraints, clinicians should view these risk categories as merely one element within a more comprehensive decision-making framework rather than the sole determinant when advising breastfeeding mothers about medication use.

9.4 First-Generation Antipsychotics (FGAs)

First-generation antipsychotics (FGAs) are generally considered compatible with breastfeeding. Although most lactation safety data derive from case reports and observational studies published than controlled trials, the collective evidence demonstrate that these medications appear in minimal concentrations in breast milk and rarely cause adverse events in exposed infants (Klinger et al. 2013; Pacchiarotti et al. 2016; Larsen et al. 2015; Gentile 2008; McAllister-Williams et al. 2017).

9.4.1 Haloperidol

Haloperidol is regarded as one of the safest antipsychotics to use during pregnancy (). While lactation safety data is more limited, Multiple reviews examining haloperidol secretion into breast milk and potential infant effects have concluded that haloperidol is compatible with breastfeeding (). Evidence from observational studies—including several case reports and a prospective observational study—suggests no acute adverse effects in breastfed infants (Whalley et al. 1981; Mendhekar and Andrade 2011; Yoshida et al. 1998a). Only small amounts of haloperidol are excreted into breast milk ().

In one case report, a mother started on 10 mg/day of haloperidol immediately after birth and discontinued therapy after 6 weeks all while breastfeeding her infant (Whalley et al. 1981). The infant showed no signs of sedation and was feeding well. Follow-up assessments indicated normal development.

In another report, a mother took haloperidol (7.5–15 mg/day) and trihexyphenidyl during three pregnancies and throughout the postpartum periods (Mendhekar and Andrade 2011). She breastfed all three infants for 6–8 months. All children met developmental milestones at the time of report (ages 16 months to 8 years).

In a small prospective study on the long-term effects of antipsychotics in breastfed infants, a decline in developmental scores was found at 12–18 months of age in 2 of 4 infants of mothers taking both haloperidol and chlorpromazine. The other 2 infants and all infants exposed to either drug alone developed normally (Yoshida et al. 1998a).

A breastfeeding mother with schizophrenia took risperidone (1.5 mg) and later added haloperidol, which was increased from 0.8 to 1.5 mg/day due to recurring symptoms. Three days after the increase, her infant experienced excessive sedation, poor feeding, and motor slowing, which resolved within 5 days after breastfeeding was discontinued, suggesting the drug combination was the cause (Uguz 2019).

9.4.2 Chlorpromazine

Multiple reviews of studies that examined the secretion of chlorpromazine into breast milk and potential adverse effects in infants have concluded that chlorpromazine may be compatible with breastfeeding (Klinger et al. 2013; Pacchiarotti et al. 2016; Drugs and Lactation Database (LactMed®) 2006e). Excretion in breast milk appears to be in small amounts (Yoshida et al. 1998a), with an estimated relative infant dose of 0.03–1.3% (Klinger et al. 2013; Odhejo et al. 2017). Older studies have noted drowsiness and placidity in infants (Yoshida et al. 1998b; Wiles et al. 1978).

In a study of four mother-infant pairs, chlorpromazine doses ranged from 50 to 600 mg/day. While no acute negative effects were observed aside from possible drowsiness, developmental delays were noted in infants exposed to both chlorpromazine and haloperidol (Yoshida et al. 1998b). In another study, two breastfed infants were observed: one exhibited drowsiness and lethargy, potentially linked to chlorpromazine, while the other showed no adverse effects. Breast milk chlorpromazine concentrations were 92 ng/mL in the affected infant's mother and 7 ng/mL in the unaffected infant's mother (Wiles et al. 1978).

Seven infants were breastfed for 3–4 months while their mothers took chlorpromazine (50–150 mg daily at bedtime) (Kris and Carmichael 1957). Five of the infants were later evaluated at ages up to 4–5 years, showing no noticeable issues with behavior, emotions, or mental health (Kris and Gross 1962). Thus, while levels in breast milk and adverse effects of exposure to chlorpromazine are low, close supervision with attention to drowsiness and development in the infant is recommended.

Other FGAs, such as trifluoperazine and perphenazine, are compatible with breastfeeding (Klinger et al. 2013). Again, data are limited but suggest low levels of medication found in the breast milk and no acute adverse effects (Klinger et al. 2013).

9.5 Second-Generation Antipsychotics (SGAs)

Second-generation antipsychotics have increasingly become the preferred first-line treatment in the treatment of mood, anxiety, and psychotics disorders compared to FGAs given a decreased risk of extrapyramidal side effects and their prolactin-sparing properties. Although evidence supporting the reproductive safety of these medications has expanded over the past two decades, data regarding their safety during lactation remains significantly less robust and continues to evolve.

9.5.1 Olanzapine

Of the SGAs, olanzapine has been the most widely studied with respect to breastfeeding and is considered a reasonable choice for women who require a second-generation antipsychotic while nursing (Klinger et al. 2013; Pacchiarotti et al. 2016; Larsen et al. 2015; Uguz 2016). The bulk of the current evidence suggests that olanzapine is compatible with breastfeeding (Drugs and Lactation Database (LactMed®) 2006f, g). The reported relative infant dose of olanzapine ranges from 0.3% to 4% of the weight-adjusted maternal dose (Gardiner et al. 2003; Kirchheiner et al. 2000; Ambresin et al. 2004; Lutz et al. 2008; Croke et al. 2002).

Several observational studies provide evidence that olanzapine use during breastfeeding does not adversely affect infants. A review of 10 studies (total $n = 64$ infants exposed to olanzapine) found that somnolence was observed in three infants (5%), slow weight gain in two (3%), and developmental delay in three (5%) (Klinger et al. 2013).

A prospective study found that adverse events were comparable for breastfeeding infants whose mothers were taking olanzapine (3/22 infants, 14%), non-breastfeeding infants of mothers taking olanzapine (1/15, 7%), and breastfeeding infants whose mothers were taking a drug known to be safe during lactation (4/51, 8%) (Gilad et al. 2011).

A study examining the manufacturer's safety registry, which included spontaneously reported adverse events in mothers who used olanzapine during pregnancy and/or breastfeeding, found no adverse events were reported in 84/102 breastfed infants (82.3%). The most common adverse events associated with exposure were nonspecific, such as somnolence (4%), irritability (2%), tremor (2%), and insomnia (2%) (Brunner et al. 2013).

Several studies of serum assays of infants (total $n = 12$) exposed to olanzapine via breast milk have not detected the drug (McAllister-Williams et al. 2017; Gilad et al. 2011). The mechanism may be due to low absorption and distribution of the drug in the large amounts of fat in children. However, one case report described an infant who had a serum concentration that was approximately 40 percent of the maternal level; subsequent infant serum concentrations were very low or undetectable (Reis and Källén 2008).

9.5.2 Risperidone and Paliperidone

The evidence suggests that risperidone and its active metabolite, paliperidone, are compatible with breastfeeding (Klinger et al. 2013; Pacchiarotti et al. 2016; Larsen et al. 2015; Uguz 2016; Risperidone 2006). The relative infant dose for risperidone ranges from 2.3% to 9.1% of the weight-adjusted maternal dose (Klinger et al. 2013; Ilett et al. 2004). In three case report studies, infant serum assays (total $n = 4$ infants) found that risperidone and its active metabolite were only detected in one infant in which the metabolite was present at minimal concentrations (Ilett et al. 2004; Aichhorn et al. 2005; Weggelaar et al. 2011). Additionally, the reported M/P ratios were all below 0.5 (Ilett et al. 2004). In a separate study, concentration of the metabolite in breastmilk itself has also found to be low consistent with these findings (Hill et al. 2000). Risperidone has been found to cause elevated prolactin serum levels (Bray and Karri 2022) However, high levels of prolactin alone may not affect a mother with established lactation's ability to breastfeed (Risperidone 2006).

Two case studies (total $n = 3$ infants) found no acute adverse effects occurred in breastfed infants (Ilett et al. 2004; Aichhorn et al. 2005). In mothers prescribed up to 6 mg/day, no adverse effects have been reported in infants (Hill et al. 2000; Bray and Karri 2022). One study of two mothers on 4 mg/day and 6 mg/day while breastfeeding found no long-term developmental abnormalities of infants at 9 months and 12 months of age, respectively (Ratnayake and Libretto 2002) Another study of a mother on 1 mg/day found no physical or neurological abnormalities at 3 months of age (Weggelaar et al. 2011).

In one recent study of a mother who started risperidone 1 mg/daily on postpartum day 12 for psychiatric episodes, researchers concluded that her preterm infant's two episodes of respiratory depression were likely caused by the drug (Pasi et al. 2023). A recent 26 year follow-up of a woman who took 4–5 mg/day of risperidone and 2 mg/day of trihexyphenidyl while breastfeeding all five of her children for 20–24 months each, found that all children are or have done well academically and the oldest three completed their education and were gainfully employed (Mendhekar and Andrade 2024).

9.5.3 Quetiapine

Most studies suggest that quetiapine is compatible with breastfeeding (Klinger et al. 2013; Pacchiarotti et al. 2016; Larsen et al. 2015; Uguz 2016; Drugs and Lactation Database (LactMed®) 2006a). Quetiapine demonstrates low excretion into breast milk (Drugs and Lactation Database (LactMed®) 2006a). Case series report that quetiapine was not secreted into breast milk at all at maternal daily doses <75 mg, and for higher maternal doses, infant dose was calculated to be less than 0.01 mg/kg (Misri et al. 2006; Aydin et al. 2015; Rampono et al. 2007). The reported relative infant dose ranges from 0.07% to 0.1%, which is extremely low (Klinger et al. 2013). Quetiapine has been found to have minimal effects on prolactin levels (Maguire 2002).

One case report of a mother on 200 mg/day of quetiapine for bipolar disorder reported no adverse effects in her breastfed infant (Uguz 2017). In another study, the infant of a mother taking 300 mg/day during the last 3 months of pregnancy and continuing post-partum was developing normally with no apparent adverse effects (Pastol et al. 2022). Several other studies report no adverse effects in breastfed infants of mothers taking quetiapine and other combinations of drugs including sodium valrpoate (Aydin et al. 2015), venlafaxine (Newport et al. 2009), and lamotrigine (Sharma and Sommerdyk 2016).

In the Misri et al. series of case reports, two infants of six were found to have mild developmental delays at age 12 months, but the persistence of these findings into later childhood remains unknown (Misri et al. 2006). In a prospective cohort study in India, two infants exposed to quetiapine in breastmilk had no short-term adverse events, however one who was also exposed in utero had motor and mental delays at 3 months (Sinha et al. 2021).

9.5.4 Aripiprazole

Although definitive data regarding the use of aripiprazole during breastfeeding are limited to case reports, the available evidence is generally reassuring, showing minimal concentrations in breast milk with a relative infant dose estimated at 0.7–6.44% (Aripiprazole 2006; Nordeng et al. 2014; Lutz et al. 2010). Additionally, no significant adverse effects have been observed in breastfed infants (Klinger et al. 2013; Pacchiarotti et al. 2016; Uguz 2016; Nordeng et al. 2014; Lutz et al. 2010; Cuomo et al. 2018; Watanabe et al. 2011).

The primary concern regarding aripiprazole during breastfeeding stems from multiple case reports linking it to inadequate milk production and premature lactation cessation (Mantilla Reyes et al. 2020; Sahoo et al. 2023; Naughton et al. 2023; Yskes et al. 2018; Walker et al. 2019; Gentile 2014). Since aripiprazole functions as both a partial dopamine agonist and antagonist, it can reduce serum prolactin levels in a dose-dependent manner, potentially leading to insufficient milk production by inhibiting prolactin release (Nordeng et al. 2014; Lutz et al. 2010). However, this effect is not consistently observed across all patients. Nevertheless, certain risk classification systems suggest that an alternate medication might be more appropriate (Uguz 2021; Aripiprazole 2006) or use with caution (Hale's Medications and Mothers' Milk 2026). In addition, available reports suggest no issues with infant growth and development in the short term (Nordeng et al. 2014; Lutz et al. 2010). A separate case report involving a mother using injectable aripiprazole while breastfeeding indicated normal developmental progression in her child through 3 years of age (Fernández-Abascal et al. 2021).

9.5.5 Clozapine

Clozapine stands out as the only antipsychotic generally contraindicated during breastfeeding due to the risk for agranulocytosis (Drugs and Lactation Database (LactMed®) 2006b). Although its RID is below 2%, its use would necessitate regular monitoring of the infant with white blood cell counts and careful observation for sedation effects, creating practical barriers to its safe use during lactation (Klinger et al. 2013; Pacchiarotti et al. 2016; Larsen et al. 2015; Uguz 2016; Gentile 2008; McAllister-Williams et al. 2017; Payne 2021; Uguz 2021; Drugs and Lactation Database (LactMed®) 2006b).

If breastfeeding is undertaken by a mother who is taking clozapine, close monitoring of the infant for hematologic effects (as is standard in adults taking clozapine) is highly recommended. Case reports suggest that clozapine tends to accumulate readily in breast milk in a dose-dependent manner (Barnas et al. 1994; Dev and Krupp 1995), however it does not appear to influence maternal prolactin levels (Maguire 2002; Bergemann et al. 2005). The relative infant dose for clozapine is approximately 1.4% of the weight-adjusted maternal dose, but concerns about adverse effects remain significant (Klinger et al. 2013).

A review of two observational studies (total $n = 5$ infants exposed to clozapine) found that one baby suffered agranulocytosis, one baby manifested lethargy, and one had speech delay (Klinger et al. 2013). In a separate case study, an infant exposed during both pregnancy and breastfeeding through 1 year of age had noticeable delay in speech acquisition though no other neurocognitive or motor deficits were reported (Mendhekar 2007).

In a recent case report, a woman with schizophrenia breastfed during two pregnancies while taking clozapine (Uygur and Uygur 2019). No adverse effects were reported after the first. During the second, under psychiatric care, she delivered while on clozapine 100 mg daily, which was tapered as olanzapine was started and increased to 20 mg daily. Due to ongoing hallucinations, clozapine was resumed at 50 mg daily while breastfeeding continued. After a year of pediatric follow-up, no agranulocytosis, seizures, or neurodevelopmental issues were observed in the infant (Uygur and Uygur 2019).

Another case report described a woman with schizophrenia who took 75 mg of clozapine daily during pregnancy and postpartum while breastfeeding (extent unspecified) (Uguz 2020). Her infant, monitored monthly with biweekly blood tests for 6 months, showed no hematologic or other adverse effects (Uguz 2020). However, these findings are based on a very small sample size and limited recent data.

The consensus in the medical literature recommends to avoid clozapine during breastfeeding (Klinger et al. 2013; Pacchiarotti et al. 2016; Larsen et al. 2015; Uguz 2016, 2021; Hale 2004; Gentile 2010; Drugs and Lactation Database (LactMed®) 2006b). Recently, lactation safety scoring systems developed have also categorized the safety of clozapine as "very low" and therefore, not recommended with breastfeeding (Uguz 2021). However, if breastfeeding is undertaken, since clozapine has not been considered an absolute contraindication to breastfeeding, close monitoring of the infant is warranted (Uguz 2020).

9.5.6 Amisulpride

Data on infant exposure to amisulpride via breastfeeding is lacking (Fortinguerra et al. 2009; Uguz 2016; Drugs and Lactation Database (LactMed®) 2006c) and excretion of amisulpride into breastmilk is higher than with other pharmacologically similar drugs (Drugs and Lactation Database (LactMed®) 2006c). Two case reports show high transfer of amisulpride into breast milk with maternal dose of 200 mg/day and 400 mg/day, resulting in a relative infant dose of 6.7–10.7%, respectively (Ilett et al. 2010; Teoh et al. 2011).

These infants, however, experienced no side effects from amisulpride exposure and had normal development at follow-up. O'Halloran et al. (2016) assessed one mother-infant pair with amisulpride exposure in breast milk and found the concentration to be 12-fold higher than simultaneous serum concentration (O'Halloran et al. 2016). The infant plasma concentration was about 10.5% of the maternal plasma concentration. Given the lack of quality studies, amisulpride's compatibility with breastfeeding remains largely unknown, and its use in breastfeeding should be evaluated on a case-by-case basis.

9.5.7 Ziprasidone

Data for ziprasidone during breastfeeding are very limited (Drugs and Lactation Database (LactMed®) 2006d). In one woman receiving a dose of 160 mg/day postpartum, drug levels in milk were undetectable (Schlotterbeck et al. 2009). The milk-to-plasma ratio was estimated to be 0.06, with a relative infant dose estimated at 1.2% (Schlotterbeck et al. 2009). A separate case report found that infant exposure to ziprasidone through breast milk resulted in no acute adverse effects, and the infant was healthy with normal growth and development at 6 months of age (Werremeyer 2009).

9.5.8 Newer Second-Generation Antipsychotics

No substantial data are available on the use of asenapine (2006), brexpiprazole (2006), cariprazine (2006), iloperidone (2006), lumateperone (2006), or lurasidone (2006) during breastfeeding. However, insufficient data does not automatically imply that a medication is "unsafe" or incompatible with nursing.

9.6 Comprehensive Risk-Benefit Assessment Framework

Clinical decision-making regarding antipsychotic use during breastfeeding requires careful consideration of multiple factors. An individualized assessment tailored to each mother-infant pair's specific circumstances, including psychiatric history, medication response, and infant health status is recommended. Informed decision-making involves engaging mothers in the process with complete information about benefits, as well as known and unknown risks. Throughout this process, the mother's own preferences regarding breastfeeding should be considered as a critical component. An assessment framework is presented below:

9.6.1 Assessment of Maternal Factors and Infant Factors

Maternal mental health must be prioritized, as untreated psychiatric illness poses greater risks to both mother and infant than medication exposure through breast milk (Miller et al. 2023). While breastfeeding offers important benefits, delaying necessary psychiatric medications only to continue breastfeeding can have serious consequences including deteriorating mental health symptoms, prolonged periods without treatment, and negative effects on both maternal and infant well-being. Women who have remained stable on a psychotropic regimen during pregnancy should generally maintain their regimen postpartum, as changing medications solely for the purpose of breastfeeding is not recommended (Miller et al. 2023).

For patients who are initiating treatment with an antipsychotic during the postpartum period, medication selection should be guided by what has been effective in the past. If a medication is started de novo, the patient's symptomatology and severity of symptoms should guide medication selection. A family history of a good response to a particular medication may also help guide medication choice.

The decision to breastfeed while taking medications is more complicated when a baby is premature or medically compromised (Nonacs et al. 2016; Llewellyn and Stowe 1998). The infant's gestational age significantly impacts medication metabolism, as premature infants have reduced metabolic capacity compared to full-term infants. Since most psychotropic medications are metabolized by the liver, there is lower capacity for hepatic drug metabolism (one-third to one-fifth of adult capacity) during the first few weeks of a full-term infant's life (Verstegen et al. 2022; Begg et al. 2002; Kelsey 2016). This capacity increases dramatically over the first few months, and by about 2–3 months of age actually surpasses that of adults. In premature infants or in infants with signs of compromised hepatic function (e.g., hyperbilirubinemia), breastfeeding is typically deferred because these infants are less able to metabolize drugs and may be more susceptible to experience adverse events (Verstegen et al. 2022; Begg et al. 2002; Kelsey 2016).

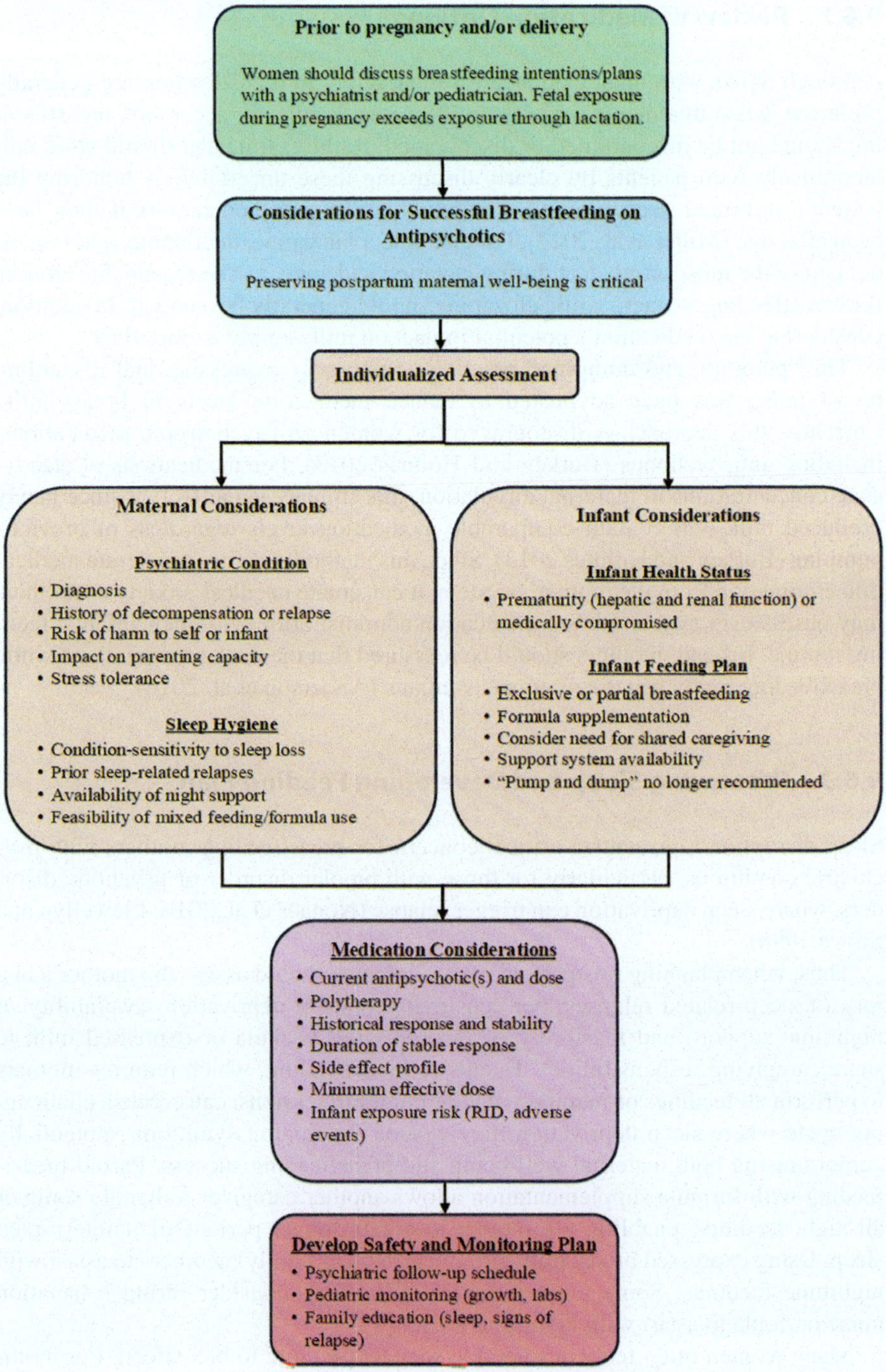
Prior to pregnancy and/or delivery
Women should discuss breastfeeding intentions/plans with a psychiatrist and/or pediatrician. Fetal exposure during pregnancy exceeds exposure through lactation.
Considerations for Successful Breastfeeding on Antipsychotics
Preserving postpartum maternal well-being is critical
Individualized Assessment
Maternal Considerations
Psychiatric Condition
• Diagnosis
• History of decompensation or relapse
• Risk of harm to self or infant
• Impact on parenting capacity
• Stress tolerance
Sleep Hygiene
• Condition-sensitivity to sleep loss
• Prior sleep-related relapses
• Availability of night support
• Feasibility of mixed feeding/formula use
Infant Considerations
Infant Health Status
• Prematurity (hepatic and renal function) or medically compromised
Infant Feeding Plan
• Exclusive or partial breastfeeding
• Formula supplementation
• Consider need for shared caregiving
• Support system availability
• "Pump and dump" no longer recommended
Medication Considerations
• Current antipsychotic(s) and dose
• Polytherapy
• Historical response and stability
• Duration of stable response
• Side effect profile
• Minimum effective dose
• Infant exposure risk (RID, adverse events)
Develop Safety and Monitoring Plan
• Psychiatric follow-up schedule
• Pediatric monitoring (growth, labs)
• Family education (sleep, signs of relapse)

9.6.2 Review of Medication Options

Although SGAs with most evidence for their safety in breastfeeding are generally preferred, when treatments with less evidence are medically necessary, breastfeeding should not be discontinued or discouraged. Rather, clinicians should work collaboratively with patients by clearly discussing these uncertainties, honoring the patient's informed decision, and continuing pregnancy medications if they have been effective (Miller et al. 2023). For example, olanzapine, quetiapine, and risperidone have the most safety data during lactation and appear to be reasonable choices for breastfeeding women, while clozapine should generally be avoided. In addition, considering the medication's potential impact on milk supply is important.

The "pumping and dumping" practice (temporarily expressing and discarding breast milk) was once advocated to reduce medication levels in breast milk. Currently, this approach is discouraged for women on psychotropic medications, including antipsychotics (Burkey and Holmes 2013). For medications at steady-state concentrations in maternal circulation, this strategy is ineffective since newly produced milk will contain comparable medication levels regardless of previous pumping (Burkey and Holmes 2013). Since this method does not accelerate medication elimination from the mother's system, it can create needless anxiety as mothers may obsess over synchronizing medication administration with their infant's feeding routine. Instead, mothers should be reassured that the use of medications while breastfeeding rarely negatively impacts infants (Anderson et al. 2016).

9.6.3 Preserving Sleep and Developing Feeding Plan

Sleep disruption represents a critical concern for breastfeeding mothers with psychiatric conditions, particularly for those with bipolar disorder or psychotic disorders, where sleep deprivation can trigger relapse (Nonacs et al. 2016; Llewellyn and Stowe 1998).

Thus, when planning postpartum care, clinicians should assess the mother's history of sleep-related relapses, her sensitivity to sleep deprivation, availability of nighttime support, and feasibility of incorporating formula or expressed milk to share caregiving responsibilities. Exclusive breastfeeding, which requires mothers to perform all feedings or maintain regular pumping sessions, can create a challenging cycle where sleep deprivation may worsen psychiatric symptoms, potentially compromising both maternal well-being and breastfeeding success. Partial breastfeeding with formula supplementation allows another caregiver to handle some or all-night feedings, enabling the mother to obtain longer periods of uninterrupted sleep. Using expressed breast milk allows partners or family members to assist with nighttime feedings. Some mothers and families may consider hiring a lactation nurse or doula to assist with nighttime feedings.

Many women often feel considerable societal pressure to breastfeed. For mothers with bipolar disorder or psychotic disorders, for whom sleep disruption is a particularly significant trigger for relapse, prioritizing sleep protection is essential to preventing relapse and minimizing psychiatric morbidity. Therefore, forgoing breastfeeding may be in the best interest of the mother-infant dyad. Clinicians should be aware of the potential psychological distress and maternal guilt surrounding such feeding decisions, and stress the overarching clinical principle that maternal well-being supports infant well-being.

9.6.4 Maternal and Infant Monitoring

Maternal monitoring should include evaluation of psychiatric symptoms, medication side effects, and impact on milk supply. For infants, standardized monitoring protocols remain absent. Routine and regular pediatric assessments for growth, developmental milestones, feeding patterns, alertness, sleep, and behavior are recommended. Any change in the infant's behavior from baseline should be investigated further. If a medication exposure is suspected of causing an adverse effect, temporarily suspending breastfeeding allows for evaluation. In a clinical scenario of a mother breastfeeding on an SGA with no to minimal safety data, close monitoring is recommended.

Measuring drug levels in the breastfeeding baby is generally not recommended since in most instances, antipsychotic levels are low or non-detectable in the infant serum. However, if there is a meaningful change in the infant's behavior (e.g., sedation, irritability, feeding problems), an infant's serum level may be helpful.

It is also important for the treating psychiatrist and the infant's pediatrician to work collaboratively in supporting the mother's decision to breastfeed or not. Ideally, it is advisable for the mother to discuss her plans to breastfeed with her psychiatrist and pediatrician *prior* to delivery. Such a discussion ensures an interdisciplinary team approach that can respond nimbly with any changes in circumstances.

9.7 Resources for Clinicians on Medication Safety During Breastfeeding

Resources for clinical decision making have expanded significantly. Breastfeeding mothers and their healthcare providers can access several comprehensive, evidence-based resources on medication safety during lactation. These highly reputable references provide up-to-date information to support informed clinical decisions. While not exhaustive, the following represent key professional resources available for consultation:

LactMed® (www.ncbi.nlm.nih.gov/books/NBK501922) is a free online resource maintained by the National Library of Medicine that serves as the most comprehensive and frequently updated online database for medication safety during lactation. It provides detailed information about maternal and infant drug levels, potential effects on infants, impacts on milk production, and suggested alternatives when available. There is also a free smartphone app, **LactRx**, designed for healthcare providers and breastfeeding mothers. This app provides quick access to information about medication safety during lactation using the LactMed database in a mobile-friendly format, allowing users to search for medications and review their compatibility with breastfeeding.

MotherToBaby (https://mothertobaby.org/pregnancy-breastfeeding-exposures) is a service of the non-profit Organization of Teratology Information Specialists (OTIS) and is one of the leading authorities and most trusted source of evidence-based information on the safety of medications and other exposures during pregnancy. MotherToBaby provides Q&A format medication fact sheets in both English and Spanish, making it an invaluable tool for patient education. These materials cover a wide range of medications and their use during both pregnancy and lactation, presenting complex medical information in an accessible format. In addition, they also offer "Ask and Expert" service via live chat which offers free, personalized, and confidential exposure information for both patients and clinicians.

The **InfantRisk Call Center at the Texas Tech Health Sciences Center** https://www.infantrisk.com (1-806-352-2519; M-F 8 am-3 pm CST) offers current information regarding medication safety for breastfeeding mothers. Staffed by nurses with specialized training from Drs. Hale and Krutsch, the center serves as an important free resource for both healthcare providers and patients seeking guidance on medications during lactation. Additionally, the center conducts ongoing research in this field and welcomes mother volunteers who wish to participate in their studies.

Hale's Medications & Mothers' Milk 2025–2026 (21st Edition) by Thomas W. Hale, RPh, PhD & Kaytlin Krutsch, PhD, PharmD, MBA, BCPS is an authoritative textbook on medication safety during lactation, trusted by healthcare professionals worldwide for years. It provides evidence-based analysis of over 1200 medications, current pharmacokinetic data and milk transfer information, clear risk categorization for clinical decision-making, and practical alternatives for high-risk medications. There is also a digital access platform available through **HalesMeds.com** for real-time updates between print editions. This is a paid subscription service.

The Food and Drug Administration (FDA) Pregnancy and Lactation Labeling Rule

The FDA Pregnancy and Lactation Labeling Rule (PLLR) (https://www.fda.gov/drugs/labeling-information-drug-products/pregnancy-and-lactation-labeling-resources) represents a significant improvement in medication safety information by replacing the previous A, B, C, D, X categorization system. This new approach requires that drug labels provide detailed, narrative summaries of available research addressing effects on women, fetuses, infants, and milk production, along with clinical considerations for minimizing exposure. While demanding more careful analysis from clinicians rather than offering simple categorical recommendations, the PLLR provides more accurate and nuanced guidance for clinical decision-making regarding drug use during pregnancy and lactation.

9.8 Conclusion and Future Directions

The overwhelming evidence, although limited, suggests that most first-generation and second-generation antipsychotics are compatible with breastfeeding, with the notable exception of clozapine. Medication choice should be individualized based on maternal history, infant health status, mother's preferences, clinical needs, and available lactation safety data. Throughout the decision-making process, maternal health and well-being must be prioritized while implementing appropriate measures to minimize infant exposure and thoroughly monitor infant growth and development. These objectives should not be viewed as competing priorities, but rather as interconnected elements of a comprehensive approach to care. Providers can use the risk assessment framework in this chapter to guide their clinical decisions (Table 9.1). Future research priorities should focus on systematic evaluation of newer antipsychotics, long-term neurobehavioral outcomes, and the development of standardized infant monitoring protocols. Additionally, emerging evidence suggesting that combination medication therapy during breastfeeding may be safer than previously believed is promising and warrants further study.

Table 9.1 Expert recommendations based on scientific evidence and clinical experience

Prioritize maternal well-being: Women who are taking an antipsychotic should not be discouraged from breastfeeding. However, sacrificing a mother's mental well-being in favor of breastfeeding is never recommended
Guidance of FGAs: Haloperidol and chlorpromazine are generally compatible with breastfeeding. Other FGAs may also be compatible but have less evidence
Guidance of SGAs: Olanzapine, quetiapine, and risperidone have the most safety data during lactation and appear to be reasonable choices for breastfeeding women. Clozapine should generally be avoided during breastfeeding due to risks of agranulocytosis and seizures in infants. Aripiprazole warrants careful consideration, particularly regarding its effects on prolactin and potential impacts on milk supply
Polytherapy: The co-administration of more than one antipsychotic and/or complex psychotropic regimen (>2 psychotropics) should not necessarily be discouraged during lactation, but close monitoring of infant is recommended
Risk-benefit assessment: The decision to use antipsychotics during breastfeeding should be individualized, considering the mother's psychiatric history, medication response, potential for relapse, support systems, sleep management, and infant factors (age, developmental stage, health status) and should be discussed collaboratively with a psychiatrist, physician, and the patient
Infant safety and monitoring: Infants exposed to an antipsychotic through breast milk should be carefully monitored for adverse events including any changes in infant behavior, alertness, feeding, or sleep

References

Aichhorn W, Stuppaeck C, Whitworth AB. Risperidone, and breast-feeding. J Psychopharmacol. 2005;19(2):211–3. https://doi.org/10.1177/0269881105049044.

Ambresin G, Berney P, Schulz P, Bryois C. Olanzapine excretion into breast milk: a case report. J Clin Psychopharmacol. 2004;24(1):93–5. https://doi.org/10.1097/01.jcp.0000106225.36344.58.

Anderson PO, Manoguerra AS, Valdés V. A review of adverse reactions in infants from medications in breastmilk. Clin Pediatr (Phila). 2016;55(3):236–44. https://doi.org/10.1177/0009922815594586.

Aripiprazole. In: Drugs and Lactation Database (LactMed®). National Institute of Child Health and Human Development; 2006. Accessed March 22, 2025. http://www.ncbi.nlm.nih.gov/books/NBK501016/

Asenapine. In: Drugs and Lactation Database (LactMed®). National Institute of Child Health and Human Development; 2006. Accessed March 4, 2025. http://www.ncbi.nlm.nih.gov/books/NBK501684/

Aydin B, Nayir T, Sahin S, Yildiz A. Olanzapine, and quetiapine use during breastfeeding: excretion into breast milk and safe breastfeeding strategy. J Clin Psychopharmacol. 2015;35(2):206–8. https://doi.org/10.1097/JCP.0000000000000291.

Baldessarini R, Henk H, Sklar A, Chang J, Leahy L. Psychotropic medications for patients with bipolar disorder in the United States: polytherapy and adherence. Psychiatr Serv. 2008;59(10):1175–83. https://doi.org/10.1176/ps.2008.59.10.1175.

Barnas C, Bergant A, Hummer M, Saria A, Fleischhacker WW. Clozapine concentrations in maternal and fetal plasma, amniotic fluid, and breast milk. Am J Psychiatry. 1994;151(6):945. https://doi.org/10.1176/ajp.151.6.945.

Begg EJ, Duffull SB, Hackett LP, Ilett KF. Studying drugs in human milk: time to unify the approach. J Hum Lact. 2002;18(4):323–32. https://doi.org/10.1177/089033402237904.

Bergemann N, Mundt C, Parzer P, et al. Plasma concentrations of estradiol in women suffering from schizophrenia treated with conventional versus atypical antipsychotics. Schizophr Res. 2005;73(2–3):357–66. https://doi.org/10.1016/j.schres.2004.06.0135.

Bray B, Karri M. Abstract #1165627: risperidone induced hyperprolactinemia levels-never seen before. Endocr Pract. 2022;28(5, Supplement):S105. https://doi.org/10.1016/j.eprac.2022.03.251.

Brexpiprazole. In: Drugs and Lactation Database (LactMed®). National Institute of Child Health and Human Development; 2006. Accessed March 4, 2025. http://www.ncbi.nlm.nih.gov/books/NBK500749/

Brunner E, Falk DM, Jones M, Dey DK, Shatapathy CC. Olanzapine in pregnancy and breastfeeding: a review of data from global safety surveillance. BMC Pharmacol Toxicol. 2013;14:38. https://doi.org/10.1186/2050-6511-14-38.

Burkey BW, Holmes AP. Evaluating medication use in pregnancy and lactation: what every pharmacist should know. J Pediatr Pharmacol Ther. 2013;18(3):247–58. https://doi.org/10.5863/1551-6776-18.3.247.

Cariprazine. In: Drugs and Lactation Database (LactMed®). National Institute of Child Health and Human Development; 2006. Accessed March 4, 2025. http://www.ncbi.nlm.nih.gov/books/NBK500757/

Center for Disease Control and Prevention. Breastfeeding Report Card United States, 2022. Accessed March 4, 2025. https://www.cdc.gov/breastfeeding-data/media/pdfs/2024/06/2022-Breastfeeding-Report-Card-508.pdf

Cohen LS, Altshuler LL, Harlow BL, et al. Relapse of major depression during pregnancy in women who maintain or discontinue antidepressant treatment. JAMA. 2006;295(5):499–507. https://doi.org/10.1001/jama.295.5.499.

Croke S, Buist A, Hackett LP, Ilett KF, Norman TR, Burrows GD. Olanzapine excretion in human breast milk: estimation of infant exposure. Int J Neuropsychopharmacol. 2002;5(3):243–7. https://doi.org/10.1017/S1461145702003012.

Cuomo A, Goracci A, Fagiolini A. Aripiprazole use during pregnancy, peripartum and lactation. A systematic literature search and review to inform clinical practice. J Affect Disord. 2018;228:229–37. https://doi.org/10.1016/j.jad.2017.12.021.

Dev V, Krupp P. Adverse event profile and safety of clozapine. Rev Contemp Pharmacother. 1995;6:197–208.

Drugs and Lactation Database (LactMed®). Bethesda (MD): National Institute of Child Health and Human Development; 2006a. Quetiapine. 2024 Oct 15.

Drugs and Lactation Database (LactMed®). Bethesda (MD): National Institute of Child Health and Human Development; 2006b. Clozapine. 2024 Oct 15.

Drugs and Lactation Database (LactMed®). Bethesda (MD): National Institute of Child Health and Human Development; 2006c. Amisulpride. 2023 Nov 15.

Drugs and Lactation Database (LactMed®). Bethesda (MD): National Institute of Child Health and Human Development; 2006d. Ziprasidone. 2024 Aug 15.

Drugs and Lactation Database (LactMed®). Bethesda (MD): National Institute of Child Health and Human Development; 2006e. Chlorpromazine. 2024 Sep 15.

Drugs and Lactation Database (LactMed®). Bethesda (MD): National Institute of Child Health and Human Development; 2006f. Olanzapine. 2025 Jan 15.

Drugs and Lactation Database (LactMed®). Bethesda (MD): National Institute of Child Health and Human Development; 2006g. Haloperidol. 2023 Aug 15.

Fernández-Abascal B, Recio-Barbero M, Sáenz-Herrero M, Segarra R. Long-acting injectable aripiprazole in pregnant women with schizophrenia: a case-series report. Ther Adv Psychopharmacol. 2021;11:2045125321991277. https://doi.org/10.1177/2045125321991277.

Fortinguerra F, Clavenna A, Bonati M. Psychotropic drug use during breastfeeding: a review of the evidence. Pediatrics. 2009;124(4):e547–56. https://doi.org/10.1542/peds.2009-0326.

Galbally M, Frayne J, Watson SJ, Snellen M. Psychopharmacological prescribing practices in pregnancy for women with severe mental illness: a multicentre study. Eur Neuropsychopharmacol. 2019;29(1):57–65. https://doi.org/10.1016/j.euroneuro.2018.11.1103.

Gardiner S, Kristensen J, Begg E, et al. Transfer of olanzapine into breast milk, calculation of infant drug dose, and effect on breast-fed infants. Am J Psychiatry. 2003;160:1428–31. https://doi.org/10.1176/appi.ajp.160.8.1428.

Gentile S. Infant safety with antipsychotic therapy in breast-feeding: a systematic review. J Clin Psychiatry. 2008;69(4):666–73. https://doi.org/10.4088/jcp.v69n0421.

Gentile S. Antipsychotic therapy during early and late pregnancy. A systematic review. Schizophr Bull. 2010;36(3):518–44. https://doi.org/10.1093/schbul/sbn107.

Gentile S. A safety evaluation of aripiprazole for treating schizophrenia during pregnancy and puerperium. Expert Opin Drug Saf. 2014;13(12):1733–42. https://doi.org/10.1517/14740338.2014.951325.

Gilad O, Merlob P, Stahl B, Klinger G. Outcome of infants exposed to olanzapine during breastfeeding. Breastfeed Med. 2011;6(2):55–8. https://doi.org/10.1089/bfm.2010.0027.

Hale TW. Pharmacology review: drug therapy and breastfeeding: antidepressants, antipsychotics, antimanics, and sedatives. NeoReviews. 2004;5(10):e451–6. https://doi.org/10.1542/neo.5-10-e451.

Hale's Medications & Mothers' Milk 2025–2026. Accessed March 18, 2025. https://www.springerpub.com/hale-s-medications-mothers-milk-2025-2026-9780826100207.html?srsltid=AfmBOooplQLcJs41HQbXtEuDWXB-9bGvfoC4hS4jO4qQAVGsKjDeau86

Hill RC, Mcivor RJ, Wojnar-Horton RE, Hackett LP, Ilett K. Risperidone distribution and excretion into human milk: case report and estimated infant exposure during breast-feeding. J Clin Psychopharmacol. 2000;20(2):285–6. https://doi.org/10.1097/00004714-200004000-00036.

Ilett KF, Hackett LP, Kristensen JH, Vaddadi KS, Gardiner SJ, Begg EJ. Transfer of risperidone and 9-hydroxyrisperidone into human milk. Ann Pharmacother. 2004;38(2):273–6. https://doi.org/10.1345/aph.1D326.

Ilett KF, Watt F, Hackett LP, Kohan R, Teoh S. Assessment of infant dose through milk in a lactating woman taking amisulpride and desvenlafaxine for treatment-resistant depression. Ther Drug Monit. 2010 Dec;32(6):704–7. https://doi.org/10.1097/FTD.0b013e3181f88f70.

Iloperidone. In: Drugs and Lactation Database (LactMed®). National Institute of Child Health and Human Development; 2006. Accessed March 4, 2025. http://www.ncbi.nlm.nih.gov/books/NBK501699/

Jones I, Craddock N. Bipolar disorder and childbirth: the importance of recognising risk. Br J Psychiatry. 2005;186:453–4. https://doi.org/10.1192/bjp.186.6.453.

Kelsey JJ. Drug Principles in Lactation. American College of Clinical Pharmacy; 2016. https://www.accp.com/docs/bookstore/psap/p2016b3_sample.pdf55.

Kendell RE, Chalmers JC, Platz C. Epidemiology of puerperal psychoses. Br J Psychiatry. 1987;150:662–73. https://doi.org/10.1192/bjp.150.5.662.

Kirchheiner J, Berghöfer A, Bolk-Weischedel D. Healthy outcome under olanzapine treatment in a pregnant woman. Pharmacopsychiatry. 2000;33(2):78–80. https://doi.org/10.1055/s-2000-7974.

Klinger G, Stahl B, Fusar-Poli P, Merlob P. Antipsychotic drugs and breastfeeding. Pediatr Endocrinol Rev. 2013;10(3):308–17.

Kris EB, Carmichael DM. Chlorpromazine maintenance therapy during pregnancy and confinement. Psychiatry Q. 1957;31(1):690–5. https://doi.org/10.1007/BF01568760.

Kris EB, Gross M. Children born to mothers maintained on pharmacotherapy during pregnancy and postpartum. In: Wortis J, editor. Recent advances in biological psychiatry: volume IV: the proceedings of the sixteenth annual convention and scientific program of the Society of Biological Psychiatry, vol. 4. Atlantic City: Springer US; 1962. p. 180–7. https://doi.org/10.1007/978-1-4684-8306-2_18.

Larsen ER, Damkier P, Pedersen LH, et al. Use of psychotropic drugs during pregnancy and breastfeeding. Acta Psychiatr Scand Suppl. 2015;445:1–28. https://doi.org/10.1111/acps.12479.

Llewellyn A, Stowe ZN. Psychotropic medications in lactation. J Clin Psychiatry. 1998;59(Suppl 2):41–52.

Lumateperone. In: Drugs and Lactation Database (LactMed®). National Institute of Child Health and Human Development; 2006. Accessed March 4, 2025. http://www.ncbi.nlm.nih.gov/books/NBK582100/

Lurasidone. In: Drugs and Lactation Database (LactMed®). National Institute of Child Health and Human Development; 2006. Accessed March 4, 2025. http://www.ncbi.nlm.nih.gov/books/NBK501728/

Lutz UC, Wiatr G, Orlikowsky T, Gaertner HJ, Bartels M. Olanzapine treatment during breast feeding: a case report. Ther Drug Monit. 2008;30(3):399–401. https://doi.org/10.1097/FTD.0b013e31816850e2.

Lutz UC, Hiemke C, Wiatr G, Farger G, Arand J, Wildgruber D. Aripiprazole in pregnancy and lactation: a case report. J Clin Psychopharmacol. 2010;30(2):204–5. https://doi.org/10.1097/JCP.0b013e3181d27c7d.

Maguire GA. Prolactin elevation with antipsychotic medications: mechanisms of action and clinical consequences. J Clin Psychiatry. 2002;63(Suppl 4):56–62.

Mantilla Reyes M, De Embun X, Ferrer I, Roca LA. Aripiprazole and hypogalactorrhea in postpartum. Eur Psychiatry. 2020;63:s488. https://doi.org/10.1192/j.eurpsy.2020.6.

McAllister-Williams RH, Baldwin DS, Cantwell R, et al. British Association for Psychopharmacology consensus guidance on the use of psychotropic medication preconception, in pregnancy and postpartum 2017. J Psychopharmacol. 2017;31(5):519–52. https://doi.org/10.1177/0269881117699361.

Meek JY, Noble L, Section on Breastfeeding. Policy statement: Breastfeeding and the use of human milk. Pediatrics. 2022;150(1):e2022057988. https://doi.org/10.1542/peds.2022-057988.

Mendhekar DN. Possible delayed speech acquisition with clozapine therapy during pregnancy and lactation. J Neuropsychiatry Clin Neurosci. 2007;19(2):196–7. https://doi.org/10.1176/jnp.2007.19.2.196.

Mendhekar DN, Andrade C. Uneventful use of haloperidol and trihehexyphenidyl during three consecutive pregnancies. Arch Womens Ment Health. 2011;14(1):83–4. https://doi.org/10.1007/s00737-010-0192-0.

Mendhekar D, Andrade C. A 26-year follow-up of a woman with 5 consecutive children exposed to risperidone during pregnancy and breastfeeding. Prim Care Companion CNS Disord. 2024;26(1):23cr03660. https://doi.org/10.4088/PCC.23cr0366.

Miller ES, Metz T, Simas TAM, Hoffman MC, Byatt N, Roussos-Ross K. Treatment and management of mental health conditions during pregnancy and postpartum: ACOG clinical practice guideline no. 5. Obstet Gynecol. 2023;141(6):1262–88. https://doi.org/10.1097/AOG.0000000000005202.

Misri S, Corral M, Wardrop AA, Kendrick K. Quetiapine augmentation in lactation: a series of case reports. J Clin Psychopharmacol. 2006;26(5):508–11. https://doi.org/10.1097/01.jcp.0000236656.70544.f3.

Naughton S, O'Hara K, Nelson J, Keightley P. Aripiprazole, brexpiprazole, and cariprazine can affect milk supply: advice to breastfeeding mothers. Australas Psychiatry. 2023;31(2):201–4. https://doi.org/10.1177/10398562231159510.

Newport DJ, Ritchie JC, Knight BT, Glover BA, Zach EB, Stowe ZN. Venlafaxine in human breast milk and nursing infant plasma: determination of exposure. J Clin Psychiatry. 2009;70(9):1304–10. https://doi.org/10.4088/JCP.08m05001.

Nonacs R, Wang B, Viguera A, Cohen L. Psychiatric illness during pregnancy and the post-partum period. In: Stern T, Fava M, Wilens T, Rosenbaum J, editors. The Massachusetts General Hospital comprehensive clinical psychiatry. 2nd ed. London: Elsevier; 2016.

Nordeng H, Gjerdalen G, Brede WR, Michelsen LS, Spigset O. Transfer of aripiprazole to breast milk: a case report. J Clin Psychopharmacol. 2014;34(2):272–5. https://doi.org/10.1097/JCP.0000000000000079.

O'Halloran SJ, Wong A, Joyce DA. A liquid chromatography-tandem mass spectrometry method for quantifying amisulpride in human plasma and breast milk, applied to measuring drug transfer to a fully breast-fed neonate. Ther Drug Monit. 2016;38:493–8.

Odhejo YI, Jafri A, Mekala HM, et al. Safety and efficacy of antipsychotics in pregnancy and lactation. J Alcohol Drug Depend. 2017;05(03) https://doi.org/10.4172/2329-6488.1000267.

Pacchiarotti I, León-Caballero J, Murru A, et al. Mood stabilizers and antipsychotics during breast-feeding: focus on bipolar disorder. Eur Neuropsychopharmacol. 2016;26(10):1562–78. https://doi.org/10.1016/j.euroneuro.2016.08.008.

Pasi R, Appikatla MB, Babu TA. Risperidone-induced respiratory depression in a neonate through breast milk. Indian J Pharmacol. 2023;55(3):185–6. https://doi.org/10.4103/ijp.ijp_645_22.

Pastol J, Le Marois M, Guilhaumou R, Blin O, Belzeaux R. Measuring drug concentrations in breast milk to improve therapeutic monitoring and patient adherence in bipolar disorder: a case report. Aust N Z J Psychiatry. 2022;56(1):96. https://doi.org/10.1177/00048674211010340.

Payne JL. Psychiatric medication use in pregnancy and breastfeeding. Obstet Gynecol Clin N Am. 2021;48(1):131–49. https://doi.org/10.1016/j.ogc.2020.11.006.

Rampono J, Kristensen JH, Ilett KF, Hackett LP, Kohan R. Quetiapine and breast feeding. Ann Pharmacother. 2007;41(4):711–4. https://doi.org/10.1345/aph.1H555.

Ratnayake T, Libretto SE. No complications with risperidone treatment before and throughout pregnancy and during the nursing period. J Clin Psychiatry. 2002;63(1):76–7. https://doi.org/10.4088/jcp.v63n0114c.

Reis M, Källén B. Maternal use of antipsychotics in early pregnancy and delivery outcome. J Clin Psychopharmacol. 2008;28(3):279–88. https://doi.org/10.1097/JCP.0b013e318172b8d5.

Risperidone. In: Drugs and Lactation Database (LactMed®). National Institute of Child Health and Human Development; 2006. Accessed March 7, 2025. http://www.ncbi.nlm.nih.gov/books/NBK501095/

Sachs HC, Committee On Drugs. The transfer of drugs and therapeutics into human breast milk: an update on selected topics. Pediatrics. 2013;132(3):e796–809. https://doi.org/10.1542/peds.2013-1985.

Sadowski A, Todorow M, Yazdani Brojeni P, Koren G, Nulman I. Pregnancy outcomes following maternal exposure to second-generation antipsychotics given with other psychotropic drugs: a cohort study. BMJ Open. 2013;3(7):e003062. https://doi.org/10.1136/bmjopen-2013-003062.

Sahoo MK, Biswas H, Grover S. Safety profile of aripiprazole during pregnancy and lactation: report of 2 cases. Turk Psikiyatri Derg. 2023;34(2):133–5. https://doi.org/10.5080/u26681.

Santucci AK, Singer LT, Wisniewski SR, et al. One-year developmental outcomes for infants of mothers with bipolar disorder. J Clin Psychiatry. 2017;78(8):1083–90. https://doi.org/10.4088/JCP.15m10535.

Schlotterbeck P, Saur R, Hiemke C, et al. Low concentration of ziprasidone in human milk: a case report. Int J Neuropsychopharmacol. 2009;12(3):437–8. https://doi.org/10.1017/S1461145709009936.

Shao P, Ou J, Peng M, Zhao J, Chen J, Wu R. Effects of clozapine, and other atypical antipsychotics on infants development who were exposed to as fetus: a post-hoc analysis. PLoS One. 2015;10(4):e0123373. https://doi.org/10.1371/journal.pone.0123373.

Sharma V, Sommerdyk C. Lamotrigine in the prevention of bipolar II postpartum depression. Prim Care Companion CNS Disord. 2016;18(6) https://doi.org/10.4088/PCC.16l01964.

Sinha SK, Kishore MT, Thippeswamy H, Kommu JVS, Chandra PS. Adverse effects and short-term developmental outcomes of infants exposed to atypical antipsychotics during breastfeeding. Indian J Psychiatry. 2021;63(1):52–7. https://doi.org/10.4103/psychiatry.IndianJPsychiatry_45_20.

Teoh S, Ilett KF, Hackett LP, Kohan R. Estimation of rac-amisulpride transfer into milk and of infant dose via milk during its use in a lactating woman with bipolar disorder and schizophrenia. Breastfeed Med. 2011;6:85–8.

Uguz F. Second-generation antipsychotics during the lactation period: a comparative systematic review on infant safety. J Clin Psychopharmacol. 2016;36(3):244–52. https://doi.org/10.1097/JCP.0000000000000491.

Uguz F. Prophylactic use of olanzapine and quetiapine from pregnancy to the postpartum period in women with bipolar disorder: a case series. J Matern Fetal Neonatal Med. 2017;30(21):2569–71. https://doi.org/10.1080/14767058.2016.1256991.

Uguz F. Adverse events in a breastfed infant exposed to risperidone and haloperidol. Breastfeed Med. 2019;14(9):683–4. https://doi.org/10.1089/bfm.2019.0093.

Uguz F. The use of clozapine during pregnancy and lactation: a case report. Psychiatry Clin Psychopharm. 2020;30(2):193. https://doi.org/10.5455/PCP.20200502080433.

Uguz F. A new safety scoring system for the use of psychotropic drugs during lactation. Am J Ther. 2021;28(1):e118–26. https://doi.org/10.1097/MJT.0000000000000909.

Uygur ÖF, Uygur H. Neurodevelopmental and growth follow-up of the baby exposed to antipsychotics during pregnancy and lactation: a case report. Psychiatry Clin Psychopharm. 2019;29(4):744–7. https://doi.org/10.1080/24750573.2019.1627695.

Verstegen RHJ, Anderson PO, Ito S. Infant drug exposure via breast milk. Br J Clin Pharmacol. 2022;88(10):4311–27. https://doi.org/10.1111/bcp.14538.

Viguera AC. Polypharmacy for perinatal mood and anxiety disorders. Lancet Psychiatry. 2024;11(8):575–7. https://doi.org/10.1016/S2215-0366(24)00215-3.

Viguera AC, Cohen LS, Bouffard S, Whitfield TH, Baldessarini RJ. Reproductive decisions by women with bipolar disorder after Prepregnancy psychiatric consultation. AJP. 2002;159(12):2102–4. https://doi.org/10.1176/appi.ajp.159.12.2102.

Viguera AC, Whitfield T, Baldessarini RJ, et al. Risk of recurrence in women with bipolar disorder during pregnancy: prospective study of mood stabilizer discontinuation. Am J Psychiatry. 2007a;164(12):1817–24. https://doi.org/10.1176/appi.ajp.2007.06101639.

Viguera AC, Newport DJ, Ritchie J, et al. Lithium in breast milk and nursing infants: clinical implications. Am J Psychiatry. 2007b;164(2):342–5. https://doi.org/10.1176/ajp.2007.164.2.342.

Viguera AC, Cohen LS, Whitfield T, Reminick AM, Bromfield E, Baldessarini RJ. Perinatal use of anticonvulsants: differences in attitudes and recommendations among neurologists and psychiatrists. Arch Womens Ment Health. 2010;13(2):175–8. https://doi.org/10.1007/s00737-009-0130-1.

Viguera AC, Tondo L, Koukopoulos AE, Reginaldi D, Lepri B, Baldessarini RJ. Episodes of mood disorders in 2,252 pregnancies and postpartum periods. Am J Psychiatry. 2011;168(11):1179–85. https://doi.org/10.1176/appi.ajp.2011.11010148.

Viguera AC, Vanderkruik R, Gaccione P, et al. Breastfeeding practices among women taking second-generation antipsychotics: findings from the National Pregnancy Registry for atypical antipsychotics. Arch Womens Ment Health. 2022;25(2):511–6. https://doi.org/10.1007/s00737-021-01162-z.

Walker T, Coursey C, Duffus ALJ. Low dose of Abilify (aripiprazole) in combination with Effexor XR (venlafaxine HCl) resulted in cessation of lactation: a case report. Clin Lactation. 2019;10(2):56–9. https://doi.org/10.1891/2158-0782.10.2.56.

Watanabe N, Kasahara M, Sugibayashi R, et al. Perinatal use of aripiprazole: a case report. J Clin Psychopharmacol. 2011;31(3):377–9. https://doi.org/10.1097/JCP.0b013e318218c400.

Weggelaar NM, Keijer WJ, Janssen PKC. A case report of risperidone distribution and excretion into human milk: how to give good advice if you have not enough data available. J Clin Psychopharmacol. 2011;31(1):129–31. https://doi.org/10.1097/JCP.0b013e318206c218.

Werremeyer A. Ziprasidone and citalopram use in pregnancy and lactation in a woman with psychotic depression. Am J Psychiatry. 2009;166(11):1298. https://doi.org/10.1176/appi.ajp.2009.09060765.

Whalley LJ, Blain PG, Prime JK. Haloperidol secreted in breast milk. Br Med J (Clin Res Ed). 1981;282(6278):1746–7. https://doi.org/10.1136/bmj.282.6278.1746.

Wiles DH, Orr MW, Kolakowska T. Chlorpromazine levels in plasma and milk of nursing mothers. Br J Clin Pharmacol. 1978;5(3):272–3. https://doi.org/10.1111/j.1365-2125.1978.tb01639.x.

Yoshida K, Smith B, Craggs M, Kumar R. Neuroleptic drugs in breast-milk: a study of pharmacokinetics and of possible adverse effects in breast-fed infants. Psychol Med. 1998a;28(1):81–91. https://doi.org/10.1017/s0033291797005965.

Yoshida K, Kumar RC, Smith B, Craggs M. Psychotropic drugs in breast milk: no evidence for adverse effects on prepulse modulation of startle reflex or on cognitive level in infants. Dev Psychobiol. 1998b;32(3):249–56.

Yskes R, Thomas R, Nagalla ML. A case of decreased milk production associated with aripiprazole. Prim Care Companion CNS Disord. 2018;20(6):18l02303. https://doi.org/10.4088/PCC.18l02303.

Mood Stabilizers in Pregnancy 10

Anne-Laure Sutter-Dallay and Florence Gressier

10.1 Introduction

For 7% of women presenting a bipolar disorder (BD), their first episode occurred in the context of the perinatal period (Viguera et al. 2011). In women with bipolar disorder prior to pregnancy, the risk of relapse may reach up to 20% during pregnancy (Van der Lugt et al. 2012) and is between 50% and 70% post-partum (Jones and Craddock 2005; Viguera et al. 2011). Conversely, bipolar disorders themselves seem to have a possible influence on the course of pregnancy: the review of Mohamed et al. (2023) suggests that the risk of obstetric complications would be higher in bipolar patients—treated or not—than in the general population. The recent work of Chan et al. (2024) is along the same lines, finding that in a population-based cohort of 465,069 women—including 302 women with a diagnosis of BD, of whom 168 had one or more prescriptions for mood stabilizers during pregnancy (treated BD) and 134 were not exposed to mood stabilizers during pregnancy (untreated BD)—BD was significantly associated with an increased risk of gestational diabetes (ORa: 1.75 [95% CI: 1.15–2.70]) and maternal somatic hospitalization ≤90 days after discharge from the index delivery (2.12 [1.19–3.90]); in treatment status-stratified analyses, treated BD women had a significantly increased

A.-L. Sutter-Dallay (✉)
Department of Perinatal Psychiatry, University Department of Child and Adolescent Psychiatry, Charles Perrens Hospital, Bordeaux, France

Bordeaux Population Health INSERM 1219 Research Center, HEALTHY Team, Bordeaux University, Bordeaux, France
e-mail: alsutter@ch-perrens.fr

F. Gressier
Department of Psychiatry, Faculté de Médecine Paris-Saclay, CESP, Inserm U1018, Bicêtre University Hospital, Assistance Publique-Hôpitaux de Paris, Hôpitaux Universitaires Paris Saclay, Université Paris-Saclay, Le Kremlin Bicêtre, France

F. Uguz, L. Orsolini (eds.), *Perinatal Psychopharmacology*,
https://doi.org/10.1007/978-3-031-99720-4_10

rate of gestational diabetes (2.09 [1.21–3.70]) compared with controls (non-BD and not exposed to mood stabilizers during pregnancy).

A preventive and multidisciplinary approach is therefore essential for women with BD. If pregnancy is not yet planned, contraceptive methods should be discussed with the patient, as certain anticonvulsant mood stabilizers are potent enzyme inducers that reduce the efficacy of oral contraceptives or progestogen-releasing implants (e.g., carbamazepine, oxcarbazepine and topiramate) (Ernst and Goldberg 2002). Conversely, ethinyl oestradiol/levonorgestrel combined oral contraceptives increase lamotrigine clearance (Clark et al. 2013; Gaffield et al. 2011). Women should also be informed about the effects of these treatments on their fertility, particularly regarding valproate, which is likely to be associated with increased testosterone levels and hyperandrogenism in women with BD (Zhang et al. 2016). In addition, women should be informed about the risk of unintended pregnancy when discontinuing hyperprolactinemia-inducing antipsychotics used as mood stabilizers. As far as pregnancy is concerned, the specificities of managing BD in the perinatal period can be addressed in the context of gynaecological and/or psychiatric care, and well before pregnancy in the case of a pre-existing diagnosis. Indeed, the ethical dimension of weighing up the benefits and risks of each pregnancy is crucial and must take into account the risk of relapse, the potential effects of mood stabilizers on embryonic and foetal development, and the wishes of the woman and the couple, which is a time-consuming issue for parents. Faced with a planned or ongoing pregnancy on mood stabilizers, the patient and her partner must be supported throughout the risk-benefit analysis, based on a multiprofessional approach combining psychiatric, obstetric, and paediatric knowledge for each molecule, taking into account the specific evolutionary features of each patient's disorder and her wishes.

Data on mood stabilizers in pregnancy are still relatively scarce, although they are increasing rapidly. Unfortunately, most studies do not take into account the influence of maternal somatic disorders on foetal development and pregnancy, such as malnutrition, obesity, diabetes, gynaecological infections, or the influence of environmental factors such as unhealthy lifestyles or domestic violence. Bearing these general limitations in mind, a summary of the current literature allows a general prescriptive framework to be defined.

Table 10.1 presents expert recommendations based on scientific evidence and clinical experience on the use of mood stabilizers during pregnancy.

10.2 Lithium

10.2.1 Placental Transfer

The first works of Newport et al. (2005) about placental transfer of lithium combined the results of a prospective sample of 10 women with 32 cases of neonatal dosages identified in the literature and suggested that placental transfer of lithium was complete and that the balance between maternal and foetal circulation (average child/mother plasma lithium ratio = 1.05 ratio) is as between the different fluid

Table 10.1 Expert recommendations based on scientific evidence and clinical experience

Regarding the increased risk of bipolar disorder episodes during pregnancy clinicians have to be able to prescribe after weighing the risks of a maternal relapse vs. the risks of antenatal exposure to the drug
To date the available limited data suggest that there is no contraindication regarding the use of lamotrigine
The available limited data suggest that there is no longer absolute contraindication regarding the use of lithium during the first trimester of pregnancy
Valproate must be avoided because of the increased risk of defects and developmental disorders for the child
Carbamazepine may increase birth defects, and impact some developmental axes
Bipolar women must be treated during pregnancy, to avoid risk-taking behavior and deterioration in the prognosis of the disorder over the long term as well as the risks for the fetus of the effects of prenatal stress, increased smoking or poor nutritional intake

compartments of an individual. Another study (van der Lugt et al. 2012) found neonatal blood lithium levels above 0.8 mEq/l in 2 of the 30 exposed children, one of which presented signs of neonatal distress. A recent retrospective observational cohort study (Imaz et al. 2024) including 66 women with BD and stable with lithium in late pregnancy for whom it was discontinued 12 h before a scheduled caesarean section or induction, or at admission day to hospital birth and restarted 6–12 hours post birth, found a mean (SD) umbilical cord/mother intrapartum lithemia ratio of 1.10 (0.17), mean lithemia were 0.178 mEq/L higher in infant with hypotonia than in those without ($p = 0.028$). However, there was an early postpartum relapse for 6% of the mothers.

Finaly, the recent paper by Molenaar et al. (2024) on 233 maternal lithium blood level measurements—55 (23.6%) in the week before delivery and 178 (76.4%) in the week after—found no association between time and lithium blood level/dose ratio (Pearson correlation coefficient − 0.03, $P = 0.63$). In addition, 29 neonates who had a lithium measurement within 24 h of birth showed that maternal and neonatal lithium blood levels were strongly correlated and that there was no association between neonatal lithium blood levels at birth and neonatal outcomes. Based on these findings, authors do not recommend lowering the dosage or discontinuation of lithium prior to delivery, as stable dosing can prevent subtherapeutic lithium serum levels, which is especially important in the postpartum period when relapse risks are highest.

Note that the co-prescription of other psychotropic drugs is not taken into account in any of these studies.

10.2.2 Embryonic Period: Organogenesis

The first studies on lithium teratogenicity are animal studies dating from the end of the nineteenth century. In animals exposed antenatally to doses used for treatment in human beings, no increase in teratogenic risk has been noticed. With very high doses, some studies reveal different types of malformations (central nervous system, skeletal, craniofacial...), while others did not find any link between prenatal exposure to lithium and birth defects (Giles and Bannigan 2006). The first data on lithium's teratogenicity in humans are issued from the "Register of Lithium Babies ", which collected retrospectively the pregnancy outcomes of patients treated by lithium in Scandinavia, the United States, and Canada. The first publication reported 118 cases of Scandinavian children whose mothers had taken lithium during the first trimester of pregnancy (Schou et al. 1973). Nine of them (7.6%) presented birth defects, among which 6 were related to the cardiovascular system, including 1 Ebstein anomaly (severe malformation of the tricuspid valve). By adding other data from the United States and Canada, the number of cases reported increased to 143. In this second sample, cardiovascular malformations accounted for 77% of congenital defects, against 12.5% in the general population. Ebstein's anomaly was largely over-represented with 40% of the babies from the registry presenting with this pathology against 1.25% in the general population. The final publication (Weinstein and Goldfield 1975) included 225 observations (with at least 3 children who were also exposed to other treatments), among which 11% ($n = 25$) of the children presented congenital malformations (against 2% in the general population). Three-quarters of these malformations were cardiovascular ($n = 18$) and 33% ($n = 6$) were Ebstein anomalies. The retrospective collection of data in this register represents a major bias, since it is likely that pathological cases have been more frequently reported than normal births. Subsequent retrospective studies used more strict data collection methods, and did not reveal statistically significant relation between the use of lithium during pregnancy and the occurrence of cardiac malformations in the newborn, nor specific links between Ebstein's anomaly and prenatal exposure to lithium (Nora et al. 1974; Kozma 2005). For example, the review of 59 cases of Ebstein diseases found no cases of children exposed to lithium in early pregnancy (Zalzstein et al. 1990).

Thereafter, the study by Patorno et al. (2017), which showed an adjusted risk ratio of cardiac malformations in lithium-exposed infants compared with unexposed infants of 1.65, highlights also that the risk ratio was 1.11 for a daily dose of 600 mg or less, 1.60 for 601 to 900 mg, and 3.22 for more than 900 mg, suggesting a dose-response relationship.

Prospective studies remain rare to date and mainly do not show a statistically significant link with birth defects, although some note the existence of sporadic cases of Ebstein's anomaly. For example, the prospective, comparative observational study of Diav-Citrin et al. (2014) followed up 183 lithium-exposed pregnancies of women who contacted the Israeli Teratology Information Service (90.2% in the first trimester) and were compared with 72 disease-matched and 748 nonteratogenic-exposed pregnancies. The rate of major congenital anomalies was not significantly different between the groups (lithium-exposed in the first trimester: 8/123 [6.5%]; bipolar: 2/61 [3.3%]; nonteratogenic: 19/711 [2.7%]). Cardiovascular anomalies occurred more frequently in the lithium group exposed during the first trimester when compared with the nonteratogenic exposure group (5/123 [4.1%] compared with 4/711 [0.6%]) but not after excluding anomalies that spontaneously resolved (3/123 [2.4%] compared with 2/711 [0.3%]).

Case-control studies have failed to demonstrate a significant association between birth defects and in utero exposure to lithium (Zalzstein et al. 1990; Gentile 2012) when case reports in the literature indicate both heart defects, sometimes with Ebstein's anomaly, other types of defects, including neural tube defects (Gentile 2012).

Finally, a meta-analysis (McKnight et al. 2012) about general toxicity of lithium concluded that the risk of congenital malformation after early in-utero exposure to lithium is "uncertain", and that the benefit-risk balance of a decrease or a discontinuation of treatment during pregnancy should be weighed for each clinical situation. Facing a probably slight increased risk of heart defects in this population, it is therefore recommended that all women receiving lithium during pregnancy should undergo fetal echocardiography and a level-2 (anatomic scan) ultrasound examination between 18 and 20 weeks of gestation (Bergink and Kushner 2014).

A recent systematic review and network meta-analysis of congenital malformations and prenatal outcomes exploring the comparative safety of antipsychotic medications and mood stabilizers during pregnancy in 18,334 potential records, and 22 studies, involving 3,042,997 pregnant women, found that, compared with the unexposed group, lithium (OR, 1.61; 95% credible interval (CrI) 1.07–2.30), risperidone (OR, 1.43; 95% CrI 1.18–1.77), olanzapine (OR, 1.33; 95% CrI 1.11–1.64), aripiprazole (OR, 1.30; 95% CrI 1.10–1.65), and quetiapine [odds ratio (OR), 1.19; 95% CrI, 1.01–1.39] were associated with a slightly increased risk of congenital malformations.

From a cardiological perspective, a recent meta-analysis of risk factors for congenital heart disease (CHDs) (Lemieux et al. 2024) compiling 131 articles, associations between antenatal exposure to psychotropic drugs and CHDs a positive association was observed between severe CHDs and lithium, but with a very wide CI encompassing the null effect (OR of 3.11 (95% CI, 0.32–30.22) and with high heterogeneity (I2 = 54.3%)), when the association with maternal antidepressants exposure was stronger (OR, 1.23; 95% CI, 1.09–1.38).

Boyle et al. (2017), in a study describing the epidemiology of Ebstein's anomaly in Europe and its association with maternal health and medication exposure during pregnancy through population-based data, reported that cases exposed to maternal mental health conditions/medications had an increased adjusted odds ratio risk of 2.64 compared with cardiac controls rather than lithium. The authors therefore emphasize that changing or stopping medication to avoid foetal exposure in the first trimester may not be preventive for either the mother or the foetus.

10.2.3 Foetal and Neonatal Periods

Lithium use during the foetal period is likely to lead to a significant increase in birth weight (Diav-Citrin et al. 2014). In a recent systematic review including 28 studies—10 of which meeting the criteria for inclusion in a meta-analysis—and exploring 1402 newborn babies and 2595 women exposed to lithium, the review found slightly increased adverse pregnancy outcomes for women taking lithium for both the first trimester only and any time during pregnancy, while the meta-analysis found increased odds for preterm birth, and a large size for gestational age with lithium at any time during pregnancy (Callovini et al. 2024). In the retrospective observational cohort study of Imaz et al. (2024), 56% of neonates presented transient acute complications with neonatal hypotonia being the most frequent outcome ($N = 15$).

Thus, paediatricians should carefully monitor babies during the first 48 h for foetal goitre, hypotonia, bradycardia, arrhythmias, systolic murmur, hypothermia, cyanosis, tachypnoea, and poor sucking reflex (Newport et al. 2005), although most of the reports described full recovery of the infants (Iqbal et al. 2001; Sutter-Dallay et al. 2015). The recommendation is therefore to refer these patients to maternity hospitals with day and night neonatal paediatric resources, in a collaborative network involving perinatal psychiatrists and trained obstetric teams (Belzeaux et al. 2024).

10.2.4 Child Development

The question of an effect on foetal brain development in the long term remains, as brain structures develop throughout pregnancy and may be particularly susceptible to the impact of psychotropic drugs. To date, the extreme paucity of data does not allow any conclusions. An animal study reported long-term effects with “anxious” persistent behaviour in pups of dams treated (Youngs et al. 2006). Results at 5 (Schou et al. 1973) and 15 years of age (Van Der Lugt et al. 2012) suggest no distinctive features of these babies as they mature. A more recent study (Forsberg et al. 2018) exploring a small clinical cohort showed no significant association between mothers’ prenatal exposure to lithium or mood disorders and offspring’s IQ. Finally, the latest systematic review from Haskey and Galbally (2017) concluded that the existing data on lithium are reassuring, but are of limited quality, indicating that further research is still required.

10.2.5 Maternal Management

The increase in the distribution volume and in renal excretion rates among pregnant women usually leads to an increase of doses during pregnancy, to maintain blood levels as low as possible within the therapeutic range. Note that this recommendation is applicable to all psychotropic substances. A study providing the kinetic of lithium blood levels during pregnancy, showed decrease in the first trimester (−24%), reached a nadir in the second trimester (−36%), increased in the third trimester (−21%) and were still slightly increased postpartum (+9%) (Wesseloo et al. 2017a). Given these variations, it is recommended to perform serum assays every 4 weeks up to 36 weeks of gestation, and then weekly until birth (NICE 2020). After birth, the decline of distribution volume will lead to a decrease in doses because of the risk of overdosage. Thereafter, requirements will be adapted according to standard protocols, while maintaining special vigilance in the first 15 days postpartum. Note that some authors (Newport et al. 2005; NICE 2020) propose to achieve a therapeutic window in 24–48 ours before delivery when scheduled, or upon start of delivery, with reintroduction immediately after birth.

10.3 What to Do

Lithium is no longer really contraindicated during the first trimester of pregnancy and is certainly not in itself an indication for termination of pregnancy today. The risk of birth defects must also consider in light of the availability of ultrasound screening and the progress in paediatric cardiac surgery. Here, even more than with other psychotropic drugs, assessing the benefit/risk ratio for each patient is essential. Viguera et al. (2000, 2007) have emphasized the importance of mood stabilization during pregnancy when necessary: women who stop their lithium treatment during pregnancy have a risk of postnatal recurrence twice as high as non-pregnant patients, and this recurrence may occur 4 times more rapidly and last 5 times longer. If the choice is to stop treatment, discontinuation must be progressive, even if the embryo is exposed, because the teratogenic risk is currently considered to be less than that of decompensation generated by abrupt cessation (Burt and Rasgon 2004). If treatment is continued throughout the pregnancy, the marked variation in blood volume and the increased rate of renal excretion during pregnancy make regular monitoring of maternal plasma and erythrocyte levels of lithium necessary. Progressive decrease in dose in the days preceding birth is proposed by some authors to avoid an overdose in the immediate postpartum period. In this perspective, proper hydration must be maintained during labour to avoid neonatal overdosing. In the postpartum, regular assays of plasma and erythrocyte lithium should be performed and dosage adjusted until the appropriate balance is obtained.

To conclude and in line with the expert consensus paper of Fiorillo et al. (2023), it is important to notice that there is "a discrepancy between evidence-based recommendations and clinical practice in using lithium treatment for patients with bipolar disorder (…). It is necessary to reinvigorate the clinical and academic discussion about the efficacy of lithium, to counteract the decreasing prescription trend of one of the most effective drugs available in the whole medicine".

10.4 Antiepileptic Drugs

With regard to knowledge on prenatal exposure to antiepileptic drugs, the main difficulty remains that of the effects of the underlying pathology, since the vast majority of publications examine epileptic disorders and not their prescription in bipolar disorders. A very recent systematic review and meta-analysis of the risks of adverse pregnancy outcomes associated with antiseizure medications (ASMs) for any indication (Berry-Noronha et al. 2025) explored 16,941,373 pregnancies or live births (14,437,221 pregnancies with maternal outcome data and 14,938,972 live births with foetal/neonatal outcome data). Compared with pregnancies in unaffected women, those exposed to ASMs had increased odds of several adverse outcomes including preterm birth (OR 1.30, 95% CI 1.09–1.54), caesarean section (OR 1.43, 95% CI 1.13–1.81), gestational diabetes (OR 1.44, 95% CI 1.07–1.94), induction of labour (OR 1.46, 95% CI 1.15–1.86), preeclampsia (OR 1.33, 95% CI 1.02–1.72), spontaneous miscarriage (OR 1.42, 95% CI 1.01–2.01), and spontaneous fetal loss (OR 2.54, 95% CI 1.04–6.24). Comparison of outcomes between untreated women with the same ASMs indications and unaffected women showed that some differences (preterm birth, caesarean section, gestational diabetes, and preeclampsia) were largely attributable to the underlying condition, particularly epilepsy. With regard to the use of antiepileptic drugs for their mood-stabilizing indication, there are virtually no data to draw any conclusions at present.

10.4.1 Placental Transfer

The work of Bank et al. (2017) found mean umbilical-to-maternal ratios for total concentrations ranging from 0.79 for carbamazepine to 1.20 for valproic acid, and mean umbilical-to-maternal ratios for free concentrations ranging from 0.86 for valproic acid to 1.42 for carbamazepine, indicating complete placental passage. However, in this study, neither umbilical cord concentrations nor umbilical-to-maternal ratios were associated with adverse neonatal outcomes.

10.4.2 Carbamazepine

10.4.2.1 Embryonic Period: Organogenesis

Data about the use of carbamazepine during pregnancy thus mainly concern women with epilepsy and reports about women with psychiatric disorders are extremely rare, although this antiepileptic drug is indicated for bipolar disorder. Either the Food and Drug Administration (FDA) or the European Medicine Agency (EMA) does not contraindicate it to date for use during pregnancy for epileptic patients, but consider, as stipulated by the ANSM (Agence Nationale de Sécurité du Médicament et des produits de santé) that carbamazepine is a teratogenic drug as the risk of malformation is up to 5.9%, which is 2–3 times higher than in the general population (ANSM, https://ansm.sante.fr/actualites/carbamazepine-et-grossesse-renforcement-de-linformation-des-femmes-pour-les-sensibiliser-aux-risques-encourus-par-les-enfants-a-naitre? 13/12/2024).

10.4.2.2 Foetus Neonate and Child Development

Increased risks of small head circumference and low birth weight for gestational age have been reported (Galbally et al. 2010; Veiby et al. 2014). The enzyme-inducing effect of carbamazepine must also be considered in the neonatal care of the baby.

Most studies of its effect on child cognitive development report a slight impact, specifically on verbal abilities (Baker et al. 2015; Van Der Pol et al. 1991). More recently, a cohort of 3,182,773 children, of which 17,495 were exposed to ASMs in pregnancy issued from routinely collected primary care data from the UK and nationwide Swedish registries, authors found that children exposed to carbamazepine were 1.25 times more likely to be diagnosed with autism (95% CI: 1.05–1.48) and 1.30 times more likely to be diagnosed with intellectual disability (95% CI: 1.01–1.69) (Madley-Dowd et al. 2024).

10.4.2.3 What to Do

If the prescription of carbamazepine is unavoidable, the risk of congenital malformations necessitates supplementation with folic acid for 2 months before and after conception to prevent neural tube defects (Gedzelman et al. 2012). Ultrasound monitoring is recommended along with a possible assay of maternal serum levels of alpha-fetoprotein before the 18th week of gestation (Galbally et al. 2010), underlying the absolute necessity for these women to be followed by obstetric and paediatric teams that are trained and able to manage complications. Lastly, regular care and monitoring in a neonatal paediatric department is recommended for the child.

10.4.3 Valproates

10.4.3.1 Embryonic Period: Organogenesis

The prescription of valproates is contraindicated during the first trimester of pregnancy. The teratogenic risk is significant, with a global malformation rate around 10% (four times higher than with other antiepileptic drugs), mainly of the central nervous system (1–2% compared to 0.1% in the general population) (Ernst and Goldberg 2002; Galbally et al. 2010; Hernández-Díaz et al. 2012). In cases of exposure in early pregnancy, some authors consider that the risk of teratogenesis outweighs that of mood decompensation and advocate rapid cessation. Specific ultrasound to screen for malformations is required as early as possible, and abortion counselling must be offered if they are suspected.

10.4.3.2 Fetus and Neonate

Valproate may lead to a haemorrhagic syndrome in the newborn, although its cause is still unclear (possibly a combination of impaired platelet aggregation, thrombocytopenia, and decreased fibrinogen). Monitoring of haemostasis is thus required in the mother before delivery and in the neonate at birth. The baby also appears to be at risk of hepatocellular insufficiency. Some studies have described a risk of neonatal hypoglycaemia (Galbally et al. 2010). Another important concern is the risk of impaired cognitive development in infants of mothers treated with valproates (Eriksson et al. 2005; Haskey and Galbally 2017). The EMA issued a warning against prescribing these drugs to women and girls of childbearing age (http://www.ema.europa.eu/ema/index.jsp?curl=pages/medicines/human/referrals/Valproate_and_related_substances/human_referral_prac_000032.jsp&mid=WC0b01ac05805c516f). The French national agency of medications banned the prescription of valproates in women of childbearing age (Casassus 2017).

Recently, Madley-Dowd et al. (2024)—previously mentioned—showed that children exposed to valproate were more likely to receive a diagnosis of autism, intellectual disability, and ADHD, when compared to children not exposed to ASMs.

10.4.3.3 What to Do

In view of the clear increase in the risk of congenital malformations and developmental disorders caused using valproates during pregnancy, switching to a different molecule before pregnancy—or as soon as pregnancy is discovered—is the first-line recommendation. In case of antenatal exposure, supplementation with folic acid from 2 months before to 2 months after conception is essential to help to the prevention of neural tube defects (Gedzelman et al. 2012).

Monitoring by special ultrasonography is strongly recommended, together with a possible assay of maternal serum levels of alpha-fetoprotein before the 18th week of gestation. During pregnancy and after childbirth, maternal and child coagulation and hepatic functions and maternal blood concentrations of valproate should all be monitored regularly.

Note that the prescription of valproates is now contraindicated in women of childbearing age unless alternative treatments are ineffective or not tolerated (WHO 2023, https://www.who.int/news/item/02-05-2023-use-of-valproic-acid-in-women-and-girls-of-childbearing-potential).

10.4.4 Lamotrigine

10.4.4.1 Embryonic Period: Organogenesis

The recent systematic review and network meta-analysis of congenital malformations and prenatal outcomes (Wang et al. 2025) exploring 3,042,997 showed that pregnant women taking lamotrigine did not show significant differences compared with the unexposed group in terms of congenital malformations (OR, 1.21; 95% CrI 0.86–1.64). However, some studies suggested a possible dose-effect relation with cleft palate, not confirmed to date (Campbell et al. 2014; Vajda et al. 2025). On the other hand, analysis of 490 pregnancies treated with lamotrigine monotherapy and 214 pregnancies in women with epilepsy who were not exposed to antiepileptic drugs during at least the first half of pregnancy showed that there was a foetal malformation rate of 4.49% in the LTG-exposed pregnancies and 3.27% in the untreated group (risk ratio = 1.37; 95% C.I. 0.60, 3.16). Logistic regression provided no evidence that the lamotrigine-associated risk of malformations was related to lamotrigine dose, although the body regions affected by malformations tended to differ between lamotrigine-treated and untreated pregnancies. Nevertheless, the authors emphasize that if the foetal malformation rates of lamotrigine monotherapy are used as a comparator to assess the risk of foetal malformation associated with other antiepileptic drugs, the results may suggest falsely reassuring results.

10.4.4.2 Fetus and Neonate

In 2018, a review concluded that "it is not clear that fetuses of lamotrigine-exposed pregnant women are at higher risk of malformation or neurodevelopmental delay" (Kong et al. 2018). A recent review and meta-analysis on neurodevelopmental outcomes after prenatal exposure to lamotrigine monotherapy in women with epilepsy found that lamotrigine monotherapy is not statistically associated with neurodevelopmental disorders as a whole, language disorders or delay, diagnosis or risk of ASD and diagnosis or risk of ADHD. However, the meta-analyses found an increased risk of psychomotor developmental disorders or delay and cognitive developmental delay in less than 3 years old children. Finally, the authors underline that these findings were exclusively based on possible biased observational studies of a limited number of children (Peron et al. 2024).

10.4.4.3 What to Do

Lamotrigine was found as not being inferior to lithium in the prevention of severe postpartum episodes, suggesting that lamotrigine could be a reasonable alternative treatment option for bipolar disorder during pregnancy in patients with vulnerability for depression and may prevent severe episodes postpartum (Wesseloo et al. 2017b). In view of the persistent doubts about the safety of antenatal exposure in terms of teratogenesis, prescribers must always bear in mind the rule of seeking the minimum effective dose. In this context, blood tests can guide decisions.

10.5 Conclusion

Table 10.1 summarizes key points.

One of the most important features of the perinatal period is the real possibility of preventive care to protect the health of both mother and child. Psychiatrists must always be aware of the importance of discussing pregnancy plans with women of childbearing age with bipolar disorder, preferably before they become pregnant.

If pregnancy occurs, regular follow-up by a specialist team should be offered whenever possible. Management needs to be embedded in a multidisciplinary network to anticipate specific postnatal care, such as prolongation of maternity stay, home help, community-based interventions or any other type of specific care foreseen by local or national perinatal mental health policies. Given the complexity of the treatment, the psychiatrist must ensure close interdisciplinary care, if possible in the form of a liaison and consultation service; it is particularly important that all involved are aware of the effects of medication on the mother, the embryo and the foetus, including the effects that vary according to gestational age.

References

Baker GA, Bromley RL, Briggs M, Cheyne CP, Cohen MJ, García-Fiñana M, Gummery A, Kneen R, Loring DW, Mawer G, Meador KJ, Shallcross R, Clayton-Smith J, Liverpool and Manchester Neurodevelopment Group. IQ at 6 years after in utero exposure to antiepileptic drugs: a controlled cohort study. Neurology. 2015;84:382–90.

Bank AM, Stowe ZN, Newport DJ, Ritchie RJ, Pennell PB. Placental passage of antiepileptic drugs at delivery and neonatal outcomes. Epilepsia. 2017;58:e82–6.

Belzeaux R, Gressier F, Boudieu L, Arnould A, Moreau E, Pastol J, Tzavara E, Sutter-Dallay AL, Samalin L. French Society for Biological Psychiatry and Neuropsychopharmacology and French-speaking Marcé society guidelines for the management of mood disorders in women before, during, and after pregnancy. Arch Womens Ment Health. 2024;27(4):595–605.

Bergink V, Kushner SA. Lithium during pregnancy. Am J Psychiatry. 2014;171:712–5.

Berry-Noronha A, Manoleehakul P, Rottler A, McGuiness G, Chen Z, Kuhn R, Vajda FJ, Perucca E, Antonic-Baker A, Perucca P. Risk of adverse pregnancy outcomes associated with Antiseizure medications and their indications: a systematic review and meta-analysis. Neurology. 2025;104(3):e210233.

Boyle B, Garne E, Loane M, Addor MC, Arriola L, Cavero-Carbonell C, Gatt M, Lelong N, Lynch C, Nelen V, Neville AJ, O'Mahony M, Pierini A, Rissmann A, Tucker D, Zymak-Zakutnia N, Dolk H. The changing epidemiology of Ebstein's anomaly and its relationship with maternal mental health conditions: a European registry-based study. Cardiol Young. 2017;27:677–85.

Burt VK, Rasgon N. Special considerations in treating bipolar disorder in women. Bipolar Disord. 2004;6:2–13.

Callovini T, Montanari S, Bardi F, Barbonetti S, Rossi S, Caso R, Mandracchia G, Margoni S, Brugnami A, Paolini M, Manfredi G, Giudice LL, Segatori D, Zanzarri A, Onori L, Calderoni C, Benini E, Marano G, Massetti M, Fiaschè F, Di Segni F, Janiri D, Simonetti A, Moccia L, Grisoni F, Ruggiero S, Bartolucci G, Biscosi M, Ferrara OM, Bernardi E, Monacelli L, Giannico AM, De Berardis D, Battisti G, Ciliberto M, Brisi C, Lisci FM, D'Onofrio AM, Restaino A, Di Benedetto L, Anesini MB, Boggio G, Specogna E, Crupi A, De Chiara E, Caroppo E, Ieritano V, Monti L, Chieffo DPR, Rinaldi L, Camardese G, Cuomo I, Brugnoli R, Kotzalidis GD, Sani G, Mazza M. Obstetric outcomes in women on lithium: a systematic review and meta-analysis. J Clin Med. 2024;18(13):4872.

Campbell E, Kennedy F, Russell A. Malformation risks of antiepileptic drug monotherapies in pregnancy: updated results from the UK and Ireland epilepsy and pregnancy register. J Neurol Neurosurg Psychiatry. 2014;85:1029–34.

Casassus B. France bans sodium valproate use in case of pregnancy. Lancet. 2017;390(10091):217.

Chan JKN, Hung SC, Lee KCK, Cheung KW, Seto MT, Wong CSM, Lin J, Chang WC. Risk of adverse pregnancy, delivery and neonatal outcomes associated with bipolar disorder and prenatal use of mood stabilizers: a population-based cohort study. Psychiatry Res. 2024;339:116050. Epub 2024

Clark CT, Klein AM, Perel JM, Helsel J, Wisner KL. Lamotrigine dosing for pregnant patients with bipolar disorder. Am J Psychiatry. 2013;170:1240–7.

Diav-Citrin O, Shechtman S, Tahover E. Pregnancy outcome following in utero exposure to lithium: a prospective, comparative, observational study. Am J Psychiatry. 2014;171:785–94.

Eriksson K, Viinikainen K, Mönkkönen A, Aikiä M, Nieminen P, Heinonen S, Kälviäinen R. Children exposed to valproate in utero – population based evaluation of risks and confounding factors for long-term neurocognitive development. Epilepsy Res. 2005;65:189–200.

Ernst CL, Goldberg JF. The reproductive safety profile of mood stabilizers, atypical antipsychotics, and broad-spectrum psychotropics. J Clin Psychiatry. 2002;63(Suppl 4):42–55.

Fiorillo A, Sampogna G, Albert U, Maina G, Perugi G, Pompili M, Rosso G, Sani G, Tortorella A. Facts and myths about the use of lithium for bipolar disorder in routine clinical practice: an expert consensus paper. Ann Gen Psychiatry. 2023;22(1):50. https://doi.org/10.1186/s12991-023-00481-y. PMID: 38057894; PMCID: PMC10702081.

Forsberg L, Adler M, Römer Ek I, Ljungdahl M, Naver L, Gustafsson LL, Berglund G, Chotigasation A, Hammar U, Böhm B, Wide K. Maternal mood disorders and lithium exposure in utero were not associated with poor cognitive development during childhood. Acta Paediatr. 2018;107:1379–88.

Gaffield ME, Culwell KR, Lee CR. The use of hormonal contraception among women taking anticonvulsant therapy. Contraception. 2011;83:16–29.

Galbally M, Snellen M, Walker S, Permezel M. Management of antipsychotic and mood stabilizer medication in pregnancy: recommendations for antenatal care. Aust N Z J Psychiatry. 2010;44:99–108.

Gedzelman E, Kimford J, Meador MD. Antiepileptic drugs in women with epilepsy during pregnancy. Ther Adv Drug Safe. 2012;3:71–87.

Gentile S. Lithium in pregnancy: the need to treat, the duty to ensure safety. Expert Opin Drug Saf. 2012;11:425–37.

Giles JJ, Bannigan JG. Teratogenic and developmental effects of lithium. Curr Pharm Des. 2006;12:1531–41.

Haskey C, Galbally M. Mood stabilizers in pregnancy and child developmental outcomes: a systematic review. Aust N Z J Psychiatry. 2017;51:1087–97.

Hernández-Díaz S, Smith CR, Shen A, Mittendorf R, Hauser WA, Yerby M, Holmes LB, North American AED Pregnancy Registry; North American AED Pregnancy Registry. Comparative safety of antiepileptic drugs during pregnancy. Neurology. 2012;78:1692–9.

Imaz ML, Torra M, Langohr K, Arca G, Soy D, Hernández AS, García-Esteve L, Vieta E, Martin-Santos R. Peripartum lithium management: early maternal and neonatal outcomes. J Affect Disord. 2024;1(366):326–34.

Iqbal MM, Sohhan T, Mahmud SZ. The effects of lithium, valproic acid, and carbamazepine during pregnancy and lactation. J Toxicol Clin Toxicol. 2001;39:381–92.

Jones I, Craddock N. Bipolar disorder and childbirth: the importance of recognising risk. Br J Psychiatry. 2005;186:453–4.

Kong L, Zhou T, Wang B, Gao Z, Wang C. The risks associated with the use of lamotrigine during pregnancy. Int J Psychiatry Clin Pract. 2018;22:2–5.

Kozma C. Neonatal toxicity and transient neurodevelopmental deficits following prenatal exposure to lithium: another clinical report and a review of the literature. Am J Med Genet. 2005;132A(4):441–4.

Lemieux A, Khalilipalandi S, Lauzon-Schnittka J, Taillefer V, Tousignant A, Perreault L, Rego K, Dubois M, Watelle L, Roy LO, Dallaire F. Meta-analysis of risk factors for congenital heart disease: part 2, maternal medication, reproductive technologies, and familial and fetal factors. Can J Cardiol. 2024;40(12):2496–511.

Madley-Dowd P, Ahlqvist VH, Forbes H, Rast JE, Martin FZ, Zhong C, Barry CS, Berglind D, Lundberg M, Lyall K, Newschaffer CJ, Tomson T, Davies NM, Magnusson C, Rai D, Lee BK. Antiseizure medication use during pregnancy and children's neurodevelopmental outcomes. Nat Commun. 2024;15(1):9640.

Mcknight RF, Adida M, Budge K, Stockton S, Goodwin GM, Geddes JR. Lithium toxicity profile: a systematic review and meta-analysis. Lancet. 2012;379:721–8.

Mohamed M, Elhelbawy A, Khalid M, AbdAllatif L, Lialy HE. Effects of bipolar disorder on maternal and fetal health during pregnancy: a systematic review. BMC Pregnancy Childbirth. 2023;23(1):617.

Molenaar NM, Poels EMP, Robakis T, Wesseloo R, Bergink V. Management of lithium dosing around delivery: an observational study. Focus (Am Psychiatr Publ). 2024;22(1):120–5.

Newport DJ, Viguera AC, et al. Lithium placental passage and obstetrical outcome: implications for clinical management during late pregnancy. Am J Psychiatry. 2005;162:2162–70.

NICE Guidelines. Antenatal and postnatal mental health: clinical management and service guidance [CG192], 2020.

Nora JJ, Nora AH, Toews WH. Lithium, Ebstein's anomaly, and other congenital heart defects. Lancet. 1974;2:594–5.

Patorno E, Huybrechts KF, Bateman BT, Cohen JM, Desai RJ, Mogun H, Cohen LS, Hernandez-Diaz S. Lithium use in pregnancy and the risk of cardiac malformations. N Engl J Med. 2017;376:2245–54.

Peron A, Picot C, Jurek L, Nourredine M, Ripoche E, Ajiji P, Cucherat M, Cottin J. Neurodevelopmental outcomes after prenatal exposure to lamotrigine monotherapy in women with epilepsy: a systematic review and meta-analysis. BMC Pregnancy Childbirth. 2024;24:103.

Schou M, Goldfield MD, Weinstein MR, Villieneuve A. Lithium and pregnancy. I. Report from the register of lithium babies. BMJ. 1973;2:135–6.

Sutter-Dallay AL, Bales M, et al. Impact of prenatal exposure to psychotropic drugs on neonatal outcome in infants of mothers with serious psychiatric illnesses. J Clin Psychiatry. 2015;76:967–73.

Vajda FJ, Vajda SRL, Eadie MJ. Is lamotrigine a teratogen? Seizure. 2025;126:1–5.

Van der Lugt NM, Van de Maat JS, Van Kamp IL, Knoppert-van der Klein EA, Hovens JG, Walther FJ. Fetal, neonatal and developmental outcomes of lithium-exposed pregnancies. Early Hum Dev. 2012;88:375–8.

Van der Pol MC, Hadders-Algra M, Huisjes HJ, Touwen BC. Antiepileptic medication in pregnancy: late effects on the children's central nervous system development. Am J Obstet Gynecol. 1991;164:121–8.

Veiby G, Daltveit AK, Engelsen BA, Gilhus NE. Fetal growth restriction and birth defects with newer and older antiepileptic drugs during pregnancy. J Neurol. 2014;261:579–88.

Viguera AC, Nonacs R, et al. Risk of recurrence of bipolar disorder in pregnant and nonpregnant women after discontinuing lithium maintenance. Am J Psychiatry. 2000;157:179–84.

Viguera AC, Whitfield T, et al. Risk of recurrence in women with bipolar disorder during pregnancy: prospective study of mood stabilizer discontinuation. Am J Psychiatry. 2007;164:1817–24.

Viguera AC, Tondo L, Koukopoulos AE, Reginaldi D, Lepri B, Baldessarini RJ. Episodes of mood disorders in 2252 pregnancies and postpartum periods. Am J Psychiatry. 2011;168:1179–85.

Wang E, Liu Y, Wang Y, Han X, Zhou Y, Zhang L, Tang Y. Comparative safety of antipsychotic medications and mood stabilizers during pregnancy: a systematic review and network meta-analysis of congenital malformations and prenatal outcomes. CNS Drugs. 2025;39(1):1–22.

Weinstein MR, Goldfield M. Cardiovascular malformations with lithium use during pregnancy. Am J Psychiatry. 1975;132:529–31.

Wesseloo R, Wierdsma AI, van Kamp IL, Munk-Olsen T, Hoogandijk WJG, Kushner SA, Bergink V. Lithium dosing strategies during pregnancy and the postpartum period. Br J Psychiatry. 2017a;211:31–6.

Wesseloo R, Liu X, Clark CT, Kushner SA, Munk-Olsen T, Bergink V. Risk of postpartum episodes in women with bipolar disorder after lamotrigine or lithium use during pregnancy: a population-based cohort study. J Affect Disord. 2017b;218:394–7.

Youngs RM, Chu MS, Meloni EG, Naydenov A, Carlezon WA Jr, Konradi C. Lithium administration to preadolescent rats causes long-lasting increases in anxiety-like behavior and has molecular consequences. J Neurosci. 2006;26:6031–9.

Zalzstein E, Koren G, Einarson T, Freedom RM. A case-control study on the association between first trimester exposure to lithium and Ebstein's anomaly. Am J Cardiol. 1990;65:817–8.

Zhang L, Li H, Li S, Zou X. Reproductive and metabolic abnormalities in women taking valproate for bipolar disorder: a meta-analysis. Eur J Obstet Gynecol Reprod Biol. 2016;202:26–31.

Mood Stabilizers During Lactation

11

Sandeep Grover, Devakshi Dua, and Nidhi Yadav

11.1 Introduction

Bipolar disorder (BD) usually starts in the late teens and early twenties and because of this, women suffering from this ailment remain at risk of an episode throughout their reproductive life (Yonkers et al. 2005). Further, available data suggests that most of the affective disorders, which are post-partum in onset, usually turn out to be BD in the longitudinal course (Munk-Olsen et al. 2012).

Mood stabilizers (MS) form an integral part of the management of BD. Due to the severity of the illness, many women continue on MS during pregnancy, which is carried through into the post-partum period. MS is also often started in the immediate post-partum period in women in whom these medications were withheld during the pregnancy or at the time of delivery. These medications are also often considered for post-partum onset BD. Continuation or discontinuation of MS during pregnancy and lactation requires appropriate knowledge about the risks and benefits of these medications, both for the mother and the baby (Grover and Avasthi 2015). In this chapter, we discuss the risks and benefits of the use of MS during the post-partum period, both for the mother and the newborn.

In general, the conventional MS includes lithium, sodium valproate, and its congeners, lamotrigine, and carbamazepine. In recent times, other antiepileptic agents like gabapentin, and atypical antipsychotics like aripiprazole, olanzapine, quetiapine, risperidone, ziprasidone, lurasidone, etc. have also been considered to have mood stabilizing properties (Smith and Dubovsky 2017). Medications like clonazepam, calcium channel blockers, etc., have also been evaluated as MS. In this

S. Grover (✉) · N. Yadav
Department of Psychiatry, Postgraduate Institute of Medical Education and Research, Chandigarh, Punjab, India

D. Dua
Midlands Partnership Foundation Trust, Stafford, UK

F. Uguz, L. Orsolini (eds.), *Perinatal Psychopharmacology*,
https://doi.org/10.1007/978-3-031-99720-4_11

chapter, we will mainly focus on the conventional agents, as information on other agents is presented in other chapters. Issues related to the use of MS during pregnancy and delivery are not addressed in this chapter.

Available data suggests that there is a high risk of relapse during pregnancy (Freeman et al. 2002; Jones and Craddock 2005; Viguera et al. 2007b) and the early post-partum period for BD (Kendell et al. 1987; Terp and Mortensen 1998; Viguera et al. 2000). While the risk of relapse during pregnancy has been estimated to be 50% or more (Freeman et al. 2002; Jones and Craddock 2005; Viguera et al. 2007b), with 2.3 times higher risk of recurrence on discontinuation of MS. A prospective study showed that compared to women who continued the MS during the pregnancy, those who stopped the MS during pregnancy spent about 5 times longer duration (8.8% versus 40%) of their pregnancy, in the episode (Viguera et al. 2007b). The risk of episodes during the post-partum period has been estimated to be 40–70% higher among women with untreated BD (Jefferson et al. 1987) and the risk is higher in those who discontinue prophylactic treatment (Viguera et al. 2000). Among the various risk factors for relapse, the rate of discontinuation of MS is an important marker, with higher risk of relapse associated with rapid discontinuation of MS (Viguera et al. 2007b). A recent systematic review and meta-analysis that included data from 37 studies involving 5700 deliveries in 4023 patients estimated the risk of post-partum relapse to be 35% (95% CI = 29 to 41) (Wesseloo et al. 2016). Another systematic review that included data from 16 studies involving 6064 deliveries of 3977 women estimated the overall risk of post-partum relapse to be 36.77% (Javier Conejo-Galindo 2022). It was further shown that the risk of relapse during the post-partum period was significantly higher among those who were medication-free during pregnancy (66%, 95% CI = 57 to 75) than those who used prophylactic medication (23%, 95% CI = 14 to 37) (Wesseloo et al. 2016). In terms of clinical variables, available data suggests that the risk of post-partum episodes is higher when the age of onset of BD is lower, a longer duration of the episode, a history of prior episodes of similar polarity, a family history of BD, history of psychiatric hospitalizations before the pregnancy and absence of prophylaxis (Javier Conejo-Galindo 2022).

Considering these facts, the selection of appropriate MS for women of reproductive age group, especially during pregnancy and post-partum, requires weighing all the pros and cons of the use of these drugs. The treating clinicians often face the challenge of minimizing the risk to the fetus along with minimizing the impact of maternal morbidity. Clinicians often have to consider either using or not using MS and determine the reasonable risk with both strategies. It is suggested that considering something as a reasonable risk during pregnancy involves shared responsibility between the patient and the treating clinician, but it is important to remember that the final decision about treatment lies with the informed patient.

11.2 Beneficial Effects of Breastfeeding

The post-partum period is associated with the additional clinical dilemma of lactation and breastfeeding. The beneficial effect of breastfeeding for both infant and mother cannot be underscored. Breast milk is considered an ideal form of nutrition, which confers many advantages to the newborn. As per the American Academy of Paediatrics, besides being an important contributor to the establishment of emotional bonds and attachment between the mother and the infant (Britton et al. 2006), breast milk is known to reduce the incidence and/or severity of a wide range of infectious diseases (Department of Health and Human Service Office on Women's Health 2003), post-neonatal infant mortality rates, sudden infant death syndrome in the first year of life, the incidence of insulin-dependent (type 1) and non–insulin-dependent (type 2) diabetes mellitus, hematological malignancies (i.e., lymphoma, leukemia, Hodgkin disease), overweight and obesity, hypercholesterolemia and asthma in older children and adults (Britton et al. 2006). Breastfeeding has also been reported to be associated with slightly better performance on tests of cognitive development (Horta et al. 2018). In terms of maternal benefits, breastfeeding has been reported to decrease post-partum bleeding, lead to faster uterine involution, decrease menstrual blood loss, child spacing by lactational amenorrhea, earlier return to pre-pregnancy weight, reduce in the risk of breast and ovarian cancer, and possibly decreased risk of hip fractures and osteoporosis in the postmenopausal period (Gartner et al. 2005). Considering these benefits, in general, breastfeeding is recommended for all newborns, with very few absolute contraindications. The use of medications and drug use are considered as relative contraindications for breastfeeding (Lawrence 2013).

Accordingly, continuing or discontinuing breastfeeding while continuing MS is often associated with an ethical dilemma and difficult decision-making. The risk-benefit should be evaluated by considering physiological and psychological benefits of breastfeeding, the potential negative impact of untreated maternal mental illness on the infant, maternal-child bonding, the negative consequences of MS on the cognitive and behavioral development of the newborn, and the consequences of untreated mental illness on the mother (Burt et al. 2001). In general, all efforts must be made to continue breastfeeding, while minimizing the negative consequences of the use of MS and other psychotropics. This requires some understanding of physiology of the breast milk secretion.

11.3 Understanding the Physiological Aspects of Breast Milk Secretion and Use of MS During Lactation

Breast milk secretion can be broadly understood as fore milk and hind milk. Fore milk is expressed during the first half of a feed and has lower lipid content, whereas hind milk, that is secreted during the second half of a feed, is rich in lipid content. Due to higher lipid content, hind milk contains a higher quantity of lipid-soluble psychotropic medications compared to the milk secreted in the first half (Burt et al.

2001). Additionally, the exposure of newborns to medications is influenced by the rate of absorption of medications into the maternal circulation, diffusion of medications from the maternal circulation to the breast milk, and absorption of the medications in the infant. It is important to understand that the concentration of a medication in breast milk depends on the non-protein-bound concentration of the drug in maternal plasma. Accordingly, the factors are taken into account to determine the concentration of the medication in breast milk, plasma protein binding, the volume of distribution, lipid solubility, molecular weight, and pka-pH. Medications that have high plasma protein binding will have low secretion in breast milk, for example, selective serotonin reuptake inhibitors (SSRIs) have high plasma protein binding, whereas venlafaxine has low plasma protein binding. Accordingly, the concentration of venlafaxine is expected to be more than that of SSRIs. Medications that have large volumes of distribution will get sequestered in different fluid compartments leading to low maternal plasma levels and thus low levels of breast milk. Medications that have high lipid solubility, such as majority of the psychotropic medications, easily pass through the alveolar cells and thus have more secretion into breast milk. Drugs with higher molecular weight have a slower diffusion rate and transfer into the breast milk. The pKa-pH value of a particular drug is the pH at which the medication is equally ionic and nonionic. Ion trapping occurs when pKa is more than 7.2, leading to high concentrations in breast milk (Ito and Lee 2003).

In clinical and research practice, the relative infant dose is an estimate of the amount of drug dose of the breastfeeding infant. Usually, milk to plasma ratio is considered an indicator of the secretion of the medication in the breast milk. The relative infant dose is calculated as dose in the infant in mg/kg/d/dose in the mother in mg/kg/d. Dose in an infant is the concentration of the medication in the breast milk divided by the volume of breast milk consumed daily. Practically relative infant dose of <10% is considered acceptable, whereas drugs that have a relative infant dose of>25% are considered to have a therapeutic effect if absorbed and are accordingly unacceptable (Ito and Lee 2003). However, it is important to remember that absorption of medication also depends on the oral bioavailability in the infant. Limited data is available on the oral bioavailability of drugs in infants. In addition, inadequate information is available regarding how much infant plasma concentration has the potential to harm (Grover and Avasthi 2015).

Factors that influence the quantity of medications in breast milk include serum albumin, lactose, lysozyme, and other enzymes, prolactin levels, and minerals like calcium and phosphates (Burt et al. 2001). It is also important to understand the factors that influence the excretion of various medications from the body of the neonates. Neonatal cytochrome P-450 activity is about half of that seen in adults. Most of the neonates take about 2 weeks to develop from minimal levels to almost adult levels, the capability to conjugate various compounds (Beath 2003). The kidneys of the neonates are also functionally immature, hence, various medications that are primarily eliminated through kidneys tend to accumulate. Effects of various medications on the brain also depend on the blood-brain barrier (BBB) and it is well known that, compared to adults, the BBB in neonates is also immature, which leads to a higher concentration of lipid-soluble agents (10–30 times) in the CSF than in serum. Additionally, compared to older infants, fat storage sites are relatively lower in neonates. This leads to a higher concentration of lipid-soluble substances in the central nervous system of newborns (Burt et al. 2001). Accordingly, all these facts must be considered when recommending breastfeeding in a newborn.

11.4 MS and Lactation

11.4.1 Lithium

There is limited data in terms of the effect of continuation of lithium during the post-partum period and continuation of breastfeeding. Studies have estimated the serum lithium levels in infants, whose mothers have been taking lithium in the dose of 600 mg to 1500 mg/day during breastfeeding and these have reported the levels among infants to vary from 0% to 30% of the maternal levels (Bogen et al. 2012; Moretti et al. 2003). However, a recent case report estimated infant serum lithium levels to be 58% of the maternal levels (Frew 2015). Another study evaluated the maternal level, levels of lithium in breast milk, and levels in the infants of 10 mothers taking lithium in the dose of 600 mg/day to 1200 mg/day. The maternal levels varied from 0.43 to 1.31 mmol/liter, the levels in the breast milk were found to be 0.19 to 0.48 mmol/liter, and infant levels were found to be 0.08 to 0.25 mmol/liter (Viguera et al. 2007a). A review of literature that included data from 39 mother-child dyads in which the infants were breastfed for a mean duration of 58.9 (83.3) days was obtained from 13 case reports/series. The mother's serum lithium dose was 904 (SD: 293) mg/day with serum lithium levels of 0.73(SD:0.26) mEq/L, breast milk lithium concentration was 0.84 (SD:0.14) mEq/L, and the mean infant lithium plasma/serum concentration of 0.23(SD: 0.26) mEq/L. The majority (80%) of the infants did not experience adverse effects and their serum lithium concentration was $\leq$0.30 mEq/L and a small proportion (20%) had a transient adverse event (i.e., acute toxicity or thyroid alterations) (Imaz et al. 2019). A recent retrospective study included data from 25 infant-mother dyads and analyzed the data by dividing the sample into a high exposure group (HEG, lithium concentrations $\geq$ 0.6 meq/l) and a low exposure group (LEG, <0.6 meq/l). The median serum lithium level at birth in the HEG and LEG was 0.90 meq/l and 0.40 meq/l, respectively. The difference persisted between the two groups at follow-up (0.20 meq/l vs 0.06 meq/l, $p < 0.05$), despite the reduction in maternal dose. The rate of neonatal symptoms in the HEG was nearly twice that of the LEG group (85.7% vs 41.2; $p = 0.08$) at birth and was about two and half times (28.6% vs 11.8%; $p = 0.55$) at follow-up at a mean of 24 days. The symptoms at birth included central nervous symptoms (jitteriness, agitation, lethargy), jaundice, respiratory symptoms (apnea, need for continuous positive airway pressure and/or ventilation), renal symptoms (increased plasma creatinine levels), and thyroid symptoms (increased levels of thyroxine). There was no statistically significant difference between the two groups for symptoms in different organ systems. In terms of the need for inpatient care, 28.6% of infants in HEG and only 5.9% in LEG ($p = 0.19$) required admission. All infants with symptoms at follow-up were either in the HEG or exposed to additional psychotropic medication. Both in terms of neonatal outcomes and outcomes at follow-up, children of mothers treated with additional psychotropics experienced more adverse outcomes (Whaites Heinonen et al. 2023). Another retrospective study evaluated 30 (21 girls and 9 boys) infants exposed to lithium through breastmilk. The median serum lithium level was 0.10 mmol/L in the second week of life (range < 0.05–0.7 mmol/L), 0.08 in weeks 2–4 (range < 0.05–1.2), 0.06 in the second month of life (range < 0.05–0.2) and 0.07 after 2 months of age (range < 0.05–0.2). Unexpectedly high lithium concentrations were found in two infants in the first month of life. Apart from poor weight gain, no adverse effects were noted (Heinonen et al. 2022). In terms of neonatal side effects, occasional reports have documented adverse effects like hypothermia, hypotonia, lethargy, and T-wave modifications on electrocardiogram (ECG) among neonates whose mothers were taking lithium during the post-partum period. There is some data to suggest a possible association between feeding difficulties with maternal use of lithium during post-partum, but the evidence for this is inconclusive (Bogen et al. 2012; Imaz et al. 2021a, b). Available data from small sample size studies suggests a lack of acute growth or developmental delays with exposure to lithium in neonates or infants (Imaz et al. 2021a, b).

Based on the available literature, the British Association for Psychopharmacology (BAP) recommends that if lithium is continued during pregnancy, serum lithium levels should be monitored at monthly intervals up to 36 weeks and then weekly till delivery. Lithium should be stopped for 24–48 h before a planned cesarean section or induction of labor. Serum lithium levels should be measured 12 h after the last dose. If serum lithium levels do not exceed the therapeutic range, lithium should be restarted on day 1 postnatal and the levels should be checked again after 1 week (McAllister-Williams et al. 2017).

11.4.2 Valproate

Available data suggests that valproate is minimally secreted in breast milk. A small sample size study, which estimated the valproate level in 6 breastfed mother-infant pairs, reported infants serum valproate levels in the range of 0.9–2.3% of the mother's serum level (Piontek et al. 2000). Another study, which was limited to 2 infants whose breast-feeding mothers were taking valproate, reported valproate levels in the infants to be 1.5 and 6%, respectively (Wisner and Perel 1998). A recent study that involved 30 nursing mothers suffering from epilepsy showed that with the mean valproic acid levels of 39 (SD: 16.7) mg/L in the maternal serum, the level of the same in milk was 1.6 (SD: 3.9 mg/L) and mean of 4.3 (SD: 4.3) mg/L in the infant serum. The ratio of milk/maternal serum levels ranged from <0.03 to 0.25 (mean: 0.03; SD: 0.06), and the infant/maternal serum level ratio ranged from <0.03 to 0.61 (mean: 0.11; SD: 0.13). Overall, about two-thirds of the milk and one-third of the infant valproate concentrations were below the quantification limit. The authors did not find any significant correlation between maternal serum and milk levels or between maternal and infant serum levels. Based on their findings, the authors concluded that there is a very small level of transfer of valproate from the mother to the breastfeeding infant (Ivana Kacirova 2019). Based on all these findings, it can be said that valproate/valproic acid use during lactation is safe. American Academy of Neurology (AAN) and American Academy of Pediatrics (AAP) support breastfeeding if the mother is taking valproate (Harden et al. 2009; Sachs and Drugs 2013). However, it is important to remember that occasional case reports have documented side effects in the form of anemia, reticulocytosis, and thrombocytopenic purpura in infants whose mother was treated with valproic acid during the postpartum period. These side effects disappeared when the mother stopped breastfeeding (Stahl et al. 1997).

11.4.3 Carbamazepine

Most of the data on carbamazepine in breastfeeding infants have been based on an assessment of offspring of mothers who took the drug during pregnancy. The concentration of carbamazepine has been estimated to be 6–65% of maternal levels among infants (Chaudron and Jefferson 2000). However, it is important to note that there are occasional case reports of transient hepatic dysfunction (Frey et al. 1990; Merlob et al. 1992) in infants whose mothers were taking carbamazepine during breastfeeding (Frey et al. 1990; Merlob et al. 1992). The neonate developed transient cholestasis with pale stools and marked elevations of glutamyltransferase (322 U/L), conjugated bilirubin (3.5 mg/dL), and bile acids (78.5 μ g/mL), raised transaminases levels (AST 112 U/L, ALT 56 U/L) with normal coagulation profile between the third and seventh week of life (Frey et al. 1990).

A recent study that included data from 66 mother-infant dyads assessed the carbamazepine levels in mothers, breast milk, and infant serum. The carbamazepine levels in maternal serum varied from 1.4 to 10.4 mg/L (median 4.5 mg/L), varied from 0.5 to 6.7 mg/L (mean 2.1 mg/L) in breast milk, and varied from 0.5 to 2.6 mg/L (median 0.5 mg/L) in infant serum. The carbamazepine-10,1-epoxide ranged from 0.3 to 5.4 mg/L (median 0.9 mg/L), 0.3 to 3.7 mg/L (median 0.5 mg/L), and from 0.3 to 0.6 mg/L (median 0.3 mg/L) in maternal serum, breast milk and infant serum, respectively, when measured between the 6th and 29th postnatal day (median 7 days). There was a significant correlation between the maternal serum and the breast milk carbamazepine and carbamazepine-10,1-epoxide levels. There was a correlation between breast milk carbamazepine levels and infant serum levels. There was no significant correlation between maternal and infant serum levels. In only 7% of the cases, the milk carbamazepine levels were in the reported therapeutic range, and 65% of the infants had carbamazepine levels that were below the therapeutic range (Kocirova et al. 2021). Both AAN and AAP support breastfeeding if the mother is taking carbamazepine (Harden et al. 2009; Sachs and Drugs 2013).

11.4.4 Oxcarbazepine

Oxcarbazepine, a congener of carbamazepine, has been used for the treatment of BD. There is a lack of data on the use of oxcarbazepine during breastfeeding. A case report suggests a low milk plasma ratio (0.5) and a low concentration in human milk (<11 μg/mL) with a low relative infant dose (1.5–1.7%) (Lutz et al. 2007). A case report documented normal development in the infant exposed to oxcarbazepine through breast milk during the first month of life (Gentile 2003).

11.4.5 Lamotrigine

Available data in the form of case reports and case series suggests mean milk/plasma ratios for lamotrigine to range from 0.40 to 0.61 (Liporace et al. 2004; Ohman et al. 2000; Page-Sharp et al. 2006; Rambeck et al. 1997). A study that involved 30 breastfeeding mothers receiving lamotrigine (50–800 mg/d; mean = 386.5) and their infants reported a mean milk/plasma ratio of 41.3% with a range of 5.7 to 147%. Lamotrigine concentrations were higher in the breast milk 4 hours after the intake of the drug by the nursing mother, although the finding was not statistically significant. Infant plasma concentrations were 18.3% of that reported for nursing mothers. However, except for mild thrombocytosis in 7 out of 8 infants, no other adverse events were observed (Newport et al. 2008). A case report documented multiple episodes of apnea in the newborn while the mother was receiving lamotrigine, which improved completely when breastfeeding was terminated (Nordmo et al. 2009). A recent relatively large sample size study, which included data from 158 women and 143 breastfed newborns collected between the second and fifth postnatal days, showed that the median lamotrigine concentrations in mg/L were 2.7, 1.4, and 1.7 in maternal serum, milk, and newborn serum, respectively. The median milk/maternal serum concentration ratio and newborn/maternal serum concentration ratio were 0.6, and the median newborn serum/milk concentration ratio was 1.00. A significant correlation was observed between milk and maternal serum concentrations and between newborn serum and milk concentrations, maternal serum concentrations, maternal daily dose, and dose-related to maternal body weight. Based on these findings, the authors concluded that exposure to lamotrigine among breastfed newborns was lower than that exposure during pregnancy (Kocirova et al. 2022). LactMed considers the use of lamotrigine during breastfeeding to be relatively safe and recommends evaluating the plasma levels and monitoring the platelet count of infants.

11.4.6 Topiramate

A small sample study involving 5 mother-infant pairs reported very low topiramate concentrations in the infants, with no adverse effects seen among the infants (Ohman et al. 2002). The mean milk/maternal plasma concentration ratio was 0.86 (range,

0.67–1.1) at 2–3 weeks and 1 month and 0.69 at 3 months after delivery. Two out of the 3 infants who were breastfed had detectable topiramate levels, i.e., >0.9 microM concentrations, however, this was lower than the limit of quantification (2.8 microM), and one infant had an undetectable concentration (Ohman et al. 2002). There are other case reports of safe use of topiramate during lactation (Gentile 2009). However, a case report documented the association of diarrhea with topiramate, while breastfed by a mother who was receiving topiramate (Westergren et al. 2014).

11.4.7 Gabapentin

The mean milk/maternal plasma concentration ratio of gabapentin in milk has been estimated to be 1 (range, 0.7–1.3) from 2 weeks to 3 months. Accordingly, the mean infant dose is reported to be 0.2–1.3 mg/kg/day, which is much lower (1.3–3.8%) than the maternal dose. In terms of plasma concentrations, plasma concentration in breast-fed infants has been estimated to be 12% of the mother's plasma levels. No adverse effects were observed with low plasma concentration in the breastfed infants (Ohman et al. 2005). In a case report, the relative infant dose was estimated to be 2.34%, with the absolute infant dose being approximately 3% of the recommended children's dose for gabapentin, and the infant plasma level was 0.4 mg/L, which was about 6% of the maternal plasma drug concentration. No adverse events were reported in the infant (Kristensen et al. 2006).

11.5 Recommendations for Use of MS During Puerperium and Lactation

Table 11.1 summarizes expert recommendations on the use of MS during the lactation period. There is a high risk of relapse among patients with BD during the puerperium. Hence, reinitiating the MS in the immediate post-partum period is

Table 11.1 Expert recommendations based on scientific evidence and clinical experience

High risk of relapse in the post-partum period
Initiation and continuation of MS must be considered
The decision to breastfeed the newborn must consider the risks & benefits
Baseline and regular evaluation of the newborn by a pediatrician is a must, with close monitoring for side effects
The lowest effective dose of MS should be used
Medications must be timed according to the neonates' feeding pattern
Valproate is considered safe; monitoring of infant liver function test is recommended
Breastfeeding should be done with caution in mothers receiving lithium; regular monitoring of electrocardiogram, lithium levels, and blood counts to be done; information to be given to parents regarding warning signs in the newborn
Lamotrigine is considered safe, however, data is sparse
Carbamazepine may be used with caution and monitoring

recommended for patients at high risk of relapse. Available data suggests that the use of lithium as a prophylactic agent in the post-partum period brings down the relapse rate from nearly 50% to less than 10% (Cohen et al. 1995).

Starting an MS during the post-partum period for the first episode of hypomania/mania/mixed episode is a tricky one, and this must be based on the consideration of the severity of symptoms and risk of continuation of symptoms to the mother and the fetus, including mother-child bonding. If the symptoms are severe enough, the use of MS needs to be considered.

If the MS is started, then whether to allow breastfeeding or not should take the risk and benefits into account. The risk-benefit analysis should take into consideration the benefits of breastfeeding (both physiological and psychological), the desires of the mother, the risk of infant exposure to the medication, and the possibility of refusal to treatment by a severely ill mother in favor of giving up breastfeeding (Gartner et al. 2005).

If the decision is made to continue breastfeeding while using MS, the newborn should be evaluated at the baseline and also must be monitored closely to minimize the risk. The newborn should be examined by a pediatrician for baseline behavior and other parameters like sleep, feeding, and alertness. The newborn should be evaluated from time to time by the pediatrician to ensure normal development. The parents need to be informed about the possible side effects of the medication being used.

Certain physiological changes that occur during infancy must be remembered, which can help minimize the negative effects of MS on the infant, who is continuing breastfeeding. Older infants metabolize and eliminate various drugs more efficiently than younger infants, and they generally sleep for longer durations. The long duration of sleep can help in planning the dosing of the mother. It is generally recommended to administer the dose to the mother immediately after breastfeeding and just prior to the baby's longest sleep interval (Grover and Avasthi 2015). While allowing breastfeeding, a close liaison needs to be maintained with the pediatrician and the discussions need to include sharing information about potential side effects of medication exposure to the newborn and possible drug interactions with other commonly prescribed medications to infants (e.g., antibiotics, nonsteroidal anti-inflammatory agents, acetaminophen).

If the MS is used during breastfeeding, the dose must be kept at the lowest effective dose. However, such an attempt must not lead to ineffective dosing, poor symptom control, and resultantly unnecessary exposure to the neonate.

In terms of selection of the MS, valproate is considered to be safer than lithium. AAN and AAP support breastfeeding if the mother is taking valproate (Harden et al. 2009; Sachs and Drugs 2013). However, monitoring of liver function tests and blood counts for the newborn is recommended. Accordingly, if a clinician needs to start MS for the first time during the post-partum period and parents/mothers wish to continue breastfeeding, valproate needs to be considered as the preferred agent.

The American College of Obstetricians and Gynecologists (ACOG) categorizes the risk of continuing psychotropic medications during lactation into five categories (L1 = Safest; L2 = Safer; L3 = Moderately safe; L4 = Possibly hazardous;

L5 = Contraindicated). Among the currently available MS divalproex (L2), and carbamazepine (L2) are considered to be safer than other options. Lithium is placed in the L4 category and lamotrigine is placed in the L3 category. Among the antipsychotics olanzapine is placed in the L2 category; risperidone, aripiprazole, and clozapine are placed in the L3 category, and quetiapine and ziprasidone are placed in the L4 category (ACOG Clinical Practice Guideline 2007).

Another categorization of medications according to the lactation risk includes the Hales categorization. According to this categorization, the available medications are divided into five categories, i.e., L1- Safest; L2- Safer; L3-Moderately Safe; L4-Possibly Hazardous; and L5- Contraindicated. This categorization is updated every 2 years. According to this, carbamazepine and valproate are placed in the L2 category. Lithium is placed in the L4 category and lamotrigine is placed in the L3 category. Among the antipsychotics, olanzapine and quetiapine are placed in the L2 category; risperidone and clozapine are placed in the L3 category, and quetiapine and ziprasidone are placed in the L4 category.

Accordingly, if someone has to start a MS for the first time during the post-partum period, valproate and carbamazepine are considered to be most compatible with breastfeeding. However, it is important to note that it is recommended to monitor the liver function tests of newborn while using valproate. Among the antipsychotics, olanzapine and quetiapine are considered to be most compatible with breastfeeding. In recent times data has also emerged on the safety of lurasidone during lactation. However, this is only in the form of case reports and not sufficient to make any specific recommendations.

According to the recommendations of AAP, breastfeeding should be done with caution while using lithium in mothers, and if this is permitted then the breastfed infant needs to be monitored for serum lithium levels, ECG, and complete blood counts from time to time (Sachs and Drugs 2013). Accordingly, lithium needs to be used when this has been used during pregnancy or the patient has a past history of response to lithium. If there are no contraindications, the mother may be given an option to switch to valproate. It is important to remember that mothers may require lower doses of lithium during the post-partum period when compared to those required during pregnancy. Hence, the maternal lithium dose needs to be reduced to the pre-pregnancy level, immediately after delivery, and serum lithium levels must be monitored. Further, the mother must be informed to monitor the newborn for signs of dehydration, lethargy, and feeding problems. The newborn must be screened for thyroid and renal functions, and maternal and infant serum lithium levels must be done if clinically indicated. The renal functions of the newborn must be monitored closely, especially during the first 6 weeks of life. The newborn must also be monitored for subtle neurological signs and needs to be referred for early intervention when indicated (Viguera et al. 2007b; Ugaz and Sharma 2016).

Lamotrigine is also considered safe during breastfeeding. However, it should be used during lactation when other safer options are not available. If carbamazepine is used, then the infant should be monitored closely for jaundice, drowsiness, adequate weight gain, and developmental milestones (Davanzo et al. 2013). LactMed database also recommends similar monitoring of breastfeeding infants, whose mothers are receiving carbamazepine. Data for other anticonvulsants is cursory.

11.6 Conclusion

The issue of the safety of the use of MS during lactation is far from being resolved. Accordingly, the decision to prescribe while continuing breastfeeding should be taken in the light of the severity of mental disease, and MS should be considered only when the potential risk to the fetus from exposure to medication outweighs the risk of untreated maternal mental disorder. The selection of the medication depends on the balance between safety and efficacy profile. Whenever MS is started during lactation, the newborn must be monitored closely.

References

American College of Obstetricians and Gynecologists. ACOG practice bulletin no. 87 November 2007: use of psychiatric medications during pregnancy and lactation. Obstet Gynecol. 2007;110(5):1179–98.

Beath SV. Hepatic function and physiology in the newborn. Semin Neonatol. 2003;8:337–46.

Bogen DL, Sit D, Genovese A, Wisner KL. Three cases of lithium exposure and exclusive breastfeeding. Arch Womens Ment Health. 2012;15:69–72.

Britton JR, Britton HL, Gronwaldt V. Breastfeeding, sensitivity, and attachment. Pediatrics. 2006;118:1436–43.

Burt VK, Suri R, Altshuler L, Stowe Z, Hendrick VC, Muntean E. The use of psychotropic medications during breast-feeding. Am J Psychiatry. 2001;158:1001–9.

Chaudron LH, Jefferson JW. Mood stabilizers during breastfeeding: a review. J Clin Psychiatry. 2000;61:79–90.

Cohen LS, Sichel DA, Robertson LM, Heckscher E, Rosenbaum JF. Postpartum prophylaxis for women with bipolar disorder. Am J Psychiatry. 1995;152:1641–5.

Conejo-Galindo J, Sanz-Giancola A, Alvarez-Mon MA, Ortega MA, Gutierrez-Rojas L, Lahera G. Postpartum relapse in patients with bipolar disorder. J Clin Med. 2022;11:3979.

Davanzo R, Dal Bo S, Bua J, Copertino M, Zanelli E, Matarazzo L. Antiepileptic drugs and breastfeeding. Ital J Pediatr. 2013;39:50–4.

Department of Health and Human Service Office on Women's Health. Benefits of breastfeeding. Nutr Clin Care. 2003;6:125–31.

Freeman MP, Smith KW, Freeman SA, McElroy SL, Kmetz GE, Wright R, Keck PE Jr. The impact of reproductive events on the course of bipolar disorder in women. J Clin Psychiatry. 2002;63:284–7.

Frew JR. Psychopharmacology of bipolar I disorder during lactation: a case report of the use of lithium and aripiprazole in a nursing mother. Arch Womens Ment Health. 2015;18:135–6.

Frey B, Schubiger G, Musy JP. Transient cholestatic hepatitis in a neonate associated with carbamazepine exposure during pregnancy and breast-feeding. Eur J Pediatr. 1990;150:136–8.

Gartner LM, Morton J, Lawrence RA, Naylor AJ, O'Hare D, Schanler RJ. Breastfeeding and the use of human milk. Pediatrics. 2005;115:496–506.

Gentile S. Oxcarbazepine in pregnancy and lactation. Clin Drug Investig. 2003;23:687.

Gentile S. Topiramate in pregnancy and breastfeeding. Clin Drug Investig. 2009;29:139–41.

Grover S, Avasthi A. Mood stabilizers in pregnancy and lactation. Indian J Psychiatry. 2015;57(Suppl 2):S308–23.

Harden CL, Hopp J, Ting TY, Pennell PB, French JA, Allen Hauser W, et al. Management issues for women with epilepsy-focus on pregnancy (an evidence-based review): I. Obstetrical complications and change in seizure frequency: report of the quality standards subcommittee and therapeutics and technology assessment Subcommittee of the American Academy of neurology and the American Epilepsy Society. Epilepsia. 2009;50:1229–36.

Heinonen E, Tötterman K, Bäck K, Sarman I, Svedenkrans J, Forsberg L. Lithium use during breastfeeding was safe in healthy full-term infants under strict monitoring. Acta Paediatr. 2022;111(10):1891–8.

Horta BL, de Sousa BA, de Mola CL. Breastfeeding and neurodevelopmental outcomes. Curr Opin Clin Nutr Metab Care. 2018:112–5.

Imaz ML, Torra M, Soy D, García-Esteve L, Martin-Santos R. Clinical lactation studies of lithium: a systematic review. Front Pharmacol. 2019;10:1005.

Imaz ML, Langohr K, Torra M, Soy D, García-Esteve L, Martin-Santos R. Neonatal feeding trajectories in mothers with bipolar disorder taking lithium: pharmacokinetic data. Front Pharmacol. 2021a;12:752022.

Imaz ML, Soy D, Torra M, García-Esteve L, Soler C, Martin-Santos R. Case report: clinical and pharmacokinetic profile of lithium monotherapy in exclusive breastfeeding. A follow-up case series. Front Pharmacol. 2021b;12:647414.

Ito S, Lee A. Drug excretion into breast milk – overview. Adv Drug Deliv Rev. 2003;55:617–27.

Jefferson JW, Greist J, Ackermann D. Lithium encyclopaedia for clinical practice. 2nd ed. Washington: American Psychiatric Press; 1987. p. 504–25.

Jones I, Craddock N. Bipolar disorder and childbirth: the importance of recognising risk. Br J Psychiatry. 2005;186:453–4.

Kacirova I, Grundmann M, Brozmanova H. Valproic acid concentrations in nursing mothers, mature milk, and breastfed infants in monotherapy and combination therapy. Epilepsy Behav. 2019;95:112–6.

Kacirova I, Grundmann M, Brozmanova H. Therapeutic monitoring of carbamazepine and its active metabolite during the 1st postnatal month: influence of drug interactions. Biomed Pharmacother. 2021;137:111412.

Kacirova I, Grundmann M, Brozmanova H. Monitoring of lamotrigine concentrations in mothers, colostrum, and breastfed newborns during the early postpartum period. Biomed Pharmacother. 2022;151:113167.

Kendell RE, Chalmers JC, Platz C. Epidemiology of puerperal psychoses. Br J Psychiatry. 1987;150:662–73.

Kristensen JH, Ilett KF, Hackett LP, Kohan R. Gabapentin and breastfeeding: a case report. J Hum Lact. 2006;22:426–8.

Lawrence RM. Circumstances when breastfeeding is contraindicated. Pediatr Clin N Am. 2013;60:295–318.

Liporace J, Kao A, D'Abreu A. Concerns regarding lamotrigine and breast-feeding. Epilepsy Behav. 2004;5:102–5.

Lutz UC, Wiatr G, Gaertner H-J, Bartels M. Oxcarbazepine treatment during breast-feeding: a case report. J Clin Psychopharmacol. 2007;27:730–2.

McAllister-Williams RH, Baldwin DS, Cantwell R, Easter A, Gilvarry E, Glover V, Green L, Gregoire A, Howard LM, Jones I, Khalifeh H. British Association for Psychopharmacology consensus guidance on the use of psychotropic medication preconception, in pregnancy and postpartum 2017. J Psychopharmacol. 2017;31(5):519–52.

Merlob P, Mor N, Litwin A. Transient hepatic dysfunction in an infant of an epileptic mother treated with carbamazepine during pregnancy and breastfeeding. Ann Pharmacother. 1992;26:1563–5.

Moretti ME, Koren G, Verjee Z, Ito S. Monitoring lithium in breast milk: an individualized approach for breast-feeding mothers. Ther Drug Monit. 2003;25:364–6.

Munk-Olsen T, Laursen TM, Meltzer-Brody S, Mortensen PB, Jones I. Psychiatric disorders with postpartum onset: possible early manifestations of bipolar affective disorders. Arch Gen Psychiatry. 2012;69:428–34.

Newport DJ, Pennell PB, Calamaras MR, Ritchie JC, Newman M, Knight B, Viguera AC, Liporace J, Stowe ZN. Lamotrigine in breast milk and nursing infants: determination of exposure. Pediatrics. 2008;122:e223–31.

Nordmo E, Aronsen L, Wasland K, Småbrekke L, Vorren S. Severe apnea in an infant exposed to lamotrigine in breast milk. Ann Pharmacother. 2009;43:1893–7.

Ohman I, Vitols S, Tomson T. Lamotrigine in pregnancy: pharmacokinetics during delivery, in the neonate, and during lactation. Epilepsia. 2000;41:709–13.

Ohman I, Vitols S, Luef G, Söderfeldt B, Tomson T. Topiramate kinetics during delivery, lactation, and in the neonate: preliminary observations. Epilepsia. 2002;43:1157–60.

Ohman I, Vitols S, Tomson T. Pharmacokinetics of gabapentin during delivery, in the neonatal period, and lactation: does a fetal accumulation occur during pregnancy? Epilepsia. 2005;46:1621–4.

Page-Sharp M, Kristensen JH, Hackett LP, Beran RG, Rampono J, Hale TW, Kohan R, Ilett KF. Transfer of lamotrigine into breast milk. Ann Pharmacother. 2006;40:1470–1.

Piontek CM, Baab S, Peindl KS, Wisner KL. Serum valproate levels in 6 breastfeeding mother-infant pairs. J Clin Psychiatry. 2000;61:170–2.

Rambeck B, Kurlemann G, Stodieck SR, May TW, Jürgens U. Concentrations of lamotrigine in a mother on lamotrigine treatment and her newborn child. Eur J Clin Pharmacol. 1997;51:481–4.

Sachs HC, Drugs CO. The transfer of drugs and therapeutics into human breast milk: an update on selected topics. Pediatrics. 2013;132:e796–809.

Smith B, Dubovsky SL. Pharmacotherapy of mood disorders and psychosis in pre- and post-natal women. Expert Opin Pharmacother. 2017;18:1703–19.

Stahl MM, Neiderud J, Vinge E. Thrombocytopenic purpura and anemia in a breast-fed infant whose mother was treated with valproic acid. J Pediatr. 1997;130:1001–3.

Terp IM, Mortensen PB. Post-partum psychoses. Clinical diagnoses and relative risk of admission after parturition. Br J Psychiatry. 1998;172:521–6.

Uguz F, Sharma V. Mood stabilizers during breastfeeding: a systematic review of the recent literature. Bipolar Disord. 2016 Jun;18(4):325–33.

Viguera AC, Nonacs R, Cohen LS, Tondo L, Murray A, Baldessarini RJ. Risk of recurrence of bipolar disorder in pregnant and nonpregnant women after discontinuing lithium maintenance. Am J Psychiatry. 2000;157:179–84.

Viguera AC, Newport DJ, Ritchie J, Stowe Z, Whitfield T, Mogielnicki J, Baldessarini RJ, Zurick A, Cohen LS. Lithium in breast milk and nursing infants: clinical implications. Am J Psychiatry. 2007a;164:342–5.

Viguera AC, Whitfield T, Baldessarini RJ, Newport DJ, Stowe Z, Reminick A, et al. Risk of recurrence in women with bipolar disorder during pregnancy: prospective study of mood stabilizer discontinuation. Am J Psychiatry. 2007b;164:1817–24.

Wesseloo R, Kamperman AM, Munk-Olsen T, Pop VJ, Kushner SA, Bergink V. Risk of postpartum relapse in bipolar disorder and postpartum psychosis: a systematic review and meta-analysis. Am J Psychiatry. 2016;173:117–27.

Westergren T, Hjelmeland K, Kristoffersen B, Johannessen SI, Kalikstad B. Probable topiramate-induced diarrhea in a 2-month-old breast-fed child –a case report. Epilepsy Behav Case Rep. 2014;2:22–3.

Whaites Heinonen E, Tötterman K, Bäck K, Sarman I, Forsberg L, Svedenkrans J. High lithium concentration at delivery is a potential risk factor for adverse outcomes in breastfed infants: a retrospective cohort study. Int J Bipolar Disord. 2023;11(1):36.

Wisner KL, Perel JM. Serum levels of valproate and carbamazepine in breastfeeding mother-infant pairs. J Clin Psychopharmacol. 1998;18:167–9.

Yonkers KA, Wisner KL, Stowe Z, Leibenluft E, Cohen L, Miller L, Manber R, Viguera A, Suppes T, Altshuler L. Management of bipolar disorder during pregnancy and the postpartum period. Focus. 2005;3:266–79.

Benzodiazepines and Z-Drugs in Pregnancy

12

Cesario Bellantuono

12.1 Introduction

Psychiatric disorders during pregnancy and postpartum are common and often need to be treated with psychotropic drug treatment. Benzodiazepines (BDZs), together with the so-called hypnotic Z-drugs, are one of the most widely prescribed psychotropic treatments, not only in psychiatric practice but also in several medical fields, for the treatment of several psychopathological conditions, particularly concerning acute anxiety and relevant sleep disorders. It has been estimated that from 5% to 15% of the adult general population have received a prescription of BDZs and Z-drugs, in many cases even for a long period of time (Galbally et al. 2014). It was documented that approximately 50% of adults report a difficulty in initiating or maintaining sleep or having unrefreshing sleep, whereas upwards of 20% of adults meet strict diagnostic criteria for a diagnosis of clinically relevant insomnia. Insomnia is also the most prevalent sleep disorder experienced in women during pregnancy, affecting a significant number of pregnant women. The prevalence of insomnia during pregnancy is usually high from the start, and two-thirds of pregnant women suffer from insomnia in the later months of their pregnancy. Results emerging from a recent meta-analysis confirm that the prevalence of insomnia is higher during pregnancy, particularly in the third trimester; the overall prevalence during the antenatal period was estimated to be 38% (Sedov et al. 2021). It is well established that insomnia is related to several potential maternal and infant health risks, such as adverse pregnancy outcomes (e.g., hypertension, gestational diabetes mellitus). Disturbed sleep in early and late pregnancy may also increase the risk of cardio-metabolic disorders, which are associated with maternal and infant morbidity.

C. Bellantuono (✉)
DeGra Clinic for Perinatal Mental Disorders, Verona, Italy;
http://www.depressionegravidanza.it

F. Uguz, L. Orsolini (eds.), *Perinatal Psychopharmacology*,
https://doi.org/10.1007/978-3-031-99720-4_12

Insomnia is also frequently related during pregnancy and postpartum to several psychiatric disorders, such as major depression, general anxiety, and post-traumatic stress disorders. In addition, sleep loss during pregnancy has been associated to fetal intrauterine growth retardation and longer duration of delivery (Wang et al. 2020). During the last two decades, with a parallel increased focus in the clinical research and development of newer antidepressants and antipsychotics, we assisted to a reduced interest in BDZs, generating therefore the false impression that these drugs represent an outdated issue in the field of clinical psychopharmacology, despite their current widespread utilization in general population. On the other hand, the prescription of anxiolytic and sleep-promoting drugs may be responsible for their uncontrolled, long-term use, with a higher potential for abuse, misuse, and dependence, particularly among polysubstance users (Walton et al. 2016). However, it should also be said that the above-mentioned risks need to be always carefully balanced with the clinical benefits that many patients may experience with a short or intermittent use of these drugs taken at therapeutic dosages.

Many expert opinions support the use of BDZs and Z-drugs as treatments of choice for acute situational anxiety, anxiety disorders associated with depressive episode, insomnia, and alcohol withdrawal syndromes. Tolerance can develop to sedation and possibly to psychomotor impairment, but not to the anxiolytic effect. Moreover, in contrast to commonly held opinion, BDZs are not frequently misused or at risk of misuse of other substances in patients without substance use disorders who are prescribed these drugs for appropriate indications and at lowest effective therapeutic doses with regular clinical monitoring by the attending physician (Dubovsky and Marshall 2022). It is also well known that BDZs and Z-drugs are usually not lethal in overdose, except when ingested with other substances, such as alcohol, opioids, and CNS depressant drugs. The mechanism of action of BDZ at CNS level is clearly delineated as well as their pharmacokinetic properties, metabolic pathways, and risk of drug interaction, allowing for greater precision in their routine clinical use. Moreover, the continued widespread use of antianxiety and hypnotic medication for several clinical conditions testifies their usefulness for many patients, but at same time strongly recommend that these drugs must be prescribed and used in agreement with the rules of good clinical practice.

The common assertion that the prescription of these drugs leads by default to the abuse of other substances or misuse seems therefore not supported by clinical experience and observational studies. In any case, considering the current widespread prescriptions of BDZs and Z-drugs both in general practice and in specialist psychiatric and non-psychiatric setting, it is advisable for an appropriate use to encourage the implementation of specific training interventions concerning their prescriptions in clinical setting; this strategy is considered a useful tool to minimize the risk of abuse and/or misuse by some patients as well as the risk of malpractice by physicians' prescribers. Finally, it is worthwhile to remember that since 2–3% of pregnant women take a BDZ and/or a Z-drug, the issue concerning their prescription in the perinatal period is not trivial, still remaining a topic for future clinical and epidemiological studies (Bellantuono et al. 2014; Bais et al. 2020).

12.2 Pharmacological Profile of Benzodiazepines and Z-Drugs

Benzodiazepines (BDZs) are a pharmacological class of drugs including agents that work on the CNS, by selectively acting on gamma-aminobutyric acid alfa-receptors (GABA-$_A$). GABA is a neurotransmitter that inhibits or reduces the activity of neurons within the brain, particularly in the amygdala and prefrontal cortex. BDZs open GABA-activated chloride channels and allow chloride ions to enter the neurons. This makes the neuron negatively charged and resistant to excitation. Even though all BDZs work in a similar way at CNS level, there are relevant differences in the way in which a specific BDZ acts on different GABA-$_A$ receptor subtypes. In addition, some BDZs are more "potent" than others and are eliminated from the plasma more slowly than others; some BDZs can also generate active metabolites, as in the case of diazepam, which generates the desmethyl-diazepam, also called "nordiazepam". Since the introduction of the first BDZ, the *chlordiazepoxide* in 1962, many other compounds were introduced into the pharmaceutical market. These drugs have been usually classified according to their length of elimination plasma half-life ($t_{½}$), hepatic metabolic pathways, the formation of active metabolites, and the interactions with other drugs. All BDZs are commonly considered very safe drugs, as no fatalities have been associated in patients taking these drugs in overdoses; symptoms observed after overdose of BDZs alone include usually deep drowsiness, sedation, and muscle relaxation. Moreover, BDZs do not cause in huge overdosages severe respiratory, cardiovascular, and CNS depression. Their side effects profile is well known (e.g., mild worsening of psychomotor performance and sleepiness), and it is dose-dependent, therefore these drugs must be prescribed in each patient using the lowest effective dosage for the treatment of anxiety conditions as well as sleep problems (Bellantuono et al. 1980). This is particularly relevant to avoid or minimize a withdrawal reaction in newborns exposed to such medication during pregnancy. Table 12.1 summarizes the most relevant pharmacological characteristics of BDZs.

Z-Drugs are a non-benzodiazepine class of drugs commonly prescribed in clinical practice for the short-term treatment of insomnia. Z-drugs, also defined as "*hypnotic benzodiazepine receptor agonists*" (HBRA), include the following agents: *zolpidem, zopiclone,* and *zaleplon*. HBRA binds to the BDZ receptor subunit of the GABA-$_A$ receptor. The peak plasma concentration is attained 1–2 h after intake. These agents are metabolized by the liver, have a short elimination half-life ranging from 2 to 6 h, are generally well tolerated by the patients, and are usually considered to be less addictive and/or habit-forming than BDZs. However, a number of cases of dependence, abuse, and misuse have also been reported in many patients treated with these drugs for a long time.

Overall, it is worthwhile to remember that each BDZ can act at different dosages as an anxiolytic (low dose) or hypnotic (high dose). Therefore, in routine clinical practice, the dosage must always be "individualized" in each patient to find the lowest

Table 12.1 Pharmacokinetic, metabolic pathways, interactions of BDZs

A. BDZs with medium-long plasma half-life
Drug name *Pro-nordiazepam-like BDZs*: Prazepam, clobazam, desmetil-diazepam, flurazepam, chlordiazepoxide, diazepam, ketazolam, medazepam, pinazepam, quazepam *Nitro-BZDs*: Nitrazepam, flunitrazepam
Pharmacokinetic features *Plasma half-life*: More than 24 (24–100 hours) including active metabolites with long half-life *Metabolism*: Demethylation to nordiazepam, hydroxylation, and conjugation by glucuronic acid
Interactions: SSRIs, oral contraceptives, can decrease hepatic hydroxylation and increase plasma levels of these BZDs. Sedative effect hypotension when combined with alcohol or CNS depressant drugs.
B. BZDs with short/ultra-short plasma half-life
Drug name: Alprazolam, bromazepam, brotizolam, estazolam, triazolam
Pharmacokinetic features (a) *Plasma half-life*: 2–6 h for triazolam, brotizolam, lormetazepam; 12–24 h for other BZDs (b) *Metabolism*: Hydroxylation and conjugation with glucuronic acid; no production of active metabolites
Interactions: SSRIs and oral contraceptives can inhibit hepatic hydroxylation and can increase Plasma levels of these BDZs Sedative effects and hypotension when combined with alcohol or CNS depressant drugs
C. BZDs with short/ultrashort plasma half-life
Drug name: *Oxazepam-like BZDs:* Camazepam, lorazepam, lormetazepam, oxazepam, temazepam)
Pharmacokinetic features (a) *Plasma half-life*: 12–24 h (b) *Metabolism*: Conjugation with glucuronic acid; no production of active metabolites
Interactions: No relevant pharmacokinetic drug interactions. Sedative effect and hypotension when combined with alcohol or CNS depressant drugs

effective anxiolytic and/or hypnotic dose. This is particularly important during the gestational period to avoid/minimize a neonatal withdrawal reaction after delivery.

12.3 Use of BDZs and Z-Drugs in Pregnancy

Pregnancy is a period of physical and psychological changes, to the extent that some women have difficulties in handling their mixed feelings of happiness and fear or concern for their future life. Epidemiological studies have documented that most psychopathological conditions may arise or worsen during the gestational period, which may require timely drug treatment and/or psychotherapy and social support. Consequently, it is important not to underestimate the occurrence of prodromal symptoms like tension, sadness, emotional distress, irritability, and sleep difficulties affecting a pregnant woman, as these symptoms could represent predictive *warning signs* of a psychiatric disorder.

Anxiety disorders and insomnia are frequently reported during pregnancy, with prevalence rates which varies widely according to different epidemiological studies. These psychopathological conditions can be moderate but persistent and, in many pregnant women, can lead to relevant levels of distress and impairment of their quality of life. It is well known that both severe anxiety disorders and persistent insomnia can occur in comorbidity with major depressive disorders or other psychopathological conditions (Goodman et al. 2014; Okun et al. 2015).

Psychiatric disorders during pregnancy and postpartum are common, and about 15% of women experience peripartum depressive disorders frequently associated with severe anxiety and sleep difficulties. Drug utilization studies are needed to better understand not only the rate and trend of anxiolytic and hypnotic drug prescriptions during pregnancy and post-partum but also their pattern of use, i.e., dosage, length of treatment, drugs used in association, and the diagnostic indication that made the prescription necessary.

Recently, a meta-analysis of 32 studies coming from 28 country and including more than 7 million of pregnancies confirmed that BDZ and Z-drugs use before, during, and after pregnancy is prevalent. The worldwide prevalence of prescriptions of these drugs during pregnancy was 1.9%; the highest prevalence rate was found in the third trimester (3.1%); lorazepam was the most frequently prescribed drug among BDZs.

Given the substantial proportion of newborns exposed in utero to BDZ and Z-drugs, future research should continue to study their safety profile during the perinatal period. Moreover, it would be desirable that the prescription of such medications should always be shared with the patient and her partner in order to explain the potential risk of an untreated psychopathological condition as well as the risks and benefits of the drug treatment (Betcher and Wisner 2020).

12.4 Risk of Congenital Major Malformations

12.4.1 Benzodiazepines

The fetal safety of BDZs during pregnancy was investigated since the first publications which date back more than 20 years ago. In a meta-analysis, including 3 cohort and 6 case-control studies, BDZs as a class were considered at risk of major congenital malformations, particularly concerning some birth defects such as cleft lip and/or cleft palate (oral cleft) (Dolovich et al. 1998). As well, even an overview including studies published from 1966 to 2000 confirmed such teratogenic risk for the BDZs advising against its use in early pregnancy (Iqbal et al. 2002). A meta-analysis of 9 cohort studies, with over 1 million of analysed pregnancies, including about 4500 newborns exposed in utero, reported some years later different results documenting that BDZs do not carry any risk of increase of major malformations in women exposed in the first trimester of pregnancy (Enato et al. 2011). Recent investigations, systematic reviews, and metanalytic studies indicate that the prescription of BZDs in the first trimester of pregnancy should not be considered contraindicated anymore, even though in clinical practice their utilization always needs a careful risk/benefit assessment and regular clinical monitoring of the patient undergoing treatment.

A large cohort study conducted in the UK on about 2000 pregnant women exposed to BDZs in the first trimester reported reassuring results about their risk of teratogenicity. Overall, the prevalence of malformations was 2.7% in 1159 children of mothers prescribed diazepam, 2.9% in 379 children with temazepam, 2.5% in 406 children with zopiclone, and 2.7% in 19,193 children whose mothers had diagnosed depression and/or anxiety but were not exposed to BDZs. When compared with 2.7% in 351,785 children with no diagnosed depression/anxiety nor medication use, the adjusted odds ratios were 1.02 (99% CI. 0.63–1.64) for diazepam, 1.07 (CI, 0.49–2.37) for temazepam, 0.96 (CI, 0.42–2.20) for zopiclone and 1.27 (CI, 0.43–3.75) for other anxiolytic/hypnotic drugs and 1.01 (CI, 0.90–1.14) for unmedicated depression/anxiety. These findings clearly confirm that the risks of system-specific birth defects were generally similar in children exposed and not exposed to anxiolytic and hypnotic drugs considered in the study, The authors' conclusions were that no evidence of increased risk of malformations, associated with antenatal drug exposure to diazepam, temazepam, zopiclone and other anxiolytic/hypnotic drugs, were found in their study. These data strongly support that the exposure to BDZs and Z-drugs during early pregnancy may be considered safe as far as the risk of major malformations is concerned (Ban et al. 2014).

A meta-analysis of 8 cohort studies evaluated the risk of major malformations in neonates of 5195 exposed women to BDZs vs more than 2 million unexposed women. BDZs were not associated with a statistically significant risk of malformations in 8 studies or cardiac malformations in 4 studies. However, it was found a statistically significant relative risk of malformations only when BDZs were associated with an antidepressant drug (Grigoriadis et al. 2019).

These results, however, have been questioned from a methodological point of view in a recent paper by Andrade, whose conclusions suggest that "*gestational exposure to BDZs is a marker of risk for major and cardiac malformations and importantly, that first trimester exposure to BDZs may not be associated with much increase in risk, if at all*" (Andrade 2019a). More recently in a nationwide cohort study of approximately 3 million pregnancies conducted in South Korea, first-trimester BDZ use was associated with a modest increase in risk of malformations, particularly concerning heart defects. The risk of primary outcomes increased with a higher mean daily dose of BDZs (more than 2.5 mg/day of lorazepam-equivalent dose), suggesting a dose–response relationship. Although the risks were similar between short- and long-acting BDZs, a small but statistically significant increase in relative risk (RR, 1.08 to 2.43) was found with some specific agents including midazolam, diazepam, flunitrazepam, and chlordiazepoxide (Noh et al. 2022). Although the relative risk found in this study was small, the potential low risks should be always evaluated against the efficacy of BDZs in many patients and above all, that BDZs must be prescribed in each patient using the "lowest effective dosage", particularly in early pregnancy as, according to such study, the risk might be dose-dependent.

It should be noted, however, that so far this is the only study in which a dose-dependent risk of malformation in newborns exposed to BDZs in pregnancy has been found. It is reasonable to conclude from most of data published and according to most the best original studies, overviews and recent guidelines, that fetal exposure of BDZs and

Z-drugs during first trimester of pregnancy, at therapeutic dosages, should be considered safe, at least in terms of risk of major congenital birth defects (McAllister-Williams et al. 2017; Bellantuono et al. 2013). Recently, a large population-based cohort study conducted in Taiwan using data from a national database has not confirmed the risk of malformations associated with BDZ and antidepressant drugs exposure in early pregnancy (Chuang et al. 2024). This study included 2.634,021 singleton pregnancies, and 8599 patients (0.3%) were concomitant users of antidepressants and BDZs during the first trimester. The results did not identify an increased relative risk for overall malformations, heart defects, or any of the other organ-specific birth defects, except for digestive system malformations. In terms of absolute risk (AR), the rate of overall malformations was 3.81 per 100 pregnancies with exposure, as compared with an AR of 2.87 per 100 pregnancies without drug exposure. The lack of an increased risk for overall malformations associated with concomitant use of antidepressants and BDZs was also supported by the analyses controlling for confounding by indication and sibling-matched comparisons.

12.4.2 Z-Drugs

The information on the fetal and neonatal safety of the Z-drugs has been so far quite scarce. Only for zolpidem there are few studies focusing on its use in early pregnancy. A first prospective study carried out on 45 pregnant women who used zolpidem in comparison with a group of untreated pregnant women did not report any congenital malformation in 90 newborns exposed in utero, including 17 who were exposed during the first trimester of pregnancy (Juric et al. 2009). As well a cohort study did not find a statistically significant difference in rates of major malformations between a group of pregnant women who were treated during early pregnancy with zolpidem and an untreated control group (Wang et al. 2010).

A recent study including a small sample of pregnant women, including 84 cases exposed to zolpidem and 46 controls, was conducted using data from two multi-site case-control studies. Seven defects had sufficient sample size to calculate adjusted odds ratios, which ranged from 0.76 for cleft lip to 2.18 for gastroschisis. Four defects had odds ratios > 1.8; all confidence intervals included the null. The authors' conclusions were that the results do not support a large increase in risk, but smaller increases in risk for certain birth defects cannot be ruled out as the sample of patients was small (Howley et al. 2024). Data from the Swedish Medical Birth Registry from 1995 up to 2007 were used to identify 1318 women who reported the use of HBRAs in early pregnancy. They gave birth to 1340 infants. Maternal characteristics and the presence of congenital malformations were compared with all other women who gave birth (n = 1,106,001) and all other infants (n = 1,125,734) born during the study period. The probability of using HBRAs increased in women who had had 3 or more earlier miscarriages or 5 or more years of involuntary childlessness. An excess use of other drugs and above all psychoactive drugs was seen in women reporting use of HBRAs. The authors' conclusions were that maternal use of HBRAs in early pregnancy does not seem to increase the risk of major congenital malformations (Wikner and Källén 2011). In the above-mentioned study by Ban which compared the safety of anxiolytic and hypnotic drugs during first trimester of pregnancy, a rate of 2.5% of newborns with major malformation was reported in 406 cases exposed to zopiclone, as compared to a rate of 2.7% reported in 19,193 infants whose mothers had an untreated depression and/or anxiety disorders during pregnancy. No significant difference was found in the risk of malformations in newborns exposed to BDZ as well as in Z-drugs in early pregnancy (Ban et al. 2014).

Overall, it could be concluded that data on the safety of zolpidem and zopiclone seems quite reassuring as far as the risk of major birth defects in newborns exposed in the first trimester of pregnancy is concerned. However, more studies are needed to confirm this reassuring data, as insomnia and sleep difficulties are common complaints during pregnancy. Notwithstanding, despite the importance of sleep during pregnancy, current understanding of the prevalence of prenatal insomnia and associated risk and protective factors is limited. Estimates of the prevalence of insomnia symptoms vary from 20% to 60% depending on the sample, the assessment measure used in the investigations as well as the population investigated.

12.5 Perinatal Complications

12.5.1 Benzodiazepines and Z-Drugs

Since a relevant number of pregnant women take a BDZ or a Z-drug during the perinatal period, the question of their gestational and neonatal safety is not trivial. BZDs and Z-drug exposure during pregnancy have been associated in some studies with gestational and neonatal complications, such as preterm birth, low birth weight, low Apgar score, spontaneous abortion, and a neonatal withdrawal or abstinence syndrome (NWS). However, data published on these important topics have reported contradictory results.

NWS is a condition affecting about 25% of newborns exposed late in pregnancy, including signs such as somnolence, irritability, hypoglycaemia difficulties with sucking, tremors, tachypnoea, gastrointestinal upset, hypoglycaemia, and hyperreflexia. The symptoms generally appear within a week after birth and can last from few days up to 3/4 weeks. It has been suggested that gradually tapering the daily dose of BZDs some weeks before delivery could be useful to minimize the neonatal withdrawal symptoms, even though this strategy has not been shown to be helpful in many cases of exposed newborns. In addition, a BZD discontinuation could induce a withdrawal reaction in pregnant woman, especially among those who have been taking higher doses of BZDs for several weeks during gestation. However, most newborns presenting withdrawal symptoms improve and recover usually after few days or weeks, without any long-lasting sequelae.

The use of BDZs, especially at high dosage, in most cases through intravenous route before delivery has been associated with an "*infant floppy syndrome*" (IFS), which is characterized by floppiness or general muscular hypotonia at birth or in early life, affecting the limbs, trunk, and the cranial-facial musculature. However, the IFS can be also induced by a variety of neuromuscular and central nervous system disorders, including genetic and/or metabolic deficits, therefore its association with exposure to BZDs at high dose before delivery needs to be better investigated. A recent population-based cohort study including mother-child pairs from 2001 to 2018 in Hong Kong compared gestationally exposed and nonexposed children to BDZs and Z-drugs to investigate the risk of preterm birth, small for gestational age, autism spectrum disorder (ASD), and attention-deficit/hyperactivity disorder (ADHD) through logistic/Cox proportional hazards regression. Sibling-matched analyses and negative control analyses were applied.

No statistically significant differences were found for all outcomes investigated when comparing children whose mothers took BDZs and/or Z-drugs during pregnancy to children whose mothers took such drugs before, but not during pregnancy. In their discussion, the author indicates that many studies on this topic may be limited by small sample sizes, poor representativeness of data, recall bias, inadequate adjustment of confounders such as indication (i.e., anxiety and/or sleep disorders) and unmeasured variables such as illicit drug use (Chan et al. 2023). In the above-mentioned retrospective cohort study by Jurich, 45 pregnant women who took zolpidem were more likely to have gestational hypertension and anaemia, as well as a greater chance of a caesarean delivery compared to the untreated group. Rates of preterm delivery and low birth weight were 26.7% and 15.6% respectively in the zolpidem-exposed group versus 13.3% and 4.4% in the matched comparator group, but no significant differences were found. It was also found that zolpidem crosses the human placenta and rapidly clears the fetal circulation; the degree of placental passage in this sample was highly variable, with cord concentrations of zolpidem ranging from 48% to 275% of maternal concentrations (Juric et al. 2009).

A large study was conducted in Norway to establish whether exposure to BDZs or Z-hypnotics in pregnancy was associated with greater risk of negative immediate pregnancy outcomes compared with non-exposed group. The main outcomes were gestational age at delivery, risk of preterm delivery, birth weight, risk of being small for head circumference, low Apgar score, and risk of neonatal respiratory distress. It was found that children born to mothers who were exposed to these drugs in pregnancy had slightly lower birth weight and had slightly higher to moderately risk of preterm birth compared with children without exposure. In their conclusions, the authors rightly pointed out that while the magnitudes of the associations were not necessarily clinically significant, BDZs and Z-drugs are not first-line treatment for anxiety disorders and therefore should only be used in pregnancy after an accurate evaluation of the benefits and risks for the mother and child *(*Huitfeldt et al. 2020*)*. A large, case-control study found that, after adjusting for measured confounds, early gestational exposure to BDZ was associated with a nearly doubled risk of spontaneous abortion; the risks were higher with higher daily doses prescribed.

However, it must be observed according to Andrade that these findings indicate that BDZs are probably a marker since the results of the study are not evidence for a cause-effect relationship, because analyses in studies such as this adjust for only "measured" confounds; therefore, unmeasured, inadequately measured and unknown confounds will continue to contaminate the interpretation of findings. Innovative research in this field should be considered, such as the examination of risk associated with BDZ exposure in the year before pregnancy, examination of risk in previously unexposed pregnancies as well of risk in discordant sibling pairs, and examination of risk associated with paternal exposure. Such studies have the potential to indirectly partially address unmeasured and unknown confounds, including those related to genetics and the family environment (Andrade 2019b).

A recent study has been conducted in Norway exploring the association between prenatal exposure to BDZs and Z-drugs and risk of ADHD in childhood (Sundbakk et al. 2022). In total, 681 offspring (0.8%) in the full sample and 468 offspring (2.4%) in the mental health sample were prenatally exposed to these medications. The results of this clearly indicate that there is no increase in risk of childhood ADHD associated with prenatal exposure to BDZs and/or Z-hypnotics. An original large cohort study including 1.138732 mothers with 1.516846 live births was recently published to assess the risk of ADHD and ASD in children exposed in utero to anxiolytic and hypnotic drugs (Chin-Hung Chen et al. 2022). No statistically significant differences were found with unexposed sibling controls during the same time frame for ADHD and ASD. Similar findings were also noted in the stratification analysis of short-acting and long-acting BDZs. To our knowledge, no prior studies have examined such an association using a sibling control method. The discordance in results between population and sibling comparisons suggests that maternal psychological or physical conditions may be potential "unmeasured" confounders for poorer neurodevelopmental outcomes among offspring. These conditions might include other maternal anxiety and sleep disorders recognized to be associated with neurodevelopmental problems among children. According to the authors it is plausible to believe that rather than simply attributing neurodevelopmental disorders as a direct consequence of neonatal BDZs exposure during pregnancy, it can be more important to reduce neurodevelopmental disorders by identifying mothers "at risk".

As appropriately suggested by Andrade in a recent comment of this study, "*the associations between gestational exposure to BDZs and Z-drugs and ASD or ADHD in offspring may be due to maternal and parental genetic factors, to family environmental variables, and to confounding by indication, rather than to such drugs exposure itself*" (Andrade 2023). A recent systematic review including 19 selected studies on this topic also confirms that it is currently not possible to conclude, with a reasonable degree of certainty, whether prenatal exposure to BZDs and/or z-drugs is associated with neurodevelopmental outcomes in offspring. This uncertainty mainly originates from a remarkable scarcity and quality of overall research on this important topic and therefore high-quality studies on the safety of BZD and Z-drug use during different stages on fetal brain development are urgently needed (Wang et al. 2022).

Overall, even though reassuring findings have been documented in the studies recently published on the risk of gestational and neonatal complications in women exposed in utero to BDZs and Z-drugs, further studies focusing on short and long-term infant adverse outcomes are still needed, particularly those focusing on the neurodevelopment disorders in children, as these disorders most likely have a multifactorial genesis.

12.6 Conclusions

According to the recent cohort studies, overviews, and guidelines, BDZs and Z-drugs exposure during early pregnancy seems not to be associated with an increased relative risk of congenital major malformations. However, it should be observed that in a few case-control studies but not in most cohort studies and meta-analysis a statistically significant association between these drugs and major birth defects was found. To explain the discrepancy in the results of such studies, it is worthwhile to consider that most of the first original investigations suffer from a number of methodological flaws, such as the lack of a careful report of BDZs and Z-drugs patterns of use in pregnancy (i.e., time of exposure, dosages, reasons for drug prescription, etc.), possible influences of recall biases (linked to case-control design), and the lack of control of several confounding factors (i.e., the presence of a severe psychiatric and /or organic disorder, alcohol abuse, smoking, and concomitant medications).

The BZDs exposure during the second and/or third trimester of pregnancy was found in some studies associated with an increased risk of neonatal and gestational complications, particularly preterm birth, low birth weight, and low Apgar score. However, even in this case, most of the above-mentioned adverse events were not observed in well-designed clinical investigations which controlled for confounding factors. On the other hand, there is a general agreement that BDZs could induce a neonatal withdrawal or abstinence syndrome, but only when used in the last two trimesters of pregnancy at high dosages, and particularly in the case of very/extremely preterm newborns. No increased risk concerning infant neurodevelopment and/or cognitive impairment has so far been well established in the majority of studies and reviews focusing on the safety of BDZs and/or Z-drugs exposure during pregnancy. However, there is still a need to perform further prospective cohort studies, based on adequate large samples, enrolling and following women from the first prenatal visit to the end of pregnancy and postpartum period, with a regular clinical monitoring of their psychopathological conditions and drug treatment. Also, a long term standardized assessment of infants exposed to BZs during the perinatal period is crucial.

It is thus recommended to treat pregnant women with anti-anxiety and/or hypnotic drugs, only in the case of severe insomnia and/or acute anxiety, where other effective therapeutic options, particularly psychological treatment, have failed. Among the BDZs, it should be preferred as a first-line option, those drugs with a short-medium elimination half-life and with no active metabolites.

The dosage and length of an anxiolytic/hypnotic treatment should be individualized in each pregnant woman, with the aim to prescribe the "lowest but effective dose". Such clinical practice is clinically relevant to prevent or minimize neonatal adverse effects, particularly the risk of withdrawal reactions. There is a need for those working in the field of perinatal mental health to improve their knowledge in this matter, thinking that perinatal psychiatry as well as perinatal psychopharmacology are not merely new or emerging specialties but everyone's business (Freeman 2014; Humphrey et al. 2016). Table 12.2 provides recommendations on the use of BDZs and Z-drugs in routine clinical practice during pregnancy, according to the recent evidence-based information and clinical experience.

Table 12.2 Expert recommendation based on scientific evidence and clinical experience

BDZs and Z-drugs during pregnancy should be prescribed to women affected by acute anxiety symptoms and severe insomnia, where non-pharmacological treatments have failed or are not effective enough to relieve such clinical conditions
BDZs are not indicated in monotherapy to treat women with general anxiety disorders, panic disorders, obsessive-compulsive disorder, and major depression; in such psychopathological conditions second-generation antidepressants, particularly SSRI, are usually recommended as a first-line pharmacological option in pregnancy
BDZs and Z-drugs should not be used for several months, but shortintermittent use is better to avoid potential risk of dependence, tolerance, or misuse; the discontinuation must always be carried out gradually, according to the dosage taken by the patient and the length of treatment she is taking
When considering the risks and benefits of anxiolytic and hypnotic drugs, clinicians should also consider the risks of an untreated severe insomnia and/or acute anxiety in pregnancy, which may lead to adverse biological effects as well as a reduced level of self-care, worsening mood, and impaired functioning
BDZs and Z-drugs are no longer considered at risk of inducing major congenital malformation as recent original studies and systematic reviews do not support such increased risk in newborns exposed in the first trimester of pregnancy as compared with newborns of unexposed pregnant women
Exposure to BDZs during gestation was considered in some studies responsible for gestational complications, particularly spontaneous abortion and preterm delivery. These findings however have not been replicated in recent original controlled studies. BDZ may be responsible in some newborns of withdrawal reactions also called "abstinence-like syndrome" which in the most cases improve in few days or a week, even though in preterm neonates could be longer (2/3 weeks), but without any long-lasting sequelae. This syndrome has been most frequently reported when the mother has been treated with high doses of BDZs during the last trimester of pregnancy
In pregnant women who are treated with high doses of BDZs an infant clinical monitoring by a paediatrician during the first month after birth is strongly recommended
The woman and her partner should be informed on the potential risks of the drug prescribed and those concerning the non-treatment of severe anxiety and insomnia. Moreover, the clinicians must be sure that all the information provided has been clearly understood
Informed signed consent should also be collected by the mother and her partner before prescribing BDZs or Z-drugs, as in the case of other psychotropic treatment
The dosage and length of drug treatment must be accurately individualized in each woman to better establish the lowest but effective therapeutic dosage
Among BDZs, drugs with short or medium elimination half-life and no active metabolites (oxazepam-like agents) should be preferred as a first-line choice for their better pharmacokinetic and metabolic profile for the foetus and the pregnant
Women treated with BDZ and Z-drugs during pregnancy, as well as other psychotropic drugs, should be advise to give birth in a general hospital where there is a neonatal intensive care unit, in order to provide effective and timely treatment in case of neonatal severe adverse reactions; this is particularly important in case of extremely preterm births (< 28 weeks of gestational age)

References

Andrade C. Gestational exposure to Benzodiazepoines:2. The risk of congenital malformations examined through the Prisma of compatibility intervals. J Clin Psychiatry. 2019a;80(5):19f13081.

Andrade C. Gestational exposure to benzodiazepines: the risk of spontaneous abortion examined through the prism of research design. J Clin Psychiatry. 2019b;80(5):19f13076.

Andrade C. Gestational exposures to BDZs and Z- hypnotic and the risk if autism spectrum disorder and attention deficit/hyperactive disorder in offspring. J Clin Psychiatry. 2023;83(2):23f14863.

Bais B, Molenaar NM, Bijma HH, Hoogendijk WJG, Mulder CL, Kamperman AM. Prevalence of benzodiazepines and benzodiazepine-related drugs exposure before, during and after pregnancy: a systematic review and meta-analysis. J Affect Disorders. 2020;269:18–27.

Ban L, West J, Gibson JE, Fiaschi L, Sokal R, Doyle P, Hubbard R, Smeeth L, Tata LJ. First trimester exposure to anxiolytic and hypnotic drugs and the risks of major congenital anomalies: a United Kingdom population-based cohort study. PLoS One. 2014;9(6)

Bellantuono C, Reggi V, Tognoni G, Garattini S. Benzodiazepines: clinical pharmacology and therapeutic use. Drugs. 1980;19(3):195–219.

Bellantuono C, Tofani S, Di Sciascio G, Santone G. Benzodiazepine exposure in pregnancy and risk of major malformations: a critical overview. Gen Hosp Psychiatry. 2013;35:3–8.

Bellantuono C, Balestrieri M. Psicofarmacoterapia. In: Balestrieri M, et al., editors. Manuale di Psichiatria. 2nd ed. Roma: Il Pensiero Scientifico Editore; 2014.

Betcher HK, Wisner KL. Psychotropic treatment during pregnancy: research synthesis and clinical care principles. J Women's Health. 2020;29(3):310–8.

Chan AYL, Gao L, Howard L, Simonoff E. Maternal benzodiazepines and Z-drugs use during pregnancy and adverse birth and neurodevelopmental outcomes in offspring: a population-based cohort study. Psychoter Psychosomatic. 2023;92:113–23.

Chin-Hung Chen V, Shu-I W, Lin C-F, Mong-Liang L, Chen Y-L, Stewart R. Association of prenatal exposure to benzodiazepines with development of autism spectrum and attention-deficit/hyperactivity disorders. JAMA Netw Open. 2022;5(11)

Chuang HM, Meng LC, Lin CW, Chen WW, Chen YY, Shang CY, Chen LK, Hsiao FY, et al. Concomitant use of antidepressants and benzodiazepines during pregnancy and associated risk of congenital malformations: a population-based cohort study in Taiwan. Lancet Psychiatry. 2024;11(8):601–10. https://doi.org/10.1016/S2215-0366(24)00176-7.

Dolovich RL, Addis A, Vaillancourt J, Koren G, Einarson TR. Benzodiazepine use in pregnancy and major malformations or oral cleft: meta-analysis of cohort and case-control studies. BMJ. 1998;317:839–43.

Dubovsky SL, Marshall D. Benzodiazepines remain important therapeutic options in psychiatric practice. Psychother Psychosom. 2022;91:307–34.

Enato E, Moretti M, Koren G. The fetal safety of benzodiazepines: an updated meta-analysis. J Obstet Gynaecol Can. 2011;33(1):46–8.

Freeman PL. Perinatal psychiatry: an emerging specialty. J Clin Psychiatry. 2014;75(10):1086–7.

Galbally M, Snellen M, Lewis A, editors. Psychopharmacology and pregnancy. Treatment efficacy, risks and guidelines. Springer; 2014.

Goodman JH, Chenausky KL, Freeman MP. Anxiety disorders during pregnancy: a systematic review. J Clin Psychiatry. 2014;75(10):e 1153-84.

Grigoriadis S, Graves L, Peer M, Mamisashvili L, Dennis CL, Vigod SN. Benzodiazepine use during pregnancy alone or in combination with an antidepressant and congenital malformations: systematic review and meta-analysis. J Clin Psychiatry. 2019;80(4):18r12412.

Howley MM, Worker MM, Fisher SC. Maternal exposure to zolpidem and risk of specific birth defects. J Sleep Research. 2024;33(1):e13958.

Huitfeldt A, Sundbakk LM, Handal M, Nordeng H. Associations of maternal use of benzodiazepines or benzodiazepine-like hypnotics during pregnancy with immediate pregnancy outcomes in Norway. JAMA Netw Open. 2020;3(6):e205860.

Humphrey J, et al. Perinatal psychiatry: a new specialty or everyone's business? Br J Psych Adv. 2016;22(6):363–72.

Iqbal MM, Sobhan T, Ryals T. Effects of commonly used benzodiazepines on the foetus, the neonate and the nursing infant. Psychiatr Serv. 2002;53:39–49.

Juric S, Newport DJ, Ritchie JC, Galanti M, Stowe ZN. Zolpidem (Ambien) in pregnancy: placental passage and outcome. Arch Women's Mental Health. 2009;12:441–6.

McAllister-Williams RH, Baldwin DS, Cantwell R, et al. British Association for Psychopharmacology consensus guidance on the use of psychotropic medication preconception, in pregnancy and postpartum; (BAP guidelines). J Psychopharmacol. 2017;31:1–34.

Noh Y, Ile H, Choi A, et al. First-trimester exposure to benzodiazepines and risk of congenital malformations in offspring: a population-based cohort study in South Korea. PLoS Med. 2022;19(3):1–15.

Okun ML, Ebert R, Saini B. A review of sleep-promoting medications used in pregnancy. Am J Obstetr Gynecol. 2015;212(4):428–41.

Sedov ID, Anderson NJ, Dhillon AK, et al. Insomnia symptoms during pregnancy: a meta analysis. J Sleep Res. 2021;30(1):e13207.

Sundbakk LM, Gran JM, Wood EM. Association of prenatal exposure to benzodiazepines and Z-hypnotics with risk of ADHD in childhood. JAMA Net Open. 2022;5(12):e2246889.

Walton GR, Hayashi K, Bach P, Dong H, Kerr T, Ahamad K, Milloy MJ, Montaner J, Wood E. The impact of benzodiazepine uses on mortality among polysubstance users in Vancouver, Canada. Public Health Rep. 2016;131(3):491–9.

Wang LH, Lin HC, Lin CC, Chen YH, Lin HC. Increased risk of adverse pregnancy outcomes in women receiving zolpidem during pregnancy. Clin Pharm Therapy. 2010;88:369–74.

Wang WJ, Hou CL, Yan-Ping J. Prevalence and associated risk factors of insomnia among pregnant in China. Compr Psychiatry. 2020;98:152168.

Wang X, Zhang T, Ekheden I, Chang Z, Hellner C, et al. Prenatal exposure to benzodiazepines and Z-drugs in humans and risk of adverse neurodevelopmental outcomes in offspring: a systematic review. Neurosci Biobehav Rev. 2022;137:104647.

Wikner BN, Källén B. Are hypnotic benzodiazepine receptor agonists teratogenic in humans? J Clin Psychopharmacol. 2011;31:356–9.

Benzodiazepines and Z-Drugs During Lactation

13

Betül Bakay and Faruk Uguz

13.1 Introduction

Puerperium is an important period in women, during which the onset and exacerbation of psychiatric disorders may be observed. Anxiety disorders in this period are frequent and affect up to 39% of women (Goodman et al. 2016). In some mothers with anxiety disorders, the high severity of anxiety symptoms or the comorbid depression can be very challenging. In addition, these symptoms can significantly interfere with the establishment of a healthy mother-infant relationship and may have a negative impact on the future social, cognitive, and emotional development of the child. Therefore, the mother may need medical treatment (Meades et al. 2024). Although antidepressants are first-line drugs used in clinical practice for the treatment of these patients, the use of benzodiazepines for a short period is not rare. On the other hand, many postpartum women experience sleep disturbances including poor sleep quality and insomnia (Ko et al. 2012). In addition to antidepressants and benzodiazepines, nonbenzodiazepine hypnotics (Z-drugs) are important pharmacological options in patients with insomnia (Wilt et al. 2016).

Breastfeeding is one of the major challenges in the treatment of women with psychiatric disorders. In a retrospective study published in 2020, at least 4-week follow-up records of 263 postpartum breastfeeding mothers were analyzed. In this study, it was shown that continuation of breastfeeding during pharmacological treatment of mothers with depression and anxiety disorders was not associated with serious infant problems (Uguz et al. 2020). It is well known that breast milk is the gold standard for infant nutrition and has indispensable lifetime benefits.

B. Bakay
Medical Faculty of Medicine, Department of Psychiatry, KTO Karatay University, Konya, Turkey

F. Uguz (✉)
Department of Psychiatry, Medova Hospital, Faculty of Medicine, KTO Karatay University, Konya, Türkiye

F. Uguz, L. Orsolini (eds.), *Perinatal Psychopharmacology*,
https://doi.org/10.1007/978-3-031-99720-4_13

Breastfeeding is associated with reduced morbidity, mortality, and occurrence of illnesses via factors including gastrointestinal mucosal maturation, decrease in the incidence of infection, alteration in the gut microflora, as well as immunomodulatory and anti-inflammatory factors, hormones, growth factors, and cytokines (Oddy 2002; Kronenfeld et al. 2017). Therefore, pharmacological agents that are recommended for postpartum women should be safe and not interfere with breastfeeding as much as possible. The milk-plasma ratio (M/P) is often used to determine the amount of drug excreted in breast milk and a ratio below 1 is preferred. However, this ratio may be misleading as it does not reflect the total daily dose received. Therefore, using the drug concentration in breast milk and the relative infant dose (RID) as a more definitive indicator would be more useful in determining exposure in breastfed infants. The RID is an indicator that estimates the amount of drug ingested in breast milk by breastfed infants and is considered safe at less than 10% in the literature (Eleftheriou et al. 2024). Considering that psychotropic medications may be excreted into the breast milk to at variable degrees, safety data on psychotropic drugs during lactation is essential to minimize infant exposure and subsequent adverse effects (Uguz and Sharma 2016).

13.2 Benzodiazepines

Benzodiazepines, especially diazepam and lorazepam, are frequently used not only for the treatment of maternal anxiety disorders but also for the management of acute neonatal seizures and status epilepticus in children, or as prophylactic drugs for the management of febrile seizure in children (Kanhere 2014; Wu et al. 2016; Offringa et al. 2017). Despite a long history of clinical usage, data so far published on the safety of benzodiazepines in breastfeeding women are limited. However, the available scientific evidence does not demonstrate any contraindication for breastfeeding during maternal use of these medications (Kronenfeld et al. 2017). BZDs have generally high binding to plasma proteins, high lipophilicity, and low molecular weight. The excretion rate into milk and half-life of each BZD vary according to their differences in these parameters (Furugen et al. 2019). In general, shorter-acting agents such as alprazolam and lorazepam are preferred to longer-acting agents such as diazepam and clonazepam that show a high risk of accumulation in infants through breast milk. In addition, among breastfeeding women with psychiatric diagnoses, it is recommended a brief and intermittent usage of benzodiazepines at low doses. Moreover, repeated doses should be avoided, if possible (Davanzo et al. 2013; Orsolini et al. 2016; Kronenfeld et al. 2017). Table 13.1 summarizes the recommendations by this paper regarding the use of benzodiazepines during breastfeeding.

It has been reported that the most commonly used benzodiazepines in the lactation period are lorazepam (52%), clonazepam (18%), and midazolam (15%) (Kelly et al. 2012). A recent study on the pharmacological management of depression during breastfeeding, including 22 case series examining the use of BZDs and Z-drugs, demonstrated that the RID values of alprazolam, clonazepam, diazepam, lorazepam, flunitrazepam, oxazepam, zolpidem, zaleplon, and zopiclone were less than 10%, and the majority were less than 5%. In this study, among 145 newborns

Table 13.1 Expert recommendations based on scientific evidence and clinical experience

Due to its tremendous beneficial effects, continuation of breastfeeding should be the main goal in clinical practice
The available limited data suggest that there is no clear contraindication regarding the use of benzodiazepines and Z-drugs during the lactation period
Benzodiazepines and Z-drugs should be used for a short term, with intermittent and as low doses as possible
Shorter-acting benzodiazepines are preferred to longer-acting ones
Infants exposed to benzodiazepines via breast milk should be carefully monitored with respect to CNS depression and feeding problems
Among benzodiazepines, lorazepam owns the largest data on safety in breastfed infants
Clonazepam should not be used during breastfeeding if it is not necessary
The best safety profile of benzodiazepines frequently used in breastfeeding women is presented by: midazolam > lorazepam > oxazepam/alprazolam > diazepam > clonazepam

exposed to BZD and Z drugs during breastfeeding, sedation and lethargy associated with alprazolam in two infants and sedation and poor milk intake due to diazepam in one infant were demonstrated (Eleftheriou et al. 2024). Recently, data from 124 breastfeeding mothers in the Motherisk program at the Hospital of Sick Children in Toronto, Ontario have suggested that only 1.6% of infants exposed to benzodiazepines had central nervous system (CNS) depression defined as sleepiness, poor latching, not waking up for breastfeeding, limpness, or lack of response to stimuli. The authors also noted that the infant sedation rate in their study was similar to that previously reported with exposure to acetaminophen (Kelly et al. 2012). It has been reported that adverse events such as sedation, lethargy, feeding difficulties or weight loss, drowsiness, apnea, restlessness and irritability were observed in a considerable proportion (17–50%) of infants exposed to benzodiazepines, particularly if the mothers used the drugs for a long period (Iqbal et al. 2002; Rubin et al. 2004; Orsolini et al. 2016). These adverse effects are mostly resolved within two weeks following discontinuation of the medication (Rubin et al. 2004). In addition, some withdrawal symptoms (e.g., tremor of the extremities, diarrhea and vomiting, restlessness, inconsolable crying, irritability, growth retardation due to feeding problems, sleep disturbances, and tendency for convulsions) may be observed in infants of women who discontinue after a long-term usage of benzodiazepines (Iqbal et al. 2002; Orsolini et al. 2016). These symptoms can appear within a few days to 3 weeks after the discontinuation and their resolution may take weeks (Iqbal et al. 2002). Therefore, benzodiazepines used for a long-term period by breastfeeding women should not be discontinued suddenly.

13.2.1 Diazepam

Safety data of approximately 20 cases using diazepam have been published in the literature (Rubin et al. 2004; Kelly et al. 2012; Kronenfeld et al. 2017). The available data suggest that diazepam is excreted in small amounts into breast milk (Orsolini et al. 2016). It is usually undetectable in the plasma of most infants. Milk to plasma ratio (M/P ratio) and relative infant dose (RID) for diazepam have been reported to be 0.2–0.58 and 3–7%, respectively (Borgatta et al. 1997; Davanzo et al. 2013; Orsolini et al. 2016; Kronenfeld et al. 2017). Adverse events have been rarely reported (Kronenfeld et al. 2017). Accumulation risk in infants due to the long half-life of diazepam is an important restrictive factor for its usage during the lactation period. A recently developed scoring system pertaining to the compatibility and safety of psychotropic drugs during breastfeeding has indicated that diazepam exhibits a low level of safety and should be employed with caution (Uguz 2021). Additionally, long-term use by nursing mothers can result in sedation and lethargy that may lead to severe feeding problems and weight loss in the infants. Therefore, use of diazepam chronically and/or at high doses should be avoided, and breastfed infants should be carefully monitored for feeding, weight, and sedation (Iqbal et al. 2002; Orsolini et al. 2016).

13.2.2 Clonazepam

Available data indicate that the use of clonazepam during the lactation period was about two-fold higher than diazepam (Kronenfeld et al. 2017). Limited available data suggest that it has similar safety features as diazepam such as a low M/P ratio (0.33), RID value (2.5%), usually undetectable plasma levels, and a high accumulation risk in the infants (Birnbaum et al. 1999; Rubin et al. 2004; Orsolini et al. 2016; Kronenfeld et al. 2017). According to available data, clonazepam has been shown to have low safety profile for breastfeeding women and should be used with caution (Uguz 2021). On the other hand, a descriptive study based on the French Pharmacovigilance Database reported that 3.7% ($n = 5$) of drug-induced adverse reactions via breastfeeding were related to the use of clonazepam (Soussan et al. 2014). Infants exposed to this benzodiazepine should be carefully monitored for CNS depression, because adverse effects in infants, especially apnea and sedation, have been reported with this medication (Iqbal et al. 2002; Kronenfeld et al. 2017). Long-term use of clonazepam is not recommended; usage should be either a single dose and/or few doses as possible with caution (Uguz 2017).

13.2.3 Alprazolam

There are 24 cases that reported the use of alprazolam in breastfeeding women in the literature (Oo et al. 1995; Kelly et al. 2012; Rubin et al. 2004; Kronenfeld et al. 2017). Oo et al. (1995) reported that the mean M/P ratio and RID value for alprazolam were 0.36 and 3%, respectively. The authors also noted that infant plasma levels of this agent were below the detection limits. Although there are some adverse events reported in infants including CNS depression (Kelly et al. 2012), irritability, sleep disturbances, sedation, and drowsiness (Rubin et al. 2004; Kronenfeld et al. 2017) in the literature, their incidence is low. According to the findings of recent studies, alprazolam has been reported to be moderately safe and appropriate for use during breastfeeding. Although alprazolam is considered less favorable than lorazepam, it is more advantageous compared to diazepam and clonazepam during breastfeeding (Uguz 2021). However, if used long term, the breastfed infant should be monitored as closely as possible for CNS effects on the infants. It is recommended that usage should be either a single dose and/or as few doses as possible; however, long-term use and/or high doses are possible with caution (Uguz 2017).

13.2.4 Lorazepam

In women experiencing severe anxiety or insomnia who do not exhibit risk factors for substance abuse, the short-term use of BZDs, such as lorazepam, during breastfeeding constitutes a significant component of treatment (Thorsness et al. 2018). Lorazepam is an intermediate-acting benzodiazepine that has the largest reported data ($n = 87$) in the literature (Kelly et al. 2012; Kronenfeld et al. 2017). M/P ratio is 0.15–0.26, and the RID value has been reported to be 10% in one patient (Orsolini et al. 2016; Kronenfeld et al. 2017). It has been shown that lorazepam is excreted into breast milk in low concentrations (Iqbal et al. 2002). Kelly et al. (2012) reported no CNS depression in infants of 64 breastfeeding women taking lorazepam. Lorazepam has been shown to be moderately safe and suitable for use during breastfeeding (Uguz 2021). When it is considered that lorazepam does not have any accumulation problem in the infants and that the exposure via breast milk is not associated with adverse effects on the infants (Iqbal et al. 2002), lorazepam appears to be most preferable benzodiazepine in the lactation period. Using this drug in a single dose and/or in a low dose is acceptable; however, long-term use and/or high doses are possible with caution (Uguz 2017).

13.2.5 Oxazepam

Half-life of oxazepam in maternal plasma is shorter than alprazolam and lorazepam. Its passage into breast milk is relatively low as shown by its reported M/P ratio (0.1–0.3) and RID value (0.7%). Moreover, to date, no adverse effects have been observed in the infants. However, the availability of safety data from very few cases in the literature ($n = 4$) is a major issue deterring the prescription of oxazepam during the lactation period (Kronenfeld et al. 2017). For this reason, usage should be either a single dose and/or as few doses as possible; however, long-term use and/or high doses are possible with caution. Oxazepam has been reported to have low safety during breastfeeding and should be used with caution (Uguz 2021).

13.2.6 Midazolam

Although midazolam is one of benzodiazepines that is frequently used during lactation, its usage in patients with psychiatric diagnosis is very rare (Uguz 2017). Incidence of adverse events in the infants is low. Midazolam has been shown to be safe and suitable for use during the breastfeeding period (Uguz 2021). Other advantages of this drug are a short half-life, being undetectable in the plasma of most infants, low M/P (0.2) ratio, and RID value (<1%) (Nitsun et al. 2006; Kronenfeld et al. 2017). Although midazolam may be used as a single dose with caution in patients with severe agitation, it does not appear to be appropriate for long-term usage since it is an intravenous anesthetic agent (Nitsun et al. 2006).

13.3 Z-Drugs

The Z-drugs including zaleplon, zopiclone, eszopiclone, and zolpidem are defined as non-benzodiazepine hypnotics and are currently more frequently prescribed compared to benzodiazepines for the treatment of insomnia (Okun et al. 2015). Since few studies have suggested their relative safety in breastfed infants, these agents may be alternative medications to benzodiazepines for the treatment of primary insomnia during lactation (Orsolini et al. 2016).

There is one study with small sample size regarding the use of zaleplon ($n = 5$), zolpidem ($n = 5$), and zopiclone ($n = 12$) in the literature. Darwish et al. (1999) reported that M/P ratio for zaleplon was 0.50 and the infant dose was below 1% of the maternal dose. These data indicate that transfer of zaleplon via breast milk to the infant was in a very small quantity that was unlikely to be clinically important. Similarly, the excretion of zolpidem in human milk was reported to be very low (M/P ratio = 0.13) (Pons et al. 1989). The average M/P ratio and weight-adjusted infant dose for zopiclone were found to be 0.51 and 1.4%, respectively (Matheson et al. 1990). Zopiclone has a relatively safe profile for use during breastfeeding, and zaleplon and zolpidem are not appropriate pharmacologic options (Uguz 2021). However, the clinical effects of these medications on breastfed infants remain unclear. Therefore, these medications should be used with caution in breastfeeding women with insomnia.

13.4 Conclusion

The corpus of data in the literature on the safety of psychotropic medications in breastfed infants does not correlate with the frequency of their usage. The utilization of BZDs in the treatment of sleep disorders and anxiety symptoms in breastfeeding mothers is proposed, with the caveat that the safety of this approach is contingent upon the preference for drugs with the least active metabolite and short half-life (e.g., lorazepam, oxazepam), with the objective of minimizing the drug's effects on the infant (Eleftheriou et al. 2024). Although the available reports do not suggest a clear contraindication for the use of benzodiazepines, their long-term effects on the breastfed infants remain unclear. Therefore, decisions concerning these medications during the lactation period should be made on the basis of the need to treat the mother and their potential side effects in the infants. Single administration or short-term usage at low doses seems to be compatible with breastfeeding. The exposed infants should be carefully monitored by the mother and pediatricians during maternal use of benzodiazepines. Short-acting drugs, especially lorazepam, are more preferable compared to long-acting ones. Limited available data suggest that among the Z-drugs, zopiclone may be an alternative to benzodiazepines in breastfeeding women with primary insomnia.

References

Birnbaum CS, Cohen LS, Bailey JW, Grush LR, Robertson LM, Stowe ZN. Serum concentrations of antidepressants and benzodizepines in nursing infants: a case series. Pediatrics. 1999;104:e11.

Borgatta L, Jenny RW, Gruss L, Ong C, Barad D. Clinical significance of methohexital, meperidine, and diazepam in breast milk. Clin Pharmacol. 1997;37:186–92.

Darwish M, Martin PT, Cevallos WH, Tse S, Wheeler S, Troy SM. Rapid disappearance of zaleplon from breast milk after oral administration to lactating women. J Clin Pharmacol. 1999;39:670–4.

Davanzo R, Bo SD, Copertino M, Zanelli E, Matarazzo L. Antiepileptic drugs and breastfeeding. Ital J Pediatr. 2013;39:50.

Eleftheriou G, et al. Consensus panel recommendations for the pharmacological management of breastfeeding women with postpartum depression. Int J Env Res Public Health. 2024;21:551.

Furugen A, Nishimura A, Kobayashi M, Umazume T, Narumi K, Iseki K. Quantification of eight benzodiazepines in human breastmilk and plasma by liquid-liquid extraction and liquid-chromatography tandem mass spectrometry: application to evaluation of alprazolam transfer into breastmilk. J Pharm Biomed Anal. 2019;168:83–93.

Goodman JH, Watson GR, Stubbs B. Anxiety disorders in postpartum women: a systematic review and meta-analysis. J Affect Disord. 2016;203:292–331.

Iqbal MM, Sobhan T, Ryals T. Effects of commonly used benzodiazepines on the fetus, the neonate, and the nursing infant. Psychiatr Serv. 2002;53:39–49.

Kanhere S. Recent advances in neonatal seizures. Indian J Pediatr. 2014;81:917–25.

Kelly LE, Poon S, Madadi P, Koren G. Neonatal benzodiazepines exposure during breastfeeding. J Pediatr. 2012;161:448–51.

Ko HS, Shin J, Kim MY, Kim YH, Lee J, Kil KC, Moon HB, Lee G, Sa-Jin K, Kim BI. Sleep disturbances in Korean pregnant and postpartum women. J Psychosom Obstet Gynecol. 2012;33:85–90.

Kronenfeld N, Berlin M, Shaniv D, Berkovitch M. Use of psychotropic medications in breastfeeding women. Birth Defects Res. 2017;109:957–97.

Matheson I, Sande HA, Gaillot J. The excretion of zopiclone into breast milk. Br J Clin Pharmacol. 1990;30:267–71.

Meades R, Moran PM, Hutton U, Khan R, Maxwell M, Cheyne H, Delicate A, Shakespeare J, Hollins K, Pisavadia K, Doungsong KP, Edwards RT, Sinesi A, Ayers S. Acceptability of identification and management of perinatal anxiety: a qualitative interview study with postnatal women. Front Public Health. 2024;12:1466150.

Nitsun M, Szokol JW, Saleh J, Murphy GS, Vender JS, Luong L, Raikoff K, Avram MJ. Pharmacokinetics of midazolam, propofol, and fentanyl transfer to human berast milk. Clin Pharmacol Ther. 2006;79:549–57.

Oddy WH. Long-term health outcomes and mechanisms associated with breastfeeding. Expert Rev Pharmacoecon Outcomes Res. 2002;2:161–77.

Offringa M, Newton R, Cozijnsen MA, Nevitt SJ. Prophylactic drug management for febrile seizures in children. Cochrane Database Syst Rev. 2017;2:CD003031.

Okun ML, Ebert R, Saini B. A review of sleep-promoting medications used in pregnancy. Am J Obstet Gynecol. 2015;212:428–41.

Oo CY, Kuhn RJ, Desai N, Wright CE, McNamara PJ. Pharmacokinetics in lactating women: prediction of alprazolam transfer into milk. Br J Clin Pharmacol. 1995;40:231–6.

Orsolini L, Valchera A, Bellantuono C. Antidepressants and anxiolytics during lactation. In: Uguz F, editor. Psychiatric disorders during the postpartum period in light of current advances. New York: Nova Science Publishers, Inc.; 2016. p. 115–42.

Pons G, Francoual C, Guillet P, Moran C, Hermann P, Bianchetti G, Thiercelin JF, Thenot JP, Olive G. Zolpidem excretion in breast milk. Eur J Clin Pharmacol. 1989;37:245–8.

Rubin ET, Lee A, Ito S. When breastfeeding mothers need CNS-acting drugs. Can J Clin Pharmacol. 2004;11:e257–66.

Soussan C, Gouraud A, Portolan G, Jean-Pastor MJ, Pecriaux C, Montastruc JL, Damase-Michel C, Lacroix I. Drug-induced adverse reactions via breastfeeding: a descriptive study in the French pharmacovigilance database. Eur J Clin Pharmacol. 2014;70:1361–6.

Thorsness KR, Watson C, LaRusso EM. Perinatal anxiety: approach to diagnosis and management in the obstetric setting. Am J Obst Gynecol. 2018;219:326–45.

Uguz F. Breastfeeding and psychotropic medications. In: Uguz F, editor. Psychotropic drugs and medical conditions. New York: Nova Science Publishers Inc.; 2017. p. 209–29.

Uguz F. A new safety scoring system for the use of psychotropic drugs during lactation. Am J Ther. 2021;2021(28):e118–26.

Uguz F, Sharma V. Mood stabilizers during breastfeeding: a systematic review of the recent literature. Bipolar Disord. 2016;18:325–33.

Uguz F, Kirkas A, Aksoy ZK, Yunden S. Use of psychotropic medication during lactation in postpartum psychiatric patients: results from an 8-year clinical sample. Breastfeed Med. 2020;15:535–7.

Wilt TJ, MacDonald R, Brasure M, Olson CM, Carlyle M, Fuchs E, Khawaja IS, Diem S, Koffel E, Quelette J, Butler M, Kane RL. Pharmacologic treatment of insomnia disorder: an evidence report for a clinical practice guideline by American College of Physcians. Ann Intern Med. 2016;165:103–12.

Wu W, Zhang L, Xue R. Lorazepam or diazepam for convulsive status epilepticus: A meta-analysis. J Clin Neurosci. 2016;29:133–8.

14 Miscellaneous Drugs During Pregnancy and Lactation

Hasan Bakay

14.1 Introduction

Drug use during pregnancy and lactation has always posed a challenge for clinicians. Ensuring maternal and infant safety while determining optimal therapy requires a thorough knowledge of the pharmacokinetic and pharmacodynamic properties of drugs and their potential teratogenic or neonatal effects. Although research in this area is increasing, there are significant gaps in the literature, particularly for drugs that are not routinely included in specific safety categories.

Due to their critical role in opioid substitution therapy, drugs such as methadone and buprenorphine have been studied relatively more extensively during pregnancy and lactation (Ordean and Tubman-Broeren 2023; Suarez et al. 2022; Jansson et al. 2024). Similarly, methylphenidate, one of the most commonly used drugs in the treatment of attention deficit hyperactivity disorder (ADHD), which has a prevalence rate of approximately 3% among women of childbearing age, is also among the well-studied compounds (Baker et al. 2022; Scoten et al. 2024; di Giacomo et al. 2024). However, data on the use of buspirone and gabapentinoids for the treatment of anxiety disorders, and naltrexone, acamprosate, baclofen, and disulfiram for the treatment of alcohol use disorder in this sensitive period are limited (Freeman et al. 2022; Beau et al. 2024; Quintrell et al. 2023). Similarly, there is a significant gap in the literature regarding the use of biperiden, a drug that can effectively control the extrapyramidal side effects of antipsychotic drugs (Escobar-Vidarte et al. 2019). An increase in the incidence of restless legs syndrome (RLS), which is thought to be related to iron

H. Bakay (✉)
Department of Psychiatry, Faculty of Medicine, Necmettin Erbakan University, Konya, Türkiye
e-mail: hasan.bakay@erbakan.edu.tr

F. Uguz, L. Orsolini (eds.), *Perinatal Psychopharmacology*,
https://doi.org/10.1007/978-3-031-99720-4_14

deficiency anemia, has been reported during pregnancy. Data on pramipexole, an important drug that is used for the treatment of RLS, both during pregnancy and breastfeeding, have also remained very limited (Dostal et al. 2013).

This chapter aims to evaluate and synthesize current evidence on the safety profiles during pregnancy and lactation of clinically important drugs that are not classified into drug groups such as antidepressants, antipsychotics, benzodiazepines, and mood stabilizers. The chapter also highlights the well-documented risks along with areas where the data are insufficient. This chapter can contribute towards ensuring the best outcomes for both mothers and their babies by providing an evidence-based framework for determining the safest treatment strategy for pregnant and breastfeeding women.

14.2 Methadone, Buprenorphine, Buprenorphine/Naloxone

Methadone has been the mainstay for the management of opioid use disorder for a long time. The use of methadone during pregnancy has been associated with neonatal abstinence, decreased head circumference, agitation, movement defects, decreased interactive behavior, as well as impaired motor and cognitive functions (Daly et al. 2012; Chen et al. 2015; Kongstorp et al. 2020). Although a few studies have reported the lack of any significant increase in the risk of congenital malformations due to methadone use during pregnancy (Ordean and Tubman-Broeren 2023), there are not enough data in the literature on the long-term consequences of methadone exposure during pregnancy and lactation reported. Daly et al. (2012) reported that perinatal methadone exposure did not have a significant effect on the physical development of the animals. However, their behavioral development was affected (Daly et al. 2012). In a more recent animal study, methadone exposure in the prenatal and early postnatal period was shown to affect the development of the circadian rhythm, circadian rhythm-related gene expression, and melatonin levels in newborns (Pačesová et al. 2023). Reports suggest that very low levels of methadone are excreted into breast milk, which may be conducive to the management of opioid withdrawal in the newborn (Jansson et al. 2008).

Ordean and Tubman-Broeren (2023) reviewed the safety and efficacy of the use of buprenorphine by pregnant women, as well as neonatal and maternal outcomes from 7 different studies. The authors examined birth parameters, congenital anomalies, and neonatal withdrawal symptoms in pregnant women and reported that the buprenorphine dose ranged from 8 to 20 mg/day. Moreover, there was a significant reduction in illicit opioid use in pregnant women using buprenorphine. This review included four different newborn groups: (1) those exposed to buprenorphine/naloxone combination, (2) those exposed to other opiate replacement therapies (buprenorphine monotherapy or methadone), (3) those exposed to illicit opioids, and (4) those without opioid exposure. No significant difference was identified in birth parameters and prevalence of congenital anomalies between the four groups. However, a significant increase in neonatal opioid withdrawal was observed in the methadone-exposed newborns. Overall, the authors emphasized that buprenorphine/naloxone combination treatment was a safe and effective treatment option in pregnant women with opioid use disorder (Ordean and Tubman-Broeren 2023).

Suarez et al. (2022) investigated neonatal and maternal outcomes in a large sample of patients who used methadone and buprenorphine during pregnancy. The authors reported that 52% of the infants of pregnant women exposed to buprenorphine and 69.2% of the infants exposed to methadone had neonatal withdrawal syndrome. Fewer preterm births (14.4% vs 24.9%), small-for-gestational-age births (12.1% vs 15.3%), and miscarriages (8.3% vs 14.9%) were reported in infants exposed to buprenorphine in early pregnancy compared to those exposed to methadone. No significant difference was identified in the rate of cesarean section delivery or other serious maternal complications between the two groups. The authors therefore emphasized that buprenorphine use was associated with lower rates of neonatal complications compared to methadone (Suarez et al. 2022). Similar findings were shown in another study that also compared maternal and neonatal outcomes related to maternal exposure to buprenorphine and methadone. In addition, it was reported that the rate of illicit drug use was higher among the methadone users. A comparison of buprenorphine and buprenorphine/naloxone showed no significant differences in maternal and neonatal outcomes (Kanervo et al. 2023). In a meta-analysis including 20 studies, Kinsella et al. (2022) reported that buprenorphine was associated with higher birth weight and less risk of prematurity compared to methadone (Kinsella et al. 2022) and was the safer option during pregnancy.

Breast milk and serum samples of mothers who used buprenorphine were collected on postpartum days 2, 3, 4, 14, and 30, and serum samples of infants were collected on postpartum day 14. The levels of buprenorphine and its metabolites were generally low in maternal serum and breast milk samples and were positively correlated with the daily dose. Additionally, buprenorphine levels were reported to be low or undetectable in the serum of breastfed infants and undetectable in the serum of 14-day-old infants. In light of these data, the authors suggested that mothers who were regularly prescribed buprenorphine could continue breastfeeding (Jansson et al. 2016). In a relatively recent study, buprenorphine and its metabolites were shown to be at low levels in the serum and milk of breastfeeding mothers who were using buprenorphine/naloxone, while naloxone levels were very low or undetectable. Moreover, naloxone levels were shown to be very low or undetectable in the serum of infants (Jansson et al. 2024). However, it should be mentioned that the relatively small number of participants in these studies is an important limitation.

14.3 Naltrexone

Naltrexone is an opioid receptor antagonist that is prescribed to reduce pleasure in addiction treatment, particularly in the treatment of alcohol and opioid use disorders (Antonelli et al. 2018). Newborns exposed to naltrexone were reported to have decreased body weight and length at birth, increased duration of hospitalization, increased frequency of congenital urogenital malformations, and susceptibility to infectious diseases in childhood (Kelty and Hulse 2017a, b). In relatively more recent studies, neonates exposed to naltrexone were reported to have significantly lower rates of withdrawal symptoms and hospitalizations compared to those exposed to methadone and buprenorphine (Wachman et al. 2019; Towers et al. 2020). Considering the maternal outcomes, ectopic pregnancy and other birth complications were reported to be higher in pregnant women using naltrexone compared to unexposed women (Kelty and Hulse 2017c). On the contrary, no significant increase in maternal risk during pregnancy with naltrexone use has also been reported (Quintrell et al. 2025).

Animal studies have shown that naltrexone exposure during pregnancy was associated with weight gain in the body and organs of the offspring (McLaughlin 2002; Youngentob et al. 2012). In another important study, although an increase in offspring size and a slight decrease in birth weight were reported in subjects with long-release naltrexone implant, no change in brain morphology was detected (Farid et al. 2012). However, naltrexone exposure in the middle and late periods of pregnancy was reported to have a negative effect on testicular development, although it had no effect on sperm development (Cajú et al. 2011). Naltrexone exposure was shown to have a dose-dependent effect on locomotor activity (Quintrell et al. 2025). Some studies have suggested that naltrexone exposure can increase cortical thickness without changing the number of neurons in the brain, contribute to neuronal maturation, and may even have neuroprotective effects on ethanol-exposed offspring (Youngentob et al. 2012). Studies also suggest that naltrexone may increase the risk of preterm birth in a dose-dependent manner (Javadi-Paydar et al. 2009).

In a recent multicenter prospective cohort study, Mantri et al. (2024) compared the 1-year development of infants who were exposed to naltrexone or buprenorphine/naloxone during pregnancy and reported the lack of any statistically significant difference (Mantri et al. 2024). It should be noted that the number of participants in the naltrexone arm was very small compared to the buprenorphine/naloxone arm in this study (n = 7 vs 34). A recent systematic review and meta-analysis that compared the exposure to naltrexone, methadone, or buprenorphine in pregnancy reported that the risk of preterm birth did not increase with naltrexone exposure compared to methadone and buprenorphine exposure; moreover, neonatal withdrawal symptoms were significantly less (Atluru et al. 2024). However, it should be noted that the referred analysis had important limitations such as the relatively small number of studies as well as participants, which may significantly reduce the statistical power of the results obtained. Thus, it is imperative that the reassuring perinatal results with the use of naltrexone are confirmed in larger samples.

A relative infant dose (RID) value of 1.06% was calculated for naltrexone during breastfeeding and no adverse effects were reported for the infant (Chan et al. 2004). Thus, the use of naltrexone during breastfeeding appears to be safe; nonetheless, these data need to be supported by other independent studies.

14.4 Buspirone

Buspirone is an important drug that is frequently used for the treatment of women of childbearing age for the treatment of anxiety disorders, although its use is generally not prioritized. Freeman et al. (2022) evaluated 68 women who used buspirone in early pregnancy and evaluated 72 babies of these pregnant women at 12 weeks postpartum. The authors reported the lack of any malformations in these babies (Freeman et al. 2022). The data obtained from referred study suggest that buspirone use does not pose an increased risk for neonatal effects; however, the study sample was small and therefore the data need to be confirmed in larger samples that also include control groups.

Comprehensive studies on the passage of buspirone into breast milk and its effects on the infant during breastfeeding have not been reported to date. In a recent study, buspirone levels were found to be below 1.5 ng/mL in milk samples obtained from 9 mothers who used buspirone at doses of 15–60 mg/day (Krutsch et al. 2024). The levels of 1-pyrimidinylpiperazine, the active metabolite of buspirone, were also shown to be low. The RID value for buspirone was found to be between 0.21% and 2.17% (mean < 1%), which was within the safe range for the infant (10% or less) and no side effects were observed in infants (Krutsch et al. 2024). In light of these data, the authors suggest that the use of buspirone during breastfeeding poses minimal risk.

14.5 Gabapentinoids

Pregabalin and gabapentin, which were first developed as antiepileptics, are now widely used especially in the treatment of neuropathic pain and certain types of anxiety disorders. These drugs exert their effects by binding to voltage-coupled calcium channels and reduce presynaptic excitatory neurotransmitter release by inhibiting calcium transport. These drugs also ameliorate neuropathic pain via alpha2 adrenoreceptors (Kremer et al. 2016; Goodman and Brett 2019). A recent review reported that the prevalence of gabapentinoid use in pregnancy was less than 1%. However, there has been an increase in its use in recent years (Beau et al. 2024).

14.5.1 Pregabalin

Certain adverse neonatal outcomes such as preterm birth, stillbirth, miscarriage, and neurodevelopmental disorders were reported to be associated with exposure to pregabalin (Mostacci et al. 2018; Margulis et al. 2019; Bjørk et al. 2022). In a recent review, Richardson et al. (2023) reported a small increase (approximately 1.5-fold) in the risk of malformations in the infants of women who were exposed to pregabalin (4% vs 4.8–5.6%). However, the authors concluded that attributing this minimal increase in risk to pregabalin use could be controversial, emphasizing important methodological limitations such as concurrent use of other medications among the patients included in the study (Richardson et al. 2023). In addition, the authors examined specific malformations such as central nervous system, eye, urogenital system, orofacial defects, and craniosynostosis and reported the lack of any association between pregabalin exposure and all other identified anomalies except for nervous system anomalies. In a more recent study from Turkiye, Kaskal et al. (2024) retrospectively compared women with (n = 31) and without (n = 93) pregabalin exposure (Kaskal et al. 2024). In this study, preterm delivery rates and low birth weight rates in infants were significantly higher in women who used pregabalin. No significant difference was reported in the spontaneous abortion rates. Although a higher incidence of major malformations was observed in the pregabalin group, no statistically significant difference could be identified between the two groups (11% vs 4.5%, $p = 0.21$). In conclusion, the authors showed that maternal pregabalin use during pregnancy was associated with increased preterm birth and low birth weight in infants compared to a control group, along with an increase in the incidence of additional comorbidities (Kaskal et al. 2024).

According to data reported in a recently published and methodologically strong meta-analysis, exposure to pregabalin in the first trimester was associated with an increased risk of major congenital anomalies in the newborn (Dudukina et al. 2023). Using various sensitivity analyses, the authors reported that this association persisted even when confounding factors such as polypharmacy were controlled. Although an increase in the incidence of minor congenital anomalies such as orofacial clefts and urogenital anomalies has been reported, these data came from a relatively small number of studies and were interpreted as statistically weak data. The existing literature does not provide a clear conclusion regarding specific (minor) congenital anomalies (Blotière et al. 2019; Dudukina et al. 2023). In the context of pregnancy outcomes, exposure to pregabalin was reported to increase the risk of stillbirth, miscarriage, low birth weight, and small for gestational age (Beau et al. 2024).

Lockwood et al. (2016) reported in a case study that the amount of pregabalin measured from the breastmilk corresponded to about 7% of the dose consumed by the mother (Lockwood et al. 2016). Humerickhouse et al. (2024) determined the pregabalin levels in breast milk by using a physiologically based pharmacokinetic model simulation in which the physicochemical properties of a specific drug can be integrated with existing lactation data to predict its passage into breast milk and infant exposure. Using this method, the authors calculated a RID value of 7% in the milk of mothers receiving 300 mg/day (2 × 150 mg) of pregabalin. The simulation experiment predicted a peak level of 0.44 μg/mL in the first 2 weeks followed by a gradual decrease over time (Humerickhouse et al. 2024). Although the RID values obtained from these reports appear to be in the safe range, an animal study reported a higher risk of tumor development in the offspring exposed to pregabalin through breast milk; therefore, the use of this drug is not recommended during breastfeeding (Sauberan 2025).

14.5.2 Gabapentin

Exposure of the fetus to gabapentin due to maternal use was shown to increase the risk of preterm birth, low birth weight, and the need for neonatal intensive care (Fujii et al. 2013; Mostacci et al. 2018; Patorno et al. 2020). The risk of major congenital anomalies was found to increase by 49–77%; however, when evaluated with confounding factors, no significant increase in the risk of major malformations was identified (Patorno et al. 2020). After post-hoc analysis, the authors noted only an increase in the risk of conotruncal defect that did not reach statistical significance. A partial increase in preterm birth, small for gestational age, and the need for neonatal intensive care with exposure to gabapentin were also reported. However, based on the overall data, it was concluded that gabapentin has a safe profile for use in pregnancy. Recent studies with relatively smaller number of patients also support the lack of any significant increase in the risk of anomalies associated with gabapentin exposure in pregnancy (Vajda et al. 2018; Blotière et al. 2019; Quintrell et al. 2025). In addition, gabapentin exposure during pregnancy has not been reported to adversely affect neurodevelopment in children (Blotière et al. 2020; Bjørk et al. 2022).

Unlike clinical research, several animal studies have shown that gabapentin exposure is indeed associated with significant anomalies. These include brachygnathia, pointed nose, cataracts, limb deformities, vertebral deformities, trunk malformations, and neural tube defects (Prakash et al. 2008; Afshar and Golalipour 2008; Afshar et al. 2009; Cetinkal and Cakir 2021). However, other animal studies have also reported that exposure to low doses of gabapentin during pregnancy did not cause any neurotoxic effects in the offspring (Erisgin et al. 2019). The findings obtained from animal studies suggest that gabapentin may increase the risk of adverse effects in a dose-dependent manner.

Overall, gabapentin appears to have a safer profile compared to pregabalin; nonetheless, when evaluated together with the findings from animal studies, the current literature raises concerns about the safety of gabapentinoids in pregnancy. It is suggested that the use of gabapentinoids should be assessed in a case-by-case basis taking into account the balance of benefit and harm for both the mother and the fetus and should only be used when appropriate alternative medications are not available (Richardson et al. 2023; Beau et al. 2024).

A gabapentin level of approximately 11.1 mg/L was reported in the breast milk of a mother taking 1800 mg/day gabapentin after a 600 mg intake. The milk/plasma ratio was 0.86 and the RID value was calculated as 2.3%. In addition, no side effects were observed in the infant (Kristensen et al. 2006). Another study reported RID values of 1.3% to 3.8% in samples from 5 mothers with no adverse effects (Ohman et al. 2005). In a recently published study, Ozalp Horsanalı et al. (2024) concluded that gabapentin use may be safe for breastfeeding women (Ozalp Horsanalı et al. 2024). Although the use of gabapentin during breastfeeding is not recommended, the current literature does not report any adverse effects upon infant exposure through breastfeeding and the RID values are in the safe range.

14.6 Pramipexole

The existing literature provides very limited data on the use of pramipexole during pregnancy and breastfeeding. Benbir et al. (2014) reported the successful use of pramipexole in a 35-year-old pregnant woman with Parkinson's disease where the pregnancy was completed with a healthy baby (Benbir et al. 2014). Dostal et al. (2013) examined the safety profiles of the use of dopamine agonists during pregnancy in patients diagnosed with RLS (n = 59) (Dostal et al. 2013). These authors reported that spontaneous abortion occurred in only three of the 12 pregnant subjects who received treatment exclusively with pramipexole. In addition, nine pregnancies were successfully completed without complications, and no malformations were observed. No congenital complications or malformations were reported in three pregnant women who received a combined treatment with pramipexole and levodopa. Although these preliminary data on the safety of pramipexole in pregnancy seem promising, more studies are needed to form a definitive opinion. Pramipexole, a dopamine agonist, is currently not recommended for use during lactation as it may decrease lactation by suppressing prolactin (Benbir et al. 2014; Picchietti et al. 2015).

14.7 Methylphenidate

The prevalence of ADHD among women of childbearing age is approximately 3%. Methylphenidate is one of the most commonly used drugs in the treatment of ADHD (Koren et al. 2020; Szpunar et al. 2023; Scoten et al. 2024). One study reported that 23.3% of women diagnosed with ADHD and prescribed medication before pregnancy continued their treatment during pregnancy, while 41.8% discontinued their treatment (Bang Madsen et al. 2024). Among the latter patients, 17.7% resumed medication in the postpartum period. Methylphenidate was the most commonly prescribed medication for ADHD treatment in this study, emphasizing the significance of investigating its safety during pregnancy and breastfeeding.

Although some studies have reported a slight increase in the risk of cardiac defects (1.07% vs 1.7%, a 59% increase) with methylphenidate use during pregnancy (Koren et al. 2020; Kolding et al. 2021), the majority of studies have not shown any significant increase in the risk of congenital malformations (Bolea-Alamanac et al. 2014; Ornoy 2018; Jiang et al. 2019; Damer et al. 2021). In a recent study, 45 women who used methylphenidate during the first trimester of pregnancy were followed longitudinally. No major malformations were observed in these infants at 6 months after birth (Szpunar et al. 2023). Considering other pregnancy outcomes, some studies reported preeclampsia, preterm delivery, low birth weight, and increased need for neonatal intensive care; however, these adverse effects could not be attributed unequivocally to the drug (Scoten et al. 2024). Untreated ADHD in pregnancy may have greater adverse effects on the mother's quality of life and the developing fetus by increasing the rates of spontaneous abortion and preterm birth (Baker et al. 2022; Scoten et al. 2024). A meta-analysis of nearly 30,000 women with ADHD from 10 large studies showed no significant increase in congenital anomalies and miscarriages in the infants of mothers who received treatment with methylphenidate and atomoxetine during pregnancy compared to control groups (di Giacomo et al. 2024). The evidence from this large-sample meta-analysis provides important insights into the safety of methylphenidate during pregnancy.

Regarding the breastfeeding period, methylphenidate was reported to have very limited excretion into milk, with a RID value of less than 1% and undetectable levels in the serum of breastfed infants (Collin-Lévesque et al. 2018). No adverse effects were observed in the infants and therefore it is considered to be generally safe during breastfeeding (Bolea-Alamanac et al. 2014; Kittel-Schneider et al. 2021). Methylphenidate may lead to a decrease in prolactin levels by increasing dopamine levels; however, this decrease was not found to exert any adverse effects on lactation (Scoten et al. 2024). Consequently, clinicians should take into consideration the potential impact of treatment on lactation when prescribing medications to breastfeeding women or to women who have not yet initiated breastfeeding.

The extant literature suggests that the use of methylphenidate during both pregnancy and breastfeeding is associated with low risks. In cases where patients' functionality is significantly affected, use of the drug in the lowest possible doses and in an intermittent manner according to the patient's condition could be more appropriate.

14.8 Acamprosate

Acamprosate is a pharmaceutical agent that is commonly prescribed for the treatment of alcohol use disorder. Its mechanism of action involves the modulation of N-methyl-d-aspartic acid receptors and calcium channels (Antonelli et al. 2018). However, data available on the safety of acamprosate use during pregnancy remain limited. A study conducted on 54 women who used acamprosate during pregnancy reported no association with adverse effects in the newborn or the mother (Kelty et al. 2019). A comparison of pregnant women who used or did not use acamprosate revealed no significant differences in the rates of low birth weight, preterm birth, or congenital anomalies between the two groups. However, other studies have identified a potential association between first-trimester exposure to acamprosate and adverse outcomes, including miscarriage, premature birth, and minor facial anomalies (Quintrell et al. 2025).

Animal studies have shown that acamprosate exposure during pregnancy did not result in adverse maternal and neonatal outcomes; in fact, a neuroprotective effect against alcohol-induced neurodegeneration was observed (Quintrell et al. 2023). There is a paucity of data on the use of acamprosate during lactation, and no scientific data on its excretion into milk. Nevertheless, considering the chemical structure of acamprosate, it is likely to be excreted into breast milk. However, given its oral bioavailability of 11% (Luo et al. 2015), the excretion of acamprosate into breast milk may not be significant enough to cause systemic side effects in the infant. However, this view has yet to be substantiated by scientific data.

14.9 Disulfiram

Disulfiram exerts its pharmacodynamic effect through the inhibition of aldehyde dehydrogenase, resulting in the accumulation of acetaldehyde. In conjunction with alcohol, the accumulation of acetaldehyde can manifest in a clinical spectrum ranging from aversive reactions to life-threatening consequences, contingent on the quantity of alcohol consumed (Mutschler et al. 2016). Following the initial observations that use of dilsufiram in conjunction with alcohol use disorder exhibited teratogenic properties, the compound was subsequently deemed to be teratogenic (Mutschler et al. 2016) and no further research was conducted on it. A later study by Briggs et al. (2017) reported a high rate (28.9%) of teratogenicity associated with disulfiram. However, it is also important to note that the limited number of studies on the teratogenicity of disulfiram contained significant methodological limitations. Some animal studies reported that disulfiram exposure could lead to severe limb deformities (Johnson et al. 2007), while others reported no effects other than a decrease in brain size in the female offspring (Harding and Edwards 1993). A recent study reported that disulfiram increased reproductive capacity in mice by increasing uterine vascularization (Teng et al. 2023). However, no record of pregnancy and fetal safety is available for this study, and no data on the safety of disulfiram use during breastfeeding are currently available.

14.10 Baclofen

Baclofen, a GABA-B receptor agonist, has been approved for the treatment of alcohol use disorder for the last 20 years. However, its use for this specific disorder is not yet widespread due to questionable effectiveness (Addolorato et al. 2006; Müller et al. 2015; Reynaud et al. 2017). A case series of 4 patients associated with baclofen exposure during pregnancy reported incidents of preeclampsia in the mother and small for gestational age in the infants (Morton et al. 2009). However, no teratogenicity was reported in this patient population, although the number of patients was very low ($n = 4$). A recent case report also found no congenital anomaly in the baby of a pregnant woman who received intrathecal baclofen (Yang et al. 2024). Thus, although case reports suggest that the use of baclofen is safe during pregnancy and breastfeeding (Hara et al. 2018), the current body of research is insufficient to provide a definitive conclusion on this matter.

14.11 Other Medicines

14.11.1 Nalmefene

Nalmefene is known to be particularly effective in reducing excessive consumption in alcohol use disorder and shows an effect on opioid receptors. However, its safety during pregnancy and breastfeeding has not been reported yet.

14.11.2 Biperiden

Biperiden has been prescribed to patients during pregnancy and lactation for conditions such as neuroleptic malignant syndrome and Parkinsonism. However, there is no record of its safety during pregnancy and lactation (Tüfekçioğlu et al. 2018; Escobar-Vidarte et al. 2019).

14.12 Conclusions

Pregnancy and lactation are critical periods when cautious and careful decisions regarding treatment strategies need to be made because of exposure-related adverse effects on maternal and infant health. This chapter summarized the current evidence on the safety of the use of a number of psychopharmaceuticals other than antidepressants, antipsychotics, benzodiazepines and mood stabilizers during this period. While some medications such as buprenorphine, methadone, and methylphenidate have been studied extensively during pregnancy and lactation, others such as buspirone, gabapentinoids, biperiden, pramipexole, acamprosate, baclofen, disulfiram, and naltrexone require further research to make a definitive statement about their safety (Table 14.1).

Table 14.1 Expert recommendations based on scientific evidence and clinical experience

Strong evidence is currently lacking on the safety of prescribed psychopharmaceuticals that are not included in the category of antidepressant, antipsychotic, benzodiazepine, and mood stabilizer drugs during pregnancy and lactation
Although no significant adverse events related to methadone exposure during pregnancy have been reported, buprenorphine and buprenorphine/naloxone have a more favorable safety profile during pregnancy and lactation as they prevent possible opioid withdrawal symptoms in the newborn
Buprenorphine and buprenorphine/naloxone can be used with low risk during pregnancy and breastfeeding. Since this treatment may reduce illicit drug use, clinicians can take the initiative to start treatment. However, use of the lowest possible dose and close monitoring for possible side effects are always necessary
Although meta-analyses have reported that use of naltrexone is associated with less withdrawal symptoms as well as a low risk of anomalies in the infant, studies have indeed reported congenital urogenital anomalies upon exposure in utero. Therefore, the use of naltrexone during pregnancy is associated with moderate risk. Alternative options should be considered, especially in the first trimester if possible. Although low RID values have been reported for naltrexone, the current literature is insufficient to conclude safety during lactation
Buspirone appears to be safe during breastfeeding due to its low RID values. There are no adverse reports associated with exposure during pregnancy suggesting that drug exposure may not pose any serious risks to the mother or baby. However, further studies are needed to substantiate this claim
Gabapentinoids, which are frequently used in the treatment of neuropathic pain, are generally not associated with any serious increase in risk during pregnancy. In this regard, gabapentin can be considered to have a better safety profile than pregabalin. However, the results obtained from animal studies suggest the presence of adverse effects, which should be considered when making treatment decisions

(continued)

Table 14.1 (continued)

Gabapentinoids can be used at the lowest possible doses with low-moderate risk especially for patients for whom no other treatment options are available during pregnancy. Regarding the breastfeeding period, gabapentin may be preferred to pregabalin due to its lower RID value. Pregabalin use is not recommended during breastfeeding
No anomalies have been reported regarding exposure to pramipexol during pregnancy. However, the current data are insufficient. The use of pramipexol during lactation is not recommended as it can decrease milk production
The use of methylphenidate was reported to have a slight increase in the risk of cardiac defects. Nonetheless, the existing literature is centered around the view that the use of methylphenidate during both pregnancy and breastfeeding is associated with low risks. Methylphenidate can be used at the lowest possible doses and in an intermittent manner in patients whose functionality is significantly affected. The possibility of reducing milk secretion during breastfeeding should be kept in mind
The use of acamprosate during pregnancy is generally considered to be safe, although the current data are very limited. There are no data on the safety of use during the breastfeeding period
Data on the use of disulfram during pregnancy and breastfeeding are currently insufficient, while data from the initial studies emphasized a high risk of teratogenicity. Therefore, the use of this drug is not recommended for either period
Data from case studies indicate that the use of baclofen during pregnancy may be safe; nonetheless, the available data from pregnant and lactating women are currently insufficient to reliably support the safety of the drug during these periods
Data on the use of nalmefene and biperiden during pregnancy and breastfeeding are not available in the current published literature

References

Addolorato G, Leggio L, Agabio R, Colombo G, Gasbarrini G. Baclofen: a new drug for the treatment of alcohol dependence. Int J Clin Pract. 2006;60(8):1003–8. https://doi.org/10.1111/j.1742-1241.2006.01065.x.

Afshar M, Golalipour MJ. Teratogenic effects of gabapentin on neural tube and limb development in mice. Neurosciences (Riyadh, Saudi Arabia). 2008;13(3):321–3.

Afshar M, Hassanzadeh-Taheri MM, Moallem SA, Tamizi A, Golalipour MJ. Teratogenic effects of gabapentin on the skeletal system of Balb/C mice fetuses. Neurosciences (Riyadh, Saudi Arabia). 2009;14(3):239–44.

Antonelli M, Ferrulli A, Sestito L, Vassallo GA, Tarli C, Mosoni C, Rando MM, Mirijello A, Gasbarrini A, Addolorato G. Alcohol addiction – the safety of available approved treatment options. Expert Opin Drug Saf. 2018;17(2):169–77. https://doi.org/10.1080/14740338.2018.1404025.

Atluru S, Bruehlman AK, Vaughn P, Schauberger CW, Smid MC. Naltrexone compared with buprenorphine or methadone in pregnancy: a systematic review. Obstet Gynecol. 2024;143(3):403–10. https://doi.org/10.1097/AOG.0000000000005510.

Baker AS, Wales R, Noe O, Gaccione P, Freeman MP, Cohen LS. The course of ADHD during pregnancy. J Atten Disord. 2022;26(2):143–8. https://doi.org/10.1177/1087054720975864.

Bang Madsen K, Bliddal M, Skoglund CB, Larsson H, Munk-Olsen T, Madsen MG, Hove Thomsen P, Bergink V, Srinivas C, Cohen JM, Brikell I, Liu X. Attention-deficit hyperactivity disorder (ADHD) medication use trajectories among women in the perinatal period. CNS Drugs. 2024;38(4):303–14. https://doi.org/10.1007/s40263-024-01076-1.

Beau AB, Mo J, Moisset X, Bénévent J, Damase-Michel C. Systematic review of gabapentinoid use during pregnancy and its impact on pregnancy and childhood outcomes: a ConcePTION study. Therapie. 2024;24 https://doi.org/10.1016/j.therap.2024.10.049.

Benbir G, Ertan S, Ozekmekci S. Successful pregnancy and delivery in a patient with Parkinson's disease under pramipexole treatment. Presse Med. 2014;43(1):83–5. https://doi.org/10.1016/j.lpm.2013.01.067.

Bjørk MH, Zoega H, Leinonen MK, Cohen JM, Dreier JW, Furu K, Gilhus NE, Gissler M, Hálfdánarson Ó, Igland J, Sun Y, Tomson T, Alvestad S, Christensen J. Association of Prenatal Exposure to Antiseizure medication with risk of autism and intellectual disability. JAMA Neurol. 2022;79(7):672–81. https://doi.org/10.1001/jamaneurol.2022.1269.

Blotière PO, Raguideau F, Weill A, Elefant E, Perthus I, Goulet V, Rouget F, Zureik M, Coste J, Dray-Spira R. Risks of 23 specific malformations associated with prenatal exposure to 10 antiepileptic drugs. Neurology. 2019;93(2):e167–80. https://doi.org/10.1212/WNL.0000000000007696.

Blotière PO, Miranda S, Weill A, Mikaeloff Y, Peyre H, Ramus F, Mahmoud Z, Coste J, Dray-Spira R. Risk of early neurodevelopmental outcomes associated with prenatal exposure to the antiepileptic drugs most commonly used during pregnancy: a French nationwide population-based cohort study. BMJ Open. 2020;10(6):e034829. https://doi.org/10.1136/bmjopen-2019-034829.

Bolea-Alamanac BM, Green A, Verma G, Maxwell P, Davies SJ. Methylphenidate use in pregnancy and lactation: a systematic review of evidence. Br J Clin Pharmacol. 2014;77(1):96–101. https://doi.org/10.1111/bcp.12138.

Briggs, G. F., Towers, R. K., Craig, V., & Forinash Alicia, B. Drugs in pregnancy and lactation: a reference guide to fetal and neonatal risk. Eleventh. Lippincott Williams & Wilkins; 2017.

Cajú FM, Queiroz GCDA, Torres SM, Tenório BM, Júnior VAS. Opioid system manipulation during testicular development: results on sperm production and sertoli cells population. Acta Sci Biol Sci. 2011;33(2):219–25.

Cetinkal A, Cakir A. Does gabapentin affect neural tube development? Experimental study using an early stage chick embryo model. Turk Neurosurg. 2021;31(6):967–72. https://doi.org/10.5137/1019-5149.JTN.34412-21.3.

Chan CF, Page-Sharp M, Kristensen JH, O'Neil G, Ilett KF. Transfer of naltrexone and its metabolite 6,beta-naltrexol into human milk. J Hum Lact. 2004;20(3):322–6. https://doi.org/10.1177/0890334404266881.

Chen HH, Chiang YC, Yuan ZF, Kuo CC, Lai MD, Hung TW, Ho IK, Chen ST. Buprenorphine, methadone, and morphine treatment during pregnancy: behavioral effects on the offspring in rats. Neuropsychiatr Dis Treat. 2015;11:609–18. https://doi.org/10.2147/NDT.S70585.

Collin-Lévesque L, El-Ghaddaf Y, Genest M, Jutras M, Leclair G, Weisskopf E, Panchaud A, Ferreira E. Infant exposure to methylphenidate and duloxetine during lactation. Breastfeed Med. 2018;13(3):221–5. https://doi.org/10.1089/bfm.2017.0126.

Daly FM, Hughes RN, Woodward LJ. Subsequent anxiety-related behavior in rats exposed to low-dose methadone during gestation, lactation or both periods consecutively. Pharmacol Biochem Behav. 2012;102(2):381–9. https://doi.org/10.1016/j.pbb.2012.05.010.

Damer EA, Edens MA, van der Loos MLM, van Esenkbrink J, Bunkers I, van Roon EN, Ter Horst PGJ. Fifteen years' experience with methylphenidate for attention-deficit disorder during pregnancy: effects on birth weight, Apgar score and congenital malformation rates. Gen Hosp Psychiatry. 2021;73:9–15. https://doi.org/10.1016/j.genhosppsych.2021.09.003.

di Giacomo E, Confalonieri V, Tofani F, Clerici M. Methylphenidate and atomoxetine in pregnancy and possible adverse fetal outcomes: a systematic review and meta-analysis. JAMA Netw Open. 2024;7(11):e2443648. https://doi.org/10.1001/jamanetworkopen.2024.43648.

Dostal M, Weber-Schoendorfer C, Sobesky J, Schaefer C. Pregnancy outcome following use of levodopa, pramipexole, ropinirole, and rotigotine for restless legs syndrome during pregnancy: a case series. Eur J Neurol. 2013;20(9):1241–6. https://doi.org/10.1111/ene.12001.

Dudukina E, Szépligeti SK, Karlsson P, Asomaning K, Daltveit AK, Hakkarainen K, Hoti F, Kieler H, Lunde A, Odsbu I, Rantanen M, Reutfors J, Saarelainen L, Ehrenstein V, Toft G. Prenatal exposure to pregabalin, birth outcomes and neurodevelopment – a population-based cohort study in four Nordic countries. Drug Saf. 2023;46(7):661–75. https://doi.org/10.1007/s40264-023-01307-2.

Erisgin Z, Ayas B, Nyengaard JR, Ercument Beyhun N, Terzi Y. The neurotoxic effects of prenatal gabapentin and oxcarbazepine exposure on newborn rats. J Matern Fetal Neonatal Med. 2019;32(3):461–71. https://doi.org/10.1080/14767058.2017.1383378.

Escobar-Vidarte MF, Loaiza-Osorio S, Messa AA, Macías GE. Neuroleptic malignant syndrome in pregnancy: case report and literature review. J Matern Fetal Neonatal Med. 2019;32(14):2438–41. https://doi.org/10.1080/14767058.2018.1432591.

Farid WO, Lawrence AJ, Krstew EV, Tait RJ, Hulse GK, Dunlop SA. Maternally administered sustained-release naltrexone in rats affects offspring neurochemistry and behaviour in adulthood. PLoS One. 2012;7(12):e52812. https://doi.org/10.1371/journal.pone.0052812.

Freeman MP, Szpunar MJ, Kobylski LA, Harmon H, Viguera AC, Cohen LS. Pregnancy outcomes after first-trimester exposure to buspirone: prospective longitudinal outcomes from the MGH National Pregnancy Registry for psychiatric medications. Arch Womens Ment Health. 2022;25(5):923–8. https://doi.org/10.1007/s00737-022-01250-8.

Fujii H, Goel A, Bernard N, Pistelli A, Yates LM, Stephens S, Han JY, Matsui D, Etwell F, Einarson TR, Koren G, Einarson A. Pregnancy outcomes following gabapentin use: results of a prospective comparative cohort study. Neurology. 2013;80(17):1565–70. https://doi.org/10.1212/WNL.0b013e31828f18c1.

Goodman CW, Brett AS. A clinical overview of off-label use of Gabapentinoid drugs. JAMA Intern Med. 2019;179(5):695–701. https://doi.org/10.1001/jamainternmed.2019.0086.

Hara T, Nakajima M, Sugano H, Karagiozov K, Hirose E, Goto K, Arai H. Pregnancy and breastfeeding during intrathecal baclofen therapy – a case study and review. NMC Case Rep J. 2018;5(3):65–8. https://doi.org/10.2176/nmccrj.cr.2017-0191.

Harding AJ, Edwards MJ. Retardation of prenatal brain growth of Guinea pigs by disulfiram 1. Congenit Anom. 1993;33(3):197–202.

Humerickhouse C, Pressly M, Lin Z, Guinn D, Samuels S, Pfuma Fletcher E, Schmidt S. Informing the risk assessment related to lactation and drug exposure: a physiologically based pharmacokinetic lactation model for pregabalin. CPT Pharmacometrics Syst Pharmacol. 2024;13(11):1953–66. https://doi.org/10.1002/psp4.13266.

Jansson LM, Choo R, Velez ML, Harrow C, Schroeder JR, Shakleya DM, Huestis MA. Methadone maintenance and breastfeeding in the neonatal period. Pediatrics. 2008;121(1):106–14. https://doi.org/10.1542/peds.2007-1182.

Jansson LM, Spencer N, McConnell K, Velez M, Tuten M, Harrow CA, Jones HE, Swortwood MJ, Barnes AJ, Scheidweiler KB, Huestis MA. Maternal buprenorphine maintenance and lactation. J Hum Lact. 2016;32(4):675–81. https://doi.org/10.1177/0890334416663198.

Jansson LM, McConnell K, Velez M, Spencer N, Gomonit M, Swortwood MJ. Buprenorphine-naloxone maintenance and lactation. J Hum Lact. 2024;40(1):113–9. https://doi.org/10.1177/08903344231209304.

Javadi-Paydar M, Lesani A, Vakilipour R, Ghazi P, Tavangar SM, Hantoushzadeh S, Norouzi A, Dehpour AR. Evaluation of the tocolytic effect of morphine in a mouse model of lipopolysaccharide-induced preterm delivery: the role of nitric oxide. Eur J Obstet Gynecol Reprod Biol. 2009;147(2):166–72. https://doi.org/10.1016/j.ejogrb.2009.08.014.

Jiang HY, Zhang X, Jiang CM, Fu HB. Maternal and neonatal outcomes after exposure to ADHD medication during pregnancy: a systematic review and meta-analysis. Pharmacoepidemiol Drug Saf. 2019;28(3):288–95. https://doi.org/10.1002/pds.4716.

Johnson CS, Zucker RM, Hunter ES 3rd, Sulik KK. Perturbation of retinoic acid (RA)-mediated limb development suggests a role for diminished RA signaling in the teratogenesis of ethanol. Birth Defects Res A Clin Mol Teratol. 2007;79(9):631–41. https://doi.org/10.1002/bdra.20385.

Kanervo MM, Tupola SJ, Nikkola EM, Rantakari KM, Kahila HK. Buprenorphine-naloxone, buprenorphine, and methadone throughout pregnancy in maternal opioid use disorder. Acta Obstet Gynecol Scand. 2023;102(3):313–22. https://doi.org/10.1111/aogs.14497.

Kaskal M, Kuru B, Erkoseoglu I, Yilmaz H, Karadas B, Goren MZ. Evaluation of the teratogenic effects of pregabalin usage during pregnancy: a multicenter case-control study. Northern Clin Istanbul. 2024;11(5):460–5. https://doi.org/10.14744/nci.2024.57702.

Kelty E, Hulse G. A retrospective cohort study of birth outcomes in neonates exposed to naltrexone in utero: a comparison with methadone-, buprenorphine- and non-opioid-exposed neonates. Drugs. 2017a;77(11):1211–9. https://doi.org/10.1007/s40265-017-0763-8.

Kelty E, Hulse G. A retrospective cohort study of the health of children prenatally exposed to methadone, buprenorphine or naltrexone compared with non-exposed control children. Am J Addict. 2017b;26(8):845–51. https://doi.org/10.1111/ajad.12642.

Kelty E, Hulse G. A retrospective cohort study of obstetric outcomes in opioid-dependent women treated with implant naltrexone, oral methadone or sublingual buprenorphine, and non-dependent controls. Drugs. 2017c;77(11):1199–210. https://doi.org/10.1007/s40265-017-0762-9.

Kelty E, Tran D, Lavin T, Preen DB, Hulse G, Havard A. Prevalence and safety of acamprosate use in pregnant alcohol-dependent women in New South Wales, Australia. Addiction. 2019;114(2):206–15. https://doi.org/10.1111/add.14429.

Kinsella M, Halliday LOE, Shaw M, Capel Y, Nelson SM, Kearns RJ. Buprenorphine compared with methadone in pregnancy: a systematic review and meta-analysis. Subst Use Misuse. 2022;57(9):1400–16. https://doi.org/10.1080/10826084.2022.2083174.

Kittel-Schneider S, Quednow BB, Leutritz AL, McNeill RV, Reif A. Parental ADHD in pregnancy and the postpartum period – a systematic review. Neurosci Biobehav Rev. 2021;124:63–77. https://doi.org/10.1016/j.neubiorev.2021.01.002.

Kolding L, Ehrenstein V, Pedersen L, Sandager P, Petersen OB, Uldbjerg N, Pedersen LH. Associations between ADHD medication use in pregnancy and severe malformations based on prenatal and postnatal diagnoses: a Danish registry-based study. J Clin Psychiatry. 2021;82(1):20m13458. https://doi.org/10.4088/JCP.20m13458.

Kongstorp M, Bogen IL, Stiris T, Andersen JM. Prenatal exposure to methadone or buprenorphine impairs cognitive performance in young adult rats. Drug Alcohol Depend. 2020;212:108008. https://doi.org/10.1016/j.drugalcdep.2020.108008.

Koren G, Barer Y, Ornoy A. Fetal safety of methylphenidate-a scoping review and meta analysis. Reprod Toxicol (Elmsford, NY). 2020;93:230–4. https://doi.org/10.1016/j.reprotox.2020.03.003.

Kremer M, Salvat E, Muller A, Yalcin I, Barrot M. Antidepressants and gabapentinoids in neuropathic pain: mechanistic insights. Neuroscience. 2016;338:183–206. https://doi.org/10.1016/j.neuroscience.2016.06.057.

Kristensen JH, Ilett KF, Hackett LP, Kohan R. Gabapentin and breastfeeding: a case report. J Hum Lact. 2006;22(4):426–8. https://doi.org/10.1177/0890334406293421.

Krutsch K, Campbell L, Baker T, Datta P. Alleviating anxiety while breastfeeding: evaluating buspirone transfer into human milk. Arch Womens Ment Health. 2024;27(4):619–23. https://doi.org/10.1007/s00737-024-01445-1.

Lockwood PA, Pauer L, Scavone JM, Allard M, Mendes da Costa L, Alebic-Kolbah T, Plotka A, Alvey CW, Chew ML. The pharmacokinetics of Pregabalin in breast milk, plasma, and urine of healthy postpartum women. J Hum Lact. 2016;32(3):NP1–NP8. https://doi.org/10.1177/0890334415626148.

Luo Z, Shen Y, Liang M, Miao J, Mei Y, Wang Y, Qin Y. Pharmacokinetics and bioequivalence evaluation of acamprosate calcium tablets in healthy Chinese volunteers. Eur J Pharm Sci. 2015;79:67–72. https://doi.org/10.1016/j.ejps.2015.09.003.

Mantri S, Cheng AC, Saia K, Shrestha H, Amgott R, Bressler J, Werler MM, Carter G, Jones HE, Wachman EM. Neurobehavioral outcomes of infants exposed to buprenorphine-naloxone compared with naltrexone during pregnancy. Early Hum Dev. 2024;194:106051. https://doi.org/10.1016/j.earlhumdev.2024.106051.

Margulis AV, Hernandez-Diaz S, McElrath T, Rothman KJ, Plana E, Almqvist C, D'Onofrio BM, Oberg AS. Relation of in-utero exposure to antiepileptic drugs to pregnancy duration and size at birth. PLoS One. 2019;14(8):e0214180. https://doi.org/10.1371/journal.pone.0214180.

McLaughlin PJ. Exposure to the opioid antagonist naltrexone throughout gestation alters postnatal heart development. Biol Neonate. 2002;82(3):207–16. https://doi.org/10.1159/000063611.

Morton CM, Rosenow J, Wong C, Kirschner KL. Intrathecal baclofen administration during pregnancy: a case series and focused clinical review. PM&R. 2009;1(11):1025–9. https://doi.org/10.1016/j.pmrj.2009.07.010.

Mostacci B, Poluzzi E, D'Alessandro R, Cocchi G, Tinuper P. Adverse pregnancy outcomes in women exposed to gabapentin and pregabalin: data from a population-based study. J Neurol Neurosurg Psychiatry. 2018;89(2):223–4. https://doi.org/10.1136/jnnp-2017-316143.

Müller CA, Geisel O, Pelz P, Higl V, Krüger J, Stickel A, Beck A, Wernecke KD, Hellweg R, Heinz A. High-dose baclofen for the treatment of alcohol dependence (BACLAD study): a randomized, placebo-controlled trial. Eur Neuropsychopharmacol. 2015;25(8):1167–77. https://doi.org/10.1016/j.euroneuro.2015.04.002.

Mutschler J, Grosshans M, Soyka M, Rösner S. Current findings and mechanisms of action of disulfiram in the treatment of alcohol dependence. Pharmacopsychiatry. 2016;49(4):137–41. https://doi.org/10.1055/s-0042-103592.

Ohman I, Vitols S, Tomson T. Pharmacokinetics of gabapentin during delivery, in the neonatal period, and lactation: does a fetal accumulation occur during pregnancy? Epilepsia. 2005;46(10):1621–4. https://doi.org/10.1111/j.1528-1167.2005.00251.x.

Ordean A, Tubman-Broeren M. Safety and efficacy of buprenorphine-naloxone in pregnancy: a systematic review of the literature. Pathophysiology. 2023;30(1):27–36. https://doi.org/10.3390/pathophysiology30010004.

Ornoy A. Pharmacological treatment of attention deficit hyperactivity disorder during pregnancy and lactation. Pharm Res. 2018;35(3):46. https://doi.org/10.1007/s11095-017-2323-z.

Ozalp Horsanalı B, Yımaz H, Uyar M, Eyigör C. Gabapentinoids and lactation: review of the literature. J Turk Soc Algol. 2024;36(1):64–7. https://doi.org/10.14744/agri.2021.55531.

Pačesová D, Spišská V, Novotný J, Bendová Z. Methadone administered to rat dams during pregnancy and lactation affects the circadian rhythms of their pups. J Neurosci Res. 2023;101(11):1737–56. https://doi.org/10.1002/jnr.25236.

Patorno E, Hernandez-Diaz S, Huybrechts KF, Desai RJ, Cohen JM, Mogun H, Bateman BT. Gabapentin in pregnancy and the risk of adverse neonatal and maternal outcomes: a population-based cohort study nested in the US Medicaid analytic eXtract dataset. PLoS Med. 2020;17(9):e1003322. https://doi.org/10.1371/journal.pmed.1003322.

Picchietti DL, Hensley JG, Bainbridge JL, Lee KA, Manconi M, McGregor JA, Silver RM, Trenkwalder C, Walters AS. Consensus clinical practice guidelines for the diagnosis and treatment of restless legs syndrome/Willis-Ekbom disease during pregnancy and lactation. Sleep Med Rev. 2015;22:64–77. https://doi.org/10.1016/j.smrv.2014.10.009.

Prakash PLV, Rai R, Pai MM, Yadav SK, et al. Teratogenic effects of the anticonvulsant gabapentin in mice. Singapore Med J. 2008;49(1):47–53.

Quintrell E, Wyrwoll C, Rosenow T, Larcombe A, Kelty E. The effects of acamprosate on maternal and neonatal outcomes in a mouse model of alcohol use disorders. Physiol Behav. 2023;259:114037. https://doi.org/10.1016/j.physbeh.2022.114037.

Quintrell E, Russell DJ, Rahmannia S, Wyrwoll CS, Larcombe A, Kelty E. The safety of alcohol pharmacotherapies in pregnancy: a scoping review of human and animal research. CNS Drugs. 2025;39(1):23–37. https://doi.org/10.1007/s40263-024-01126-8.

Reynaud M, Aubin HJ, Trinquet F, Zakine B, Dano C, Dematteis M, Trojak B, Paille F, Detilleux M. A randomized, placebo-controlled study of high-dose baclofen in alcohol-dependent patients-the ALPADIR study. Alcohol Alcoholism (Oxford, Oxfordshire). 2017;52(4):439–46. https://doi.org/10.1093/alcalc/agx030.

Richardson JL, Damkier P, Diav-Citrin O, George N, Greenall AJ, Oliver AM, Stephens S, Hodson KK. A critical appraisal of controlled studies investigating malformation risks following pregabalin use in early pregnancy. Br J Clin Pharmacol. 2023;89(2):630–40. https://doi.org/10.1111/bcp.15607.

Sauberan JB. FDA Pregnancy and lactation labeling rule, considerations for population lactation section 8.2. Available at: https://www.fda.gov/media/97055/download. Accessed 04 Jan 2025.

Scoten O, Tabi K, Paquette V, Carrion P, Ryan D, Radonjic NV, Whitham EA, Hippman C. Attention-deficit/hyperactivity disorder in pregnancy and the postpartum period. Am J Obstet Gynecol. 2024;231(1):19–35. https://doi.org/10.1016/j.ajog.2024.02.297.
Suarez EA, Huybrechts KF, Straub L, Hernández-Díaz S, Jones HE, Connery HS, Davis JM, Gray KJ, Lester B, Terplan M, Mogun H, Bateman BT. Buprenorphine versus methadone for opioid use disorder in pregnancy. N Engl J Med. 2022;387(22):2033–44. https://doi.org/10.1056/NEJMoa2203318.
Szpunar MJ, Freeman MP, Kobylski LA, Rossa ET, Gaccione P, Chitayat D, Viguera AC, Cohen LS. Risk of major malformations in infants after first-trimester exposure to stimulants: results from the Massachusetts General Hospital National Pregnancy Registry for psychiatric medications. J Clin Psychopharmacol. 2023;43(4):326–32. https://doi.org/10.1097/JCP.0000000000001702.
Teng M, Luo Y, Wang C, Lei A. Effect of disulfiram on the reproductive capacity of female mice. Int J Mol Sci. 2023;24(3):2371. https://doi.org/10.3390/ijms24032371.
Towers CV, Katz E, Weitz B, Visconti K. Use of naltrexone in treating opioid use disorder in pregnancy. Am J Obstet Gynecol. 2020;222(1):83.e1–8. https://doi.org/10.1016/j.ajog.2019.07.037.
Tüfekçioğlu Z, Hanağası H, Yalçın Çakmaklı G, Elibol B, Esmeli Tokuçoğlu F, Kaya ZE, Ertan S, Özekmekçi S, Emre M. Use of anti-Parkinson medication during pregnancy: a case series. J Neurol. 2018;265(8):1922–9. https://doi.org/10.1007/s00415-018-8937-1.
Vajda FJE, O'Brien TJ, Graham J, Hitchcock AA, Lander CM, Eadie MJ. Anti-epileptic drug exposure and risk of foetal death in utero. Acta Neurol Scand. 2018;137(1):20–3. https://doi.org/10.1111/ane.12816.
Wachman EM, Saia K, Miller M, Valle E, Shrestha H, Carter G, Werler M, Jones H. Naltrexone treatment for pregnant women with opioid use disorder compared with matched buprenorphine control subjects. Clin Ther. 2019;41(9):1681–9. https://doi.org/10.1016/j.clinthera.2019.07.003.
Yang K, Mistry PD, Richeimer SH. Intrathecal baclofen pump in pregnancy: case report, literature review, and management considerations. Reg Anesth Pain Med. 2024;49(12):919–22. https://doi.org/10.1136/rapm-2024-105569.
Youngentob SL, Kent PF, Youngentob LM. Gestational naltrexone ameliorates fetal ethanol exposures enhancing effect on the postnatal behavioral and neural response to ethanol. Exp Biol Med (Maywood). 2012;237(10):1197–208. https://doi.org/10.1258/ebm.2012.012132.

Part III

Pharmacological Management of Psychiatric Disorders During the Perinatal Period

15 Major Depression

Sonya Rasminsky and Vivien K. Burt

15.1 Introduction

The treatment of pregnant and postpartum women has come to be viewed mainly as a concern of reproductive psychiatrists. However, since more than 10% of women ages 18–39 in the United States now take antidepressants (Brody 2020) and half of all pregnancies are unplanned, perinatal psychiatry has become the purview of all psychiatrists who treat women of childbearing age. Furthermore, depression during pregnancy is common, and the use of antidepressants in pregnancy has been steadily increasing over the past two decades (Mitchell et al. 2011; Huybrechts et al. 2013). The postpartum period is an especially vulnerable time for mood disorders, particularly for women with histories of perinatal depression.

After careful analysis and consideration of both the strengths and limitations of the evidence-based data on psychopharmacologic management of depression in pregnancy and the postpartum, the challenge for psychiatrists who treat women of childbearing age is to facilitate the generation of a plan that optimizes outcomes for their patients while considering possible implications for their potential offspring. Given the underlying reality of an uncertain future, treatment recommendations should be carefully individualized, taking into consideration both the most current scientific data and the patient's values and preferences.

Sensitive to the lingering stigma associated with psychiatric disorders, women who struggle with perinatal depression are often reluctant to voice their suffering to even close family or friends. The internet is replete with advice, often based on personal experiences from women who are themselves depressed; new publications about antidepressants in pregnancy garner dramatic headlines regardless of their

S. Rasminsky (✉) · V. K. Burt (✉)
Department of Psychiatry and Biobehavioral Sciences, University of California, Los Angeles, David Geffen School of Medicine, Los Angeles, CA, USA
e-mail: srasminsky@mednet.ucla.edu; vburt@mednet.ucla.edu

F. Uguz, L. Orsolini (eds.), *Perinatal Psychopharmacology*, https://doi.org/10.1007/978-3-031-99720-4_15

scientific merit. Faced with worrisome information in the media, pregnant depressed women often hesitate to seek help that may include necessary advice about medication. Since depression is often accompanied by uncertainty, poor self-esteem, and a lack of confidence, these women fear that they will be viewed as weak, flawed, or complaining. For women who struggle with perinatal depression, their sense of incompetence often contributes to a feeling of isolation and alienation.

Fortunately, women with histories of depression are increasingly requesting psychiatric consultation because they wish to plan ahead in order to maximize positive outcomes for themselves and their babies. Women present at various points: some are not currently pregnant but may become pregnant in the future; some seek treatment during different trimesters of pregnancy; some are newly postpartum or present later in the first postpartum year. Unfortunately, many women and referring clinicians have limited knowledge about treatment options in these settings, and the knowledge they do have is often tainted by misinformation and misunderstanding.

Like all patients who present for psychiatric treatment, women's needs vary based on psychiatric and medical history, psychosocial stressors, personal and partner values, and a myriad of other factors, all specific to each patient. Nevertheless, a unifying goal when treating women in the perinatal period is to maximize mental health and recognize that maternal depression impacts the entire family.

15.2 Decision-Making in the Perinatal Period

Pharmacologic treatment of depression during pregnancy has become increasingly common, with approximately 6–8% of women taking antidepressants during pregnancy (Andrade et al. 2016; Huybrechts et al. 2013). Traditionally, the decision about whether to take psychotropic medications during pregnancy has been described as a risk-benefit analysis, when it is more correctly framed as a risk-risk analysis. Since there are no randomized placebo-controlled studies on the effects of psychotropic medication and depression (or other psychiatric disorders) on pregnancy and infant outcomes, conclusions are largely based on case-control or cohort studies. Many of these are observational studies derived from clinical databases and thus are subject to confounding variables. The most troubling of these is that existing studies have not been able to analyze whether adverse outcomes are associated with antenatal psychotropic medications or the condition for which the medications have been prescribed ("confounding by indication"). It is incumbent upon clinicians to help patients sort through alternative options, while understanding the incomplete and uncertain nature of available data.

For some women, the decision may be to "watch and wait" with close psychiatric monitoring without immediate pharmacologic intervention, often with ongoing psychotherapy. For others, the choice may be an antidepressant, possibly with other psychiatric medications when needed, to relieve depression and associated symptoms. Data on various treatment approaches should be deciphered for each patient, with an understanding that no one study is perfect. Patients need to be reminded that the background risk of congenital abnormalities is 3–5% (Stallings et al. 2024).

Using an honest, empathic approach, discussion should ideally incorporate a mutual understanding that to expect perfection is to guarantee disappointment. The goal is to help each patient understand the available data (with its strengths and limitations) and then to arrive at a decision that she can most comfortably live with.

No two patients are the same. What one woman can accept in terms of risk is different from what another woman deems reasonable. How a woman has addressed stressful decisions in the past is likely to inform how she will deal with decisions regarding psychiatric treatment during pregnancy and the postpartum. Risk assessment should optimally include both the perinatal patient and her partner. A stable and supportive family and social network is critical to helping the pregnant or postpartum woman live comfortably with the treatment regimen she has chosen. It is often advisable for the treating clinician to facilitate other avenues of support (e.g., individual psychotherapy, couples' counseling, perinatal support groups). Frequently, although decisions have been made to move forward with pharmacologic treatment, doubts and new questions arise as new studies are published and reported in the popular media. Clinicians should be readily available to review existing and new data and its interpretation in ways that are clear and understandable for the patient.

15.3 Assessment of the Perinatal Patient

The treatment of perinatal depression begins with a thorough clinical and psychosocial assessment, with the goals both of assessing personal risk and also eliciting patient knowledge and preference. Because a large body of information already exists on the assessment of the general psychiatric patient, this section will focus on the unique aspects of the assessment of women who either desire to become pregnant or are currently pregnant or postpartum. For a detailed list of the components specific to assessing the perinatal patient, see Table 15.1.

The initial evaluation should include questions about the patient's feelings and expectations regarding pregnancy and motherhood. Her experience with previous pregnancies (both emotionally and obstetrically) will inform those expectations. In a woman who is not yet pregnant, an exploration of her relationship to her body, previous weight changes, and eating habits may be informative regarding how she will experience bodily changes and weight gain during pregnancy. If the patient is already pregnant, was the pregnancy planned? What are the patient's thoughts regarding plans for delivery and infant feeding (breastfeeding, pumping, or formula), and what are her resources for support during and after pregnancy?

The perinatal postpartum patient should be observed for interactions with her baby and with older children, since bonding and attachment can be compromised by maternal mental illness. Telepsychiatry, increasingly common since the COVID-19 pandemic, facilitates these observations by providing the opportunity to evaluate patients in their homes. In addition to allowing the clinician to observe the physical home environment, virtual visits provide a close-up view of mother-child and partner interactions—information that can be difficult to glean in an office setting. At

Table 15.1 Assessment of the perinatal patient: clinically significant considerations

Component	Consideration
Clinical issues	Assess for psychiatric symptoms in relation to: Pregnancy (past or present)—Including history of birth trauma or pregnancy loss Postpartum (past or present)—Include whether breast-feeding, supplementing with formula, or weaning Premenstrual mood changes History of abortion Infertility treatment Inquire about past or present symptoms or signs of eating disorder or body image perceptions that may be particularly problematic during pregnancy or the postpartum
Medications	Inquire about effectiveness: What has been helpful in the past? Is the patient taking medications now? Are they effective? Any side effects? Inquire about beliefs and understanding regarding the use of medication during pregnancy, breastfeeding
Alcohol and drug use	Inquire about past or present use of alcohol or illicit drugs Inquire about the use of cannabis Inquire about the use of painkillers Rule out possible covert use
Family psychiatric history	Include history of psychiatric instability in female family members in relation to pregnancy, postpartum
Medical history	Rule out illnesses that may emerge or exacerbate in pregnancy or postpartum (e.g., lupus, thyroiditis, fibromyalgia)
Social and developmental history	Inquire about current relationships—Is there a partner, are they supportive, psychologically aware? Note history of emotional response and level of functioning in response to past transitions, role changes, or traumatic events Assess level of economic support as this may relate to ability to get extra help if needed for child care and other responsibilities Inquire about religious or cultural views that may be relevant to interactions with the baby or may influence the patient's ability to understand and accept treatment recommendations.
Views and plans regarding pregnancy, postpartum, and parenthood	Inquire about expectations regarding pregnancy, motherhood Inquire about plans for antenatal care, delivery, postpartum preparations, childcare, breastfeeding
Evaluate level of functioning	If postpartum, observe for interactions, bonding with baby, other children (especially other children at home)
Assess for issues of safety	Inquire about thoughts of self-harm, harm to others (especially infant, if postpartum) Establish whether any thoughts of harm are ego-syntonic or ego-dystonic Connect with child welfare authorities if needed for further assessment

the same time, telepsychiatry may alert the observant clinician to the need to see a patient in person, particularly if she is too distracted at home to focus on the appointment, or if safety issues are of concern. If a clinician observes psychotic signs or symptoms, or serious behavioral aberrations that appear to impact the safety and care of the infant or other children in the home, it is essential to arrange for an in-person evaluation.

The perinatal patient should be evaluated both for thoughts of self-harm and for thoughts of harm towards infants and children. In the event that a mother has thoughts of harming her child, it is important to assess whether these thoughts are ego-syntonic or dystonic. Ego-syntonic thoughts of harming one's child suggest psychosis and invariably warrant intensive inpatient care. Ego-dystonic thoughts may be indicative of obsessive-compulsive illness that, while disabling, does not directly endanger the child. Only by carefully teasing out the nature of such thoughts can the astute clinician assess whether child-care authorities should be called for further evaluation of possible safety concerns in the home.

Newly pregnant women are at substantial risk for recurrence if they discontinue the medications that have kept them well (Cohen et al. 2006). Thus, recommendations regarding medication are based not only on the patient's current presentation, but also on her history. Of particular importance to the perinatal assessment is a detailed history of response to prior treatment regimens during past pregnancies and postpartum periods, as this may guide future interventions.

A thorough reproductive history includes eliciting timing of menarche, menstrual irregularities, history of premenstrual psychiatric symptoms and response to hormonal birth control, infertility treatments, and number and outcome of past pregnancies. Since past response to hormonal changes may be predictive of psychiatric status during the perinatal period, this information can be a useful guide. A patient who is older or has a history of prior losses, miscarriages, traumatic deliveries, or repeated assisted reproductive procedures may understand and interpret available data quite differently from a younger pregnant woman with no past obstetrical stressors and considerable time ahead in which to achieve emotional stability prior to conception.

Given the impact of alcohol and other substances on pregnancy, a substance use history is essential to the perinatal evaluation. It is well known that alcohol use during pregnancy increases the risk of miscarriage, preterm birth, stillbirth, and sudden infant death syndrome (SIDS) and is associated with lifelong behavioral, intellectual, and physical disabilities known as fetal alcohol spectrum disorders (FASDs). Less is known about the effects of cannabis, but increasing evidence suggests that gestational exposure is associated with increased risk of low birth weight, small for gestational age, preterm birth (Baia and Domingues 2024), a small but statistically significant increased risk of birth defects (Andrade 2024), and potential risk of psychiatric disorders in exposed offspring (Bassalov et al. 2024). Given the increasing availability of cannabis among the general population, and increased use due to legalization in many locations, clinicians should counsel their perinatal patients about the dearth of substantive rigorous data regarding teratogenicity and effects in breastfed infants.

Understanding the setting into which a baby is born is also essential. Social history includes a detailed understanding of the relationships within the family of origin, family of a partner (if involved), history of trauma, developmental difficulties, educational history, employment (including plans about returning to work after baby), financial means, relationship with partner, and social supports. A patient's personal history of parental figures may provide insight into her ability to function as she transitions into motherhood. A family history of mood disorders, particularly during the postpartum, increases the risk for perinatal depression. A patient's cultural and religious views of contraception, elective abortion, pregnancy, delivery, and breastfeeding should be discussed. What constitutes pathology for one patient may be a normal practice for another, and understanding the patient's core values and beliefs is integral to the collaborative decision-making process.

15.4 Risks of Untreated Maternal Disorders

Depressive symptoms are extremely common during and after pregnancy, with depression affecting 15–20% of pregnant women, with rates as high as 25% in middle and lower-income countries (Yin et al. 2021; Roddy Mitchell et al. 2023). Although pregnancy is not itself a risk factor for depression, for women who enter pregnancy euthymic and on antidepressant medication, discontinuation of their medication increases the risk for recurrence of their symptoms (Cohen et al. 2006). Depression during pregnancy carries with it significant morbidity for both the expectant mother and her developing fetus, and can have a downstream impact on risk of postpartum depression and child development. Depression during pregnancy can lead to challenges following prenatal directions and difficulty eating a balanced diet or gaining the recommended amount of weight, which can in turn have a negative effect on maternal obstetrical health and the health of the infant. Adverse effects of untreated depression during pregnancy may include hypertension, pre-eclampsia, preterm birth, spontaneous abortion, intrauterine growth retardation, and decreased breastfeeding initiation (Ghimire et al. 2021; Jarde et al. 2016).

Women who are depressed are more likely to use alcohol, tobacco, and illicit drugs to manage their symptoms, leading to deleterious effects on the developing fetus. Seriously depressed pregnant women are at risk for suicidal thinking and attempts. When depression is severe, some women contemplate abortion, even when the pregnancy was desired and planned.

Women who experience depression during pregnancy have abnormalities of cortisol secretion, which affects the maternal hypothalamic pituitary axis and intrauterine hormonal milieu (Seth et al. 2016; Reynolds et al. 2013). It is hypothesized that this dysregulation may explain some of the negative outcomes for infants of depressed women. In addition, children born to mothers who are depressed in the perinatal period are at increased risk for mood and anxiety disorders themselves, and increasing data suggests that epigenetics may play a role (Stein et al. 2014; Abrishamcar et al. 2024).

Depression during pregnancy is a major risk factor for postpartum depression, which in turn affects child development. Maternal sensitivity to infant needs is essential for the healthy development of an infant's social, cognitive, and behavioral skills. Depressed mothers often show inconsistent parenting behaviors, contributing to adverse outcomes in their children, and children exposed to early maternal depression may have increased behavioral problems and mental health symptomatology in early childhood (Park et al. 2018).

For mothers who experience depression during the postpartum, it may be difficult to meet their infant's needs for the development of a secure attachment style, rendering the child at a higher risk for poor functioning in a range of developmental domains (López Seco et al. 2016; Wan and Green 2009). Mothers with even subclinical or mild depressive symptoms report significantly impaired bonding with their babies. They report feeling resentful, angry, and distant from their babies, and have difficulty feeling happy when their infants smile or feeling confident that they can care for their babies. Poor maternal-fetal attachment during pregnancy may contribute to abnormal maternal-infant attachment in the postpartum (Delavari et al. 2018). Successful treatment of maternal depression has been shown to have a positive impact for both mothers and their children (Weissman et al. 2006).

Partners of mothers with postpartum depression are also at risk for the development of mood and anxiety symptoms (Hoffman et al. 2017). When both parents are stressed, this places further strain on the family structure and makes it more difficult to meet the infant's needs.

15.5 Treatment of Depression During Pregnancy

Patient preference is an important consideration in the treatment of perinatal depression: what one woman may regard as unacceptable (e.g., any report of possible increased risk of autism, no matter how limited the data) may be a reasonable risk to another. While there is no one-size-fits-all strategy for managing depression during pregnancy, some general principles do apply. Table 15.2 outlines discussion points throughout pregnancy, and Table 15.3 outlines general guidelines for treatment.

If a woman is experiencing severe depression and is functionally impaired, or has a history of psychosis, suicide attempts, chronic depression, or relapses following medication discontinuation, treatment with antidepressants is advisable. In these cases, the risk of untreated maternal depression generally outweighs the risks associated with antidepressant exposure in utero. Some women with even moderate depression choose to remain on the medication that keeps them well. In such cases, so long as known risks of both depression and antidepressant medication on both mother and baby are reviewed, it is reasonable to continue pharmacologic management during pregnancy.

Nonpharmacological modalities vary from first-line options for treatment of mild disease to intensive treatment for refractory and severe depression. Psychotherapy can provide much-needed support, as well as practical tools for

Table 15.2 Discussion points for the treatment of depression in pregnancy

Pre-pregnancy
Discuss options regarding medication, ideally involving partner (partner should participate in at least one visit)
Review risks of depression during pregnancy, as well as risks of medication during pregnancy and lactation
Include information about baseline risks of major malformations (3–5%) and miscarriage (20%)
Explain that it may be necessary to adjust medication regimen to lowest effective dose of the fewest medications
Coordinate with Ob/Gyn about plan for medication during pregnancy
Recommend starting prenatal vitamins
First trimester
Review choices about medication during pregnancy.
If not done previously, review risks of depression in pregnancy, as well as risks of medication during pregnancy and lactation
Discussion should focus on first trimester exposure, e.g., risk of major malformations, risk of miscarriage
Monitor depressive symptoms and adjust medication dose as needed
Elicit feelings about motherhood
Discuss social supports during pregnancy
Coordinate with Ob/Gyn
Coordinate with therapist
Second trimester
Review choices about medication during pregnancy
Provide updates about any new data since last discussion
Monitor depressive symptoms; dose may need to be increased given changing metabolism
Discuss plans for delivery, including importance of in-hospital monitoring for babies exposed to antidepressants in utero
Begin discussion of feeding choices, e.g., breastmilk, formula, combination
Coordinate with Ob/Gyn
Coordinate with therapist
Third trimester
Review choices about medication during pregnancy
Provide updates about any new data since last discussion
Review risk of neonatal abstinence syndrome (NAS)
Monitor depressive symptoms and adjust dose as needed; do not lower dose to prevent NAS
Review plans for delivery
Provide psychoeducation about postpartum depression to both patient and partner
Continue discussion of feeding choices, and make plan for protecting mother's sleep after delivery (e.g., sharing feedings, night nurse, etc.)
Encourage patient to meet with pediatrician, especially if she is planning to take medication while breastfeeding
Discuss social supports after delivery, and help patient make plans to involve supports
Discuss plans for return to work, including childcare options

(continued)

Table 15.2 (continued)

Coordinate with Ob/Gyn
Coordinate with therapist
Postpartum
Meet 1–2 weeks after delivery
Review delivery, complications, baby's APGAR scores
Monitor depressive symptoms and adjust medication dose as needed
Discuss adjustment to motherhood and assess bonding with baby
Discuss feeding and provide support for whatever mother chooses (breastfeeding or formula)
Evaluate sleep and review plans for protecting mother's sleep
Discuss support and adjust plans for help at home
Discuss plans for return to work, including childcare options
Coordinate with Ob/Gyn
Coordinate with therapist

Table 15.3 Pharmacologic treatment of perinatal depression: guidelines and considerations

1.	The best time to devise a treatment plan in women with histories of depression is before they conceive
2.	Take care to decipher the data regarding possible medications in pregnancy or the postpartum and explain the information to the patient and preferably also her partner
3.	In general, unless there are clear adverse effects for the patient or her baby, use the medication that has worked best in the past
4.	When possible, choose medication that has the most credible safety and tolerability data
5.	Although not always possible, monotherapy is preferable to polypharmacy
6.	Use the lowest *effective* dose. Do not compromise efficacy in order to adhere to a low dose
7.	Monitor the patient frequently through pregnancy and the postpartum, adjusting the dose as needed clinically. Remember that for some medications, dose adjustments may be needed due to hormonally-influenced antidepressant metabolism, drug interactions, or changes in extracellular volume
8.	Encourage the patient to try to get as much uninterrupted sleep as possible, as this is a factor that often influences antidepressant efficacy
9.	Encourage psychotherapy as this often provides benefit to the depressed patient who is being treated with medication. If needed, couples' therapy may be helpful as well
10.	Educate the patient about treatment options with regard to breastfeeding: exclusive breastfeeding, supplementing with formula, exclusive formula feeding, etc. Explain that while most antidepressants are not contraindicated in breastfeeding, sleep is often compromised when nursing, particularly if the patient is also pumping
11.	Consider hospitalization if the patient is seriously impaired, suicidal, or a threat to others, including her baby

managing symptoms and understanding the contextual changes that accompany new motherhood. Manualized therapies such as interpersonal therapy (IPT) and cognitive behavioral therapy (CBT) have shown efficacy for treating antenatal and postpartum depression (Hankin et al. 2023; Shortis et al. 2020; van Ravesteyn et al. 2017; Sockol 2018). Bright light therapy is a noninvasive treatment for antenatal depression (Li et al. 2023). An increasing body of literature suggests that transcranial magnetic stimulation (rTMS) is both safe and effective during pregnancy (Kim et al. 2019; Lee et al. 2021). On the other end of the spectrum, electroconvulsive therapy (ECT) may be used during pregnancy for treatment of severe depression that has not responded adequately to pharmacological management. While some obstetrical complications have been reported with ECT use in pregnancy, it is largely a safe and effective treatment for patients with a heavy disease burden, particularly if suicidality is involved (Ward et al. 2018).

15.5.1 General Principles of Treatment

The decision about which medication to use is determined by a number of factors, including a particular medication's safety profile, stage of gestation, symptom profile, personal history of response to particular medications, and family history.

In general, monotherapy is preferred, and dosages should be kept at the minimum necessary to promote ongoing mood stability and normal functioning. The goal is to treat with the fewest number of medications at the minimum *effective* dose. Treatment needs may also change over time, since pharmacokinetic changes during pregnancy may lead to alterations in drug or metabolite levels, with potential need for dosing adjustments (Deligiannidis et al. 2014). If new literature emerges during the course of a pregnancy, it should be carefully interpreted and shared with the patient.

15.5.2 Safety Profile

The safety profile of antidepressants in pregnancy is outlined in Chap. 20. While there are no randomized placebo-controlled trials of antidepressants in pregnant women, registry data does provide some evidence-based guidance. There is more data available for serotonin-reuptake inhibitors (SSRIs) than other antidepressants during pregnancy, and these agents are therefore generally considered first-line treatment (McAllister-Williams et al. 2017). While serotonin-norepinephrine reuptake inhibitors (SNRIs) are less well studied than SSRIs, they have increasing data associated with their use and are a viable alternative, particularly when a patient has previously responded well to these agents. Tricyclic antidepressants have a long history of use in pregnancy and may be a reasonable choice when a patient has failed a newer medication or has a history of response to a TCA. The 2014 NICE guidelines (last updated 2020) recommend treatment with an SSRI, SNRI, or TCA.

Ketamine and eskatamine have been found to be effective for patients with serious treatment-refractory psychiatric disorders. The increasingly widespread use of these agents (especially following the US Food and Drug Administration's approval of esketamine for major depressive disorder in 2020) has raised concerns that women of childbearing age who may knowingly or unknowingly be pregnant may be exposed. A recent study found that fewer than half of clinics that dispense ketamine discuss potential impacts in pregnancy (Pacilio et al. 2024). Given that the

FDA has stated that ketamine is not recommended in pregnancy due to the sparsity of data on fetal effects in humans, treatment with ketamine and esketamine should be avoided during pregnancy.

While newer antidepressants may be touted as having fewer side effects than their older counterparts, there is generally little to no literature regarding their use in pregnancy. Unless a woman has done poorly on several better-studied treatments, there is little justification for using a medication about which we have no information.

15.5.3 Symptom Profile

For the medication-naïve patient, symptom profile should guide the choice of antidepressant. For example, if a patient is particularly agitated or suffering with insomnia, a more sedating antidepressant is a reasonable first choice. If the patient has an anergic depression, a more activating antidepressant should be considered.

15.5.4 History of Response to Particular Medications

An important factor when recommending a medication during pregnancy is a patient's own history of medication response. Since the past is generally predictive, restarting a medication that was previously effective is the most rapid and direct way to achieve remission. If the medication previously used is one with minimal data in pregnancy, it is worth considering a trial of a more-studied medication, for example an SSRI. On the other hand, a trial with a new SSRI in a patient who has previously failed to respond to another SSRI may only prolong the patient's depression. Ideally, any medication change should take place prior to pregnancy, since changing medications during pregnancy results in multiple exposures. Thus, for the younger woman (e.g., less than 35 years old, who is hoping to become pregnant, and for whom there is time to try another medication), a trial of a more studied medication such as an SSRI is a reasonable approach. However, unlike the younger patient, the woman over 35, perhaps with a history of infertility or multiple pregnancy losses, may not have reproductive time ahead to experiment with a new medication. In these cases, it is prudent to continue with a medication that has been effective, but may have somewhat less data to support its use in pregnancy.

15.5.5 Dosing

Pharmacokinetic changes during pregnancy can lead to changing drug or metabolite levels, and it is therefore possible that a dose that was previously effective will no longer work for a particular patient. Since there are no dosing parameters specific to pregnancy, standard depression dosing should be used as a starting point, with adjustments made based on clinical response. A woman should be seen frequently during pregnancy and should be made aware early in treatment that dosing may need to be increased. While previous clinical guidelines recommended decreasing the dose of antidepressants in the third trimester in order to mitigate the risk of neonatal abstinence syndrome (NAS), that strategy is no longer recommended for two reasons: (1) Decreasing the dose prior to delivery leaves a woman undertreated just as she enters the vulnerable postpartum period, and (2) Research studies have not demonstrated a decrease in NAS with lower antidepressant doses (Warburton et al. 2010; Salisbury et al. 2016).

15.6 Treatment of Postpartum Depression

The postpartum is a vulnerable time for women, particularly if they have histories of depression either before or during pregnancy. Postpartum depressed women often struggle with meeting the needs of their babies and other children while taking care of their own mental health. Like depressed pregnant women, postpartum depressed women frequently feel conflicted about the "best" treatment regimen to treat their depression while safeguarding the health of their babies.

As during pregnancy, the goal of the treating clinician should be to help new mothers accept that although the information about treatment options is necessarily limited by literature that is compromised by confounders and is constantly changing, of paramount importance is the need to recover from depression in order to maximize the best possible outcome for mother, baby, and other family members. While the information regarding treatment options is limited, it is sufficient to allow clinicians to sort through treatment options with their patients, and to facilitate thoughtful decisions that will enable a healthy and gratifying outcome for new mothers and their babies.

As discussed earlier in the chapter (see "Assessment of the perinatal patient"), the treatment of postpartum depression must include a thorough assessment of both suicide risk and risk of infanticide. If a mother is deemed at high risk of harming herself or her baby, she should be hospitalized, ideally in a setting where she can continue to have contact with her infant while being supported in her recovery. It is also important to screen depressed mothers for features associated with bipolar disorder (e.g., history of mania/hypomania, family history of bipolar disorder, switches on antidepressants, early onset of mood symptoms, etc.), since postpartum depression can sometimes be the index episode of bipolar illness (Azorin et al. 2012).

In general, if a woman has responded well to a particular medication in the past (including during pregnancy), that medication should be the starting point. SSRIs are the best studied and most frequently used medications for postpartum depression. There are very few randomized controlled trials of antidepressants for postpartum depression. Pooled estimates from a 2021 Cochrane review found that SSRIs were more effective than placebo in treating postnatal depression, but the certainty of the evidence was low (Brown et al. 2021). Medication dose should be increased to an effective dose as quickly as tolerated; caution should be exercised not to underdose a woman because she is nursing.

Most postpartum women are sleep deprived due to their babies' feeding schedules, and lack of sleep is magnified significantly when mothers choose to breastfeed (often pumping around the clock to augment milk production). Even if they are totally exhausted and suffer from increasing debilitating depression, many women feel guilty even thinking about limiting or discontinuing breastfeeding. For those depressed women who find breastfeeding to be fulfilling, they worry about exposing their babies to psychiatric medications.

From a clinical standpoint, decisions about breastfeeding should be made with attention not only to medication safety, but also to the impact on maternal mental health. If a woman finds breastfeeding to be fulfilling, she should be encouraged to continue. However, if breastfeeding worsens her depression or interferes with her ability to care for herself and her baby, she should be given permission to stop.

Most antidepressants are considered compatible with breastfeeding, with weight-adjusted maternal dose delivered through breast milk falling under the 10% threshold regarded as clinically relevant. As during pregnancy, the SSRIs are better studied during lactation than other antidepressants, and sertraline is generally considered the preferred agent due to its minimal passage into breast milk (Orsolini and Bellantuono 2015). Please see Chap. 20 for details about particular antidepressants during lactation.

When discussing options regarding the treatment of postpartum depression, it is essential to address the importance of sleep. Fatigue during the postpartum period worsens depressive symptoms, and depression contributes to further insomnia (Giallo et al. 2016). Even if a woman is breastfeeding, it can be helpful to have another person (partner, relative, night nurse) assist with night feeding, in order to allow the new mother to get one uninterrupted stretch of sleep. Depression is extremely challenging to treat when a woman is significantly sleep-deprived, and adequate sleep often goes a long way toward the successful treatment of postpartum depression. Treatment of postpartum depression should also address co-morbid anxiety, which is common in new mothers and can impact both sleep and daily functioning.

While most women can be treated with psychotherapy and antidepressants, some postpartum depression is not responsive to standard treatment. The advent of neurosteroid hormones to treat postpartum depression has opened a new avenue of treatment beyond the longstanding reliance on serotonergic antidepressants. Brexanolone, an intravenous formulation of allopregnanolone—a positive allosteric modulator of γ-aminobutyric acid ($GABA_A$) receptors—was approved by the US Food and Drug Administration in 2019 to treat postpartum depression (Powell et al. 2020). Zuranolone, its oral equivalent, was approved in 2023. Brexanolone must be administered intravenously over 60 h and can cause excessive sedation, requiring patients to be hospitalized or treated in specialized settings for about 3 days. A major advantage of zuranolone is that it is taken as a single daily pill for 2 weeks, requiring no active surveillance or specialized in-patient settings. Both brexanolone and zuranolone have rapid onset, differentiating them from traditional antidepressants. Zuranolone's antidepressant efficacy was sustained through day 45 and anxiety, global, and maternal functioning were also improved. (Deligiannidis et al.

2021). There is very little data about zuranolone and breastfeeding. Although a single study in 14 patients found very little passage of zuranolone into breastmilk (1% of the maternal dose), more data is needed to assess the effect on exposed breastfed infants (Deligiannidis et al. 2024).

Although data is limited, esketamine shows promise for both treatment and prevention of postpartum depression. A recent randomized controlled study found that mothers with mild depressive symptoms at delivery who were given esketamine after childbirth had fewer depressive symptoms at week 1 postpartum and had a 75% reduction in significant depressive symptoms at postpartum day 42 (Wang et al. 2024). Furthermore, another recent meta-analysis of cesarean section patients found that those who were treated with perioperative esketamine had fewer postpartum depressive symptoms and a lower incidence of postpartum depression up to day 42 (Wen et al. 2024). While esketamine or ketamine may reduce the risk for postpartum depression, more data is needed to determine if these agents are effective treatments for postpartum depression.

Finally, it is important to remind women that postpartum depression is treatable. While a subset of women do go on to experience chronic depression, a large proportion recover. Ongoing monitoring, discussion, and collaboration can significantly improve the experience of early motherhood for women with depression.

15.7 Expert Recommendations Based on Scientific Evidence and Clinical Experience

- The overall goal of treatment is to maximize maternal wellness, since maternal well-being is intimately tied to infant and family well-being.
- Decisions about medication should be made collaboratively, ideally involving the patient, her partner, obstetrician, and psychiatrist in the decision-making process.
- The best antidepressant during pregnancy is the one that works for the patient.
- All else being equal, when treating antenatal depression it is better to choose a medication that has more data behind its use.
- Treatment during pregnancy should be with the fewest possible medications at the lowest *effective* dose.
- In the postpartum period, addressing sleep deprivation and protecting maternal sleep is an essential component of treating depression.
- Decisions about breastfeeding should be made with attention not only to medication safety, but also to the impact on maternal mental health.

References

Abrishamcar S, Zhuang BC, Thomas M, Gladish N, MacIsaac JL, Jones MJ, Simons E, Moraes TJ, Mandhane PJ, Brook JR, Subbarao P, Turvey SE, Chen E, Miller GE, Kobor MS, Hüls A. Association between maternal perinatal stress and depression and infant DNA methylation in the first year of life. Transl Psychiatry. 2024;14(1):445.

Andrade C. Towards a further understanding of meta-analysis using gestational exposure to cannabis and birth defects as a case in point. J Clin Psychiatry. 2024;85(4):24f15673.

Andrade SE, Reichman ME, Mott K, Pitts M, Kieswetter C, Dinatale M, Stone MB, Popovic J, Haffenreffer K, Toh S. Use of selective serotonin reuptake inhibitors (SSRIs) in women delivering liveborn infants and other women of child-bearing age within the U.S. Food and Drug Administration's mini-sentinel program. Arch Womens Ment Health. 2016;19(6):969–77.

Azorin JM, Angst J, Gamma A, et al. Identifying features of bipolarity in patients with first-episode postpartum depression: findings from the international BRIDGE study. J Affect Disord. 2012;136(3):710–5.

Baia I, Domingues RMSM. The effects of cannabis use during pregnancy is associated with increased risk of low birth weight and preterm birth: a systematic review and meta-analysis. Am J Perinatol. 2024;41(1):17–30.

Bassalov H, Yakirevich-Amir N, Reuveni I, et al. Prenatal cannabis exposure and the risk for neuropsychiatric anomalies in the offspring: a systematic review and meta-analysis. Am J Obstet Gynecol. 2024;231(6):574–88.

Brody DJ, Gu Q. Antidepressant use among adults: United States, 2015–2018. NCHS Data Brief, no 377. Hyattsville: National Center for Health Statistics. 2020. Retrieved from: https://www.cdc.gov/nchs/data/databriefs/db377-H.pdf

Brown JVE, Wilson CA, Ayre K, Robertson L, South E, Molyneaux E, Trevillion K, Howard LM, Khalifeh H. Antidepressant treatment for postnatal depression. Cochrane Database Syst Rev. 2021;2(2):CD013560.

Cohen LS, Altshuler LL, Harlow BI, et al. Relapse of major depression during pregnancy in women who maintain or discontinue antidepressant treatment. JAMA. 2006;295:499–507.

Delavari M, Mohammad-Alizadeh-Charandabi S, Mirghafourvand M. The relationship of maternal-fetal attachment and postpartum depression: a longitudinal study. Arch Psychiatr Nurs. 2018;32(2):263–7.

Deligiannidis KM, Byatt N, Freeman MP. Pharmacotherapy for mood disorders in pregnancy: a review of pharmacokinetic changes and clinical recommendations for therapeutic drug monitoring. J Clin Psychopharmacol. 2014;34(2):244–55.

Deligiannidis KM, Meltzer-Brody S, Gunduz-Bruce H, Doherty J, Jonas J, Sigui L, Sankoh AJ, Silber C, Campbell AD, Werneburg B, Kanes SJ, Lasser R. Effect of Zuranolone vs placebo in postpartum depression. A randomized clinical trial. JAMA Psychiatry. 2021;78(9):951–9.

Deligiannidis KM, Bullock A, Nandy I, Dunbar J, Lasser R, Witte M, Leclair B, Wald J. Zuranolone concentrations in the breast milk of healthy, lactating individuals: results from a phase 1 open-label study. J Clin Psychopharmacol. 2024;44(4):337–44.

Ghimire U, Papabathini SS, Kawuki J, Obore N, Musa TH. Depression during pregnancy and the risk of low birth weight, preterm birth and intrauterine growth restriction- an updated meta-analysis. Early Hum Dev. 2021;152:105243.

Giallo R, Gartland D, Woolhouse H, Brown S. "I didn't know it was possible to feel that tired": exploring the complex bidirectional associations between maternal depressive symptoms and fatigue in a prospective pregnancy cohort study. Arch Womens Ment Health. 2016;19(1):25–34.

Hankin BL, Demers CH, Hennessey EP, Perzow SED, Curran MC, Gallop RJ, Hoffman MC, Davis EP. Effect of brief interpersonal therapy on depression during pregnancy: a randomized clinical trial. JAMA Psychiatry. 2023;80(6):539–47.

Hoffman C, Dunn DM, Njoroge WFM. Impact of postpartum mental illness upon infant development. Curr Psychiatry Rep. 2017;19(12):100.

Huybrechts KP, Pamsten K, Mogun H, et al. National trends in antidepressant medication treatment among publicly insured pregnant women. Gen Hosp Psychiatry. 2013;35:265–71.

Jarde A, Morais M, Kingston D, Giallo R, MacQueen GM, Giglia L, Beyene J, Wang Y, McDonald SD. Neonatal outcomes in women with untreated antenatal depression compared with women without depression: a systematic review and meta-analysis. JAMA Psychiatry. 2016;73(8):826–37.

Kim DR, Wang E, McGeehan B, Snell J, Ewing G, Iannelli C, O'Reardon JP, Sammel MD, Epperson CN. Randomized controlled trial of transcranial magnetic stimulation in pregnant women with major depressive disorder. Brain Stimul. 2019;12(1):96–102.

Lee HJ, Kim SM, Kwon JY. Repetitive transcranial magnetic stimulation treatment for peripartum depression: systematic review & meta-analysis. BMC Pregnancy Childbirth. 2021;21(1):118.

Li X, Fang L, Guan L, Zhang J, Zheng M, Zhu D. The effects of light therapy on depression and sleep in women during pregnancy or the postpartum period: a systematic review and meta-analysis. Brain Behav. 2023;13(12):e3339.

López Seco F, Mundo-Cid P, Aguado-Gracia J, Gaviria-Gómez AM, Acosta-García S, Martí-Serrano S, Vilella E, Masana-Marín A. Insecure maternal attachment is associated with depression in ADHD children. Atten Defic Hyperact Disord. 2016;8(4):189–96.

McAllister-Williams RH, et al. British Association for Psychopharmacology consensus guidance on the use of psychotropic medication preconception, in pregnancy and postpartum 2017. J Psychopharmacol. 2017;31(5):519–52.

Mitchell A, Gilboa S, Wexler M, Kelley K, Louik C, Hernandez-Diaz S. Medication use during pregnancy, with particular focus on prescription drugs: 1976-2008. Am J Obstet Gynecol. 2011;205(1):51.

NICE Clinical Guideline 192. Antenatal and postnatal mental health: clinical management and service guidance; 2014, updated February 2020. Retrieved from: https://www.nice.org.uk/guidance/cg192/chapter/Recommendations#treating-specific-mental-health-problems-in-pregnancy-and-the-postnatal-period

Orsolini L, Bellantuono C. Serotonin reuptake inhibitors and breastfeeding: a systematic review. Hum Psychopharmacol. 2015;30(1):4–20.

Pacilio RM, Lopez JF, Parikh SV, Patel PD, Geller JA. Safe ketamine use and pregnancy: a nationwide survey and retrospective review of informed consent, counseling, and testing practices. J Clin Psychiatry. 2024;85(3):24m15293. https://doi.org/10.4088/JCP.24m15293.

Park M, Brain U, Grunau RE, Diamond A, Oberlander TF. Maternal depression trajectories from pregnancy to 3 years postpartum are associated with children's behavior and executive functions at 3 and 6 years. Arch Womens Ment Health. 2018;21(3):353–63.

Powell JG, Garland S, Preston K, Piszczatoski C. Brexanolone (Zulresso): finally, an FDA-approved treatment for postpartum depression. Ann Pharmacother. 2020;54(2):157–63.

Reynolds RM, Labad J, Buss C, Ghaemmaghami P, Räikkönen K. Transmitting biological effects of stress in utero: implications for mother and offspring. Psychoneuroendocrinology. 2013;38(9):1843–9.

Roddy Mitchell A, Gordon H, Lindquist A, Walker SP, Homer CSE, Middleton A, Cluver CA, Tong S, Hastie R. Prevalence of perinatal depression in low- and middle-income countries: a systematic review and meta-analysis. JAMA Psychiatry. 2023;80(5):425–31.

Salisbury A, O'Grady K, Battle C, et al. The roles of maternal depression, serotonin reuptake inhibitor treatment, and concomitant benzodiazepine use on infant neurobehavioral functioning over the first postnatal month. Am J Psychiatry. 2016;173:147–57.

Seth S, Lewis AJ, Galbally M. Perinatal maternal depression and cortisol function in pregnancy and the postpartum period: a systematic literature review. BMC Pregnancy Childbirth. 2016;16(1):124.

Shortis E, Warrington D, Whittaker P. The efficacy of cognitive behavioral therapy for the treatment of antenatal depression: a systematic review. J Affect Disord. 2020;272:485–95.

Sockol LE. A systematic review and meta-analysis of interpersonal psychotherapy for perinatal women. J Affect Disord. 2018;232:316–28.

Stallings EB, Isenburg JL, Rutkowski RE, Kirby RS, Nembhard WN, Sandidge T, Villavicencio S, Nguyen HH, McMahon DM, Nestoridi E, Pabst LJ. National Birth Defects Prevention Network. National population-based estimates for major birth defects, 2016-2020. Birth Defects Res. 2024;116(1):e2301.

Stein A, Pearson RM, Goodman SH, Rapa E, Rahman A, McCallum M, Howard LM, Pariante CM. Effects of perinatal mental disorders on the fetus and child. Lancet. 2014;384(9956):1800–19.

van Ravesteyn LM, Lambregtse-van den Berg MP, Hoogendijk WJ, Kamperman AM. Interventions to treat mental disorders during pregnancy: a systematic review and multiple treatment meta-analysis. PLoS One. 2017;12(3):e0173397.

Wan MW, Green J. The impact of maternal psychopathology on child-mother attachment. Arch Womens Ment Health. 2009;12(3):123–34.

Wang S, Deng CM, Zeng Y, Chen XZ, Li AY, Feng SW, Xu LL, Chen L, Yuan HM, Hu H, Yang T, Han T, Zhang HY, Jiang M, Sun XY, Guo HN, Sessler DI, Wang DX. Efficacy of a single low dose of esketamine after childbirth for mothers with symptoms of prenatal depression: randomised clinical trial. BMJ. 2024;385:e078218.

Warburton W, Hertzman C, Oberlander TF. A register study of the impact of stopping third trimester selective serotonin reuptake inhibitor exposure on neonatal health. Acta Psychiatr Scand. 2010;121(6):471–9.

Ward HB, Fromson JA, Cooper JJ, De Oliveira G, Almeida M. Recommendations for the use of ECT in pregnancy: literature review and proposed clinical protocol. Arch Womens Ment Health. 2018;21(6):715–22.

Weissman MM, Pilowsky DJ, Wickramaratne PJ, et al. Remissions in maternal depression and child psychopathology, a STAR*D-child report. JAMA. 2006;295(12):1389–98.

Wen Y, Mao M, Wang X, Xu C, Shi X, Li P, Tian Z, Jiang M, Yuan H, Feng S. Efficacy and safety of perioperative application of esketamine on postpartum depression: a meta-analysis of randomized controlled studies. Psychiatry Res. 2024;333:115765.

Yin X, Sun N, Jiang N, Xu X, Gan Y, Zhang J, Qiu L, Yang C, Shi X, Chang J, Gong Y. Prevalence and associated factors of antenatal depression: systematic reviews and meta-analyses. Clin Psychol Rev. 2021;83:101932. https://doi.org/10.1016/j.cpr.2020.101932.

Bipolar Disorder 16

Michael Thomson and Verinder Sharma

16.1 Introduction

This manuscript is an update of the chapter by Thomson and Sharma (2019) found in the first version of the Perinatal Psychopharmacology textbook (Uguz and Orsolini 2019).

Managing bipolar disorder (BD) during the perinatal period involves balancing the numerous risks associated with the maternal illness against potential risks that medication exposure can pose to the mother, the fetus, or the neonate. Factors that further complicate management include a lack of international consensus guidelines, differing patient priorities, little consistency in clinician practices, and the historical exclusion of pregnant and postpartum women from most clinical trials (Graham et al. 2018). To date, no randomized controlled trials (RCTs) have investigated the pharmacological management of BD in pregnant or postpartum women. BD has been associated with an increased risk of adverse obstetrical outcomes, some of which are independent of medication exposure (Boden et al. 2012).

Although the prevalence of BD in obstetrical populations has not been well established. A recent systematic review and meta-analysis found a 2.6% prevalence rate of bipolar disorder in women without a known psychiatric illness history (Masters et al. 2022). Given its high prevalence and propensity for affecting women of reproductive ages (Pedersen et al. 2014; Masters et al. 2022), knowledge of its management is imperative for clinicians providing care to women.

M. Thomson
Department of Psychiatry, Western University, London, ON, Canada
e-mail: mthoms6@uwo.ca

V. Sharma (✉)
Departments of Psychiatry and Obstetrics and Gynecology, Western University, London, ON, Canada
e-mail: vsharma@uwo.ca

F. Uguz, L. Orsolini (eds.), *Perinatal Psychopharmacology*,
https://doi.org/10.1007/978-3-031-99720-4_16

16.2 Identifying Perinatal Bipolar Disorder

BD is often a difficult clinical diagnosis to establish, and misdiagnosis is frequent. In addition to the risk of impairment and distress, the healthcare resource costs of this misdiagnosis can be significant (McIntyre et al. 2022). Symptomatically, the illness can overlap with multiple other psychiatric disorders including major depressive disorder (MDD), psychotic disorders, substance use disorders, and personality disorders, among others. Additionally, underlying medical concerns such as hypothyroidism and anemia can also present with psychiatric manifestations (Pedersen et al. 2007). The first presentation of BD is usually that of a major depressive episode (MDE) which can make the illness very difficult to distinguish from MDD. Based on the Diagnostic and Statistical Manual of Mental Disorders, fifth edition (DSM-5), BD type I or II cannot be diagnosed until a manic or hypomanic episode has occurred (American Psychiatric Association 2013). Many patients have had the illness for multiple years before the correct diagnosis (Hirschfeld et al. 2003). Although universal screening for perinatal depression has been recommended by the American College of Obstetricians and Gynecologists (2015), this generally has not included screening for BD. In both research studies and in clinical practice, the most used screening tool has been the Edinburgh Postnatal Depression Scale. This tool has a sensitivity ranging from 67% to 100% and a specificity ranging from 87% to 100% in detecting postpartum depression (O'Connor et al. 2016). Another easy-to-use questionnaire, the Mood Disorder Questionnaire (MDQ), has been validated by Sharma and Xie for the screening of BD in the postpartum period. The MDQ demonstrated a sensitivity of 87.72% and a specificity of 85.29% for the identification of BD in postpartum women when the supplementary questions were excluded (Sharma and Xie 2011).

First presentations of BD are usually MDEs which can be very difficult to distinguish from those seen in an MDD. Atypical symptoms of depression can be suggestive of BD, yet these are also frequently observed in MDD (Thomson and Sharma 2018). As BD is highly heritable, obtaining a thorough family history of psychiatric disorders is vital including specific questioning on the family history of BD and perinatal psychiatric concerns (Barnett and Smoller 2009).

It is increasingly being recognized that the postpartum period is a high-risk time for the first onset of BD (Munk-Olsen et al. 2006; Azorin et al. 2012; Sharma et al. 2014; Inglis et al. 2014). As such, clinicians should be vigilant in screening for the illness in postpartum women presenting with symptoms of a mood disorder. Although MDD and bipolar depression can be very difficult to differentiate, features that can be suggestive of bipolar depression are the onset of depressive symptoms within the first 2 weeks postpartum, a family history of BD, and atypical depressive symptoms.

16.3 The Complexity of Bipolar Disorder Management During Pregnancy

Unfortunately, most medications used in the treatment of BD can pose significant risks to both the mother and her baby. Some of the commonly used mood-stabilizing medications, e.g., valproate and carbamazepine, are well-known to have significant teratogenicity (Hernandez-Diaz et al. 2012). However, untreated maternal illness can also pose large risks including suicide, substance abuse, and lower adherence to recommended prenatal care. In many cases, these risks outweigh the risks of medication exposure. As the risks and benefits must be weighed on a case-by-case basis, it has been very difficult to establish general management guidelines for this population. Additionally, the woman's preferences in treatment are a paramount aspect that must be factored into treatment decisions. Some women may decide that preventing a relapse or optimizing control of their mood symptoms is their primary concern and in doing so are willing to tolerate a higher risk of fetal medication exposure. Others may decide that fetal safety is their top priority and are willing to accept an increased risk of BD relapse to minimize fetal exposure to medications.

Where possible, the use of medications during the perinatal period should be limited to monotherapy. Women with BD often have complex medication regimens before conception, especially in cases of more severe or treatment-resistant illness. Studies of fetal risk associated with mood stabilizer polytherapy are lacking. However, one study showed higher rates of congenital anomalies with polytherapy compared to monotherapy for the treatment of epilepsy (Holmes et al. 2011). Another study showed higher rates of adverse outcomes for both the mother and fetus when antipsychotics were combined with other psychotropic medications compared to antipsychotic monotherapy (Sadowski et al. 2013). Another factor contributing to the complexity of antenatal BD management has been a lack of consistency in the findings of adverse fetal outcomes attributed to different mood-stabilizing medications. Most systematic reviews and meta-analyses of fetal risks associated with antipsychotics have looked at the medication as a group rather than separating out data for individual antipsychotics (Coughlin et al. 2015). Studies of fetal risk using information from population-based databases may have significant confounding factors that are co-morbid to the psychiatric disorder being treated, such as higher rates of substance abuse, poorer physical health, and poorer access to prenatal care. BD itself may have a teratogenic risk as it has been associated with higher rates of microcephaly and neonatal hypoglycemia in offspring (Boden et al. 2012). Yet, an overall understanding of the risks that the illness itself poses to pregnancy is inadequate.

16.4 Risks of Untreated Bipolar Disorder

The risks associated with untreated maternal BD during pregnancy have not been well-established (Uguz et al. 2023). Multiple studies have associated untreated maternal depression with adverse markers of fetal health and adverse pregnancy outcomes (Gentile and Luigia Fusco 2016; Nulman et al. 2012). However, these findings predominately relate to major depressive disorder and may not apply to BD. A population-based study compared pregnancy outcomes for women with untreated BD to women with treated BD and women without BD. This study demonstrated increased rates of neonatal microcephaly, neonatal hypoglycemia, preterm birth, small for gestational age infants, and induced or planned cesarean section in women with BD even when the illness was untreated (Boden et al. 2012).

Women with BD who remain medication-free during the postpartum period experience significantly higher relapse rates compared to women taking mood stabilizers during this time (Wesseloo et al. 2015).

16.5 Pre-conception Planning in Bipolar Disorder

In ideal situations, women with BD are identified early and stabilized on medication for a prolonged duration before conception. This notion was supported by research by Viguera et al. (2007) which demonstrated a decreased risk of relapse in women with BD who had a prolonged period of stability before pregnancy. However, the length of time considered to be a prolonged period was not defined in the study. Women who are family planning often request a consultation with their health care providers to discuss the implications of their medication on pregnancy or inquire about the pregnancy risks associated with medication before starting it. These are opportune times for clinicians to provide education on the risks and benefits of psychotropic medications and to provide some guidance on what the medication options are should a pregnancy occur. Tapering a medication is easier to trial before a pregnancy occurs as fetal exposure is not an ongoing concern. In this situation, it is easier to attempt a slow taper, and medications can often be quickly reinstated should a relapse occur. However, given that half of all pregnancies are unplanned, and this increases to two-thirds in women with BD (Marengo et al. 2015), this ideal scenario will often not be the clinical reality. Unplanned pregnancies have been associated with significantly higher rates of relapse (Viguera et al. 2007; Doyle et al. 2012). This is likely multifactorial with psychosocial contributions in addition to some women abruptly discontinuing medications upon learning they are pregnant.

Pre-conception counseling should begin by obtaining a thorough psychiatric history. Important information to obtain includes the number of prior mood episodes, the severity of past episodes, duration of euthymic periods between episodes, past response to medications, family psychiatric history, history of suicidality, and history of psychosis (Sharma 2011). Completing a thorough psychiatric history helps with estimating both the risk of a mood episode relapse occurring and the potential severity should one occur. Family history of BD, postpartum mood disorders, and postpartum psychosis should be elicited as these have been associated with a risk of postpartum mood episodes (Sharma 2011). The woman should be counseled on the fetal risks associated with her psychotropic medications, advised of any alternative medications which may be safer, and educated on the risk of a mood episode relapse during the perinatal period. It is also important to identify co-morbid psychiatric disorders as these are usually the rule, rather than the exception, in BD. The treatment of co-morbid disorders must be taken into consideration as they bring additional complexity into treatment decisions, e.g., different medications or options for therapy. There has been little research on the prevalence of co-morbid psychiatric disorders in perinatal women with BD. However, one naturalistic study of women with BD identified lifetime co-morbidity rates of 51% for anxiety disorders, 11% for alcohol abuse, and 10% for cannabis use disorder (Driscoll et al. 2017). Identification and treatment of co-morbidities may reduce the risk of a BD relapse and reduce maternal morbidity. If present, obesity, substance use disorders, and smoking should all be addressed as they are more prevalent in individuals with BD (Yatham et al. 2018) and are associated with a higher risk of adverse maternal and neonatal outcomes.

Population-based studies have identified that discontinuation of psychotropic medication is common in women who become pregnant. A Canadian study identified that 16.2% of women filled at least one prescription for psychotropic medication in the 3 months before pregnancy. This number decreased to 6.0% during pregnancy and was 9.5% in the first 3 months postpartum. The study also identified an increase in the use of psychotropic medications before, during, and after pregnancy from 2003 to 2013. Women who were taking an anti-epileptic medication were more likely to continue their medication throughout pregnancy (18.1%) but this study did not differentiate use in epilepsy from use in BD. Only 7.8% of women taking antipsychotic medications continued them throughout pregnancy and 29.0% had intermittent use (Leong et al. 2017). Should discontinuation of mood stabilizing medications be attempted before conception or during pregnancy it is best done under medical supervision so that relapses can be quickly identified and addressed. Tapering of medications, rather than abrupt discontinuation, has been associated with a much lower risk of relapse during pregnancy. The same study demonstrated that the time to relapse was 11 times shorter in women who abruptly discontinued mood-stabilizing medication compared to gradual discontinuation (Viguera et al. 2007). Monitoring mood states without the use of medication may be appropriate in women who have had a mild lifetime illness course (e.g., no history of suicide attempts or psychosis and a historically good response to treatment). Another potential in select circumstances is the tapering of medications during the first trimester with a resumption in the second or third trimesters. This theoretically reduces fetal exposure to medications during the predominate periods of organogenesis.

As the severity of the past illness course increases (e.g., a history of suicide attempts, psychotic features, and limited past response to medications), the estimated risk of a relapse also increases. Women with a history of severe illness may require maintenance treatment throughout pregnancy given the increased risks should a relapse occur. Close follow-up is required if a woman with a history of severe illness attempts medication discontinuation. Where possible, family members should be involved in the treatment process, educated on signs of relapse, and made aware of how medical care can be accessed should a relapse occur. When reviewing psychotropic medications during pregnancy and the pre-conceptual period all the woman's psychotropic medications should be scrutinized. Women with BD are frequently prescribed antidepressant medications despite their role in the treatment of the disorder being controversial (Schneck et al. 2008; Ghaemi et al. 2000; Valenti et al. 2011; Yatham et al. 2018). A naturalistic study of pregnant women with BD identified that 9% of women with both BD I and BD II were treated with either antidepressant monotherapy or with antidepressants combined with other medications that were not guideline-concordant (Driscoll et al. 2017). The use of antidepressants in pregnant women with BD is a robust predictor of depression relapse during pregnancy (Viguera et al. 2007). Clinicians must be aware of the potential fetal safety concerns posed by antidepressant medications and be mindful that these medications may increase the risk of relapses, especially if they are unopposed following the discontinuation of mood-stabilizing medications (Viguera et al. 2007).

16.6 Management of Antenatal Bipolar Disorder

16.6.1 Acute Treatment

Whether or not to initiate medications in the treatment of acute mood episodes will depend on the severity of the episode and the woman's preferences for treatment. In milder cases, a wait-and-watch approach may be appropriate. In more severe cases, urgent intervention is often required and may include hospitalization. Severe cases include those with suicidality, psychosis, or significant functional impairment. There have been no clinical trials on the treatment of acute BD episodes in pregnancy. As such, it is reasonable to use best-evidence guidelines from non-perinatal populations with additional considerations given to the pregnancy safety profile of medications. Preference is generally given to medications that have demonstrated benefit in the woman's past treatment, however, this should be balanced with the pregnancy safety profile of the medication. When the previously used medication is associated with significant fetal risk (e.g., valproate), it is usually best to trial a medication with a better pregnancy safety profile despite the mother's response to this alternative medication potentially being unknown. Detailed discussions on the safety of different mood-stabilizing agents including lithium, anti-epileptic medications, and antipsychotics are covered elsewhere in this textbook.

Most antenatal bipolar relapses are depressive episodes (Viguera et al. 2011). Guidelines from the Canadian Network for Mood and Anxiety Treatments (CANMAT) and the International Society for Bipolar Disorders (ISBD) indicate that both lamotrigine and quetiapine are first-line medications for the acute treatment of bipolar depression (Yatham et al. 2018). These medications are thought to be among the safest mood stabilizers for use in pregnancy (Pariente et al. 2017; Ennis and Damkier 2015). If a relapse occurs despite the woman taking maintenance medications, then dosage optimization should be attempted before the addition of augmenting medications. When the maximum dose has been reached or there are intolerable side effects then augmentation can be considered. However, studies have identified additive, and potentially synergistic, increases in the risk of congenital anomalies with polypharmacy (Holmes et al. 2011; Sadowski et al. 2013). Additionally, there are no studies that have established efficacy for any augmenting agents in a pregnant population.

Any antidepressant medications that pregnant women with BD are taking should be given scrutiny. The use of antidepressant medications in women with BD is common (Driscoll et al. 2017) and their use in treating the disorder has been controversial (Yatham et al. 2018). Antidepressant use was shown to be a robust predictor of BD relapse in a study by Viguera et al. (2007). However, it cannot be excluded that the use of antidepressants in this study may have been a marker of more severe maternal illness (Viguera et al. 2007). A case-control study of infanticide noted that high rates of antidepressant use within bipolar disorder were identified in a population where infanticide has occurred (Bramanta and Di Florio 2023). Clinicians should be mindful that the observed effects of antidepressants may change if mood-stabilizing medications are discontinued resulting in the antidepressant medication becoming unopposed. 2018 CANMAT/ISBD bipolar disorder guidelines have recommended against the use of antidepressant monotherapy in bipolar I disorder (Yatham et al. 2018). It is also important to be mindful of antidepressant withdrawal as it must be differentiated from a mood disorder relapse. A thorough screening for co-morbid psychiatric disorders should be undertaken as these conditions may be benefiting from the use of antidepressants but alternative treatment options with fewer risks may also exist.

The use of psychotherapy may be an additional treatment option. Although there is no evidence supporting the use of psychotherapy in antenatal BD, some meta-analyses have shown efficacy for its use in non-perinatal BD. The 2018 CANMAT/ISBD guidelines have recommended psychoeducation as a first-line adjunctive maintenance treatment in BD (Yatham et al. 2018). Efficacy for monotherapy with social rhythm therapy without the use of medication was suggested by a small proof-of-concept study involving 17 non-perinatal patients with acute bipolar II depression. In the study, 41% of the patients achieved ≥50% symptom reduction by 12 weeks. An additional 41% of the patients dropped out or were removed which could suggest that the response rate was even an underestimation of efficacy (Swartz et al. 2009). Psychotherapy, particularly cognitive behavioral therapy (CBT), may be very helpful for women who have a co-morbid anxiety disorder (Provencher et al. 2011). The efficacy of CBT in reducing relapse risk in non-perinatal BD was seen in one RCT (Lam et al. 2003). A second, larger RCT found that CBT may help reduce relapse risks in non-perinatal BD patients who have had fewer mood episodes, but not in those who have had ≥12 past episodes (Scott et al. 2006).

An increasing body of research has suggested that lamotrigine may have one of the best pregnancy safety profiles among mood-stabilizing medications. Most studies have not identified an increased risk of congenital anomalies with lamotrigine use. A single study found an increased risk of oral-cleft defects (Dolk et al. 2008) but this was not replicated in a later meta-analysis and systematic review by Pariente et al. (2017). Lamotrigine has also been labelled as a first-line medication for both acute bipolar depression treatment and maintenance treatment in the CANMAT/ISBD guidelines (Yatham et al. 2018). Maintenance treatment efficacy with lamotrigine was demonstrated in a 2008 study by Newport et al. where 30% of women taking lamotrigine had postpartum BD relapses versus 100% of women not taking mood stabilizing medications (Newport et al. 2008). Unfortunately, studies have suggested that lamotrigine is not effective in treating mania and this medication requires slow titration given the risk of Stevens-Johnson syndrome (Guberman et al. 1999). Lamotrigine is not recommended for the treatment of mania in the CANMAT/ISBD 2018 guidelines which were developed for the general BD population (Yatham et al. 2018).

There have been no published clinical trials to guide the management of manic or mixed episodes during pregnancy and the existing literature is limited to case reports and case series. As such, treatment decisions largely rely on data extrapolated from studies using non-perinatal populations. Usually, antenatal hypomanic episodes are monitored without pharmacological intervention to see if they remit spontaneously. Addressing psychosocial factors and attempting strategies to improve sleep are often beneficial. Should significant safety concerns or significant functional impairment arise then medications can be initiated, or if currently being used, optimized. Studies in non-perinatal patients have shown haloperidol to be among the most efficacious medications for treating acute manic episodes (Cipriani et al. 2011). However, prolonged use of haloperidol may increase the risk of a depressive episode (Cipriani et al. 2011; Yatham et al. 2018). Haloperidol has a long history of use in pregnancy, and it has generally not been associated with an increased risk of congenital anomalies. A study that examined a group of pregnancies exposed to haloperidol (n = 188) and penfluridol (n = 27) did not show an increased risk of congenital anomalies compared to a control group (3.4% versus 3.8%, $p = 0.787$). However, it should be noted that a study limited to 188 cases may be underpowered for detecting smaller increases in the risk of congenital anomalies, especially when looking for specific anomalies. The group receiving haloperidol or penfluridol had higher rates of pregnancy termination (8.8% versus 3.8%, $p = 0.004$) and there was a trend towards a higher rate of miscarriage, but this did not achieve statistical significance (8.8% versus 5.5%, $p = 0.105$). The rate of stillbirths (0.0% vs 0.2%, $p = 1.00$) was comparable between the antipsychotic group and control group (Diav-Citrin et al. 2005). Quetiapine is another anti-manic medication that appears to have one of the better pregnancy safety profiles. A systematic review including 443 pregnancies exposed to quetiapine in the first trimester showed a congenital anomaly rate of 3.6% (16/443) (Ennis and Damkier 2015). The background risk for major congenital anomalies is felt to be around 3% (Egbe et al. 2015). Another study of 54 late-stage pregnancies determined that the mean concentration of quetiapine obtained from umbilical cord blood was only 24% of the maternal serum concentration. This was the lowest ratio among the antipsychotics used (n = 20 for quetiapine) (Newport et al. 2007).

16.6.2 Management of Newly Diagnosed Bipolar Disorder

Pregnancy may be the time of first onset for a mood disorder or it may be the time during which a BD is first recognized. The significant overlap between the reproductive years and the age of onset for bipolar disorders is contributory (Pedersen et al. 2014). However, the rate of first onset of BD during pregnancy has not been established (Sharma and Pope 2012). In some cases, a new diagnosis of BD may be made when a pregnant woman is referred by her general practitioner or obstetrician for psychiatric assessment during pregnancy. The diagnosis is usually made when the clinician identifies past hypomanic or manic episodes. However, this then poses the challenge of how the psychiatric disorder should be managed during the pregnancy. In this situation, a pre-conceptual trial of medication is no longer an option and starting medication poses the risk of fetal medication exposure with unknown maternal response. In cases where there are minimal concerns concerning suicidality and functional impairment, a wait-and-watch approach may be appropriate. This allows additional time for diagnostic clarification, and it allows the pregnancy to progress further before fetal medication exposure occurs. However, urgent intervention and hospitalization are usually required in situations where there is suicidality, psychosis, or significant functional impairment. When a wait-and-watch approach is pursued, it is important to educate the woman and her supports about the possibility of worsening mood symptoms and to discuss how care can urgently be accessed should this occur.

16.6.3 Maintenance Treatment

The goals of maintenance treatment are to reduce the risk of relapse during pregnancy as well as in the postpartum period. In predicting the risk of an antenatal BD relapse, it is important to understand the course of the illness during pregnancy. In the past, it was believed that pregnancy was protective against mental illness. It is now understood that the influences of pregnancy on mental illness are not clear-cut and there is currently a lack of consensus regarding the effects of pregnancy on BD specifically. Sharma and Pope (2012) analyzed studies of BD illness course in pregnancy and concluded that there is evidence from non-clinical samples, retrospective studies and studies of hospitalization rates which are suggestive of a protective effect of pregnancy on BD. However, they also note that studies have shown a high relapse rate during pregnancy when mood stabilizing medications were discontinued. In a retrospective study by Viguera et al. (2007), women who discontinued lithium during pregnancy had comparable relapse rates to non-pregnant women who discontinued lithium (52% versus 58% respectively) when both groups were followed over 40 weeks. The women in both groups relapsed more frequently than they did in the year before lithium discontinuation. A similar study by Grof et al. (2000) compared the risk of relapse in 28 pregnant women against 33 non-pregnant women. All women in the study had BD I and were responsive to lithium. Relapses occurred less frequently in the pregnant group compared to the non-pregnant group.

Women in the pregnant group also had fewer relapses during their pregnancy than they did in the 9 months preceding the pregnancy. Additionally, most of the relapses that occurred during pregnancy took place in the last 5 weeks of gestation. These studies suggest that pregnancy may have either a neutral or protective effect on the course of BD. However, the results of a study done in a lithium-responsive antenatal BD I population are not necessarily applicable to all cases of antenatal BD. A retrospective study by Viguera et al. analyzed the risk of mood episodes in 1162 women comprising 2252 pregnancies. Of the women enrolled, 283 had BD I and 338 had BD II. The risk of a BD relapse during pregnancy was 22.7% (Viguera et al. 2011). Another study by Viguera et al. (2007) compared the risk of relapse during pregnancy in women who remained on mood-stabilizing medications versus those who discontinued them. The group that remained on the medications had a relapse rate of 37.0% versus 85.5% in the group that discontinued the medications. Of the 37.0% of women who experienced a relapse during pregnancy, 18.5% experienced depressive episodes, 25.9% had hypomanic episodes, and 7.4% had manic episodes. No mixed episodes were identified in the women who continued to take maintenance medications. The relapse rate for the group of women who discontinued medications was much higher at 85.5%. The time to relapse was also four times longer in the group that continued mood-stabilizing medications (>40 weeks versus 9 weeks). However, there were some significant differences between the groups which may have caused confounding. Women from the group that discontinued the medications were more likely to be taking multiple psychotropic medications, had a longer duration of illness, were more likely to have illness onset before age 15, and had significantly higher rates of rapid cycling. All of these are indicators of increased illness severity. They were also more likely to be taking antidepressant medications (66.1% versus 18.5%), to have an unplanned pregnancy, and to be diagnosed with BD II which are all factors associated with higher relapse rates during pregnancy.

Individualized assessments of the risks and benefits of medication use must be performed when making decisions on maintenance treatment in antenatal BD. It has been well-established that discontinuing maintenance treatment is associated with an increased risk of relapse during pregnancy and an even higher risk for postpartum relapse. Yet, there are risks to both the mother and the fetus with medication exposure. Obtaining a thorough psychiatric history helps to estimate the woman's risk of having a relapse and to predict the potential severity should this happen. This risk assessment should be discussed with the woman and her views on the use of medication should be inquired about. Many pregnant women prioritize the minimization of fetal medication exposure and are willing to accept a higher risk of relapse to do so. In cases where the illness has been stable for a minimum of 4–6 months and the woman is considered to be at low risk for relapse, discontinuing medication with symptom monitoring may be the overall safest option (Yatham et al. 2018). This approach minimizes fetal exposure but does so at the cost of increasing the risk of a relapse. Where possible, family members and others involved should be engaged in the treatment planning so that they can provide additional support to the woman if needed and assist her in obtaining medical care should decompensation occur. In cases where complete discontinuation of medications poses too great of risk or multiple psychotropic medications are being used, a strategy involving the selective tapering of medications may be appropriate. In this situation, medications which pose the greatest fetal risk or those which have been the least beneficial should be considered first. Another strategy commonly used in the treatment of antenatal BD is the tapering or discontinuation of mood stabilizing medications during the first trimester with a plan to restart them in the second or third trimesters. The main benefit of this strategy is that fetal medication exposure is reduced during the time of organogenesis. This allows for prophylactic mood stabilizing medications to be re-initiated before the period of highest overall relapse risk, the postpartum period. However, a downside is that antenatal BD relapses may have a propensity for the first trimester. In the Viguera et al. (2007) study, 47% of antenatal relapses occurred during the first trimester. However, this notion conflicts with the Grof et al. (2000) study where most of the women who relapsed following lithium discontinuation did so in the late third trimester. Another factor for consideration is that a woman may not become aware of the pregnancy until after the period of highest risk for teratogenicity has already occurred.

There is a dearth of research looking at BD maintenance treatment during pregnancy. Most of the research that does exist has analyzed the risk of relapse in women who continue versus those who discontinue mood stabilizing medications. No RCTs have looked at this and studies comparing the efficacy of different medications have been minimal. Most of the existing studies have used lithium. These studies have shown lithium to be efficacious in reducing the risk of mood episode relapses both during pregnancy and in postpartum (Viguera et al. 2007; Rosso et al. 2016; Bergink et al. 2012). Lithium has also been recommended as a first-line treatment for bipolar depression, maintenance treatment, and mania in the non-perinatal BD population (Yatham et al. 2018). However, the safety of lithium during pregnancy has not been firmly established and there are conflicting opinions on its use. The National Institute for Health and Care Excellence (NICE) recommended that antipsychotic medications be used preferentially over lithium in women with BD who are pregnant or planning on becoming pregnant. It further advises that lithium be discontinued with consideration of using antipsychotics if women become pregnant while on lithium or that lithium be discontinued and then restarted in the second trimester (National Institute for Clinical Excellence 2016). The most recent large cohort study was done by Patorno et al. (2017). This study looked at 1,325,563 infants of which 663 were exposed to lithium in the first trimester. The rate of cardiac malformations in lithium-exposed infants was 2.41% compared to 1.15% in non-exposed infants and 1.39% in infants exposed to lamotrigine. After adjustment, they found a risk ratio for cardiac malformations of 1.11 for daily doses less than 600 mg, 1.60 for daily doses between 601 and 900 mg, and 3.22 for daily doses greater than 900 mg. The relative risk of malformations overall was 1.37 (95% CI 1.29–2.40) in infants exposed to lithium versus unexposed infants after adjustment.

If lithium is used in pregnancy, close monitoring of serum levels is required. Lithium excretion increases as the glomerular filtration rate increases. As such, dosage increases may be required to prevent symptom relapse. A recent study by Wesseloo et al. (2017b) monitored lithium levels obtained from 113 pregnancies.

Compared to the preconception baseline lithium levels there were changes of −24% in the first trimester, −36% in the second trimester, −21% in the third trimester, and there was an increase in lithium levels by 9% in the postpartum. This suggests that lithium clearance is highest during the second trimester and that lithium levels can increase quickly in the postpartum if not closely monitored. The authors recommended monitoring lithium levels every 3 weeks until 34 weeks of gestation and then weekly until delivery. Given the risk of lithium toxicity that can occur postpartum, especially if doses were increased during pregnancy, the authors have recommended that lithium levels be checked twice weekly for the first two postpartum weeks. They also recommended using a higher target serum lithium level (≥ 0.8 mmol/L) in the first postpartum month as this is a time of highest risk for relapse. There are mixed opinions on how lithium should be dosed in the days before delivery. Some experts have recommended holding lithium for 1–3 days as higher serum lithium levels have been associated with adverse neonatal effects. Others have felt that holding lithium before delivery is unnecessary if the woman remains well-hydrated and that doing so may increase the risk of a postpartum relapse. Anti-inflammatory medications should be avoided while taking lithium as they can increase the risk of toxicity.

Lamotrigine has shown efficacy in preventing antenatal BD relapses in small studies. Newport et al. (2008) followed a group of 26 women who were euthymic at conception and assessed for major depressive, hypomanic, or manic episodes during pregnancy. There were significantly lower rates of relapse in the women maintained on lamotrigine (30%) versus 100% in the group that discontinued mood stabilizing medications. Additionally, the time to 25% relapse was 14 times longer in the women who took lamotrigine throughout pregnancy (28.0 versus 2.0 weeks). Lamotrigine is generally thought to have a favorable pregnancy safety profile when compared to other mood stabilizing medications. A recent systematic review and meta-analysis by Pariente et al. (2017) did not find an increased risk of congenital malformations in fetuses exposed to lamotrigine when compared to a disease-matched control group (OR 1.15, 95% CI 0.62–2.16) and a control group without mood stabilizing medication exposure (OR 1.25, 95% CI 0.89–1.74). Additionally, they did not detect increased rates of preterm delivery, spontaneous abortion, stillbirth, or small for gestational age neonates after lamotrigine exposure but these outcomes were not meta-analyzed. Lamotrigine may require dosage titration throughout pregnancy to maintain a euthymic state as clearance of the medication increases. A study of serum lamotrigine concentrations in 14 pregnant women showed a progressive increase in lamotrigine clearance until it peaked at 32 weeks then declined. The peak clearance was 330% of baseline (Pennell et al. 2004). Like lithium, abrupt dosage reductions may be required immediately following delivery to avoid developing toxicity.

A single case study by Uguz (2017) has suggested that both quetiapine and olanzapine may be effective in the maintenance treatment of antenatal BD. He reported on six cases where low-dose olanzapine (5–10 mg) was used without any antenatal relapses occurring. He also reported on two cases of maintenance treatment with quetiapine, one of which experienced a relapse that resolved with re-instating the pre-pregnancy medications. Detailed discussion of the safety of antipsychotics in pregnancy is provided in Chap. 7.

16.6.4 Prophylaxis Against Postpartum Relapses in Bipolar Disorder

Prophylactic treatment against postpartum BD episodes cannot be entirely separated from prophylactic treatment of antenatal episodes. As with other areas of management in perinatal BD, studies of management in the early postpartum period are lacking. A meta-analysis by Wesseloo et al. (2015) demonstrated that women who remain on mood-stabilizing medications during pregnancy have a lower rate of postpartum relapse (23% versus 66%). Women taking prophylactic medications in the postpartum also had a significantly lower relapse rate at 29% (CI 16–47%). Of these women, 22 initiated prophylactic medications in the immediate postpartum and 38 were taking medication during pregnancy. The authors were unable to determine the relapse rate in women who initiated mood-stabilizing medications in the postpartum, but they reported on previous studies that analyzed this. One study showed a relapse rate of 30% (3/10 women) with immediate postpartum prophylaxis (Meakin et al. 1995). Another study had a relapse rate of 14% (3/21) in women who initiated postpartum lithium (Stewart et al. 1991). A recent systematic review and meta-analysis by Sharma et al. (2024) demonstrated a 58.1% rate of postpartum manic or mixed episodes in studies where medications were not used compared to a 25.9% rate in women who took medications. In an additional study, a group of 20 women who initiated prophylactic lithium in the postpartum had no relapses whereas 44% (4/9) of the women who remained medication-free did (Bergink et al. 2012). The results of these studies suggest that the risk of experiencing a postpartum BD relapse may be greatly reduced when prophylactic medication is started in the immediate postpartum even when women remain medication-free during pregnancy.

A small study by Sharma et al. suggested that there may be benefits from starting olanzapine in the immediate postpartum for women with BD who remain medication-free in pregnancy. In the open-label study a group of 11 women treated with olanzapine, with or without a mood stabilizer, had a much lower relapse rate than 14 comparison women who were treated with a mood stabilizer, an antidepressant or no medication (18.2% versus 57.1%). Only 3 of the 11 women in the olanzapine group initiated the medication before parturition (Sharma et al. 2006).

A single study has compared the efficacy of two different mood-stabilizing agents (lithium and lamotrigine) in preventing relapses requiring psychiatric hospitalization. In this study, there were no statistical differences in the hospitalization rates between the groups with 7.3% of those taking lamotrigine hospitalized versus 15.3% in those taking lithium (adjusted OR 0.83, 95% CI 0.22–3.14) (Wesseloo et al. 2017a).

A recent case series by Sharma and Wood (2025) suggested potential benefits from a multimodal treatment approach including psychoeducation, medication management, symptom monitoring using a mood diary, and management of sleep-related concerns. The use of this multimodal approach resulted in a postpartum relapse rate of only 16.7% with no hospitalizations required. In this study, medication management primarily involved the use of sedating antipsychotic medications, however, women on antidepressant medications were tapered off them.

16.7 Management of Bipolar Mood Disorder Episodes in the Postpartum Period

There is an increasing evidence base indicating that the postpartum period is a time of high risk for both first presentations and relapses of BD. Depressive episodes are the most common form of relapse that occurs, but hypomanic, manic, and mixed episodes also occur at increased frequencies (Viguera et al. 2011). There have only been two open-label studies of the acute treatment for postpartum bipolar depression, both of which used quetiapine. The study by Sharma et al. involved 18 postpartum women with BD. All the women had an onset of depression within the first 4 weeks postpartum. After treatment with quetiapine for 8 weeks (the median dose was only 75 mg), 83% of the women were reported as "much improved" or "very much improved" (Sharma et al. 2015). A second study by Misri et al. (2015) included 26 women and used doses of quetiapine XR between 50 and 300 mg. Remission of depression was achieved at an average quetiapine XR dose of 137.5 mg and sleep restoration occurred at 114.3 mg. At the 14-week point, 86.7% of the women were asymptomatic. Although these two small studies using quetiapine are promising, overall, there is a dearth of evidence to guide the management of postpartum BD. Given this, it is reasonable to extrapolate from guidelines that have been created for the non-perinatal population. In situations where the women have opted not to breastfeed, the guidelines can be followed as they would for non-postpartum women (Yatham et al. 2018). Alternatively, when women are breastfeeding, the risks of different medications to the breastfeeding infant must be given careful consideration. A detailed discussion of mood stabilizing medications during breastfeeding can be found elsewhere in this textbook. While data on the subject remains sparse and limited to case reports, there is increasing evidence suggesting that the cessation of breastfeeding can also be a trigger for emergence of a relapse in postpartum women with bipolar disorder (Sharma 2018; Schmidt et al. 2016).

16.8 Management of Postpartum Psychosis

Postpartum psychosis is a psychiatric emergency that occurs in 0.89–2.60/1000 postpartum women (VanderKruik et al. 2017). These episodes most frequently occur within the first weeks postpartum. Women who experience mania or psychosis during pregnancy are at a significantly increased risk of experiencing a postpartum episode (Perry et al. 2021). A study of 130 women with postpartum psychosis admitted to a mother-baby inpatient unit reported that the most common symptoms were irritability (73%), abnormal thought content (72%), and anxiety (71%).

Suicidal ideation was present in 19% of the women and infanticidal ideation in 8%. The most common presentation was depression (41%). A manic profile was seen in 1/3 of the women and 25% had an atypical presentation (Kamperman et al. 2017). Psychiatric hospitalization is generally required in the management of postpartum psychosis as there are usually significant functional impairments in addition to greatly increased risks for suicide and infanticide (Sit et al. 2006; Spinelli 2004). Treatment usually involves antipsychotic medications but can also involve antiepileptics, benzodiazepines, or electroconvulsive therapy (ECT) (Spinelli 2009). Previous studies on prophylaxis against postpartum psychosis have predominately used lithium and shown this medication to be efficacious (Bergink et al. 2012). A small study by Sharma et al. (2006) suggested the efficacy of olanzapine in preventing postpartum psychosis in women with BD.

To date, there have not been any RCTs in the treatment of postpartum psychosis. Most of the literature available is limited to case studies and case reports that have used various mood-stabilizing medications. The largest study completed was by Bergink et al. (2015) who composed a treatment protocol that was administered to 64 women consecutively admitted to the hospital for postpartum psychosis. The protocol had four treatment stages which were progressed through if symptom remission was not achieved at the preceding stage. A 98.4% remission rate was obtained using levels I—III. Level I of the protocol was the use of benzodiazepine monotherapy for 3 days to determine if optimizing sleep was sufficient to achieve remission. This was successful in 6.3% ($n = 4$) of the women. Step II involved augmenting the benzodiazepine with an antipsychotic, most commonly haloperidol or olanzapine. An additional 18.8% ($n = 12$) of the women achieved remission within 3 weeks of this stage. Adjunctive lithium was added to the treatment regime in stage III and the dose was titrated to achieve a serum level of 0.8–1.2 mmol/L. An additional 75% of the women achieved remission in this stage. Stage IV was ECT, but this was not used in any of the women. Following the acute treatment women were advised to remain on maintenance therapy for 9 months except for the women who remitted in stage I as they were tapered off the benzodiazepine after remission. None of the patients who remitted in stage I relapsed in the following 9 months. Fifty percent of the women who remitted in stage II and were maintained on an antipsychotic medication relapsed over the 9 months. For women who remitted in stage III, the benzodiazepine and antipsychotic were discontinued and the women had maintenance treatment with lithium (serum lithium level 0.6–0.8 mmol/L). The relapse rate at 9 months in this group was 12.8%. The overall rate of remission at 9 months was 79.7% among the 64 women. An increasing body of literature suggests that sleep disruption may be a very important factor in both the development and prevention of postpartum psychosis (Sharma and Mazmanian 2003; Lewis et al. 2018). Given this, the management of sleep-related issues should be considered a vital component of overall psychiatric management (Lewis et al. 2018).

16.9 Conclusions

Pharmacological management of perinatal BD remains a highly complex area where the risks of maternal illness must be estimated and weighed against the risks associated with mood-stabilizing medications (Table 16.1). This balancing of risks must be performed on a case-by-case basis for each woman but information about the risks associated with both the illness and the medications are lacking. Untreated maternal BD often leaves women at risk of significant morbidity, worsened obstetrical care, and impaired capacity for childcare. Yet, many of the medications

Table 16.1 Expert recommendations for the management of perinatal bipolar disorder based on scientific and clinical experience

Perinatal period	
1.	Treatment decisions in the management of perinatal bipolar disorder should be individualized
2.	Perinatal recurrences of bipolar disorder are usually characterized by depressive or mixed symptoms
3.	Treatment decisions should take into consideration the past illness course (especially during the perinatal period), current symptoms, co-morbid psychiatric disorders, family psychiatric history, and history of treatment response
4.	Management of co-morbid psychiatric disorders and medical co-morbidities (e.g., obesity, smoking, and substance abuse) are important in minimizing risks to both the mother and her baby
5.	Use of mood stabilizing medications should be limited to monotherapy where possible.
6.	Valproate should not be prescribed to women during the childbearing years
Pre-conception	
1.	Pre-conception counselling should be an integral part of the plan to manage bipolar disorder during and after pregnancy
2.	Women who have been clinically stable for at least six months and have had a mild illness course may be appropriate for tapering or discontinuing medications during pregnancy or in the pre-conception period
Pregnancy	
1.	Both mood stabilizing medications and untreated bipolar disorder can pose significant risks to the mother and fetus during pregnancy
2.	Both the mother and fetus should be closely monitored during pregnancy
3.	Lamotrigine may have the best pregnancy safety profile among mood stabilizing medications, but it lacks efficacy in managing hypomanic and manic episodes
4.	Haloperidol is a preferred medication for management of mania during pregnancy
5.	Careful balancing of risks and benefits is necessary when considering the use of lithium in pregnancy
6.	Antidepressants should be given scrutiny in pregnancy as they have associated fetal risks and may precipitate mood instability, especially if mood stabilizers are discontinued
7.	Valproate should be avoided during pregnancy because of its high teratogenic risk
Postpartum	
1.	Women with bipolar disorder require very close monitoring in the postpartum given the high rates of illness relapse during this time
2.	Women who remain medication-free during pregnancy may benefit from the initiation of prophylactic mood stabilizing medications in the immediate postpartum

commonly used to manage BD, particularly some of the anti-epileptic agents, are associated with significant risks to fetal development.

There are numerous aspects of perinatal BD pharmacology that require further study. To date, no RCTs have been completed in this population. However, these RCTs would be challenging to feasibly do given ethical concerns. Studies in the acute treatment of BD both during pregnancy and the postpartum are needed. Currently, evidence on the effectiveness of various mood-stabilizing medications must be extrapolated from studies done in non-perinatal populations, many of which specifically excluded pregnant and postpartum women. Existing perinatal literature is heavily focused on BD I as there has only been a single study with an exclusive focus on the management of perinatal BD II (Sharma et al. 2013). It is not yet known if there are significant pathophysiological differences between BD in the perinatal period versus BD in other periods of a woman's life. Should significant differences exist, this could suggest that a different approach to treatment would be indicated. Another emerging issue is a lack of pregnancy safety data for many of the newer antipsychotic medications being used to treat BD. This lack of data makes it very difficult for clinicians to discuss the risks of treatment with pregnant women which is vital in allowing them to make informed treatment decisions. Further collection of safety data on these medications will be imperative to allow women to make informed decisions about their treatment during the antenatal period.

References

American College of Obstetricians and Gynecologists Committee. American College of Obstetricians and Gynecologists Committee opinion no. 630. Screening for perinatal depression. Obstet Gynecol. 2015;125:1268–71.

American Psychiatric Association. Diagnostic and statistical manual of mental disorders: DSM-5. Washington: American Psychiatric Press; 2013.

Azorin JM, Angst J, Gamma A, Bowden CL, Perugi G, Vieta E, Young A. Identifying features of bipolarity in patients with first-episode postpartum depression: findings from the international BRIDGE study. J Affect Disord. 2012;136:710–5.

Barnett JH, Smoller JW. The genetics of bipolar disorder. Neuroscience. 2009;164:331–43.

Bergink V, Bouvy PF, Vervoort JS, Koorengevel KM, Steegers EA, Kushner SA. Prevention of postpartum psychosis and mania in women at high risk. Am J Psychiatry. 2012;169:609–15.

Bergink V, Burgerhout KM, Koorengevel KM, Kamperman AM, Hoogendijk WJ, Lambregtse-van den Berg MP, Kushner SA. Treatment of psychosis and mania in the postpartum period. Am J Psychiatry. 2015;172:115–23.

Boden R, Lundgren M, Brandt L, Reutfors J, Andersen M, Kieler H. Risks of adverse pregnancy and birth outcomes in women treated or not treated with mood stabilisers for bipolar disorder: population based cohort study. BMJ. 2012;345:e7085.

Bramanta A, Di Florio A. A case-control study of filicide/infanticide in 90 mothers. Arch Womens Ment Health. 2023;28:415. https://doi.org/10.1007/s00737-023-01401-5.

Cipriani A, Barbui C, Salanti G, Rendell J, Brown R, Stockton S, Purgato M, Spineli LM, Goodwin GM, Geddes JR. Comparative efficacy and acceptability of antimanic drugs in acute mania: a multiple-treatments meta-analysis. Lancet. 2011;378:1306–15.

Coughlin CG, Blackwell KA, Bartley C, Hay M, Yonkers KA, Bloch MH. Obstetric and neonatal outcomes after antipsychotic medication exposure in pregnancy. Obstet Gynecol. 2015;125:1224–35.

Diav-Citrin O, Shechtman S, Ornoy S, Arnon J, Schaefer C, Garbis H, Clementi M, Ornoy A. Safety of haloperidol and penfluridol in pregnancy: a multicenter, prospective, controlled study. J Clin Psychiatry. 2005;66:317–22.

Dolk H, Jentink J, Loane M, Morris J, et al. Does lamotrigine use in pregnancy increase orofacial cleft risk relative to other malformations? Neurology. 2008;71:714–22.

Doyle K, Heron J, Berrisford G, Whitmore J, Jones L, Wainscott G, Oyebode F. The management of bipolar disorder in the perinatal period and risk factors for postpartum relapse. Eur Psychiatry. 2012;27:563–9.

Driscoll KE, Sit DKY, Moses-Kolko EL, Pinheiro E, Yang A, Ciolino JD, Eng HF, Luther JF, Clark CT, Wisniewski SR, Wisner KL. Mood symptoms in pregnant and postpartum women with bipolar disorder: a naturalistic study. Bipolar Disord. 2017;19:295–304.

Egbe A, Lee S, Ho D, Uppu S. Effect of race on the prevalence of congenital malformations among newborns in the United States. Ethn Dis. 2015;25:226–31.

Ennis ZN, Damkier P. Pregnancy exposure to olanzapine, quetiapine, risperidone, aripiprazole and risk of congenital malformations. A systematic review. Basic Clin Pharmacol Toxicol. 2015;116:315–20.

Gentile S, Luigia Fusco M. Placental and fetal effects of antenatal exposure to antidepressants or untreated maternal depression. J Matern Fetal Neonatal Med. 2016;30:1189–99.

Ghaemi SN, Boiman EE, Goodwin FK. Diagnosing bipolar disorder and the effect of antidepressants: a naturalistic study. J Clin Psychiatry. 2000;61:804–8.

Graham RK, Tavella G, Parker GB. Is there a consensus across international evidence-based guidelines for the psychotropic drug management of bipolar disorder during the perinatal period? J Affect Disord. 2018;228:216–21.

Grof P, Robbins W, Alda M, Berghoefer A, Vojtechovsky M, Nilsson A, Robertson C. Protective effect of pregnancy in women with lithium-responsive bipolar disorder. J Affect Disord. 2000;61:31–9.

Guberman AH, Besag FM, Brodie MJ, Dooley JM, Duchowny MS, Pellock JM, Richens A, Stern RS, Trevathan E. Lamotrigine-associated rash: risk/benefit considerations in adults and children. Epilepsia. 1999;40:985–91.

Hernandez-Diaz S, Smith CR, Shen A, Mittendorf R, Hauser WA, Yerby M, Holmes LB. Comparative safety of antiepileptic drugs during pregnancy. Neurology. 2012;78:1692–9.

Hirschfeld RM, Lewis L, Vornik LA. Perceptions and impact of bipolar disorder: how far have we really come? Results of the national depressive and manic-depressive association 2000 survey of individuals with bipolar disorder. J Clin Psychiatry. 2003;64:161–74.

Holmes LB, Mittendorf R, Shen A, Smith CR, Hernandez-Diaz S. Fetal effects of anticonvulsant polytherapies: different risks from different drug combinations. Arch Neurol. 2011;68:1275–81.

Inglis AJ, Hippman CL, Carrion PB, Honer WG, Austin JC. Mania and depression in the perinatal period among women with a history of major depressive disorders. Arch Womens Ment Health. 2014;17:137–43.

Kamperman AM, Veldman-Hoek MJ, Wesseloo R, Robertson Blackmore E, Bergink V. Phenotypical characteristics of postpartum psychosis: a clinical cohort study. Bipolar Disord. 2017;19:450–7.

Lam DH, Watkins ER, Hayward P, Bright J, Wright K, Kerr N, Parr-Davis G, Sham P. A randomized controlled study of cognitive therapy for relapse prevention for bipolar affective disorder: outcome of the first year. Arch Gen Psychiatry. 2003;60:145–52.

Leong C, Raymond C, Chateau D, Dahl M, Alessi-Severini S, Falk J, Bugden S, Katz A. Psychotropic drug use before, during, and after pregnancy: a population-based study in a Canadian cohort (2001-2013). Can J Psychiatr. 2017;62:543–50.

Lewis KJS, Di Florio A, Forty L, Gordon-Smith K, Perry A, Craddock N, Jones L, Jones I. Mania triggered by sleep loss and risk of postpartum psychosis in women with bipolar disorder. J Affect Disord. 2018;225:624–9.

Marengo E, Martino DJ, Igoa A, Scápola M, Fassi G, Baamonde MU, Strejilevich SA. Unplanned pregnancies and reproductive health among women with bipolar disorder. J Affect Disord. 2015;178:201–5.

Masters G, Huguin J, Xu L, Ulbricht C, Moore Simas T, Ko J, Byatt N. Prevalence of bipolar disorder in perinatal women: a systematic review and meta-analysis. J Clin Psychiatry. 2022;83

McIntyre RS, Laliberte F, Germain G, MacKnight SD, Gillard P, Harrington A. The real-world health resource use and costs of misdiagnosing bipolar I disorder. J Affect Disord. 2022;316:26–33.

Meakin CJ, Brockington IF, Lynch S, Jones SR. Dopamine supersensitivity and hormonal status in puerperal psychosis. Br J Psychiatry. 1995;166:73–9.

Misri S, Abizadeh J, Eng A, Ryan D, Swift E. An open-label study of quetiapine extended-release in a sample of postpartum women with bipolar II depressive episode. Curr Psychopharmacol. 2015:16–26.

Munk-Olsen T, Laursen TM, Pedersen CB, Mors O, Mortensen PB. New parents and mental disorders: a population-based register study. JAMA. 2006;296:2582–9.

National Institute for Health and Care Excellence. Antenatal and postnatal mental health; 2016. Available from: https://www.nice.org.uk/guidance/qs115/resources/antenatal-and-postnatal-mental-health-75545299789765

Newport DJ, Calamaras MR, DeVane CL, Donovan J, Beach AJ, Winn S, Knight BT, Gibson BB, Viguera AC, Owens MJ, Nemeroff CB, Stowe ZN. Atypical antipsychotic administration during late pregnancy: placental passage and obstetrical outcomes. Am J Psychiatry. 2007;164:1214–20.

Newport DJ, Stowe ZN, Viguera AC, Calamaras MR, Juric S, Knight B, Pennell PB, Baldessarini RJ. Lamotrigine in bipolar disorder: efficacy during pregnancy. Bipolar Disord. 2008;10:432–6.

Nulman I, Koren G, Rovet J, Barrera M, Pulver A, Streiner D, Feldman B. Neurodevelopment of children following prenatal exposure to venlafaxine, selective serotonin reuptake inhibitors, or untreated maternal depression. Am J Psychiatry. 2012;169:1165–74.

O'Connor E, Rossom RC, Henninger M, Groom HC, Burda BU, Henderson JT, Bigler KD, Whitlock EP. U.S. Preventive Services Task Force evidence syntheses, formerly Systematic Evidence Reviews. Screening for depression in adults: an updated systematic evidence review for the US Preventive Services Task Force. Rockville (MD): Agency for Healthcare Research and Quality (US); 2016.

Pariente G, Leibson T, Shulman T, Adams-Webber T, Barzilay E, Nulman I. Pregnancy outcomes following in utero exposure to lamotrigine: a systematic review and meta-analysis. CNS Drugs. 2017;31:439–50.

Patorno E, Huybrechts KF, Hernandez-Diaz S. Lithium use in pregnancy and the risk of cardiac malformations. N Engl J. 2017;376:2245–54.

Pedersen CA, Johnson JL, Silva S, Bunevicius R, Meltzer-Brody S, Hamer RM, Leserman J. Antenatal thyroid correlates of postpartum depression. Psychoneuroendocrinology. 2007;32:235–45.

Pedersen CB, Mors O, Bertelsen A, Waltoft BL, Agerbo E, McGrath JJ, Mortensen PB, Eaton WW. A comprehensive nationwide study of the incidence rate and lifetime risk for treated mental disorders. JAMA Psychiatry. 2014;71:573–81.

Pennell PB, Newport DJ, Stowe ZN, Helmers SL, Montgomery JQ, Henry TR. The impact of pregnancy and childbirth on the metabolism of lamotrigine. Neurology. 2004;62:292–5.

Perry A, Gordon-smith K, Di Florio A, Craddock N, Jones L, Jones I. Mood episodes in pregnancy and risk of postpartum recurrence in bipolar disorder: the bipolar disorder research network pregnancy study. J Affect Disord. 2021;294:714–22.

Provencher MD, Hawke LD, Thienot E. Psychotherapies for comorbid anxiety in bipolar spectrum disorders. J Affect Disord. 2011;133:371–80.

Rosso G, Albert U, Di Salvo G, Scata M, Todros T, Maina G. Lithium prophylaxis during pregnancy and the postpartum period in women with lithium-responsive bipolar I disorder. Arch Womens Ment Health. 2016;19:429–32.

Sadowski A, Todorow M, Yazdani Brojeni P, Koren G, Nulman I. Pregnancy outcomes following maternal exposure to second-generation antipsychotics given with other psychotropic drugs: a cohort study. BMJ Open. 2013:3.

Schmidt KA, Palmer BA, Fyre MA. Mixed mania with cessation of breastfeeding. Int J Bipolar Disord. 2016;4:18.

Schneck CD, Miklowitz DJ, Miyahara S, Araga M, Wisniewski S, Gyulai L, Allen MH, Thase ME, Sachs GS. The prospective course of rapid-cycling bipolar disorder: findings from the STEP-BD. Am J Psychiatry. 2008;165:370–7.

Scott J, Paykel E, Morriss R, Bentall R, Kinderman P, Johnson T, Abbott R, Hayhurst H. Cognitive-behavioural therapy for severe and recurrent bipolar disorders: randomised controlled trial. Br J Psychiatry. 2006;188:313–20.

Sharma V. Considerations in the pharmacotherapy of bipolar disorder during and after pregnancy. Curr Drug Saf. 2011;6:318–23.

Sharma V. Weaning and mixed mania – a case report. J Hum Lact. 2018;34:4.

Sharma V, Mazmanian D. Sleep loss and postpartum psychosis. Bipolar Disord. 2003;5:98–105.

Sharma V, Pope CJ. Pregnancy and bipolar disorder: a systematic review. J Clin Psychiatry. 2012;73:1447–55.

Sharma V, Wood K. Effect of optimized treatment on the postpartum recurrence in women with bipolar I disorder: a case series. J Affect Disord Rep. 2025;20:100873. https://doi.org/10.1016/j.jadr.2025.100873.

Sharma V, Xie B. Screening for postpartum bipolar disorder: validation of the mood disorder questionnaire. J Affect Disord. 2011;131:408–11.

Sharma V, Smith A, Mazmanian D. Olanzapine in the prevention of postpartum psychosis and mood episodes in bipolar disorder. Bipolar Disord. 2006;8:400–4.

Sharma V, Sommerdyk C, Xie B, Campbell K. Pharmacotherapy of bipolar II disorder during and after pregnancy. Curr Drug Saf. 2013;8:246–52.

Sharma V, Xie B, Campbell MK, Penava D, Hampson E, Mazmanian D, Pope CJ. A prospective study of diagnostic conversion of major depressive disorder to bipolar disorder in pregnancy and postpartum. Bipolar Disord. 2014;16:16–21.

Sharma V, Khan M, Sommerdyk C. Quetiapine in the acute treatment of bipolar postpartum depression: a chart review. J Clin Psychopharmacol. 2015;35:733–5.

Sharma V, Wood KN, Weaver B, Mazmanian D, Thomson M. Occurrence of postpartum manic or mixed episodes in women with bipolar I disorder: a systematic review and meta-analysis. Bipolar Disord. 2024;26:240–8.

Sit D, Rothschild AJ, Wisner KL. A review of postpartum psychosis. J Women's Health. 2006;15:352–68.

Spinelli MG. Maternal infanticide associated with mental illness: prevention and the promise of saved lives. Am J Psychiatry. 2004;161:1548–57.

Spinelli MG. Postpartum psychosis: detection of risk and management. Am J Psychiatry. 2009;166:405–8.

Stewart DE, Klompenhouwer JL, Kendell RE, van Hulst AM. Prophylactic lithium in puerperal psychosis. The experience of three centres. Br J Psychiatry. 1991;158:393–7.

Swartz HA, Frank E, Frankel DR, Novick D, Houck P. Psychotherapy as monotherapy for the treatment of bipolar II depression: a proof of concept study. Bipolar Disord. 2009;11:89–94.

Thomson M, Sharma V. Weighing the risks: the management of bipolar disorder during pregnancy. Curr Psychiatry Rep. 2018;20:20.

Thomson M, Sharma V. Bipolar disorder. In: Uguz F, Orsolini R, editors. Perinatal psychopharmacology. Springer Nature; 2019. p. 239–57.

Uguz F. Prophylactic use of olanzapine and quetiapine from pregnancy to the postpartum period in women with bipolar disorder: a case series. J Matern Fetal Neonatal Med. 2017;30:2569–671.

Uguz F, Orsolini L. Perinatal psychopharmacology. Cham, Switzerland :Springer 2019.

Uguz F, Sharma S, Boyce P, Clark CT, Galbally M, Koukopoulos A, Marsh W, Stevens A, Vigeura A. Prophylatic management of women with bipolar disorder during pregnancy and the perinatal period – clinical scenario-based practical recommendations from a group of perinatal psychiatry authors. J Clin Psychopharmacol. 2023;43:434–52.

Valenti M, Pacchiarotti I, Rosa AR, Bonnin CM, Popovic D, Nivoli AM, Murru A, Grande I, Colom F, Vieta E. Bipolar mixed episodes and antidepressants: a cohort study of bipolar I disorder patients. Bipolar Disord. 2011;13:145–54.

VanderKruik R, Barreix M, Chou D, Allen T, Say L, Cohen LS. The global prevalence of postpartum psychosis: a systematic review. BMC Psychiatry. 2017;17:272.

Viguera AC, Whitfield T, Baldessarini RJ, Newport DJ, Stowe Z, Reminick A, Zurick A, Cohen LS. Risk of recurrence in women with bipolar disorder during pregnancy: prospective study of mood stabilizer discontinuation. Am J Psychiatry. 2007;164:1817–24.

Viguera AC, Tondo L, Koukopoulos AE, Reginaldi D, Lepri B, Baldessarini RJ. Episodes of mood disorders in 2,252 pregnancies and postpartum periods. Am J Psychiatry. 2011;168:1179–85.

Wesseloo R, Kamperman AM, Munk-Olsen T, Pop VJ, Kushner SA, Bergink V. Risk of postpartum relapse in bipolar disorder and postpartum psychosis: a systematic review and meta-analysis. Am J Psychiatry. 2015;173:117–27.

Wesseloo R, Liu X, Clark CT, Kushner SA, Munk-Olsen T, Bergink V. Risk of postpartum episodes in women with bipolar disorder after lamotrigine or lithium use during pregnancy: a population-based cohort study. J Affect Disord. 2017a;218:394–7.

Wesseloo R, Wierdsma AI, van Kamp IL, Munk-Olsen T, Hoogendijk WJG, Kushner SA, Begink V. Lithium dosing strategies during pregnancy and the postpartum period. Br J Psychiatry. 2017b;211:31–6.

Yatham L, et al. Guidelines for the management of patients with bipolar disorder. Bipolar Disord. 2018;2018:1–74.

Schizophrenia and Related Psychoses 17

Selma Bozkurt

17.1 Introduction

Schizophrenia is a severe psychiatric disorder which occurs in young age and affects the perception, thinking, feeling, psycho-motor activity, behavior, and cognitive functions of the patient. Schizophrenia leads to dysfunction in the areas such as learning, self-care, working, social relationships, and daily-life skills and might result to lots of problems in work and social life (Öztürk 2015). Although the prevalence of schizophrenia in general population is less than the anxiety and depressive disorders, because the onset of schizophrenia is obviously in reproductive ages, psychotic symptoms can be seen during the perinatal period (Bozkurt 2017a).

17.2 Schizophrenia and Fertility

Women with the diagnosis of schizophrenia have lower fertility rates as compared to general population. According to the findings of a society-based retrospective study conducted in Canada between 2002 and 2011, in every 1000 pregnancies there are 3 mothers with schizophrenia (Vigod et al. 2014). Howard (2005) suggests that schizophrenia is the most common psychiatric disorder which affects the reproducibility.

There are some underlying probable causes, for example, schizophrenia affects negatively keeping healthy social relationships, low marriage rates, sexual dysfunction due to illness or psychotropic medications, and suppression of ovulation due to hyperprolactinemia (Laursen and Olsen 2010). Nowadays, there are some practices supporting deinstitutionalization of patients with severe psychiatric disorders from closed clinical settings and they are supported to be in active daily social life.

S. Bozkurt (✉)
Istanbul, Turkey

F. Uguz, L. Orsolini (eds.), *Perinatal Psychopharmacology*,
https://doi.org/10.1007/978-3-031-99720-4_17

Having lower hyperprolactinemia rates with atypical antipsychotics increases the opportunity of these women becoming pregnant. Thus, according to the findings of a study conducted in the USA between 2000 and 2007, it was reported that antipsychotic drug usage was 3 in every 1000 pregnant women which increased up to 8 in every 1000 pregnancies (Toh et al. 2013).

17.3 Clinical Features and Course of Schizophrenia During the Perinatal Period

Studies about clinical features and prognosis of schizophrenia in pregnancy are insufficient, thus it doesn't show whether it's positive or negative effects. It has been reported that more than half of the patients with schizophrenia who show active symptoms do not visit psychiatrists (Howard 2005). Retrospective studies highlighted that women with diagnosis of schizophrenia have exacerbation of symptoms rather than psychotic symptoms appearing for the first time (Özdamar et al. 2014). Cessation of existing treatment or attempt to replace a currently effective drug in this period, by the concern of negative effect on the pregnancy, increases exacerbation risk even more (Robinson 2012). Result of the reviews done about this subject is that, women patients with schizophrenia whose antipsychotics are stopped have recurrence rate of 50% whereas for continued medical therapy this rate is found about 15%. In other words, patients who stopped their antipsychotic drug treatment has 2- to three-fold increased possible recurrence risk compared to continuation of treatment and in sudden drug withdrawals have increased risk of recurrence compared to gradual withdrawals (Barnes 2011).

A meta-analysis concluded that the psychotic relapse ratio of schizophrenic patients in pregnancy is 6.9%, as for postpartum 37.5% and relapsing risk is higher at postpartum period rather than pregnancy (Matevosyan 2011). According to observational studies, for more than half of the patients, psychiatric exacerbation is seen and the risk of psychotic recurrence increases approximately up to 7-folds in the first year especially in the first 3 months (Matevosyan 2011; Howard 2005). Patients with inpatient treatment history of more than 3 months and active symptoms within 6 months before pregnancy have higher risk of psychotic relapse (Solari et al. 2009). Of women diagnosed with schizophrenia, 8% have treatment in an inpatient clinic during pregnancy (Howard et al. 2002; Howard 2005).

17.4 Risks of Untreated Maternal Schizophrenia

It is reported that more than half of the patients with schizophrenia do not go to psychiatry follow-ups during their pregnancy despite the existence of active psychotic symptoms (Howard 2005). Studies about the effect of schizophrenia on pregnancy and developing fetus are increasing. While some coherent results are obtained in some studies, significant procedural differences between studies constitute an obstacle to accessing more clear information. The effects of schizophrenia on pregnancy and fetus may be direct, but there are also indirect effects with various factors such as pregnancy planning, prenatal care, nutrition, alcohol, and substance use. The risk is further increased in patients without treatment (Bülbül et al. 2014; Matevosyan 2011; Miller 1997).

It has been reported that vitamin intake during pregnancy is lower and antenatal care level is lower (Matevosyan 2011). In a community-based study, preterm birth and low birth weight ratios are reported to be about 2 times higher than those who receive adequate care in schizophrenic mothers who do not receive adequate medical care during pregnancy. Women with schizophrenia are at risk for stillbirth, premature birth, low birth weight infants, and sudden infant deaths when pregnant (Nilsson et al. 2002, 2008; Bennedsen et al. 2001; Jablensky et al. 2005).

While it is not clear enough in studies that the contribution of indirect factors and the adverse effects of which are directly related to the disorder itself, some authors suggest that the effect of maternal factors such as preterm birth, low birth weight, maternal age, parity, education level, smoking on risk of stillbirth in schizophrenia is high even if they participate in the account, thus suggesting that risk increases cannot be explained only by maternal factors (King-Hele et al. 2007, 2009; Nilsson et al. 2002).

However, studies reported that women with schizophrenia had an increased risk of complications such as preeclampsia, thromboembolism, low birth weight infant, placental insufficiency, gestational diabetes, and premature birth during pregnancy (Hoirisch-Clapauch et al. 2015; Vigod et al. 2014). In addition, a meta-analysis showed that the risk of placental abruption, postpartum hemorrhage, cesarean section, birth defects, and neonatal mortality is significantly higher in pregnant women with schizophrenia compared to healthy controls (Tang et al. 2023). Hoirisch-Claupach and colleagues (2015) noted that patients with severe mental impairment such as schizophrenia may have a low-activity tissue plasminogen activator and a procoagulant phenotype, which may contribute to placental failure. The risk of developing congenital cardiovascular anomalies in infants of women with schizophrenia is increased (Jablensky et al. 2005). There is also an increased risk of obstetric complications involving placental abnormalities and prenatal bleeds in the pregnancy of schizophrenic patients (Hoirisch-Clapauch et al. 2015; Jablensky et al. 2005). Nosarti and Froudist-Walsh (2016) reported that women who had recently been diagnosed with schizophrenia had a 1.6-fold increased risk of premature birth (Nosarti and Froudist-Walsh 2016). Studies show that LBW (low birth weight) increases 1.2–2.3-fold in infants of mothers with schizophrenia (Nilsson et al. 2002, 2008; Jablensky et al. 2005; Hoirisch-Clapauch et al. 2015; Tang et al. 2023). About 1.1% of schizophrenic mothers lose their babies in the first year and risk is 2–2.5 times more likely than controls (King-Hele et al. 2009; Nilsson et al. 2002, 2008; Webb et al. 2005; Bennedsen et al. 2001). Sudden infant death syndrome risk is reported to be 0.5% and is about 5 times higher (Hizkiyahu et al. 2010; Hoirisch-Clapauch et al. 2015; Bennedsen et al. 2001). Both clinical conditions seem to be related to schizophrenia regardless of demographic factors (Nilsson et al. 2002, 2008; Bennedsen et al. 2001).

17.5 Psychopharmacologic Treatment of Schizophrenia in the Perinatal Period

Table 17.1 presents expert recommendations on the treatment of schizophrenia during the perinatal period.

17.5.1 Pregnancy

Most women are not aware of pregnancy before four to six gestational weeks. This can lead to infant exposure to combination of many antipsychotic medications during a considerable time of the sensitive period. Therefore, women with schizophrenia during childbearing years should be advised by their psychiatrist regarding fertility and pregnancy planning (Breadon and Kulkarni 2019).

Due to several reasons, pregnancy of women with schizophrenia is considered a relative risk. Pregnancy can trigger psychophysiological decompensation for women diagnosed with schizophrenia. Certain risk factors for pregnancy in schizophrenia are realization of pregnancy with delay, having reduced prenatal care and routine follow-up visit, excessive smoking, and inability to notice and understand the start of labor. There may be patients reporting hallucinations leading to denial of pregnancy or to refusal of prenatal ultrasound examination. In these cases, the risks of having unaided labor and failure of mother-baby bond are high. For these patients, there can be either obstetric or psychiatric complications (Nilsson et al. 2008; King-Hele et al. 2009).

Routine treatment suggestions of pregnancy period are not found and with regard to developing baby's safety, it is hard to have an absolute conclusion about these treatments. Selection of antipsychotics for the treatment of pregnant women with schizophrenia, especially when it comes to application of new agents is a complicated process (Seeman 2013; Robinson 2012; Reis and Kallen 2008). Effects of treatment on the fetus should be considered besides its effects on the patient. Every pregnant woman should be evaluated by her own special condition (Robinson 2012). Regarding the ethical issues, none of the studies about drugs that have been used doesn't meet the gold standards as randomized, placebo-controlled, double-blind, crossover studies. Very few studies have been conducted by controlling patient's age, past pregnancy losses, antipsychotic dosages, timing of administration, usage of multiple drugs or illegal agents (Robinson 2012; Seeman 2013).

Single antipsychotic drug use and minimum effective dose should be preferred for pregnant women as much as possible; treatment should be given in divided doses. Later in pregnancy, as a result of weight gain, metabolism, excretion of drug. and muscle/fat ratio changes, increased doses might be needed (Robinson 2012). Still, maintenance of current stabilization in terms of mental aspect is the main subject for consideration and sometimes more than one agent can be needed. Risk/benefit argument for antipsychotic drug treatment is designed by the woman's treatment history. Selection of the most appropriate treatment course rather than right or wrong choice should be the main target. Replacement of currently effective

Table 17.1 Expert recommendations based on scientific evidence and clinical experience

1.	Considering the potential of pregnancy as much as possible, the best pharmacological treatment approach should be planned from the beginning of pregnancy. Therapeutic co-operation should be well established and non-drug treatments should be tailore
2.	Close cooperation should be ensured among all disciplines involved in perinatal care, such as psychiatry, psychology, gynecology, pediatrics, midwifery, social worker, and maternal-infant health nursing
3.	In addition to remaining untreated during the perinatal period, it should be ensured that written consent is obtained after the patient and his/her relatives have been informed in detail of the current available data on the benefits and risks of the treatment to be performed
4.	Baseline measurements of basic biological parameters compatible with mental disorders and treatment should be obtained. Measure prolactin levels in patients taking prolactin-raising antipsychotics; if raised, consider prolactin-sparing antipsychotic: Continue antipsychotic if she is likely to relapse without medication. Do not offer depot antipsychotics in women who are planning a pregnancy, pregnant, or considering breastfeeding, unless she is responding well to depot and has previous history of non-adherence to oral medication
5.	Monotherapy should be targeted as much as possible. Antipsychotic treatment should be given in a minimal effective dose. However, it should be avoided at ineffective low doses. It should not be forgotten that the fetus will be exposed to both congenital and untreated outcomes with incomplete treatment
6.	During pregnancy, fetal development, obstetric physiology, and changes in maternal mental status should be adequately monitored. Ideally, a treatment team specializing in high-risk scenarios should undertake obstetric care. Similarly, close monitoring of fetal development (preferably weekly at 28, 32, 34, 36 weeks and after weeks) is crucial for increased risks, such as low and high birth weight
7.	At the 12th week of pregnancy, an ultrasound examination of the nuchal translucency of the fetus should be performed followed by a high-resolution morphology scan at 20 weeks
.	Because of the potential for increased risk for metabolic syndrome and gestational diabetes with second-generation antipsychotics, glucose tolerance test should be performed from week to week 28 and from week 28 to the glucose uptake test
9.	At birth, close observation and careful morphological examination should be performed in terms of withdrawal symptoms, toxicity, extrapyramidal symptoms, sleepiness, or other adverse effects that may occur in the newborn
10.	Early warning signs for the relocation of existing psychiatric disorder and those to be performed for necessary care should be prescribed in case of a relapse
11.	Discussion of the risks and benefits of using certain antipsychotic medications during breastfeeding with the patients and their relatives in the prenatal period, and accordingly, advice and priorities should be given on breastfeeding. Pharmacological suppression of lactation should be avoided. Encourage breastfeeding unless patients are taking clozapine. The level of antipsychotic medication in breast milk depends on the drug

treatment with a safer drug is not recommended however, if there is a pre-existing response to a safer drug in patient's history, a modification may be considered (Solari et al. 2009; Robinson 2012). In addition, while considering secondary conditions [complications] to drug use, rather than medication, negative results of the disease [low birth weight, early labor, occurrence of problems in the long terms, a worse manifestation in lactation period, etc.] that might affect the course of pregnancy should be kept in mind (Solari et al. 2009). While detecting whether a drug is whether teratogen or not, appeared defect should have a distinctive pattern [like extremity problems that appear with Thalidomide] or should appear more than 3% which is the general ratio of defects in newborns (Robinson 2012).

In a review considering the findings of Einarson's several studies in recent years, first-generation antipsychotics (FGAs) are accepted as relatively safe (Einarson 2010). It has been reported that women taking piperidil piperazine, [fluphenazine, trifluphenazine and perphenazine], phenothiazine [chlorpromazine, thioridazine and promethazine], butyrophenone [haloperidol], tioksanten [flupentixol], dibenzoksapin or diphenylbutylpiperidine group typical antipsychotics do not have an increase in teratogenity (Einarson 2010). By now, there are no certain results that have been concluded for second-generation antipsychotics (SGAs) use in women at reproductive ages or in pregnant women. In addition, generally SGAs have better safety profiles when compared to FGAs (Dodd and Berk 2006).

Poo and Agius's report published in 2015 reports the last suggestions and updates for pregnancy and breast-feeding period of NICE treatment guide (Poo and Agius 2015; NICE Guideline 2014). In this specific period, while considering pharmacological treatment for minimizing the risks for mother and baby, encouragement of psychological trials in the first place as possible shows the broadest perspective. It's known that SGAs are related to metabolic complications like weight gain and DM II. But the relationship between antipsychotics and undesired defects and pregnancy is not shown clearly (Poo and Agius 2015).

Compared to FGAs, SGAs are more frequently used in the treatment of schizophrenia or related psychiatric disorders. The available scientific evidence shows that absolute risk for congenital malformations in pregnant women using SGAs is no or small (Habermann et al. 2013; Huybrechts et al. 2016; Wang et al. 2021; Viguera et al. 2021). Therefore, there is no clear contraindication for their usage during pregnancy. In general, olanzapine and quetiapine followed by aripiprazole and risperidone may be chosen for the treatment of schizophrenia in pregnancy (Uguz et al. 2023). For the use of newer SGAs such as lurasidone, cariprazine, asenapine, and lumateperone, the more safety data is required. Although there is a potential bone marrow suppression, clozapine should not be stopped in pregnant and postpartum women with refractory schizophrenia (Uguz et al. 2023). If necessary, long-acting injectable SGAs, especially aripiprazole, are other pharmacological options (Fernández-Abascal; Uguz et al. 2023).

According to a study based on a wide population, women with severe psychiatric disorders such as schizophrenia and bipolar disorder have increased risk of pregnancy-related complications compared to the general population (Jablensky et al. 2005). Hence, it is difficult to specify the origins of obstetric complications and neonatal results are from either disease, drugs, interfering factors, or incidentally. Also, it is difficult to specify the causative agents because these patients are frequently under the effect of polypharmacological treatment (Jablensky et al. 2005).

Robakis and Williams (2013) emphasized safety rather than effectiveness in their current review, while pediatricians and obstetricians argue on the algorhytim that guides the choice of SGA on treating pregnant women.

17.5.2 Postpartum Period

Postpartum period is one of the most dangerous periods for exacerbation of psychiatric disorders and re-hospitalize in women's life. For this reason, to prevent a potential psychotic exacerbation during pregnancy and after birth, exceptional attention is necessary. For exacerbation of disease just after the birth (or in the third trimester) or for women with schizophrenia, it might be necessary to use antipsychotic agents (Bozkurt 2017b).

A successful antipsychotic treatment during the perinatal period is a result of good multidisciplinary cooperation between obstetricians, general practitioners, and psychiatrists (Solari et al. 2009; Robinson 2012). The risk of acute psychotic exacerbation in schizophrenia is mostly seen in the first 3 months after birth (Tomruk and Saatçioğlu 2010). Physiologically, progesterone and estrogen levels are lowest in the first few days of the postpartum period. Loss of anti-dopaminergic activity of estrogen may increase the risk of decompensation for psychosis (Doucet et al. 2011). Clinical manifestation of the women with schizophrenia, exacerbation related to leaving the medical treatment, or stress factors during the postpartum period have a risk of harm to the baby (Uguz 2016; Spinelli 2009).

As impairment of a mother's psychological situation may result in breakdown of healthy mother-baby bonding, it may also effect negatively to the baby's cognitive and behavioral development. Breastfeeding must be encouraged because of not only for safe mother-baby relation but also for decreasing the risk of infection and death ratios. Breastfeeding is described as the best feeding source for the first 6 months of baby (Babu et al. 2015). Besides, as many woman desires to breastfeed their babies, they are unwilling about psychiatric disorders' treatment during the postpartum period (Getile 2008; Uguz 2016). For this reason, there is a need of safety data about antipsychotics in order to decrease unintended exposition of the baby and preserve the mother's psychiatric health ideally (Klinger et al. 2013; Sharma 2008).

During the perinatal period, psychotic exacerbation or onset of schizophrenia may increase the risk of mortality and morbidity so it is important to treat properly and with great attention. Besides, because babies of untreated mothers are less susceptible, it is reported that these children are at increased risk of physical and emotional neglect and abuse (Niemi et al. 2004; Snellen et al. 1999). Choosing an antipsychotic for the treatment of a woman with schizophrenia during the perinatal period requires considering many issues with regard to the patient and general activity profile of the antipsychotics is the best approach for personalization of the treatment. In general, if the patient has used an antipsychotic and benefits from it, it is prior to choose (Getile 2008).

All the data up to date shows that for the breastfeeding women with schizophrenia and related psychotic disorders, it is very difficult to decide risk/benefit profiles of the antipsychotics for the babies. Although there is limited data, current information shows that it's not contraindicated to use antipsychotic drugs while breastfeeding (Babu et al. 2015).

Studies that investigate the usage of FGAs during the breastfeeding period and milk/plasma ratio are determined in a consistent way as small and there are no reported toxic or adverse effects (Babu et al. 2015). According to the research results and case reports it is possible to reach outcomes of: most of the undesirable outcomes are not relevant to SGA, detected at acceptable and safe levels on breastfed babies, and mild, temporary side effects are seen. For this reason, the risk of leaving mother with psychotic disorder untreated is higher than transmission of low amount of drug to the baby (Uguz 2016).

If the woman with schizophrenia in postpartum period wants to breastfeed, single SGA should be given at low dose. According to current literature, the drug of choice for breastfeeding women should be olanzapine. Because of the very low RID values, quetiapine may be given as first- or second-line treatment but there is very limited data (Aydin et al. 2015; Uguz 2021). Risperidone has a relatively high RID value than these two drugs; it is suggested as second-line therapy while breastfeeding. Clozapine usage must be avoided as possible in the breastfeeding period. For reliable suggestion for usage of aripiprazole, ziprasidone, asenapine, cariprazine, lurasidone, and lumateperone, there is a requirement for more data (Uguz 2021; Uguz et al. 2023).

In the breastfeeding period, chlorpromazine, haloperidol, and zuclopenthixol must be given at the minimum possible doses and only with continuous monitoring (Klinger et al. 2013). In the available data about SGAs are used mostly between first week and sixth month after birth; and maternal dose range is 2.5-20 mg/g[7.52 mg/day] for olanzapine, 25–400 mg/day [med: 183.92 mg/day] for quetiapine, 1-6 mg/day [med: 3.18 mg/day] for risperidone, 10-18 mg/day [med: 14.5 mg/day] for aripiprazole, 40–160 mg/day for ziprasidone, 250–400 mg for amisulpride and 100 mg/day for clozapine (Bozkurt 2017b). It is early to talk about long-term effects of antipsychotics as these studies are less than 18 months (Uguz 2016). The longest follow-up study related to the usage of AP agents in postpartum period belongs. In this study, children of women who used clozapine during the period of pregnancy and breastfeeding period are followed up for 5 years and dwell on the latency of verbal skills. Measuring antipsychotic levels on baby's plasma or breast milk is a useful way as it is a very difficult way. As it is more practical, parents should be instructed about the negative effects of antipsychotics (respiratory problems, chill, irritability, hypoglycemia, feeding difficulties, sleeping problems, rigidity, jaundice) and should be evaluated by a pediatrician frequently (Bozkurt 2017a).

17.6 Conclusion

The pharmacological management of schizophrenia in women of reproductive age is highly complex, and requires a holistic approach in order to maximize both the maternal and child's physical and mental well-being (Poo and Agius 2015). NICE CG192 presents the current evidence on atypical antipsychotics for schizophrenia in pregnancy; and good management requires a solid understanding of the illnesses themselves and the pharmacodynamics of medications used. Although firm conclusions cannot be drawn at this stage, current studies have improved our understanding on the pharmacology and risk:benefit profile of these drugs, with each antipsychotic having varying efficacy and side effects. Each treatment option should therefore be thoroughly discussed and the decision should be based on balancing the benefits and risks, with considerations for patient preference and other patient factors. There is also a strong emphasis on continuous monitoring and modulation of drugs in order to ascertain the best possible outcome for patients. There is a need of well-designed prospective studies for the proper evaluation of development of the children of the women who used antipsychotic drugs at the perinatal period. In these studies, besides maternal psychiatric disorders, alcohol use, drug use, and exposure to drugs should be reported with certain measurements.

References

Aydin B, Nayir T, Sahin S, Yıldız A. Olanzapine and quetiapine use duringbreastfeeding: excretion into breast milk and safe breastfeeding strategy. J Clin Psychopharmacol. 2015;35:206–8.

Babu GN, Desai G, Chandra PS. Antipsychotics in pregnancy and lactation. Indian J Psychiatry. 2015;57(Suppl 2):S303–7.

Barnes TRE and the Schizophrenia Consensus Group of the British Association for Psychopharmacology. Evidence-based guidelines for the pharmacological treatment of schizophrenia: recommendations from the British Association for Psychopharmacology. J Psychopharmacol. 2011;25:567–620.

Bennedsen BE, Mortensen PB, Olesen A, Henriksen TB. Congenital malformations, stillbirths and infant deaths among children of women with schizophrenia. Arch Gen Psychiatry. 2001;58:674–9.

Bozkurt ZS. Gebelik Döneminde Şizofreni. In: Uguz F, editor. Gebelik ve Postpartum Dönemde Psikiyatrik Bozukluklar. İstanbul Medikal Yayıncılık; 2017a, p. 49–65 (in Turkish).

Bozkurt ZS. Perinatal Dönemde Antipsikotik İlaçlar. In: Uguz F, editor. Gebelik ve Postpartum Dönemde Psikiyatrik Bozukluklar. İstanbul Medikal Yayıncılık; 2017b, p. 227–257.

Breadon C, Kulkarni J. An update on medication management of women with schizophrenia in pregnancy. Expert Opin Pharmacother. 2019;20:1365–76.

Bülbül F, Çöpoglu ÜS, Demir B, Bulut M, Alpak G, Ünal A, Savaş H. Psikiyatrik hastalığı nedeniyle yatarak tedavi gören gebe hastaların klinik ve sosyodemografik özellikleri ve izlem sonuçları. Düşünen Adam J Psychiatry Neurol Sci. 2014;27:21–6. (in Turkish)

Dodd S, Berk M. The safety of medications for the treatment of bipolar disorder during pregnancy and the puerperium. Curr Drug Saf. 2006;1:25–33.

Doucet S, Jones I, Letourneau N, Dennis CL, Blackmore ER. Interventions for the prevention and treatment of postpartum psychosis: a systematic review. Arch Womens Ment Health. 2011;14:89–98.

Einarson A. Antipsychotic medication (safety/risk) during pregnancy and breastfeeding. Curr Women's Health Rev. 2010;6:34–8.

Getile S. Infant safety with antipsychotic therapy in breast-feeding: a systematic review. J Clin Psychiatry. 2008;69:666–73.

Habermann F, Fritzsche J, Fuhlbruck F, et al. Atypical antipsychotic drugs and pregnancy outcome: a prospective cohort study. J Clin Psychopharmacol. 2013;33:453–62.

Hizkiyahu R, Levy A, Sheiner E. Pregnancy outcome of patients with schizophrenia. Am J Perinatol. 2010;27:19–23.

Hoirisch-Clapauch S, Brenner B, Nardi AE. Adverse obstetric and neonatal outcomes in women with mental disorders. Thromb Res. 2015;135(Suppl 1):S60–3.

Howard LM. Fertility and pregnancy in women with psychotic disorders. Eur J Obstet Gynaecol Reprod Biol. 2005;119:3–10.

Howard LM, Kumar C, Leese M, Thornicroft G. The general fertility rate in women with psychotic disorders. Am J Psychiatry. 2002;159:991–7.

Huybrechts K, Hernandez-Diaz S, Patorno E, et al. Antipsychotic use in pregnancy and the risk for congenital malformations. JAMA Psychiatry. 2016;73:938–46.

Jablensky VA, Morgan V, Zubrick SR, Bower C, Yellachich L. Pregnancy, delivery and neonatal complications in population cohort of women with schizophrenia and major affective disorders. Am J Psychiatry. 2005;162:79–91.

King-Hele SA, Abel KM, Webb RT, Mortensen PB, Appleby L, Pickles AR. Risk of sudden infant death syndrome with parental mental illness. Arch Gen Psychiatry. 2007;64:1323–30.

King-Hele S, Webb RT, Mortensen PB, Appleby L, Pickles A, Abel KM. Risk of stillbirth and neonatal death linked with maternal mental illness: a national cohort study. Arch Dis Childhood Fet Neonat Ed. 2009;94:105–10.

Klinger G, Stahl B, Fusar-Poli P, Merlob P. Antipsychotic drugs and breastfeeding. Pediatr Endocrinol Rev. 2013;10:308–17.

Laursen TM, Olsen TM. Reproductive patterns in psychotic patients. Schizophr Res. 2010;121:234–40.

Matevosyan NR. Pregnancy and postpartum specifics in women with schizophrenia: a meta-study. Arch Gynecol Obstet. 2011;283:141–7.

Mendhekar DN. Possible delayed speech acquisition with clozapine therapy during pregnancy and lactation. J Neuropsychiatry Clin Neurosci. 2007;19(2):196–7.

Miller LJ. Sexuality, reproduction, and family planning in women with schizophrenia. Schizophr Bull. 1997;23:623–35.

National Institute for Health and Care Excellence. Antenatal and postnatal mental health: clinical management and service guidance (NICE CG192). London: National Institute for Health and Care Excellence; 2014.

Niemi L, Suvisaari J, Haukka J, Wrede G, Lonnqvist J. Cumulative incidence of mentaldisorders among offspring of mothers with psychoticdisorder. Results from the Helsinki high-risk study. Br J Psychiatry. 2004;185:11–7.

Nilsson E, Lichtenstein P, Cnattingius S, Murray RM, Hultman CM. Women with schizophrenia: pregnancy outcome and infant death among their offspring. Schizophr Res. 2002;58:221–9.

Nilsson E, Hultman CM, Cnattingius S, Olausson PO, Björk C, Lichtenstein P. Schizophrenia and offspring's risk for adverse pregnancy outcomes and infant death. Br J Psychiatry. 2008;193:311–5.

Nosarti C, Froudist-Walsh S. Alterations in development of hippocampal and cortical memory mechanisms following very preterm birth. Dev Med Child Neurol. 2016;58:35–45.

Özdamar Ö, Yılmaz O, Beyca HH, Muhcu M. Gebelik ve postpartum dönemde sık görülen ruhsal bozukluklar. Zeynep Kamil Tıp Bülteni. 2014;45:71–7. (In Turkish)

Öztürk O. Ruh Sağlığı ve Bozuklukları, 13th ed. Ankara; 2015, p. 42–48 (In Turkish).

Poo SXW, Agius M. Atypical antipsychotics for schizophrenia and/or bioplar disorder in pregnancy: current recommendations and updates in the NICE guidelines. Psychiatr Danub. 2015;27(Suppl. 1):255–60.

Reis M, Kallen B. Maternal use of antipsychotics in early pregnancy and delivery outcome. J Clin Psychopharmacol. 2008;28:279–88.

Robakis T, Williams KE. Atypical antipsychotics during pregnancy. Curr Psychiatr Ther. 2013;12:12–8.

Robinson GE. Treatment of schizophrenia in pregnancy and postpartum. J Popul Ther Clin Pharmacol. 2012;19:380–6.

Seeman MV. Clinical interventions for women with schizophrenia: pregnancy. Acta Psychiatr Scand. 2013;127:12–22.

Sharma V. Treatment of postpartum psychosis: challenges and opportunities. Curr Drug Saf. 2008;3:76–81.

Snellen M, Mack K, Trauer T. Schizophrenia, mental state, and mother-infant interaction: examining the relationship. Aust N Z J Psychiatry. 1999;33:902–11.

Solari H, Dickson KE, Miller L. Understanding and treating women with schizophrenia during pregnancy and postpartum. Can J Clin Pharmacol. 2009;16:e23–32.

Spinelli MG. Postpartum psychosis: detection of risk and management. Am J Psychiatry. 2009;166(4):405–8.

Tang W, Zhou LJ, Zhang WQ, Jia YJ, Hu FH, Chen HL. Adverse perinatal pregnancy outcomes in women with schizophrenia: a systematic review and meta-analysis. Schizophr Res. 2023;262:156–67.

Toh S, Li Q, Cheetham TC, Cooper WO, Davis RL, Dublin S, Hammad TA, Li DK, Pawloski PA, Pinheiro SP, Raebel MA, Scott PE, Smith DH, Bobo WV, Lawrence JM, Dashevsky I, Haffenreffer K, Avalos LA, Andrade SE. Prevalence and trends in the use of antipsychotic medications during pregnancy in the U.S., 2001-2007: apopulation-based study of 585,615 deliveries. Arch Womens Ment Health. 2013;16:149–57.

Tomruk NB, Saatçioğlu Ö. Treatment challenges in schizophrenia in perinatal period and infanticide. Bull Clin Psychopharmacol. 2010;20:266–8.

Uguz F. Second generation antipsychotics during the lactation period: a comparative systematic review on infant safety. J Clin Psychopharmacol. 2016;36:244–52.

Uguz F. A new safety scoring system for the use of psychotropic drugs during lactation. Am J Ther. 2021;28:2118–26.

Uguz F, Sharma V, Boyce P, Clark CT, Galbally M, Koukopoulos A, Marsh W, Stevens A, Viguera A. Prophylactic management of women with bipolar disorder during the perinatal period. Clinical scenario-based practical recommendations from a group of perinatal psychiatry experts. J Clin Psychopharmacol. 2023;43:434–52.

Vigod SN, Kurdyak PA, Dennis CL, Gruneir A, Newman A, Seeman MV. Maternal and newborn outcomes among women with schizophrenia: a retrospective population based cohort study. BJOG. 2014;121:566–74.

Viguera AC, Freeman MP, Góez-Mogollón L, et al. Reproductive safety od second-generation antipsychotics: updated data from the Massachusetts General Hospital National Pregnancy Registry for atypical antipsychotics. J Clin Psychiatry. 2021;82:20m13745.

Wang Z, Brauer R, Man KKC, et al. Prenatal exposure to antipsychotic agents and the risk of congenital malformations in children: a systematic review and meta-analysis. Br J Clin Pharmacol. 2021;87:4101–23.

Webb R, Abel K, Pickles A, Appleby L. Mortality of offspring of parents with psychotic disorders: a critical review and meta-analysis. Am J Psychiatry. 2005;162:1045–56.

Obsessive-Compulsive Disorder

18

Faruk Uguz

18.1 Introduction

Obsessive-compulsive disorder (OCD) is a relatively common psychiatric disorder frequently emerging among women in the reproductive years (Karno et al. 1988; Burke et al. 1990; Kolada et al. 1994). Its major characteristics include marked anxiety in the patients and disturbances in academic, occupational, and social functions (Bobes et al. 2001; Kıvırcık Akdede et al. 2005; Huppert et al. 2009). In addition, OCD may lead to a considerable reduction in the quality of life, often to the same extent as schizophrenia (Bobes et al. 2001).

Epidemiological studies have suggested that OCD represents the fourth most frequent psychiatric disorder following substance use disorders, mood disorders, and phobias (Karno et al. 1988). In recent years, many studies have examined whether reproductive events in women such as pregnancy and the postpartum period may be associated with OCD. Some authors have noted that female OCD patients reported pregnancy and childbirth to be precipitating events for the onset of OCD (Neziroglu et al. 1992; Maina et al. 1999). While the prevalence rate of this disorder was reported as 1.8–3.3% of women in the general population (Karno et al. 1988; Cilli et al. 2004), it was observed in 0.2–5.2% of pregnant women (Zar et al. 2002; Sutter-Dallay et al. 2004; Adewuya et al. 2006; Andersson et al. 2006; Felice et al. 2007; Uguz et al. 2007a; Borri et al. 2008; Farias et al. 2013) and 0.7–9.0% of postpartum women (Wenzel et al. 2001, 2005; Andersson et al. 2006; Navarro et al. 2008; Zambaldi et al. 2009). A meta-analysis has suggested that pregnant and postpartum women were at an increased risk of 2.07- and 2.43-fold, respectively to experience OCD compared to the general population (Russell et al. 2013). In addition, the perinatal period may affect the course of OCD in women (Labad et al.

F. Uguz (✉)
Department of Psychiatry, Medova Hospital, Faculty of Medicine, KTO Karatay University, Konya, Türkiye

F. Uguz, L. Orsolini (eds.), *Perinatal Psychopharmacology*,
https://doi.org/10.1007/978-3-031-99720-4_18

2005; Vulink et al. 2006; Guglielmi et al. 2014). On the other hand, inarguably, the newborn requires maternal attention, which emphasizes the importance of the treatment of OCD during this period.

Pharmacotherapy and psychotherapy are two main treatment regimens in OCD. Cognitive behavioral therapy (CBT) is the most effective evidence-based psychotherapy for OCD (Hirschtritt et al. 2017). Although it has been suggested that this method is as effective as pharmacotherapy (Björgvinsson et al. 2007; Franklin and Foa 2011), this chapter will not discuss CBT as a treatment method as it is not relevant to the theme of the book.

18.2 Risks of Untreated OCD

The emotional state of the mother during the perinatal period can have both short-term and long-term effects on her child (Glover 2014). Anxiety is one of the core symptoms of OCD. Studies have suggested that maternal antenatal and postnatal anxiety is associated with an increased risk of preterm birth and low birth weight, disturbances in sleep and feeding of the infant, lower maternal bonding, decreased interactions between mother and the infant, and increased risks of cognitive, emotional, and behavioral problems in the child stage (Van den Bergh et al. 2005; Talge et al. 2007; Buss et al. 2011; Leis et al. 2014; Ding et al. 2014; Kılınc and Herguner 2016). OCD may have similar negative effects on the fetus or infants. Although some authors have reported contrary data (House et al. 2016; Ferraro et al. 2017), this hypothesis has been supported by recent studies. Uguz et al. (2015) have reported that birth weight and gestational age were lower in newborns exposed to maternal OCD compared to babies who were not exposed. Two cohort studies suggested that maternal OCD was associated with adverse pregnancy (gestational diabetes, preeclampsia and placental abruption), delivery (elective and emergency cesarean), and neonatal outcomes (preterm birth, low birth weight, neonatal respiratory distress, and low Apgar score at 5 min) (Fernández de la Cruz et al. 2023). A most recent meta-analysis including eight studies has shown, in addition to these pregnancy, delivery, and neonatal complications, a significantly higher risk of major congenital malformations in fetuses of pregnant women with OCD (Aujla et al. 2024). Long-term effects of perinatal maternal OCD on the infants remain unknown. Results of a study with small sample size suggested that maternal OCD, particularly in those patients with higher maternal anxiety levels, may affect brain development of the fetus via increased neuroinflammation (Uguz et al. 2014). In addition, it was recently suggested that maternal postpartum OCD was associated with lower sensitivity during interactions with infants (Challacombe et al. 2016).

18.3 Pharmacological Treatment

The effectiveness of pharmacological treatments, including serotonergic antidepressants and their augmentation with antipsychotics, is well documented. Despite noteworthy advances in non-perinatal patients, pharmacological treatment and treatment guidelines for psychiatric disorders in perinatal patients have been largely neglected. Major issues in determining treatment regimen for OCD in women during pregnancy and lactation are possible adverse events in the fetus and breastfed infants due to psychotropic medications. In contrast, due to the potential negative effects of maternal OCD and secondary anxiety or depression on fetuses or infants, the risk of not treating this disorder during the perinatal period exists. However, to date, no study examining whether pharmacotherapy is useful in decreasing the possible negative effects of untreated OCD has been published in the literature. Therefore, recommending the safest and most effective pharmacological approach for the mother and her baby in this chapter is challenging.

18.3.1 General Considerations

The decision regarding the pharmacological treatment regimen should be based on several factors such as the risk of untreated maternal psychiatric illness, the known or unknown potential effects of psychotropic medications, benefits of pharmacological treatment, and alternative treatments to medication (Byatt et al. 2013). A careful psychiatric assessment should include individual and family history of psychiatric disorders, side effects or therapeutic effects of medications used previously, severity of the disorder, comorbid conditions, duration of remissions both on and off medication, time to relapse after previous discontinuation, time to recovery on reintroduction of medication, frequency of, and triggers for relapse, and degree of impairment in occupational, family and social areas secondary to the disorder (Yonkers et al. 2009; McAllister-Williams et al. 2017).

There are five main clinical rules in the pharmacological treatment of OCD during pregnancy and the lactation period: First, the treatment should be individualized. Second, the benefits and risks of untreated and treated OCD for the mother, her baby, and her family including other children should be discussed with the mother and her relatives. These discussions and the patient's choice should be documented. Third, all steps of the treatment should be administered in agreement with the patient and her relatives. Fourth, psychotropics with an evidence base with regard to both efficacy and safety in pregnant or lactating women should be chosen. Fifth, the clinical status and response to the treatment of the patients should be closely monitored (Uguz 2015). Other general recommendations are as follows (McAllister-Williams et al. 2017; Uguz 2017): (1) The lowest therapeutic (but not sub-therapeutic) doses should be chosen to minimize fetus/infant exposure. (2) Using a drug of known efficacy in the patient may be preferable to using one with unknown efficacy. (3) If a decision is taken to discontinue medication, this should be carried out as slowly as possible. (4) Although some patients require the use of combined antipsychotics, monotherapy is essential. If combination is inevitable, the second medication should be used as briefly as possible. (5) Older medications are preferred to newer medications, if there are inadequate data on infant safety.

Another issue in clinical practice is the decision on which patients actually need to be treated pharmacologically. There is no consensus on clinical indications for initiating pharmacological treatment in perinatal women with OCD, because there are no comparative studies on the influence of OCD untreated or treated by antidepressants in pregnant or lactating women with similar clinical features. However, pharmacological options may be considered in patients with severe depression and anxiety symptoms, a high risk of suicidal attempts, considerable feeding and sleep disturbances secondary to OCD, or OCD that is unresponsive to cognitive-behavioral therapy (Uguz 2015).

18.3.2 Treatment of Active Symptoms

18.3.2.1 First-Line Treatment

To date, clinical guidelines for the pharmacological treatment of OCD in pregnant or lactating women have not been published in the literature. In addition, it is unclear whether response to pharmacotherapy in perinatal and non-perinatal women with OCD is different (Brakoulias et al. 2020). Overall, it is assumed that these drugs are also effective in the perinatal period despite the lack of placebo-controlled studies (Uguz 2015). Moreover, none of the specific antiobsessional drugs are contraindicated for use during pregnancy and the lactation period.

Selective serotonin reuptake inhibitors (SSRIs) and clomipramine are first-line medications for OCD in the non-perinatal period (Kellner 2010). Compared to SSRIs, clomipramine has greater or equivalent efficacy in OCD; however, its lower tolerability by the patients led to a marked decrease in prescribing the drug (Fineberg et al. 2012; Hirschtritt et al. 2017). In addition, when the limited data on the safety of clomipramine during pregnancy and results of several studies suggesting increased risk of cardiac malformations and severe perinatal complications are considered, this drug does not appear to be appropriate as a first-line treatment of pregnant women with OCD. Similarly, factors such as limited available data on its safety, higher risk for propensity to convulsions. and increased risk of arrhythmia restrict its choice during lactation (Alper et al. 2007; Gentile 2014; Hirschtritt et al. 2017). The available scientific evidence on safety suggest that clomipramine should be cautiously preferred in pregnant and breastfeeding women with OCD who cannot tolerate or who have failed to respond to SSRIs (Uguz 2015; Fineberg et al. 2012).

SSRIs are recommended as first-line pharmacological agents for OCD in the perinatal period based on a relatively large database regarding their safety on the fetus and breastfed infants (McAllister-Williams et al. 2017). Some authors reported that the most commonly prescribed SSRIs in non-perinatal inpatients are sertraline, citalopram, and paroxetine (Poppe et al. 2016). The current evidence does not support the superior efficacy or tolerability of specific SSRIs to each other in OCD (Fineberg et al. 2015). The most important factors affecting the decision regarding which SSRI can be prescribed to perinatal patients with OCD are the available scientific data on the safety of each SSRI during pregnancy and lactation as well as a history of their effectivity and tolerability in the mother in the past.

Despite some negative reports, sertraline and citalopram/escitalopram seem to be more favorable as pharmacological options during pregnancy based on their safety in the fetus (Myles et al. 2013; Uguz 2015; Larsen et al. 2015; Kang et al. 2017; Shen et al. 2017; Womersley et al. 2017). However, the advantages of sertraline compared to citalopram/escitalopram are that the treatment can be continued during breastfeeding due to a high safety index, and there is much stronger evidence on efficacy in OCD (Larsen et al. 2015; Katzman et al. 2014). There is limited data in the literature on the safety of fluvoxamine; therefore, this antidepressant is not recommended during pregnancy (Larsen et al. 2015). Despite highest amount of data, clinicians have some concerns about the use of fluoxetine during pregnancy, because there is growing evidence suggesting increased risk of fetal defects and because the drug is released slowly in the body of newborns (Uguz 2015; Larsen et al. 2015). Similarly, it has been accepted that paroxetine is associated with an increased risk of congenital malformations, especially cardiac types (Myles et al. 2013; Grigoriadis et al. 2013). Owing to these features, fluoxetine and paroxetine are not appropriate for first-line treatments of OCD in pregnant women (Uguz 2015, 2020; Larsen et al. 2015; Womersley et al. 2017). However, these antidepressants show low elevation of absolute risk of birth defects and may be used in patients with OCD who cannot tolerate or do not respond sertraline, citalopram, or escitalopram (Myles et al. 2013; Grigoriadis et al. 2013; Uguz 2015).

There is a consensus in the literature on sertraline and paroxetine as first-line SSRIs during the lactation period because of adequate scientific data on their safety in breastfed infants. Citalopram/escitalopram and especially fluoxetine are less favorable. Citalopram/escitalopram do not accumulate, which is more advantageous compared to fluoxetine. Fluvoxamine should be used cautiously due to very limited data on its use during lactation (Gentile 2007; Orsolini and Bellantuono 2015; Uguz 2017, 2018).

Several studies have suggested that venlafaxine may be efficient in the treatment of OCD (Albert et al. 2002; Denys et al. 2003). Its safety profile in pregnancy appears to be similar to SSRIs (Byatt et al. 2013; Bellantuono et al. 2015; Furu et al. 2015; Lassen et al. 2016). Moreover, the fact that adverse events have been rarely reported in breastfed infants encourages the use of this antidepressant during the lactation period (Orsolini and Bellantuono 2015). On the other hand, limited available evidence of venlafaxine on efficacy in OCD and safety during pregnancy and breastfeeding are major disadvantages for its use. This paper recommends the use of venlafaxine prior to combined pharmacological options if pregnant or breastfeeding women with OCD do not respond to monotherapy with other antiobsessional antidepressants and have severe comorbid psychiatric disorders such as major depression, generalized anxiety disorder, and panic disorder.

18.3.2.2 Non-response to the First-Line Treatments

Approximately half of the patients with OCD who receive serotonergic antidepressant monotherapy at adequate doses and durations do not experience clinically significant improvement in symptoms (Kellner 2010). Initially, accuracy of the current diagnosis, possible medical or psychiatric comorbidities, degree of response, and treatment compliance in the patients should be carefully reviewed by the psychiatrist (Abudy et al. 2011; Fineberg et al. 2015; Uguz 2015). There are several pharmacological approaches in unresponsive patients: switch between antidepressants, treatment with initial SSRI at a supratherapeutic dose, combining SSRI and clomipramine, and augmentation with antipsychotics (Kellner 2010; Fineberg et al. 2015). Due to the lack of randomized controlled studies, which option is safer and effective in pregnant or breastfeeding women is currently unknown (Uguz 2018).

Switch Between Antidepressants

Despite insufficient scientific evidence, switching from one SSRI to another in patients who do not respond is an acceptable pharmacological option that is performed commonly in clinical practice (Castle et al. 2015; Fineberg et al. 2015). Several studies have suggested that about 40% of the patients experience clinically significant reduction in OCD symptoms (Denys et al. 2004; Fineberg et al. 2015). Although there are no studies conducted in the perinatal period, clinical experience implies that the switching method may be effective in a considerable number of pregnant or postpartum women with OCD. When safety in the fetus and/or breastfed infants is considered, this strategy may be more favorable as the first step in perinatal women compared to other pharmacological strategies. Switching between sertraline and citalopram/escitalopram during pregnancy, and between sertraline and paroxetine during breastfeeding may be appropriate (Uguz 2015, 2018).

SSRI Treatment at Supratherapeutic Doses

High-dose treatment with SSRIs even at 2- to three-fold of the maximum therapeutic doses is another pharmacological strategy (Ninan et al. 2006; Rabinowitz et al. 2008; Rampoloni et al. 2010; Fineberg et al. 2015). However, data supporting the benefits of this strategy is limited in non-perinatal patients (Fineberg et al. 2015). Additionally, the potential effects of SSRIs at supratherapeutic doses on the fetus or breastfed infants are unknown. Some authors reported that high doses of SSRIs (e.g., more than 40 mg/day for fluoxetine, citalopram, and paroxetine), even within the therapeutic dose limits, are associated with 2.5- to five-fold higher risk of preterm birth compared to lower daily doses (Suri et al. 2007; Roca et al. 2011; Michielsen et al. 2014). As a result, this is not a good pharmacological option in unresponsive perinatal women with OCD. If administration of such high doses indeed becomes necessary, the pregnant patient and exposed infants must be followed closely by the mother and physicians (Uguz 2015).

Combination Between Clomipramine and SSRIs

Clinicians frequently use this combinatorial method in non-perinatal women with SSRI-resistant OCD. Nevertheless, this strategy does not seem to be feasible as the first or second-line of pharmacotherapy in the pregnancy and lactation period due to the following reasons: (1) Studies examining the efficacy of this combination in OCD are few and their results are controversial (Marazziti et al. 2008; Kellner 2010; Diniz et al. 2010), (2) There are no data on safety of the fetus and/or breastfed infants in the literature, (3) This combination, especially between clomipramine and paroxetine or fluoxetine, is associated with a risk of clinically significant pharmacokinetic interactions that could lead to a dangerous build-up of clomipramine (Fineberg et al. 2015).

Augmentation with Antipsychotics

In the non-perinatal period, the most convincing evidence of treatment of SSRI-resistant OCD was with adjunctive antipsychotics (Fineberg et al. 2015). This strategy is recommended in the treatment guidelines (Kellner 2010; Katzman et al. 2014; Bandelow et al. 2023). It has been reported that adjunctive antipsychotics are prescribed in 30–40% of patients using SSRIs. The most commonly administered antipsychotics are risperidone, quetiapine, and olanzapine (Van Ameringen et al. 2014; Poppe et al. 2016). Actually, there is no clear evidence suggesting the superiority of one antipsychotic drug over others, because comparative studies between different antipsychotic augmentations are very limited.

As an augmentation treatment in nonperinatal patients, risperidone and aripiprazole are antipsychotics with the most consistent successful results (Bloch et al. 2006; Skapinakis et al. 2007; Dold et al. 2013; Veale et al. 2014; Muscatello et al. 2011; Selvi et al. 2011; Sayyah et al. 2012; Veale et al. 2014; Maiti et al. 2023). Moreover, the Canadian clinical practice guideline (Katzman et al. 2014) recommends the use of aripiprazole in addition to risperidone as the first-line adjunctive therapy. Augmentation with haloperidol was found to be effective in at least two meta-analyses in spite of being used in only one placebo-controlled study (Bloch et al. 2006; Skapinakis et al. 2007). Despite at least one positive randomized controlled trial (Fineberg et al. 2012) and one meta-analysis (Zhou et al. 2019; Fineberg et al. 2006), four meta-analyses (Bloch et al. 2006; Skapinakis et al. 2007; Dold et al. 2013; Veale et al. 2014) have suggested that augmentation with olanzapine and quetiapine was not superior to placebo. Recently, Shoja Shafti and Kaviani (2015) have suggested that treatment-resistant OCD patients may benefit more from the addition of quetiapine than aripiprazole. Additionally, quetiapine is also the single antipsychotic agent that has been studied in pregnant women with OCD. Misri and Milis (2004) suggested that 78.6% of postpartum women with OCD were responders to augmentation with quetiapine.

This strategy may be theoretically effective in some perinatal patients. Nonetheless, there are no studies examining the safety of a combination of antidepressants and antipsychotics during pregnancy and lactation in the literature (Uguz 2015). Antipsychotic augmentation is effective in approximately 30% of treatment-resistant nonperinatal patients, and it has potentially higher adverse effects on the fetus, breastfed infant, or the mother (Uguz 2015; Hirschtritt et al. 2017). Consequently, this strategy should be preferred in case there is a clinical conviction that the augmentation has higher benefits compared to untreated OCD. After the decision to augment with antipsychotics is made, the drug should be used at as low doses as possible (Uguz 2015). On the other hand, based on scientific evidences on effectivity in nonperinatal patients and safety on the fetuses and breastfed infants, an augmentation with low-dose antipsychotics (for example, 0.5–1 mg/day for risperidone, 2.5–5 mg/day for olanzapine, 100–200 mg/day for quetiapine) may be more appropriate pharmacological option compared to high-dose SSRI administration and combination between SSRI and clomipramine at therapeutic doses,

There is no clear contraindication to the use of risperidone or aripiprazole in pregnant or breastfeeding women. However, due to recent data on safety during pregnancy and on efficacy in nonperinatal patients (Freeman et al. 2021; Damkier and Videbech 2018; Gautam 2023), aripiprazole seems to be more preferable during pregnancy. On the other hand, compared to aripiprazole, risperidone has greater safety data on lactation. Therefore, compared to aripiprazole, it may be a more favorable antipsychotic in breastfeeding women with OCD (Uguz 2018, 2021). If the mother and/or the breastfed infant cannot tolerate risperidone or aripiprazole, or the patient does not respond to these adjuvant medications, alternative antipsychotics including haloperidol, quetiapine, and olanzapine should be discussed for further augmentation. If the patient has severe anxiety and markedly decreased sleep and appetite, quetiapine and olanzapine may be the first-line antipsychotics during both pregnancy and lactation periods. This option is based on their relatively good safety data on pregnant and breastfeeding women, several positive study results suggesting possible their efficacy as adjuvant in nonperinatal patients with OCD and their sedative and anxiolytic effects observed in clinical practice (Uguz 2021; Damkier and Videbech 2018; Zhou et al. 2019).

18.3.3 Prophylactic Treatment

It is well known that OCD has a chronic course in which recurrence and remission in the symptoms are observed. Studies have suggested a high symptomatic relapse after discontinuation of antiobsessional treatment (Fineberg et al. 2012). Moreover, an exacerbation in obsessive-compulsive symptoms during pregnancy is associated with significantly elevated risk of gestational diabetes and a diagnosis of major depression and/or anxiety disorder (Holingue et al. 2021). On the other hand, many women with OCD at remission apply to psychiatrists when planning for their pregnancy or determining a management strategy during pregnancy or postpartum period. Indeed, there are no guidelines in the literature regarding pharmacological prophylaxis of OCD symptoms during pregnancy or the lactation period in patients who are symptomatically in remission. An exceptional consensus among perinatal psychiatrists is that the pharmacological management should be individualized after a careful clinical evaluation including current mental status and OCD characteristics, treatment response, and symptomatic relapse in the past.

This paper recommends a treatment approach for active symptoms mentioned above if the patient has moderate or severe symptoms. In this part of the chapter, the recommendations for prophylaxis will be presented based on the following clinical scenarios:

1. *Current mental status*: Symptomatically in remission (no longer meets syndromal criteria for the disorder and has no more than minimal symptoms) (Mataix-Cols et al. 2016).
2. *Current mental status*: Symptomatically non-remitted but mild clinical severity of the symptoms.
   (a) *History of the disorder*: Severe OCD symptoms and functional impairment, low response rate and late response to pharmacotherapy, sudden symptomatic relapse following discontinuation of pharmacotherapy, and comorbidity with depression and/or anxiety disorders.
   (b) *History of the disorder*: Mild to moderate OCD symptoms and functional impairment, high response rate and immediate response to pharmacotherapy, no symptomatic relapse or relapse for a long time after the discontinuation of pharmacotherapy and no comorbidity with depression and/or anxiety disorders.

If the decision is to continue with medication, previously used psychotropics may not be discontinued since absolute risks are low even with agents that are potentially associated with increased risk of birth defects, or lack a clear contraindication regarding their use during breastfeeding. However, a switch from other anti-obsessional antidepressants to sertraline or citalopram/escitalopram in pregnancy and sertraline or paroxetine in the lactation period may be more suitable with respect to the safety of the fetus if the patients' history indicates that these drugs are effective and tolerated by the patients. Additionally, prophylaxis with an SSRI is preferred to polypharmacy due to possible higher risks in the fetus and breastfed infants exposed to multidrugs.

18.3.3.1 Pre-conceptional Phase

A reasonable period in psychiatric patients (at least 6 months) of clinical stability (mild or no symptoms) before attempting to conceive is recommended (Yonkers et al. 2009). If the patient meets this recommendation, two main strategies should be discussed with the patient and her relatives before conception: (1) the medication is gradually discontinued after the last interview, (2) the medication is continued until conception, and then discontinued as soon as the pregnancy is detected. The duration from decision to conceive to an actual pregnancy cannot be predicted. Therefore, the major disadvantage of the first option is symptomatic relapse until conception. In the second option, this risk may be prevented; however, the fetus is exposed to the medication in the 2th to 4th weeks of pregnancy. Table 18.1 summarizes the recommendations by this paper on the basis of the different scenarios mentioned above and management strategies.

Table 18.1 Management strategies recommended by this paper for prophylaxis of OCD symptoms based on clinical scenarios (please see the text for details) in the pre-conceptional phase, pregnancy, and the postpartum period

Clinical scenario	Management strategy
Pre-conceptional phase	
1a	Continue the medication until conception
1b	Gradually discontinue the medication
2a	Continue the medication until conception
2b	Continue the medication until conception
Pregnancy	
1a	Consider the following options: (1) clinical monitoring without medication until the relapse of symptoms (2) Clinical monitoring without medication for the first 12 weeks of pregnancy, after that prophylaxis with an SSRI (3) Prophylaxis with an SSRI at the lowest therapeutic dose
1b	Clinical monitoring without medication until symptomatic relapse
2a	Prophylaxis with an SSRI at the lowest therapeutic dose
2b	Clinical monitoring without medication until symptomatic exacerbation
Postpartum period	
1a	Discuss the prophylactic treatment with the patient and her family
1b	Clinical monitoring without medication until symptomatic relapse
2a	Prophylaxis with an SSRI at the lowest therapeutic dose
2b	Clinical monitoring without medication until symptomatic exacerbation

OCD obsessive-compulsive disorder, *SSRI* selective serotonin reuptake inhibitor

18.3.3.2 Pregnancy

Retrospective studies have suggested that the severity of OCD symptoms worsened in 8–46%, improved in 8–28%, and remained unchanged in 31–69% of pregnant women (Labad et al. 2005, 2010; Uguz et al. 2007a, 2011; Vulink et al. 2006; Forray et al. 2010; Guglielmi et al. 2014). A prospective study by House et al. (2016) reported that there was no significant change in the severity of preexisting OCD symptoms. Worsening of the symptoms during this period seems to be associated with a history of individual major depression, presence of major depression and an anxiety disorder at the onset of pregnancy, contamination, symmetry/exactness obsessions, and cleaning/washing and ordering/arranging compulsions in the patient (Uguz et al. 2011). These findings should be kept in mind prior to making any decision regarding management of the treatment regimen during pregnancy.

If a pregnant patient has clinical features of scenario 1b, antiobsessional drug may not be needed until the recurrence of symptoms. In scenario 1a, either prophylaxis with an SSRI, especially sertraline or citalopram/escitalopram at the lowest therapeutic dose or no medication with frequent clinical controls until the initiation of symptomatic relapse and until the end of the first trimester of pregnancy may be discussed. It is unknown whether pharmacological treatment in pregnant women with OCD with mild severity of symptoms is superior to untreated OCD with respect to neonatal outcomes. In addition, as mentioned above, at least half of the patients do not experience any exacerbation in OCD symptoms during pregnancy. Therefore, in scenario 2b, the patient may not require any prophylactic treatment. For patients that match scenario 2a based on the history of the disorder, prophylaxis with an SSRI at the lowest therapeutic dose appears to be more appropriate (Table 18.1).

18.3.3.3 Postpartum Period

It has been reported that obsessive-compulsive symptoms remain unchanged in approximately half of the patients during the postpartum period (Labad et al. 2005, 2010; Vulink et al. 2006; Forray et al. 2010; Guglielmi et al. 2014). There are two prospective studies suggesting significant reduction (Uguz et al. 2007b) or no significant change (House et al. 2016) in the severity of symptoms.

Postpartum women in scenarios 1b and 2b may not receive any prophylactic treatment. In contrast, for patients in scenario 2a, this paper recommends clinical monitoring with an SSRI, especially sertraline or paroxetine, at the lowest therapeutic dose. Prophylactic treatment should be discussed with the patient and her relatives if the patient is considered to be in scenario 1a. If no prophylaxis is decided, it is recommended that the medication be administered as soon as the symptoms are initiated (Table 18.2).

Table 18.2 Expert recommendations based on scientific evidence and clinical experience

There are risks of untreated OCD as well as the medications on the fetus or infants
Treatment decision should be based on a careful psychiatric assessment, including individual history of OCD and current mental status
The treatment should be individualized
Both the patients and the exposed fetus or infant should be closely monitored
Monotherapy and lowest therapeutic doses are preferred to combinations of medication and high daily doses
The first-line agents recommended for treating OCD are sertraline and citalopram/escitalopram during pregnancy, and sertraline and paroxetine during lactation
Switching from an SSRI to other drugs in treatment-resistant patients is favorable to other pharmacological options
As an augmentation treatment, aripiprazole during pregnancy and risperidone during lactation appear to be the most preferable antipsychotic drugs
Benzodiazepines, especially lorazepam, may be administered for a short time in pregnant or breastfeeding patients with intensive anxiety
Mirtazapine at 7.5 to 15 mg/day may be added to SSRIs in pregnant patients with severe insomnia, decreased appetite, and nausea/vomiting
OCD patients who are symptomatically non-remitted require prophylactic treatment during pregnancy and the postpartum period

OCD obsessive-compulsive disorder, *SSRI* selective serotonin reuptake inhibitor

18.4 Conclusion

Due to the possible negative effects of OCD on the fetus, infant, and pregnancy, patients should be carefully monitored during pregnancy and the postpartum period. The data on the treatment of the disorder are very limited and there are no published guidelines regarding the clinical approach to OCD in pregnant and lactating women. Therefore, it is difficult to know to decide the pharmacological options for these women. Both prophylactic medication and treatment of active symptoms should be individualized based on the history of OCD, the clinical status, and degree of impairment in social and family functions in the patient.

References

Abudy A, Juven-Wetzler A, Zohar J. Pharmacological management of treatment-resistant obsessive-compulsive disorder. CNS Drugs. 2011;25:585–96.

Adewuya AO, Ola BA, Aloba OO, Mapayi BM. Anxiety disorders among Nigerian women in late pregnancy: a controlled study. Arch Womens Ment Health. 2006;9:325–8.

Albert U, Aguglia E, Maina G, Bogetto F. Venlafaxine versus clomipramine in the treatment of obsessive-compulsive disorder: a preliminary single-blind, 12-week, controlled study. J Clin Psychiatry. 2002;63:1004–9.

Alper K, Schwartz KA, Kolts RL, Khan A. Seizure incidence in psychopharmacological clinical trials: an analysis of Food and Drug Administration (FDA) summary basis of approval reports. Biol Psychiatry. 2007;62:345–54.

Andersson L, Sundström-Poromaa I, Wulff M, Åström M, Bixo M. Depression and anxiety disorder during pregnancy and six months postpartum: a follow-up study. Acta Obstet Gynecol Scand. 2006;85:937–44.

Aujla S, Sandeep M, Aparnavi P, Padhi BK, Shamim MA, et al. Effect of maternal obsessive-compulsive disorder (OCD) on feto-matrenal outcomes: a systematic review and meta-analysis. Int J Gynaecol Obstet. 2024;167:949.

Bandelow B, Allgulander C, Baldwin DS, Costa DLDC, Denys D, Dilbaz N, et al. World Federation of Societies of Biological Psychaitry (WFSBP) guidelines for treatment of anxiety, obsessive-compulsive and posttraumatic stres disorder – version 3. Part II: OCD and PTSD. World J Biol Psychiatry. 2023;24:118–34.

Bellantuono C, Vargas M, Mandarelli G, Nardi B, Martini MG. The safety of serotonin-noradrenaline reuptake inhibitors (SNRIs) in pregnancy and breastfeeding: a comprehensive review. Hum Psychopharmacol Clin Exp. 2015;30:143–51.

Björgvinsson T, Hart J, Hefelfinger S. Obsessive-compulsive disorder: update on assessment and treatment. J Psychiatr Pract. 2007;13:362–72.

Bloch MH, Landeros-Weisenberger A, Kelmendi B, Coric V, Bracken MB, Leckman JF. A systematic review: antipsychotic augmentation with treatment refractory obsessive-compulsive disorder. Mol Psychiatry. 2006;11:622–32.

Bobes J, González MP, Bascarán MT, Arango C, Sáiz PA, Bousoño M. Quality of life and disability in patients with obsessive-compulsive disorder. Eur Psychiatry. 2001;16:239–45.

Borri C, Mauri M, Oppo A, Banti S, Rambelli C, Ramacciotti D, Montagnani MS, Camilleri V, Cortopassi S, Bettini A, Ricciardulli S, Rucci P, Montaresi S, Cassano GB. Axis I psychopathology and functional impairment at the third month of pregnancy: results from the perinatal depression-research and screening unit (PND-ReScU) study. J Clin Psychiatry. 2008;69:1617–24.

Brakoulias V, Viswasam K, Dwyer A, Raine KH, Starcevic V. Advances in the pharmacological management of obsessive-compulsive disorder in the postpartum period. Expert Opin Pharmacother. 2020;21:163–5.

Burke KC, Burke JD, Regier DA, Rae DS. Age at onset of selected mental disorders in five community populations. Arch Gen Psychiatry. 1990;47:511–8.

Buss C, Davis EP, Hobel CJ, Sandman CA. Maternal pregnancy-specific anxiety is associated with child executive function at 6-9 years age. Stress. 2011;14:665–76.

Byatt N, Deligiannidis KM, Freeman MP. Antidepressant use in pregnancy: a critical review focused on risks and controversies. Acta Psychiatr Scand. 2013;127:94–114.

Castle D, Bosanac P, Rossell S. Treating OCD: what to do when fist-line therapies fail. Aust Psychiatry. 2015;4:350–3.

Challacombe FL, Salkovskis PM, Woolgar M, Wilkinson EL, Read J, Acheson R. Parenting and mother-infant interactions in the context of maternal postpartum obsessive-compulsive disorder: effects of obsessional symptoms and mood. Infant Behav Dev. 2016;44:11–20.

Cilli AS, Telcioğlu M, Aşkın R, Kaya N, Bodur S, Kucur R. Twelve-month prevalence of obsessive-compulsive disorder in Konya, Turkey. Compr Psychiatry. 2004;45:367–74.

Damkier P, Videbech P. The safety of second-generation antipsychotics during pregnancy: a clinically focused review. CNS Drugs. 2018;32:351–66.

Denys D, van der Wee N, van Megen HJ, Westenberg HG. A double blind comparison of venlafaxine and paroxetine in obsessive-compulsive disorder. J Clin Psychopharmacol. 2003;23:568–75.

Denys D, van Megen HJ, van der Wee N, Westenberg HG. A double-blind switch study of paroxetine and venlafaxine in obsessive-compulsive disorder. J Clin Psychiatry. 2004;65:37–43.

Ding XX, Wu YL, Xu SJ, Zhu RP, Jia XM, Zhang SF, Huang K, Zhu P, Hao JH, Tao FB. Maternal anxiety during pregnancy and adverse birth outcomes: a systematic review and meta-analysis of prospective cohort studies. J Affect Disord. 2014;159:103–10.

Diniz JB, Shavitt RG, Pereira CA, Hounie AG, Pimentel I, Koren LM, Dainesi SM, Miguel EC. Quetiapine versus clomipramine in the augmentation of selective serotonin reuptake inhibitors for the treatment of obsessive-compulsive disorder: a randomized, open-label trial. J Psychopharmacol. 2010;24:297–307.

Dold M, Aigner M, Lanzenberger R, Kasper S. Antipsychotic augmentation of serotonin reuptake inhibitors in treatment resistant obsessive-compulsive diorder: a meta-analysis of double-blind, randomized, placebo-controlled trials. Int J Neuropsychopharmacol. 2013;16:557–74.

Farias DR, TdeJ P, Teofilo MM, Vilea AA, Vaz Jdos S, Nardi AE, ve ark. Prevalence of psychiatric disorders in the first trimester of pregnancy and factors associated with current suicide risk. Psychiatry Res. 2013;210:962–8.

Felice E, Saliba J, Grech V, Cox J, Calleja N. Antenatal psychiatric morbidity in maltase women. Gen Hosp Psychiatry. 2007;29:501–5.

Fernández de la Cruz L, Joseph KS, Wien Q, Stephansson O, Mataix-Cols D, Razaz N. Pregnancy, delivery, and neonatal outcomes associated with maternal obsessive-compulsive disorder. Two cohort studies in Sweden and British Columbia, Canada. JAMA Netw Open. 2023;6:e2318212.

Ferraro AA, Rohde LA, Polanczyk GV, Argeu A, Miguel EC, Grisi SJ, Fleitlich-Bilyk B. The specific and combined role of domestic violence and mental health disorders during pregnancy on new-born health. BMC Pregnancy Childbirth. 2017;17:257.

Fineberg NA, Stein DJ, Premkumar P, Carey P, Sivakumaran T, Vythilingum B, Seedat S, Westenberg H, Denys D. Adjunctive quetiapine for serotonin reuptake inhibitor-resistant obsessive-compulsive disorder: a meta-analysis of randomized controlled treatment trials. Int Clin Psychopharmacol. 2006;21:337–43.

Fineberg NA, Reghunandanan S, Brown A, Pampaloni I. Pharmacotherapy of obsessive-compulsive disorder: evidence-based treatment and beyond. Aust N Z J Psychiatry. 2012;47:121–41.

Fineberg NA, Reghunandanan S, Simpson HB, Philips KA, Richter MA, Matthews K, Stein DJ, Sareen J, Brown A, Sookman D. Obsessive-compulsive diaorder (OCD): practical strategies for pharmacological and somatic treatments in adults. Psychiatry Res. 2015;227:114–25.

Forray A, Focseneanu M, Pittman B, McDougle CJ, Epperson CN. Onset and exacerbation of obsessive-compulsive disorder in pregnancy and the postpartum period. J Clin Psychiatry. 2010;71:1061–8.

Franklin ME, Foa EB. Treatment of obsessive-compulsive disorder. Ann Rev Clin Psychol. 2011;7:229–43.

Freeman MP, Viguera AC, Góez-Mogollón L, Young AV, Caplin PS, McElheny SA, et al. Reproductive safety of aripiprazole: data from the Massachusetts general Hopital National Pregnancy Registry of atypical antipsychotics. Arch Women Ment Health. 2021;24:659–67.

Furu K, Kieler H, Haglund B, Engeland A, Selmer R, Stephansson O, Valdimarsdottir UA, Zoega H, Artama M, Gissler M, Malm H, Nørgaard M. Selective serotonin reuptake inhibitors and venlafaxine in early pregnancy and risk birth defects: population based cohort study and sibling design. BMJ. 2015;350:h1798.

Gautam M. Clinical recommendations for augmentation agents in obsessive-compulsive disorder partially responsive to serotonin reuptake inhibitors. J Clin Pharmacol. 2023;43:369–77.

Gentile S. Use of contemporary antidepressants during breastfeeding. A proposal for a sfety index. Drug Saf. 2007;30:107–21.

Gentile S. Tricyclic antidepressants in pregnancy and puerperium. Expert Opin Drug Saf. 2014;13:207–25.

Glover V. Maternal depression, anxiety and stress during pregnancy and child outcome; what needs to be done. Best Pract Res Clin Obstet Gynaecol. 2014;28:25–35.

Grigoriadis S, VonderPorten EH, Mamisashvili L, Roerecke M, Rehm J, Dennis CL, Koren G, Steiner M, Mousmanis P, Cheung A, Ross LE. Antidepressant exposure during pregnancy and congenital malformations: is there an association? A systematic review and meta-analysis of the best evidence. J Clin Psychiatry. 2013;74:e293–308.

Guglielmi V, Vulink NC, Denys D, Wang Y, Samuels JF, Nestadt G. Obsessive-compulsive disorder and female reproductive cycle events: results from the OCD and reproduction collaborative study. Depress Anxiety. 2014;31:979–87.

Hirschtritt ME, Bloch MH, Mathews CA. Obsessive-compulsive disorder. Advances in diagnosis and treatment. JAMA. 2017;317:1358–67.

Holingue C, Samuels J, Guglielmi V, Ingram W, Nestadt G, Nestadt PS. Peripartum complications associated with obsessive-compulsive disorder exacerbation during pregnancy. J Obsessive Compuls Relat Disord. 2021;29:100641.

House SJ, Tripathi SP, Knight BT, Morris N, Newport DJ, Stowe ZN. Obsessive-compulsive disorder in pregnancy and the postpartum period: course of illness and obstetrical outcome. Arch Womens Ment Health. 2016;19:3–10.

Huppert JD, Simpson HB, Nissenson KJ, Liebowitz MR, Foa EB. Quality of life and functional impairment in obsessive-compulsive disorder: a comparison of patients with and without comorbidity, patients in remission, and healthy controls. Depress Anxiety. 2009;26:39–45.

Kang HH, Ahn KH, Hong SC, Kwon BY, Lee EH, Lee JS, Oh MJ, Kim HJ. Association of citalopram with congenital anomalies: a meta-analysis. Obstet Gynecol Sci. 2017;60:145–53.

Karno M, Golding JM, Sorenson SB, Burnam A. The epidemiology of obsessive-compulsive disorder in five US communities. Arch Gen Psychiatry. 1988;45:1094–9.

Katzman MA, Bleau P, Blier P, Chokka P, Kjernisted K, Van Ameringen M. Canadian clinical practice guidelines for the management of anxiety, posttraumatic stres and obsessive-compulsive disorders. BMC Psychiatry. 2014;14(Suppl 1):S1.

Kellner M. Drug treatment of obsessive-compulsive disorder. Dialogues Clin Neurosci. 2010;12:187–97.

Kılınc S, Herguner S. Effects of maternal psychopathology on children. In: Uguz F, editor. Psychiatric disorders during the postpartum period in light of current advances. New York: Nova Science Publishers, Inc.; 2016. p. 101–14.

Kıvırcık Akdede BB, Alptekin K, Akvardar Y, Kitis A. Quality of life in patients with obsessive-compulsive disorder: relations with cognitive functions and clinical symptoms. Turk Psikiyatri Derg. 2005;16:13–9.

Kolada JL, Bland RC, Newman SC. Obsessive-compulsive disorder. Acta Psychiatr Scand. 1994;76(Suppl 3):24–35.

Labad J, Menchón JM, Alonso P, Segalàs C, Jiménez S, Vallejo J. Female reproductive cycle and obsessive-compulsive disorder. J Clin Psychiatry. 2005;66:428–35.

Labad J, Alonso P, Segalas C, Reval E, Jimenez S, Bueno B, Vallejo J, Menchon JM. Distinct correlates of hoarding and cleaning symptom dimensions in relation to onset of obsessive-compulsive disorder at menarche or perinatal period. Arch Womens Ment Health. 2010;13:75–81.

Larsen ER, Damkier P, Pedersen LH, Fenger-Gron J, Mikkelsen RL, Nielsen RE, Linde VJ, Knudsen HE, Skaarup L, Videbech P, et al. Use of psychotropic drugs during pregnancy and breast-feeding. Acta Psychiatr Scand. 2015;445:1–28.

Lassen D, Enniz ZY, Damkier P. First-trimester pregnancy exposure to venlafaxine or duloxetine and risk of major congenital major malformations: a systematic review. Basic Clin Pharmacol Toxicol. 2016;118:32–6.

Leis JA, Heron J, Stuart EA, Mendelson T. Associations between maternal mental health and child emotional and behavioral problems: does prenatal mental health matter? J Abnorm Child Psychol. 2014;42:161–71.

Maina G, Albert U, Bogetto F, Vaschetto P, Ravizza L. Recent life events and obsessive-compulsive disorder (OCD): the role of pregnancy delivery. Psychiatry Res. 1999;89:49–58.

Maiti R, Mishra A, Srinivasan A, Mishra BR. Pharmacological augmentation of serotonin reuptake inhibitors in patients with obsessive-compulsive disorder: a network meta-analysis. Acta Psychiatr Scand. 2023;148:19–31.

Marazziti D, Golia F, Consoli G, Presta S, Pfanner C, Carlini M, Mungai F, Catena D'OM. Effectiveness of long-term augmentation with citalopram to clomipramine in treatment-resistant OCD patients. CNS Spectr. 2008;13:971–6.

Mataix-Cols D, de la Cruz LF, Nordsletten AE, Lenhard F, Isomura K, Simpson HB. Towards an international expert consensus for defining treatment response, remissioni recovery and relapse in obsessive-compulsive disorder. World Psychiatry. 2016;15:80–1.

McAllister-Williams RH, Baldwin DS, Cantwell R, Easter A, Gilvarry E, Glover V, Green L, Gregoire A, Howard LM, Jones I, Khalifeh H, Lingford-Hughes A, McDonald E, Micali N, Pariante CM, Peters L, Roberts A, Smith NC, Taylor D, Wieck A, Yates LM, Young AH. British Association for Psychopharmacology consensus guidance on the use of psychotropic medication preconception, in pregnancy and postpartum. J Psychopharmacol. 2017;31:519–32.

Michielsen LA, Heijden FM, Janssen PK, Kujpers HJ. Effects of maternal psychotropic drug dosage on birth outcomes. Neuropsychiatr Dis Treat. 2014;10:13–8.

Misri S, Milis L. Obsessive-compulsive disorder in the postpartum. Open-label trial of quetiapine augmentation. Int Clin Psychopharmacol. 2004;24:624–7.

Muscatello MR, Bruno A, Pandolfo G, Micò U, Scimeca G, Romeo VM, Micò U, Scimeca G, Romeo VM, Santoro V, Settineri S, Spina E, Zoccali RA. Effect of aripiprazole augmentation of serotonin reuptake inhibitors or clomipramine in treatment-resistant obsessive-compulsive disorder: a double-blind, placebo-controlled study. J Clin Psychopharmacol. 2011;31:174–9.

Myles N, Newall H, Ward H, Matthew L. Systematic meta-analysis of individual selective serotonin reuptake inhibitor medications and congenital malformations. Aust N Z J Psychiatry. 2013;47:1002–12.

Navarro P, Garcia-Esteve L, Ascaso C, Aguado J, Gelabert E, Martin-Santos R. Non-psychotic psychiatric disorders after childbirth: prevalence and comorbidity in a community sample. J Affect Disord. 2008;109:171–6.

Neziroglu F, Anemone R, Yaryura-Tobias JA. Onset of obsessive-compulsive disorder in pregnancy. Am J Psychiatry. 1992;149:947–50.

Ninan PT, Koran LM, Kiev A, Davidson JR, Rasmussen SA, Zajecka JM, Robinson DG, Crits-Christoph P, Mandel FS, Austin C. High-dose sertraline strategy for nonresponders to acute treatment for obsessive-compulsive disorder: a multi-center double-blind trial. J Clin Psychiatry. 2006;67:15–22.

Orsolini L, Bellantuono C. Serotonin reuptake inhibitors and breastfeeding: a systematic review. Hum Psychopharmacol Clin Exp. 2015;30:4–20.

Poppe C, Müller ST, Greil W, Walder A, Grohmann R, Stübner S. Pharmacotherapy for obsessive-compulsive disorder in clinical practice. Data of 842 inpatients from the international AMSP project between 1994-2012. J Affect Disord. 2016;200:89–96.

Rabinowitz I, Baruch Y, Barak Y. High-dose escitalopram for the treatment of obsessive-compulsve disorder. Int Clin Psychopharmacol. 2008;32:49–53.

Rampoloni I, Sivakumaran T, Hawley CJ, Al Allag A, Farrow J, Nelson S, Fineberg NAl. High-dose selective serotonin reuptake inhibitors in OCD: a systematic retrospective case notes survey. J Psychopharmacol. 2010;24:1439–45.

Roca A, Garcia-Esteve LI, Imaz ML, Torres A, Hernández S, Botet F, Gelabert E, Subira S, Plaza A, Valdes M, Martin-Santos R. Obstetrical and neonatal outcomes after prenatal exposure to selective serotonin reuptake inhibitors: the relevance of dose. J Affect Disord. 2011;135:208–15.

Russell EJ, Fawcett JM, Mazmanian D. Risk of obsessive-compulsive disorder in pregnant and postpartum women: a meta-analysis. J Clin Psychiatry. 2013;74:377–85.

Sayyah M, Sayyah M, Boostani H, Ghaffari SM, Hoseini A. Effects of aripiprazole augmentation in treatment-resistant obsessive-compulsive disorder (a double blind clinical trial). Depress Anxiety. 2012;29:850–4.

Selvi Y, Atli A, Aydın A, Besiroglu L, Ozdemir P, Ozdemir O. The comparison of aripiprazole and risperidone augmentation in selective serotonin reuptake inhibitor-refractory obsessive-compulsive disorder: a single-blind, randomised study. Hum Psychopharmacol Clin Exp. 2011;26:51–7.

Shen ZQ, Gao SY, Li SX, Zhang TN, Liu CX, Lv HC, Zhang Y, Gong TT, Xu X, Ji C, Wu QJ, Li D. Sertraline use in the first trimester and risk of congenital anomalies: a systemic review and meta-analysis of cohort studies. Br J Clin Pharmacol. 2017;83:909–22.

Shoja Shafti S, Kaviani H. Aripiprazole versus quetiapine in treatment-resistant obsessive-compulsive disorder: a double-blind clinical trial. Ther Adv Psychopharmacol. 2015;5:32–7.

Skapinakis P, Papatheodorou T, Mavreas V. Antipsychotic augmentation of serotonergic antidepressants in treatment-resistant obsessive-compulsive disorder: a meta-analysis of the randomized controlled trials. Eur Neuropsychopharmacol. 2007;17:79–93.

Suri R, Altshuler L, Hellemann G, Burt VK, Aquino A, Mintz J. Effects of antenatal depression and antidepressant treatment on gestational age at birth and risk of preterm birth. Am J Psychiatry. 2007;164:1206–13.

Sutter-Dallay AL, Giaconne-Marcesche V, Glatigny-Dallay E, Verdeoux H. Women with anxiety disorders during pregnancy are at increased risk of intense postnatal depressive symptoms: a prospective survey of the MATQUID cohort. Eur Psychiatry. 2004;19:459–63.

Talge NM, Neal C, Glover V. Translational research and prevention science network: fetal and neonatal experience on child and adolescent mental health. Antenatal maternal stress and long-term effects on child neurodevelopment: how and why? J Child Psychol Psychiatry. 2007;48:245–61.

Uguz F. Pharmacotherapy of obsessive-compulsive disorder during pregnancy: a clinical approach. Revista Brasil Psiquiatr. 2015;37:334–42.

Uguz F. Breastfeeding and psychotropic medications. In: Uguz F, editor. Psychotropic drugs and medical conditions. New York: Nova Science Publishers Inc.; 2017. p. 209–29.

Uguz F. Pharmacotherapy of obsessive-compulsive disorder during breastfeeding. Am J Ther. 2018;25:e541–7.

Uguz F. Selective serotonin reuptake inhibitors and the risk of congenital anomalies: a systematic review or current meta-analyses. Expert Opin Drug Saf. 2020;19:1595–604.

Uguz F. a new safety scoring system for the use of psychotropic drugs during lactation. Am J Ther. 2021;28:e118–26.

Uguz F, Gezginc K, Zeytinci IE, Karatayli S, Karatayli R, Aksin R, Guler O, Sahin FK, Emul HM, Ozbulut O, Gecici O. Obsessive-compulsive disorder in pregnant women during the third trimester of pregnancy. Compr Psychiatry. 2007a;48:441–5.

Uguz F, Gezginc K, Zeytinci IE, Karatayli S, Karatayli R, Askin R, Guler O, Sahin FK, Emul HM, Ozbulut O, Gecici O. Course of obsessive-compulsive disorder during early postpartum period: a prospective analysis of 16 cases. Compr Psychiatry. 2007b;48:558–61.

Uguz F, Kaya V, Gezginc K, Kayhan F, Çiçek E. Clinical correlates worsening in obsessive-compulsive symptoms during pregnancy. Gen Hosp Psychiatry. 2011;33:197–9.

Uguz F, Sonmez EO, Sahingoz M, Gokmen Z, Basaran M, Gezginc K, Sonmez G, Kaya N, Yilmaz E, Erdem SS, Dulger HH, Cicekler H, Tasyurek E. Neuroinflammation in the fetus exposed to maternal obsessive-compulsive disorder during pregnancy: a comparative study on cord blood tumor necrosis factor-alpha levels. Compr Psychiatry. 2014;55:861–5.

Uguz F, Yuksel G, Karsidag C, Guncu H, Konak M. Birth weight and gestational age in newborns exposed to maternal obsessive-compulsive disorder. Psychiatry Res. 2015;226:396–8.

Van Ameringen M, Simpson W, Petterson B, Dell'Osso B, Fineberg N, et al. Pharmacological treatment strategies in obsessive-compulsive disorder: a cross-sectional view in nine international OCD centers. J Psychopharmacol. 2014;28:596–602.

Van den Bergh BR, Mulder EJ, Mennes M, Glover V. Antenatal maternal anxiety and stress and the neurobehavioral development of the fetus and child: links and possible mechanisms. A review. Neurosci Behav Rev. 2005;29:237–58.

Veale D, Miles N, Ghezai H, Goldacre B, Hodsoll J. Atypical antipsychotic augmentation in SSRI treatment refractory obsessive-compulsive disorder: a systematic review and meta-analysis. BMC Psychiatry. 2014;14:317.

Vulink NC, Denys D, Bus L, Westenberg HG. Female hormones affect symptom severity in obsessive-compulsive disorder. Int Clinl Psychopharmacol. 2006;21:171–5.

Wenzel A, Gorman LL, O'Hara MW, Stuart S. The occurence of panic and obsessive-compulsive symptoms in women with postpartum dsyphoria: a prospective study. Arch Womens Ment Health. 2001;4:5–12.

Wenzel A, Haugen EN, Jackson LC, Brendle JR. Anxiety symptoms and disorders at eight weeks postpartum. J Anxiety Disord. 2005;19:295–311.

Womersley K, Ripullone K, Agius M. What are the risks associated with different selective serotonin re-uptake inhibitors (SSRIs) to treat depression and anxiety in pregnancy? An evaluation of current evidence. Psychiatr Danub. 2017;29(Suppl 3):629–44.

Yonkers KA, Wisner KL, Stewart DE, Oberlander TF, Dell DL, Stotland N, Ramin S, Chaudron L, Lockwood C. The management of depression during pregnancy: a report from the American Psychiatric Association and the American College of Obstetricians and Gynecologists. Gen Hosp Psychiatry. 2009;31:403–13.

Zambaldi CF, Cantilino A, Montenegro AC, Paes JA, de Albuquerque TL, Sougey EB. Postpartum obsessive-compulsive disorder: prevalence and clinical characteristics. Compr Psychiatry. 2009;50:503–9.

Zar M, Wijma K, Wijma B. Relations between anxiety disorders and fear of childbirth during late pregnancy. Clin Psychol Psychother. 2002;9:122–30.

Zhou DD, Zhou XX, et al. Augmentation agents to serotonin reuptake inhibitors for treatment-resistant obsessive-compulsive disorder: a network meta-analysis. Prog Neuro-Psychopharmacol Biol Psychiatry. 2019;90:277–87.

Anxiety Disorders

19

Benyamin Daniel Daniel, Caterina Dell'Anna,
and Carlo Marchesi

19.1 Introduction

In common perception, pregnancy and motherhood are often seen as times of joyful anticipation and happiness. However, the perinatal period, which spans from conception to 1 year postpartum (O'Hara and Wisner 2014), is also marked by profound physical and psychological changes (Bellantuono et al. 2022). This period often presents a dichotomy: while it brings the joyful anticipation of motherhood, it also increases vulnerability to mental health distress. Historically, idealized notions of pregnancy and motherhood led to the belief that the perinatal period was a low-risk time for the onset or exacerbation of anxiety disorders (ADs) (Bellantuono et al. 2022).

Nevertheless, it is now widely recognized that anxiety symptoms and ADs are prevalent both during pregnancy and the postpartum period, with significant adverse outcomes for the mother, the fetus, and its development (Marchesi et al. 2014; Ross and McLean 2006).

Even when symptoms do not meet the threshold for a formal diagnosis of an AD, mild to moderate levels of distress and impairment due to subthreshold anxiety can significantly impact maternal well-being.

A broad spectrum of ADs, including generalized anxiety disorder (GAD), panic disorder (PD), and phobias, can manifest during this time.

Given the potential impact of maternal psychopathology not only on the mother but also on the child (Stein et al. 2014; Glasheen et al. 2010), addressing perinatal ADs is critical. Effective treatment can alleviate maternal distress, improve functioning during this sensitive life stage, and reduce potential negative outcomes for

B. D. Daniel (✉) · C. Dell'Anna · C. Marchesi
Treatment of Psychiatric Disorders in Perinatal Period Unit, University Hospital of Parma, Department of Mental Health, Parma Local Health Agency, University of Parma, Parma, Italy
e-mail: benyamindaniel.daniel@unipr.it; caterina.dellanna@unipr.it; carlo.marchesi@unipr.it

F. Uguz, L. Orsolini (eds.), *Perinatal Psychopharmacology*,
https://doi.org/10.1007/978-3-031-99720-4_19

the fetus. Identifying evidence-based treatments that are both safe and acceptable for women during pregnancy and breastfeeding is therefore of paramount importance.

19.2 Epidemiology and Prevalence of Perinatal Anxiety Disorders

An estimated 30% of adults experience ADs at some point in their lives (APA 2022), a rate significantly higher than that of other mental health conditions. The impact of ADs on social, emotional, and physical functioning is profound, placing a considerable burden on healthcare services (Ohayon et al. 2000; McCusker et al. 1997).

In addition to the direct public health costs associated with ADs, substantial indirect costs arise from functional impairments, such as reduced work capacity and unemployment (Greenberg et al. 1999). Women are particularly vulnerable, with a notably higher prevalence of ADs compared to men (Somers et al. 2006; Kessler et al. 2005).

In the context of the perinatal period, these conditions have historically been underestimated and under-investigated (Bellantuono et al. 2022). Earlier meta-analyses estimated that ADs affected between 8.5% (Goodman et al. 2016) and 15.2% (Dennis et al. 2017) of women during pregnancy, and 9.9% (Dennis et al. 2017) during the postpartum period. However, a more recent meta-analysis (Fawcett et al. 2019) reported an overall prevalence of 20.7% during the perinatal period. Additionally, Fawcett and colleagues (Fawcett et al. 2019) found that 1 in 20 women (5.5%) met the criteria for at least two ADs. Regarding the prevalence of specific ADs, a study (Goodman et al. 2016) identified GAD, obsessive-compulsive disorder (OCD), and PD as the most common ADs during the postpartum period. In contrast, a more recent study (Fawcett et al. 2019) found specific phobia, GAD, and social phobia to be the most prevalent perinatal disorders. It is worth noting that OCD is no longer classified as an AD under DSM-5.

Anxiety can manifest both as a disorder, characterized by chronic and persistent levels of worry that significantly impairs daily functioning and quality of life, and as a symptom, occurring in physiological or para-physiological contexts and within distinct psychopathological trajectories that differ from true ADs. From a psychopathological perspective, the distinction lies in the chronicity, severity, and impact on daily life. During pregnancy, somatic symptoms such as palpitations, breathing difficulties, muscle tension, gastrointestinal discomfort, and dizziness may overlap with those of ADs, making diagnosis more complex and increasing the risk of mistaking normal physiological responses for pathological anxiety. Furthermore, anxiety symptoms can significantly affect quality of life, often co-occurring with other psychological or somatic conditions and negatively impacting relationships, work performance, and overall well-being.

Significant variations in perinatal anxiety prevalence are evident across different geographical regions and cultural contexts, with perinatal anxiety prevalence reported at 17.4% in China (Yang et al. 2023) and 28.2% in Africa (Umuziga et al.

2020). These variations likely stem from differences in assessment methods, diagnostic criteria, timing of evaluations, and populations studied.

Global events also play a crucial role in shaping prevalence rates. During the SARS-CoV-2 pandemic, clinically elevated anxiety symptoms were reported in 57% of pregnant women (Lebel et al. 2021), highlighting the influence of extraordinary circumstances on perinatal mental health.

In conclusion, perinatal anxiety and perinatal ADs represent a critical global public health issue. Variability in prevalence across populations, cultures, and contexts underscores the need for culturally sensitive, evidence-based approaches to screening, prevention, and treatment. As understanding of perinatal anxiety evolves, addressing these conditions remains a central focus in maternal mental healthcare worldwide.

19.3 Diagnostic Challenges, Classification, and Clinical Presentation

19.3.1 Limitations of Current Diagnostic Criteria (DSM-5)

Diagnosing ADs during the perinatal period presents various challenges. While the DSM-5 includes the specifier "with onset in the peripartum" for mood disorders, it does not provide a similar designation for ADs (Bellantuono et al. 2022). This omission reflects the historical focus of clinical research on perinatal depression, leaving ADs during this critical period underexplored (Marchesi et al. 2014).

The current lack of a peripartum specifier for ADs creates several diagnostic hurdles. GAD, characterized by excessive and uncontrollable worry that significantly impairs daily functioning, is among the most common ADs during the perinatal period. However, the absence of the DSM specifier "with peripartum onset" creates several issues. Specifically, applying DSM-5 criteria designed for the general population to pregnant or postpartum women may exclude individuals experiencing excessive worry for less than 6 months. To address this limitation, some authors suggest adapting the criteria for perinatal GAD by reducing the required duration to 1 month, provided other DSM criteria are met (Misri et al. 2015; Buist and Gotman 2011; Wenzel et al. 2003).

Another significant issue in diagnosing ADs during the perinatal period lies in the overlap between the physical symptoms of some ADs, such as fatigue, irritability, tension, concentration difficulties, and insomnia, and the common physiological changes of pregnancy and postpartum (Davis et al. 2004). Furthermore, distinguishing between normal pregnancy-related worries and pathological anxiety can be particularly challenging, especially for primiparous women during the first trimester (Bellantuono et al. 2022).

19.3.2 Pregnancy-Specific Anxiety Versus General Anxiety Disorders

Anxiety symptoms during the perinatal period can be classified as common general ADs, as defined by the DSM-5, or as abnormal anxiety states specific to the context of pregnancy (Bellantuono et al. 2022). Some authors (Brockington et al. 2006) argue that perinatal ADs share the same characteristics as classic ADs seen in the general population, but with a distinct focus on concerns such as fetal abnormalities, fetal death, maternal inadequacy, childbirth, and lack of support.

Conversely, other authors have emphasized the need to differentiate general ADs from pathological anxiety specific to the perinatal period. Studies have shown that anxiety symptoms during this time are primarily associated with worries about bodily changes and fears for the child's health (Huizink et al. 2014), negative expectations about motherhood (Hart and McMahon 2006), or fears of inadequacy in fulfilling maternal responsibilities (Huizink et al. 2014; Heron et al. 2004).

Regardless of their specific focus, ADs during the perinatal period can cause significant functional impairment. Although not exclusive to pregnancy or postpartum, individuals with anxiety are more likely to experience suicidal ideation and attempts than those without anxiety (Kanwar et al. 2013). ADs are strong predictors of postpartum depression (Robertson et al. 2004), often co-occur with perinatal depression (Falah-Hassani et al. 2017), and have been linked to adverse pregnancy outcomes, such as preterm birth and low birth weight (Ossola et al. 2021; Ding et al. 2014). Additionally, they have been associated with behavioral problems in offspring (Schreier et al. 2008).

19.3.3 The Concept of Pregnancy-Related Anxiety (PrA)

The concept of a perinatal-specific AD, referred to as pregnancy-related anxiety (PrA), has been proposed since the 1950s (Levin 1991; Standley et al. 1979; Pleshette et al. 1956). PrA is characterized by specific dimensions of anxiety, such as concerns about pregnancy, childbirth, and hospitalization. Over time, numerous measures of PrA and distress have been developed (Somerville et al. 2014; DiPietro et al. 2008; Lobel et al. 2008; Huizink et al. 2004; Cote-Arsenault 2003), and several literature reviews have been conducted on the subject (Brunton et al. 2015; Alderdice et al. 2012; Dunkel Schetter and Tanner 2012). A central tenet of these studies is that PrA extends beyond merely describing pregnant women's concerns, positing it as a distinct clinical entity with both construct and discriminant validity. A prospective longitudinal study evaluated the hypothesis that PrA represents a distinct clinical phenotype, separate from general anxiety and depression. PrA levels were assessed using specialized questionnaires alongside measures of general anxiety and depression. The findings demonstrated that PrA is distinct from general anxiety and depression, with a specific focus on pregnancy-related concerns, including the health of the baby, childbirth, and future parenthood. These results support the construct and discriminant validity of PrA as a unique clinical entity (Blackmore et al. 2016). Furthermore, a review (Williams and Koleva 2018) found that two-thirds of pregnant women express concerns about their unborn child, body image, or relationship with their partner. When these worries become excessive and interfere with daily functioning, they are classified as perinatal ADs.

19.4 Risk Factors for Perinatal Anxiety Disorders

Although not extensively studied, several potential risk factors for perinatal ADs can be identified. These include: (1) socio-demographic factors, such as a low socio-cultural background, limited education, ethnic minority status, young maternal age (<25 years), financial insecurity (Shariatpanahi et al. 2023; Bellantuono et al. 2022; Barcelona de Mendoza et al. 2016; Kane 2016); (2) psychosocial factors, including a history of childhood or recent trauma, lack of partner or familiar support, relationship tensions, being a single mother, low self-esteem, high perceived stress (Bellantuono et al. 2022; Dunkel Schetter and Tanner 2012; Blackmore et al. 2011); (3) biological factors, such as elevated cortisol levels, imbalances in polyunsaturated fatty acids, and increased pro-inflammatory cytokines (Bellantuono et al. 2022; Karlsson et al. 2017; Glover 2015; Glover et al. 2018); (4) pregnancy-related factors, including unintended pregnancies, high-risk pregnancies, delivery complications, negative birth experiences, and preterm births (Shariatpanahi et al. 2023); (5) a history of depression (van der Zee-van den Berg et al. 2021; Marchesi et al. 2014); (6) a history of ADs, which is a particularly strong predictor of anxiety during pregnancy, regardless of other risk factors (Marchesi et al. 2014).

19.5 Risks of Untreated Perinatal Anxiety Disorders

As outlined in this section, untreated perinatal ADs can lead to a range of negative consequences for both mothers and fetus/infant, with potential long-term effects on the offspring.

For mothers, perinatal ADs are associated with an increased risk of postpartum depression (Heron et al. 2004), frequently co-occur with perinatal depression (Falah-Hassani et al. 2017), suicidal behavior (Farias et al. 2013), pre-eclampsia (Winkel et al. 2015), fear of childbirth (Rubertsson et al. 2014), lower odds of breastfeeding (Grigoriadis et al. 2018), and poor coping strategies (George et al. 2013).

In terms of infant health, perinatal ADs are associated with a variety of negative outcomes, including preterm birth (Ding et al. 2014; Sanchez et al. 2013), low Apgar scores (Uguz et al. 2013), fetal hyperactivity, and irregular fetal heart rate (Uguz et al. 2019). Other complications include polyhydramnios (Bánhidy et al. 2006), a 1.6-fold increased risk of congenital abnormalities (Uguz et al. 2013), small head circumference, and being small for gestational age (Grigoriadis et al. 2018; Chen et al. 2010), as well as low birth weight (Ding et al. 2014; Teixeira et al. 1999). Interestingly, one study (Ossola et al. 2021) found a significant correlation between the severity of anxiety symptoms and birth weight, showing a “dose-response” effect. Higher levels of anxiety were linked to lower birth weight, with the difference between the least and most anxious women corresponding to a decrease of more than 600 grams. This impact on birth weight may stem from both biological and behavioral mechanisms. Maternal anxiety, through adrenergic stimulation, might affect blood pressure and cortisol levels, which are known to contribute to low birth weight (Fan et al. 2016, 2018). Furthermore, anxiety in mildly depressed subjects (Ossola et al. 2018) may limit healthy behaviors and foster undesirable life habits linked to negative pregnancy outcomes (Bae et al. 2010).

Moreover, perinatal ADs can also cause long-term developmental issues for offspring. Infants may experience difficulties with sleeping, feeding, and activity as well as poorer attention, hyperactivity, behavioral and emotional problems (Uguz et al. 2019), including irritability (Van den Bergh and Marcoen 2004), attention deficit hyperactivity disorder (ADHD) (Martini et al. 2010), internalizing difficulties, a tendency to social withdrawal and depression (Rees et al. 2019). Regarding the risk of depression in offspring, alterations in neuroendocrine pathways, particularly the hypothalamic-pituitary-adrenal (HPA) axis, have been observed in children born to anxious mothers. One study (Van den Bergh et al. 2008) highlighted the role of the HPA axis in the link between prenatal maternal anxiety and the development of depressive symptoms in post-pubertal female adolescents.

Perinatal ADs may also impact the child’s neurodevelopment. One study found that prolonged maternal GAD during pregnancy affects the circulating brain-derived neurotrophic factor (BDNF) in the fetus. BDNF plays a crucial role in neuronal development, and lower levels of circulating BDNF have been observed as a result (Uguz et al. 2013).

A systematic review (Adamson et al. 2019) summarized the existing literature linking prenatal maternal anxiety with neuroimaging measures of the child’s brain structure and function. The results revealed increased brain activation and reduced cortical thickness in the frontal, temporal, and limbic regions of the brain. These areas are typically associated with emotional and behavioral regulation, and their alterations may underlie the behavioral and mental health difficulties more commonly observed in children born to mothers with prenatal anxiety.

19.6 Pharmacological Treatment

19.6.1 General Considerations

As highlighted throughout this chapter, anxiety during pregnancy is a condition that warrants serious consideration due to its potential adverse effects on both maternal and fetal health. However, the decision to use pharmacological treatments for ADs during pregnancy or breastfeeding poses a considerable challenge in clinical practice. This difficulty often stems from physicians’ concerns regarding the safety profile of psychotropic medications, despite numerous studies assessing the risks associated with in utero and breastfeeding exposure to these drugs. It is worth noting that a comprehensive analysis of the safety of psychotropic medications during the perinatal period falls beyond the scope of this chapter.

When treating perinatal ADs, two primary intervention strategies are available: pharmacotherapy and psychotherapy. According to the guidelines set forth by the National Institute for Health and Care Excellence (NICE 2020), pharmacological intervention may be deemed appropriate for perinatal ADs when symptoms are moderate to severe, psychological interventions are insufficient, anxiety coexists with depression, or there is an elevated risk of suicidal behavior. Conversely, in instances of mild to moderate symptoms, psychotherapeutic approaches, particularly cognitive behavioral therapy (CBT), should be prioritized. Given the focus of this chapter, however, the discussion will center on pharmacological interventions.

The American College of Obstetricians and Gynecologists (2023) offers similar recommendations for managing ADs throughout pregnancy and the postpartum period. ACOG acknowledges both psychotherapy and pharmacotherapy as valid treatment options for perinatal anxiety and emphasizes that treatment decisions should be individualized. Factors influencing this decision include the severity of symptoms, the patient's preferences, and the potential risks and benefits associated with each treatment option. ACOG generally recommends CBT for mild to moderate symptoms, while indicating that psychopharmacotherapy is warranted in severe cases or when psychotherapy alone proves insufficient. Additionally, ACOG underscores the importance of continuous mental health monitoring during pregnancy and postpartum to provide timely and adequate support.

For women with a history of ADs, ACOG guidelines recommend that medications should not be halted or discontinued solely due to pregnancy or breastfeeding. Decisions regarding the continuation or adjustment of pharmacological treatment must be tailored to the individual, taking into account the severity of symptoms, the patient's medical history, and the associated risks and benefits of the therapy. Generally, it is advisable for most patients to continue psychotropic pharmacotherapy throughout pregnancy and breastfeeding, as discontinuation may pose a significant risk of relapse or worsening of symptoms. If necessary, a gradual tapering of medication may be implemented alongside psychological interventions. Alternatively, switching to a drug with a lower risk of adverse effects can be considered if the current medication causes significant side effects.

Once the decision to initiate or continue pharmacotherapy has been reached, careful attention to optimal dosing is paramount to prevent undertreatment (ACOG 2023). While it is crucial to consider the individual severity of the patient's condition and past psychiatric history, broad principles of psychopharmacotherapy during pregnancy include the following recommendations:

1. Use the lowest effective dose: The objective of any treatment regimen is to administer the lowest effective dose of medication required to achieve the desired clinical outcome. Following the implementation of the initial treatment plan, regular monitoring of the patient's symptoms is essential to assess efficacy. If necessary, the dosage should be adjusted or titrated to ensure optimal symptom management and facilitate remission.

2. Prioritize monotherapy: It is generally preferred to achieve symptom remission with a single pharmacological agent.
3. Minimize medication switching: A thorough assessment of the efficacy of prior medications is critical. If side effects are manageable, it is advisable to optimize the current dosage before considering a transition to another medication.
4. Consider untreated or inadequately treated mental health disorders as an exposure: While the risks associated with any psychopharmacological agent should be considered in the clinical decision-making process, healthcare professionals must also acknowledge the risks associated with inadequate treatment of mental health conditions.

Table 19.1 summarizes these recommendations. Similar recommendations are outlined in the Maudsley guidelines (Maudsley 2021).

In terms of pharmacological options, current guidelines advocate for the use of selective serotonin reuptake inhibitors (SSRIs) as a first-line treatment for perinatal ADs, when appropriate. This recommendation is supported by a substantial body of evidence detailing their safety for use during pregnancy and breastfeeding (McAllister-Williams et al. 2017). Alternatively, serotonin-norepinephrine reuptake

Table 19.1 Expert recommendations based on scientific evidence and clinical experience

There are risks associated with both untreated anxiety disorders and the medications used to treat them in terms of fetal or infant exposure (ACOG 2023; NICE 2020)
Treatment decisions should be based on a careful psychiatric assessment (NICE 2020)
The treatment should be individualized (ACOG 2023; NICE 2020)
Both the patients and the exposed fetus or infant should be closely monitored (NICE 2020)
Choose an antidepressant that has worked before. For patients who are antidepressant-naive, medication selection should be based on the recommendations below, with careful consideration of patient preference, as antidepressants generally exhibit similar efficacy and side effect profiles (ACOG 2023; NICE 2020)
If a patient with pre-existing anxiety disorders is well-managed on an antidepressant, do not switch it during pregnancy or lactation (ACOG 2023)
Minimize exposure to both illness and medication (ACOG 2023; NICE 2020): Untreated/inadequately treated illness is an exposure Use lowest effective doses Minimize switching of medications Monotherapy is preferred, when possible
The first-line agents recommended for treating anxiety disorders during pregnancy are sertraline and escitalopram (ACOG 2023) The first-line agents recommended for treating anxiety disorders during lactation are sertraline and paroxetine (Uguz 2021)
Benzodiazepines should be avoided or prescribed sparingly as a treatment for perinatal anxiety (ACOG 2023; Maudsley 2021; NICE 2020)
Mirtazapine at 7.5 to 15 mg/day may be added to SSRIs for pregnant patients with severe insomnia, decreased appetite and nausea/vomiting (Uguz 2013)
Tricyclics, such as imipramine, and SNRI, such as Venlafaxina, are similarly efficacious but exhibit a comparatively lower safety profile, thus limiting their use to the second line or in cases of non-response to SSRIs (Uguz 2021; Uguz et al. 2014, 2016)

inhibitors (SNRIs) are also considered viable options. ACOG discourages the use of benzodiazepines, recommending their sparing use or, where possible, their complete avoidance during the perinatal period.

The most significant factors influencing the selection of a specific SSRI or SNRI for patients with perinatal ADs include the available scientific evidence regarding the safety of each.

The selection of a specific SSRI or SNRI is primarily guided by the available evidence on its safety profile during pregnancy and breastfeeding, alongside the mother's previous history of response and tolerability to treatment. For women who have previously experienced effective management of symptoms with an antidepressant of any class (e.g., SSRI or SNRI), the same medication should typically be considered as the first-line pharmacotherapy. Most experts recommend starting treatment with SSRIs or SNRIs at approximately half the lowest recommended dose to minimize the likelihood of early side effects such as anxiety, agitation, or insomnia (Thorsness et al. 2018). Additionally, the treatment of anxiety and related conditions often requires up-titration to doses higher than those commonly prescribed for depression. Finally, individuals receiving treatment for anxiety or anxiety-related conditions are generally advised to remain in remission for an extended period before any consideration is given to tapering or discontinuing pharmacotherapy.

19.6.2 General Considerations for Pharmacological Treatment in Pregnancy

In terms of pharmacological management, the ACOG (2023) recommends that treatment for ADs during pregnancy be individualized, taking into account any prior response to therapy when applicable. In cases where there is no history of pharmacotherapy, sertraline or escitalopram are considered appropriate first-line options due to their efficacy and tolerability profiles (ACOG 2023; Cipriani et al. 2009) (Table 19.1). Citalopram is also deemed a favorable choice, supported by its established fetal safety profile (Womersley et al. 2017; Larsen et al. 2015; Uguz 2015; Myles et al. 2013). Fluoxetine has a prolonged half-life and active metabolites (Weissman et al. 2004); while this does not imply fluoxetine should be excluded from treatment, especially for patients with a history of successful outcomes on the medication, its use during pregnancy requires a careful assessment of the potential benefits to the mother versus the risks to the fetus. Paroxetine is associated with an increased risk of congenital malformations, particularly septal heart defects (Grigoriadis et al. 2013; Myles et al. 2013). In light of these characteristics, neither fluoxetine nor paroxetine is recommended as first-line treatments for ADs in pregnant women (Womersley et al. 2017; Larsen et al. 2015; Uguz 2015). Nevertheless, both antidepressants present a low absolute risk of birth defects and remain viable options for patients with AD in pregnancy who cannot tolerate or do not respond to sertraline, citalopram, or escitalopram (Uguz 2015; Grigoriadis et al. 2013; Myles et al. 2013).

TCAs, particularly imipramine and clomipramine, may also be considered an additional pharmacological option, although the available data on their safety during pregnancy are more limited compared to SSRIs. As such, TCAs are generally regarded as second-line options for psychopharmacological therapy (Uguz et al. 2014, 2016) (Table 19.1).

Mirtazapine, another potential pharmacological choice, appears to have a favorable safety profile during pregnancy, as noted in a systematic review (Smit et al. 2016); one case report (Uguz 2013) presented the successful use of low-dose mirtazapine, also highlighting its effectiveness in reducing severe symptoms of nausea and vomiting during the first gestational weeks in two cases. Another case report presented the beneficial effect of low-dose mirtazapine added to SSRIs in treating symptoms of severe nausea, insomnia, and loss of appetite that accompany ADs during pregnancy (Uguz 2013) (Table 19.1).

If benzodiazepines are prescribed, they should be used transiently as a bridge until SSRIs or SNRIs achieve the expected response (ACOG 2023); their routine use is not recommended unless "severe anxiety and/or agitation" occurs (NICE) (Table 19.1). However, benzodiazepines may have a clinical role in the pharmacological management of ADs in specific clinical settings. As ACOG suggests, they are often used to manage acute symptoms until the benefits of SSRIs or SNRIs take effect. They may also be considered when first-line treatment options have proven ineffective. Although their use as primary treatment of anxiety is not recommended due to side effects and risk for dependence, benzodiazepines have a limited but overall relatively acceptable perinatal safety profile (Wikner et al. 2007).

19.6.3 General Considerations for Pharmacological Treatment During Breastfeeding

For women with ADs, it is crucial not to discourage them from breastfeeding if it is their preferred method of feeding the baby. Furthermore, if the woman has maintained a stable drug regimen throughout pregnancy, psychopharmacotherapy should not be altered in the postpartum period unless significant contraindications arise. As in pregnancy, drugs with more extensive safety data are preferred, though the individual's history must also be taken into account in clinical decision-making (ACOG 2023; Gentile 2008; Eberhard-Gran et al. 2006). Measures such as the relative infant dose (RID) should be evaluated to assess the infant's exposure to a medication through breast milk relative to the maternal dose. Factors influencing the RID include lipid solubility, half-life, oral bioavailability, molecular weight, drug ionization, and protein binding. Generally, an RID of less than 10% is considered compatible with breastfeeding; however, medication-specific data should also be considered. Additionally, the infant's age and preterm birth should be accounted for, as immature metabolic pathways can reduce drug clearance. A consensus has emerged from existing research regarding the use of certain SSRIs during breastfeeding, particularly sertraline and paroxetine, which are supported by extensive scientific data on their safety in breastfed infants (Uguz 2021; Pogliani et al. 2019; Schoretsanitis et al. 2019; Molenaar et al. 2018; McAllister-Williams et al. 2017) (Table 19.1). Due to their low levels in breast milk, the amounts of sertraline and paroxetine ingested by infants are minimal and typically undetectable in serum. However, the weakly active metabolite norsertraline (desmethylsertraline) may occasionally be detected at low levels in the infant's serum. Most authors consider sertraline and paroxetine among the preferred antidepressants during breastfeeding, thus constituting first-line therapy (Uguz 2021; Grzeskowiak et al. 2018; Molenaar et al. 2018; McAllister-Williams et al. 2017; Weissman et al. 2004).

Citalopram, escitalopram, and particularly fluoxetine are less recommended during breastfeeding. Fluoxetine tends to have a higher average concentration in breast milk compared to other SSRIs (Pogliani et al. 2019). Furthermore, the long-acting active metabolite norfluoxetine has been detected in the serum of most breastfed infants during the first 2 months postpartum and, in some cases, beyond. Adverse effects, including colic, agitation, and drowsiness, have been observed in some breastfed infants. Nonetheless, if fluoxetine is necessary for the mother, especially if it was taken during pregnancy or if other antidepressants are ineffective, its use, while not first-line, is considered compatible with breastfeeding (Uguz 2021; Amir et al. 2011; Berle and Spigset 2011; Lanza di Scalea and Wisner 2009).

Citalopram and escitalopram, although not first-line SSRIs during lactation, are less prone to accumulation and may be more favorable than fluoxetine (Uguz 2021; Pogliani et al. 2019; Uguz et al. 2018; Gentile and Fusco 2017; Orsolini and Bellantuono 2015). As with pregnancy, the use of mirtazapine during breastfeeding is also considered compatible, with evidence indicating low levels in milk and minimal risk of adverse effects in breastfed infants, particularly those older than 2 months (Uguz 2021).

With regard to TCAs, both imipramine and clomipramine are generally compatible with breastfeeding (Uguz 2021; Schafer and Genna 2015; Davanzo et al. 2011; Lanza di Scalea and Wisner 2009), although there are some differences. Imipramine and its metabolite exhibit low levels in breast milk and have not been detected in the serum of breastfed infants, making its use unlikely to cause adverse effects, especially if the infant is older than 2 months (Uguz 2016; Birnbaum et al. 1999; Misri and Sivertz 1991). In fact, according to a safety scoring system, imipramine is considered appropriate for use during breastfeeding (Uguz 2021). However, other agents may be preferred when large doses are required or when breastfeeding a preterm infant (Davanzo et al. 2011).

Clomipramine, while acceptable during lactation, requires caution according to a safety scoring system (Uguz 2021; Yoshida et al. 1997; Misri and Sivertz 1991). Safer alternatives may be preferable, especially during the neonatal period and in cases of prematurity. Therefore, TCAs should generally not be considered first-line treatments during breastfeeding.

Regarding the use of benzodiazepines during breastfeeding, the main guidelines (ACOG 2023; Maudsley 2021; NICE 2020) recommend caution, as these drugs can be transferred to the infant through breast milk, posing a risk of adverse effects (Table 19.1). If benzodiazepine use is considered necessary, it is advisable to select those with a short half-life, such as lorazepam, with the lowest effective dose being administered (Rowe et al. 2013), particularly during the neonatal period and in cases of prematurity (Sachs 2013). Conversely, benzodiazepines with a long half-life, such as diazepam, should be avoided to minimize the risk of drug accumulation in the infant (Borgatta et al. 1997; Dusci et al. 1990; Wesson et al. 1985; Brandt 1976; Cole and Hailey 1975; Patrick et al. 1972). With these precautions in mind, the occasional, low-dose use of benzodiazepines is generally considered compatible with breastfeeding (Kelly et al. 2012; Iqbal et al. 2002; Hägg and Spigset 2000; McElhatton 1994; Kanto 1982). In particular, expert authors regard the use of some benzodiazepines, including lorazepam, brotizolam, midazolam, and oxazepam, as safe or very likely safe during breastfeeding (Nishimura et al. 2021; Saito et al. 2021; Uguz 2021; Kelly et al. 2012; Wretlind 1987).

19.7 Treatment of Panic Disorder (PD)

PD is a relatively common psychiatric condition characterized by recurrent, spontaneous panic attacks. This disorder is observed twice as frequently in women compared to men, with the average age of onset typically coinciding with the childbearing years in women. Consequently, it is expected that a proportion of women in the perinatal period may experience PD. According to a recent review, the estimated prevalence of PD during pregnancy varies across studies, ranging from 0.2% to 7.0% (Al-Awabdeh et al. 2024). Moreover, pregnancy can affect the severity of pre-existing PD symptoms, with up to 33% of patients experiencing exacerbation during pregnancy (Uguz 2016; Bandelow et al. 2006).

When deciding on pharmacological treatment of perinatal PD, it is important to consider the potential neonatal outcomes if the disorder is left untreated. A study (Uguz et al. 2018) found that infants born to untreated pregnant patients had significantly lower birth weight and gestational age at delivery, compared to infants of healthy pregnant women or pregnant women pharmacologically treated. Additionally, the infants of untreated patients had a higher rate of hospitalization in the neonatal care unit. These findings suggest that pharmacological treatment of PD during pregnancy should not be overlooked, as it may have beneficial effects in reducing the risk of negative neonatal outcomes related to maternal PD.

Even though there is no unanimous consensus on the clinical indications for using anti-panic medications during the perinatal period, specific clinical features outlined by Uguz (2016) may serve as potential criteria for initiating pharmacological treatment for PD during this time. These include:

- Severe PD leading to significant impairment in work, social, or family functioning.
- Comorbidity with severe major depressive disorder or other ADs.
- Severe maternal weight loss and/or metabolic disturbances attributable to PD.
- High maternal suicide risk.
- Uncontrolled medical conditions exacerbated by elevated anxiety levels.
- A temporal relationship between the onset of intrauterine growth restriction in the fetus and maternal PD symptoms.

- A history of ineffective psychotherapy or poor adherence to treatment.

19.7.1 General Consideration on Perinatal PD Pharmacological Treatment

Currently, no evidence-based guidelines or placebo-controlled studies specifically address the pharmacological treatment of PD during the perinatal period.

However, pharmacological agents demonstrated to be effective in the general population are generally considered equally efficacious during pregnancy and lactation. SSRIs, imipramine, clomipramine, venlafaxine, and benzodiazepines are established as effective treatments for PD. Additionally, mirtazapine may also be a viable treatment option (Uguz et al. 2016; Serretti et al. 2011; Batelaan et al. 2012; Marchesi 2008; Bandelow and Rüther 2004).

When selecting pharmacological agents during pregnancy, considerations should include the patient's history of response to specific medications and any previous adverse drug reactions, thus ensuring the most appropriate therapeutic choice.

19.7.2 Clinical Practice Suggestions for the Pharmacological Treatment of PD in Pregnancy

SSRIs should be the preferred pharmacological option for PDs during pregnancy. Specifically, sertraline, citalopram, and escitalopram are recommended as first-line medications due to their favorable fetal safety profile (Womersley et al. 2017; Marchesi et al. 2016; Larsen et al. 2015; Uguz 2015; Myles et al. 2013). A recent retrospective study (Uguz 2020) assessing the efficacy of citalopram in 22 pregnant women diagnosed with PD found that a dosage of 20 mg/day of citalopram was effective in treating PD during pregnancy. Regarding other SSRIs, paroxetine is associated with an increased risk of congenital malformations, particularly those affecting the heart (septal defects) (Grigoriadis et al. 2013; Myles et al. 2013). Fluoxetine is also associated with birth defects, albeit to a lesser extent than paroxetine (Weissman et al. 2004); however, due to the long half-life of its active metabolites, it carries a reduced risk of neonatal withdrawal syndrome. As a result, neither of these two SSRIs is recommended as a first-line treatment (Myles et al. 2013). However, they may be considered for pregnant women with PD who have not responded to other antidepressant treatments.

TCAs represent an alternative pharmacological option, though safety data on their use during pregnancy remain more limited compared to SSRIs. Pregnant patients with PD treated with imipramine (Uguz et al. 2014; Ware and DeVane 1990) have benefited from pharmacotherapy, reporting remission of panic symptoms. Specifically, a study involving 16 pregnant women with panic attacks found low-dose imipramine (10–40 mg/day) to be effective, with 75% of participants experiencing a statistically significant reduction in the mean number of weekly panic attacks (Uguz et al. 2014).

Venlafaxine, an established treatment for PD, is widely used as a first-line agent in non-pregnant women (Batelaan et al. 2012). However, during pregnancy, it is generally regarded as a second-line option due to the relatively limited safety data compared to SSRIs. A 2019 observational study involving 281 pregnancies exposed to venlafaxine found no conclusive evidence linking its use to risks of adverse pregnancy or fetal outcomes (Richardson et al. 2019).

In cases of partial response to first-line therapy, the combination of SSRIs and mirtazapine may be a viable alternative. Case reports have supported the adjunctive use of low-dose mirtazapine (7.5–15 mg/day) with SSRIs in pregnant women experiencing severe nausea, insomnia, and reduced appetite associated with PD (Uguz 2013) (Table 19.1).

Benzodiazepines remain an effective and widely used treatment for PD (Marchesi 2008). Despite their rapid onset of action, these medications present several disadvantages, including the potential for physical dependence, abuse, withdrawal symptoms, and the possibility of cognitive impairment in patients (Marchesi 2008). Moreover, some authors have indicated that the concomitant use of benzodiazepines and antidepressants is associated with an elevated risk of birth defects. Consequently, benzodiazepines should be reserved for short-term use at the lowest possible dosage, either as a bridge until antidepressants achieve the expected response or in cases of "severe anxiety and/or agitation" (ACOG 2023; Marchesi 2008). When their use is necessary, short half-life agents, such as lorazepam, are preferred (Rowe et al. 2013).

19.7.3 Clinical Practice Suggestions for the Pharmacological Treatment of PD During Breastfeeding

Most authors consider sertraline and paroxetine among the preferred antidepressants for use during breastfeeding (Uguz 2021; Grzeskowiak et al. 2018; Molenaar et al. 2018; McAllister-Williams et al. 2017; Weissman et al. 2004), as both exhibit undetectable or low infant plasma concentrations and a RID of 0.5–2.8% (paroxetine) and 0.5–3% (sertraline) (NICE 2020; Pogliani et al. 2019; Uguz et al. 2016; Berle and Spigset 2011; Weissman et al. 2004; Begg et al. 1999).

Among other SSRIs, escitalopram presents undetectable or low infant plasma concentrations, with a RID ranging from 3% to 8.3% (NICE 2020; Neuman et al. 2014; Bellantuono et al. 2012; Berle and Spigset 2011). Citalopram, while excreted into breast milk in small amounts, has occasionally been reported to reach an RID exceeding 10% (NICE 2020; Pogliani et al. 2019; Heikkinen et al. 2002). Fluoxetine is excreted into human milk in small to moderate amounts, yet its relative dose (>10%) may be higher than that of other antidepressants in the same SSRI group (NICE 2020; Pogliani et al. 2019; Epperson et al. 2003; Hendrick et al. 2001b). Therefore, while these SSRIs may be considered compatible with breastfeeding under certain circumstances, they should not be regarded as first-line treatments. In particular, fluoxetine use requires careful consideration due to its higher RID.

With regard to TCAs, a study (Uguz et al. 2016) presented the results of 6 patients with PD treated with low doses of imipramine (dosages ranging from 25 to 35 mg/day) during breastfeeding. The level of anxiety symptoms significantly decreased after treatment; in fact, the response rate was 66.7%, with all participants reporting a reduction in symptoms to varying degrees. These findings suggest that low doses of imipramine may serve as a pharmacological alternative to paroxetine and sertraline for breastfeeding women with PD.

19.8 Treatment of Generalized Anxiety Disorder (GAD)

Perinatal GAD has a high prevalence, ranging from 8.5% to 10.5% during pregnancy and 4.4% to 10.8% in the postpartum period (Buist and Gotman 2011; Sutter-Dallay et al. 2004). Despite its significant impact on the patient's functioning, this potentially debilitating mental health condition is often underdiagnosed. A key challenge in perinatal GAD diagnosis lies in differentiating between normal and pathological worry. Given its potential to negatively influence neonatal outcomes, early detection and timely intervention are essential.

19.8.1 General Consideration on Perinatal GAD Pharmacological Treatment

Treatment approaches for perinatal GAD vary depending on the severity of the condition. CBT is considered the first-line treatment for mild to moderate perinatal GAD. However, for moderate to severe cases, pharmacotherapy should be considered (Misri et al. 2015). SSRIs and SNRIs are the primary pharmacological options for managing GAD. The use of SSRIs/SNRIs in the management of perinatal GAD should be determined on an individual basis. Patients with a prior history of SSRI/SNRI use should continue their prescribed medication to minimize the risk of relapse, with the possible exception of paroxetine due to its potential cardiac risks to the fetus. For women initiating pharmacological treatment for the first time, an SSRI/SNRI with established efficacy for GAD should be selected. Furthermore, preference may be given to those agents with low accumulation in breast milk, a proven safety profile during pregnancy, and a low drug concentration ratio in the umbilical cord and serum (Misri et al. 2015).

19.8.2 Clinical Practice Suggestions for the Pharmacological Treatment of GAD in Pregnancy

According to guidelines, pharmacotherapy may be indicated for pregnant women with moderate to severe, treatment-resistant GAD. Over the past decade, the use of SSRIs during pregnancy has become increasingly common in clinical practice. Recent studies indicate that the safety profile of SSRIs, including their use during the first trimester, is generally reassuring (Huybrechts et al. 2014; Jimenez-Solem et al. 2013; Reis and Källén 2010). However, we recommend prescribing sertraline and citalopram as first-line options due to their extensive study and established safety profile in pregnancy.

Regarding SNRIs, venlafaxine may be considered as a potential treatment option during early pregnancy for women with severe GAD who have previously demonstrated a favorable response to this medication (Bellantuono et al. 2015). More specifically, venlafaxine may be considered for use early in pregnancy in the following clinical situations: (1) women with a documented history of recurrent, severe GAD who are currently receiving venlafaxine for long-term maintenance; and (2) women experiencing a severe new episode of GAD who have previously responded successfully to venlafaxine treatment (Bellantuono et al. 2015).

BDZs remain effective for the rapid treatment of short-term anxiety, particularly for alleviating somatic symptoms. Given that antidepressants typically require several weeks to show therapeutic effects, BDZs may be used for brief treatment to provide an immediate anxiolytic response. As noted, lorazepam may be preferred over other BDZs due to its lower accumulation in fetal tissue (Misri et al. 2015).

19.8.3 Clinical Practice Suggestions for the Pharmacological Treatment of GAD During Breastfeeding

The available data regarding the effects of SSRIs on breastfeeding infants are on the whole reassuring, and breastfeeding should generally not be discouraged in women using these medications. A review (Rowe et al. 2015) showed that the transfer of sertraline, fluvoxamine, and paroxetine into human milk is low, with even lower levels of uptake by the infant. To date, minimal or no adverse effects have been reported following the use of these three SSRIs in breastfeeding mothers. Regarding SNRIs, few but encouraging data have emerged from limited studies on the neonatal safety of venlafaxine and duloxetine during breastfeeding (Bellantuono et al. 2015; Boyce et al. 2011; Briggs et al. 2009; Newport et al. 2009; Berle et al. 2004; Ilett et al. 2002; Hendrick et al. 2001a). Adverse events in infants breastfed by mothers using these medications have been reported only occasionally (Orsolini and Bellantuono 2015). When benzodiazepines are considered, a short-acting formulation should be selected, and the lowest effective dose should be administered for the shortest duration to minimize infant exposure.

19.9 Treatment of Specific and Social Phobias

The existing literature on the treatment of both specific and social phobias during the perinatal period is notably limited, with a lack of studies specifically addressing the postpartum phase (Nath et al. 2020). The available data on the prevalence of these disorders during the perinatal period are as follows:

- Prevalence rates for specific phobia range from 3.2% to 19.9% (Nath et al. 2020; Fairbrother et al. 2016; Goodman et al. 2014).
- For social phobia, prevalence rates across five studies vary from 0.2% to 5.1% (Wisner et al. 2013; Navarro et al. 2008; Wenzel et al. 2005).
- For agoraphobia, the prevalence rates reported in two studies were 0% and 0.6% (Navarro et al. 2008; Wenzel et al. 2005).

Specific phobias, such as emetophobia (fear of vomiting) and blood-injection phobia (including needle phobia), are particularly relevant in the context of pregnancy (Patel and Hollins 2015). These disorders can have significant consequences; emetophobia has been associated with pregnancy avoidance, termination of pregnancy, and the avoidance of surgical procedures or general anesthesia due to a fear of vomiting (Veale and Lambrou 2006). Additionally, in cases of severe needle phobia, women may delay seeking antenatal care and avoid necessary blood tests and injections (McAllister et al. 2012). A study has shown that pregnant women with needle phobia are at higher risk for adverse obstetric and neonatal outcomes, including prematurity, low birth weight, and neonatal morbidity (Lilliecreutz et al. 2010). In recent years, there has been growing interest in the phenomenon of birth phobia, also known as tocophobia. The intensity of this phobia can lead to avoidance of pregnancy or a preference for cesarean section (Demšar et al. 2018).

To date, research focused on the treatment of phobias in the perinatal period has largely concentrated on non-pharmacological interventions, which fall outside the scope of this chapter.

19.10 Conclusion

As elucidated throughout this chapter, ADs during the perinatal period are prevalent yet often underestimated. The ramifications of these disorders, when left unrecognized or inadequately addressed, are significant and multifaceted. They pose considerable risks not only to the pregnant woman or new mother—heightening the likelihood of postpartum depression, suicidal ideation, pre-eclampsia, fear of childbirth, diminished breastfeeding, maladaptive coping mechanisms, and substance misuse (e.g., alcohol)—but also to neonatal health outcomes. Such adverse effects may encompass preterm birth, low Apgar scores, fetal hyperactivity, irregular fetal heart rates, polyhydramnios, small size for gestational age, and low birth weight. The implications of untreated perinatal anxiety are not confined to the immediate perinatal period; they extend into the long term, potentially contributing to a range of challenges in offspring, such as sleep disturbances, feeding difficulties, activity issues during infancy, and an increased risk of attention deficits, hyperactivity, and emotional or behavioral disorders throughout childhood.

To date, no placebo-controlled studies have directly compared the outcomes of women with perinatal anxiety disorders receiving pharmacological treatment to those remaining untreated. As such, deriving definitive conclusions about the most effective treatment strategies during this critical period remains a challenge.

However, it is paramount to recognize that existing evidence suggests that pregnant women and new mothers, along with their healthcare providers, should prioritize the potential consequences of untreated ADs over the risks associated with appropriately managed and monitored pharmacotherapy.

Current literature indicates that sertraline, escitalopram, and citalopram are among the most favorable antidepressants for the management of perinatal ADs, offering a favorable balance of efficacy and safety. In contrast, TCAs, SNRIs, and mirtazapine have not been studied as extensively as SSRIs. Should a short-term regimen of benzodiazepines be deemed necessary, it should be prescribed with careful consideration. In the context of breastfeeding, there is a growing consensus endorsing sertraline and paroxetine as first-line pharmacotherapies. In conclusion, the determination of the optimal pharmacological strategy for women facing perinatal ADs remains a complex endeavor. Nevertheless, the available safety data regarding specific medications, particularly SSRIs, provide reassurance. Therefore, when pharmacological treatment is indicated—especially in cases of severe ADs or when less invasive interventions have failed—it should be strongly considered. Such therapeutic decisions must be individualized, weighting the patient's history of ADs, current clinical status, severity, and overall functional impairment to ensure both maternal and fetal well-being.

References

ACOG. Treatment and Management of Mental Health Conditions during Pregnancy and Postpartum: ACOG clinical practice guideline no. 5. Obstet Gynecol. 2023;141(6):1262–88.

Adamson B, Letourneau N, Lebel C. Prenatal maternal anxiety and children's brain structure and function: a systematic review of neuroimaging studies. J Affect Disord. 2019;253:111–20.

Al-Awabdeh E, Abu Shaikha L, Salameh A, Alshraideh JA. Panic disorder during pregnancy: a scoping review. Heliyon. 2024;10(7):e28999.

Alderdice F, Lynn F, Lobel M. A review and psychometric evaluation of pregnancy-specific stress measures. J Psychosom Obstet Gynaecol. 2012;33(1):62–77.

American Psychiatric Association. Anxiety disorders. In: Diagnostic and statistical manual of mental disorders. 5th ed. Arlington: American Psychiatric Association; 2022. p. 215–23.

Amir LH, Pirotta MV, Raval M. Breastfeeding – evidence based guidelines for the use of medicines. Aust Fam Physician. 2011;40(9):684–90.

Bae HS, Kim SY, Ahnv HS, Cho YK. Comparison of nutrient intake, lifestyle variables, and pregnancy outcomes by the depression degree of pregnant women. Nutr Res Pract. 2010;4(4):323–31.

Bandelow B, Rüther E. Treatment-resistant panic disorder. CNS Spectr. 2004;9(10):725–39.

Bandelow B, Baldwin DS, Dolberg OT, Andersen HF, Stein DJ. What is the threshold for symptomatic response and remission for major depressive disorder, panic disorder, social anxiety disorder, and generalized anxiety disorder? J Clin Psychiatry. 2006;67(9):1428–34.

Bánhidy F, Acs N, Puhó E, Czeizel AE. Association between maternal panic disorders and pregnancy complications and delivery outcomes. Eur J Obstet Gynecol Reprod Biol. 2006;124(1):47–52.

Barcelona de Mendoza V, Harville E, Theall K, Buekens P, Chasan-Taber L. Effects of acculturation on prenatal anxiety among Latina women. Arch Womens Ment Health. 2016;19(4):635–44.

Batelaan NM, Van Balkom AJ, Stein DJ. Evidence-based pharmacotherapy of panic disorder: an update. Int J Neuropsychopharmacol. 2012;15(3):403–15.

Begg EJ, Duffull SB, Saunders DA, et al. Paroxetine in human milk. Br J Clin Pharmacol. 1999;48(2):142–7.

Bellantuono C, Bozzi F, Orsolini L, Catena-Dell'Osso M. The safety of escitalopram during pregnancy and breastfeeding: a comprehensive review. Hum Psychopharmacol. 2012;27(6):534–9.

Bellantuono C, Vargas M, Mandarelli G, Nardi B, Martini MG. The safety of serotonin-noradrenaline reuptake inhibitors (SNRIs) in pregnancy and breastfeeding: a comprehensive review. Hum Psychopharmacol. 2015;30(3):143–51.

Bellantuono C, De Berardis D, Valchera A, Vecchiotti R. Manuale di psichiatria perinatale. Roma (Italy): Giovanni Fioriti Editore; 2022. p. 107–24.

Berle JO, Spigset O. Antidepressant use during breastfeeding. Curr Womens Health Rev. 2011;7(1):28–34.

Berle JØ, Steen VM, et al. Breastfeeding during maternal antidepressant treatment with serotonin reuptake inhibitors: infant exposure, clinical symptoms, and cytochrome p450 genotypes. J Clin Psychiatry. 2004;65(9):1228–34.

Birnbaum CS, Cohen LS, Bailey JW, Grush LR, Robertson LM, Stowe ZN. Serum concentrations of antidepressants and benzodiazepines in nursing infants: a case series. Pediatrics. 1999;104(1):e11.

Blackmore ER, Côté-Arsenault D, Tang W, et al. Previous prenatal loss as a predictor of perinatal depression and anxiety. Br J Psychiatry. 2011;198(5):373–8.

Blackmore ER, Gustafsson H, Gilchrist M, Wyman C, O'Connor TG. Pregnancy-related anxiety: evidence of distinct clinical significance from a prospective longitudinal study. J Affect Disord. 2016;197:251–8.

Borgatta L, Jenny RW, Gruss L, Ong C, Barad D. Clinical significance of methohexital, meperidine, and diazepam in breast milk. J Clin Pharmacol. 1997;37(3):186–92.

Boyce PM, Hackett LP, Ilett KF. Duloxetine transfer across the placenta during pregnancy and into milk during lactation. Arch Womens Ment Health. 2011;14(2):169–72.

Brandt R. Passage of diazepam and desmethyldiazepam into breast milk. Arzneimittelforschung. 1976;26(3):454–7.

Briggs GG, Ambrose PJ, Ilett KF, Hackett LP, Nageotte MP, Padilla G. Use of duloxetine in pregnancy and lactation. Ann Pharmacother. 2009;43(11):1898–902.

Brockington IF, Macdonald E, Wainscott G. Anxiety, obsessions and morbid preoccupations in pregnancy and the puerperium. Arch Womens Ment Health. 2006;9(5):253–63.

Brunton RJ, Dryer R, Saliba A, Kohlhoff J. Pregnancy anxiety: a systematic review of current scales. J Affect Disord. 2015;176:24–34.

Buist A, Gotman N. Generalized anxiety disorder: course and risk factors in pregnancy. J Affect Disord. 2011;131:277–83.

Chen YH, Lin HC, Lee HC. Pregnancy outcomes among women with panic disorder: do panic attacks during pregnancy matter? J Affect Disord. 2010;120(1–3):258–62.

Cipriani A, Furukawa TA, Salanti G, Geddes JR, Higgins JP, Churchill R, et al. Comparative efficacy and acceptability of 12 new-generation antidepressants: a multiple-treatments meta-analysis. Lancet. 2009;373:746–58.

Cole AP, Hailey DM. Diazepam and active metabolite in breast milk and their transfer to the neonate. Arch Dis Child. 1975;50(9):741–2.

Cote-Arsenault D. The influence of perinatal loss on anxiety in multigravidas. J Obstet Gynecol Neonatal Nurs. 2003;32:623–9.

Davanzo R, Copertino M, De Cunto A, Minen F, Amaddeo A. Antidepressant drugs and breastfeeding: a review of the literature. Breastfeed Med. 2011;6(2):89–98.

Davis EP, Snidman N, Wadhwa PD, Glynn LM, Schetter CD, Sandman CA. Prenatal maternal anxiety and depression predict negative behavioral reactivity in infancy. Infancy. 2004;6(3):319–31.

Demšar K, Svetina M, Verdenik I, Tul N, Blickstein I, Globevnik VV. Tokophobia (fear of childbirth): prevalence and risk factors. J Perinat Med. 2018;46(2):151–4.

Dennis CL, Falah-Hassani K, Shiri R. Prevalence of antenatal and postnatal anxiety: systematic review and meta-analysis. Br J Psychiatry. 2017;210(5):315–23.

Ding XX, Wu YL, Xu SJ, et al. Maternal anxiety during pregnancy and adverse birth outcomes: a systematic review and meta-analysis of prospective cohort studies. J Affect Disord. 2014;159:103–10.

DiPietro JA, Christensen AL, Costigan KA. The pregnancy experience scale-brief version. J Psychosom Obstet Gynaecol. 2008;29:262–7.

Dunkel Schetter C, Tanner L. Anxiety, depression and stress in pregnancy: implications for mothers, children, research, and practice. Curr Opin Psychiatry. 2012;25:141–8.

Dusci LJ, Good SM, Hall RW, Ilett KF. Excretion of diazepam and its metabolites in human milk during withdrawal from combination high dose diazepam and oxazepam. Br J Clin Pharmacol. 1990;29(1):123–6.

Eberhard-Gran M, Eskild A, Opjordsmoen S. Use of psychotropic medications in treating mood disorders during lactation: practical recommendations. CNS Drugs. 2006;20:187–98.

Epperson CN, Jatlow PI, Czarkowski K, Anderson GM. Maternal fluoxetine treatment in the postpartum period: effects on platelet serotonin and plasma drug levels in breastfeeding mother-infant pairs. Pediatrics. 2003;112(5):e425.

Fairbrother N, Janssen P, Antony MM, Tucker E, Young AH. Perinatal anxiety disorder prevalence and incidence. J Affect Disord. 2016;200:148–55.

Falah-Hassani K, Shiri R, Dennis CL. The prevalence of antenatal and postnatal co-morbid anxiety and depression: a meta-analysis. Psychol Med. 2017;47:2041–53.

Fan F, Zou Y, Tian H, et al. Effects of maternal anxiety and depression during pregnancy in Chinese women on children's heart rate and blood pressure response to stress. J Hum Hypertens. 2016;30(3):171–6.

Fan F, Zou Y, Zhang Y, et al. The relationship between maternal anxiety and cortisol during pregnancy and birth weight of Chinese neonates. BMC Pregnancy Childbirth. 2018;18(1):265.

Farias DR, Pinto Tde J, Teofilo MM, et al. Prevalence of psychiatric disorders in the first trimester of pregnancy and factors associated with current suicide risk. Psychiatry Res. 2013;210(3):962–8.

Fawcett EJ, Fairbrother N, Cox ML, White IR, Fawcett JM. The prevalence of anxiety disorders during pregnancy and the postpartum period: a multivariate Bayesian meta-analysis. J Clin Psychiatry. 2019;80(4):18r12527.

Gentile S. Infant safety with antipsychotic therapy in breastfeeding: a systematic review. J Clin Psychiatry. 2008;2008(69):666–73.

Gentile S, Fusco ML. Placental and fetal effects of antenatal exposure to antidepressants or untreated maternal depression. J Matern Fetal Neonatal Med. 2017;30(10):1189–99.

George A, Luz RF, De Tychey C, Thilly N, Spitz E. Anxiety symptoms and coping strategies in the perinatal period. BMC Pregnancy Childbirth. 2013;13:233.

Glasheen C, Richardson GA, Fabio A. A systematic review of the effects of postnatal maternal anxiety on children. Arch Womens Ment Health. 2010;13:61–74.

Glover V. Prenatal stress and its effects on the fetus and the child: possible underlying biological mechanisms. Adv Neurobiol. 2015;10:269–83.

Glover V, O'Donnell KJ, O'Connor TG, Fisher J. Prenatal maternal stress, fetal programming, and mechanisms underlying later psychopathology – a global perspective. Dev Psychopathol. 2018;30(3):843–54.

Goodman JH, Chenausky KL, Freeman MP. Anxiety disorders during pregnancy: a systematic review. J Clin Psychiatry. 2014;75:1153–84.

Goodman JH, Watson GR, Stubbs B. Anxiety disorders in postpartum women: a systematic review and meta-analysis. J Affect Disord. 2016;203:292–331.

Greenberg PE, Sisitsky T, Kessler RC, et al. The economic burden of anxiety disorders in the 1990s. J Clin Psychiatry. 1999;60(7):427–35.

Grigoriadis S, VonderPorten EH, Mamisashvili L, et al. Antidepressant exposure during pregnancy and congenital malformations: is there an association? A systematic review and meta-analysis of the best evidence. J Clin Psychiatry. 2013;74(4):e293–308.

Grigoriadis S, Graves L, Peer M, et al. Maternal anxiety during pregnancy and the association with adverse perinatal outcomes: systematic review and meta-analysis. J Clin Psychiatry. 2018;79(5):17r12011.

Grzeskowiak LE, Leggett C, Costi L, et al. Impact of serotonin reuptake inhibitor use on breast milk supply in mothers of preterm infants: a retrospective cohort study. Br J Clin Pharmacol. 2018;84:1373–9.

Hägg S, Spigset O. Anticonvulsant use during lactation. Drug Saf. 2000;22(6):425–40.
Hart R, McMahon CA. Mood state and psychological adjustment to pregnancy. Arch Womens Ment Health. 2006;9(6):329–37.
Heikkinen T, Ekblad U, Kero P, Ekblad S, Laine K. Citalopram in pregnancy and lactation. Clin Pharmacol Ther. 2002;72(2):184–91.
Hendrick V, Altshuler L, Wertheimer A, Dunn WA. Venlafaxine and breast-feeding. Am J Psychiatry. 2001a;158(12):2089–90.
Hendrick V, Stowe ZN, Altshuler LL, et al. Fluoxetine and norfluoxetine concentrations in nursing infants and breast milk. Biol Psychiatry. 2001b;50(10):775–82.
Heron J, O'Connor TG, Evans J, Golding J, Glover V. The course of anxiety and depression through pregnancy and the postpartum in a community sample. J Affect Disord. 2004;80(1):65–73.
Huizink AC, Mulder EJH, Buitelaar JK. Prenatal stress and risk for psychopathology: specific effects or induction of general susceptibility? Psychol Bull. 2004;130(1):115–42.
Huizink AC, Menting B, Oosterman M, Verhage ML, Kunseler FC, Schuengel C. The interrelationship between pregnancy-specific anxiety and general anxiety across pregnancy: a longitudinal study. J Psychosom Obstet Gynaecol. 2014;35(3):92–100.
Huybrechts KF, Palmsten K, Avorn J, et al. Antidepressant use in pregnancy and the risk of cardiac defects. N Engl J Med. 2014;370(25):2397–407.
Ilett KF, Kristensen JH, Hackett LP, Paech M, Kohan R, Rampono J. Distribution of venlafaxine and its O-desmethyl metabolite in human milk and their effects in breastfed infants. Br J Clin Pharmacol. 2002;53(1):17–22.
Iqbal MM, Sobhan T, Ryals T. Effects of commonly used benzodiazepines on the fetus, the neonate, and the nursing infant. Psychiatr Serv. 2002;53(1):39–49.
Jimenez-Solem E, Andersen JT, Petersen M, et al. Prevalence of antidepressant use during pregnancy in Denmark, a nation-wide cohort study. PLoS One. 2013;8(4):e63034.
Kane JB. Marriage advantages in perinatal health: evidence of marriage selection or marriage protection? J Marriage Fam. 2016;78(1):212–29.
Kanto JH. Use of benzodiazepines during pregnancy, labour and lactation, with particular reference to pharmacokinetic considerations. Drugs. 1982;23(5):354–80.
Kanwar A, Malik S, Prokop LJ, Sim LA, Feldstein D, Wang Z, Murad MH. The association between anxiety disorders and suicidal behaviors: a systematic review and meta-analysis. Depress Anxiety. 2013;30:917–29.
Karlsson L, Nousiainen N, Scheinin NM, et al. Cytokine profile and maternal depression and anxiety symptoms in mid-pregnancy – the FinnBrain birth cohort study. Arch Womens Ment Health. 2017;20(1):39–48.
Kelly LE, Poon S, Madadi P, Koren G. Neonatal benzodiazepines exposure during breastfeeding. J Pediatr. 2012;161(3):448–51.
Kessler RC, Berglund P, Demler O, Jin R, Merikangas KR, Walters EE. Lifetime prevalence and age-of-onset distributions of DSM-IV disorders in the National Comorbidity Survey Replication. Arch Gen Psychiatry. 2005;62(6):593–602.
Lanza di Scalea T, Wisner KL. Antidepressant medication use during breastfeeding. Clin Obstet Gynecol. 2009;52(3):483–97.
Larsen ER, Damkier P, Pedersen LH, et al. Use of psychotropic drugs during pregnancy and breast-feeding. Acta Psychiatr Scand Suppl. 2015;445:1–28.
Lebel C, MacKinnon A, Bagshawe M, Tomfohr-Madsen L, Giesbrecht G. Elevated depression and anxiety symptoms among pregnant individuals during the COVID-19 pandemic. J Affect Disord. 2021;279:377–9.
Levin JS. The factor structure of the pregnancy anxiety scale. J Health Soc Behav. 1991;32(4):368–81.
Lilliecreutz C, Josefsson A, Sydsjö G. An open trial with cognitive behavioral therapy for blood- and injection phobia in pregnant women – a group intervention program. Arch Womens Ment Health. 2010;13(3):259–65.
Lobel M, Cannella DL, Graham JE, DeVincent C, Schneider J, Meyer BA. Pregnancy-specific stress, prenatal health behaviors, and birth outcomes. Health Psychol. 2008;27:604–15.

Marchesi C. Pharmacological management of panic disorder. Neuropsychiatr Dis Treat. 2008;4(1):93–106.

Marchesi C, Ampollini P, Paraggio C, et al. Risk factors for panic disorder in pregnancy: a cohort study. J Affect Disord. 2014;156:134–8.

Marchesi C, Ossola P, Amerio A, Daniel BD, Tonna M, De Panfilis C. Clinical management of perinatal anxiety disorders: a systematic review. J Affect Disord. 2016;190:543–50.

Martini J, Knappe S, Beesdo-Baum K, Lieb R, Wittchen HU. Anxiety disorders before birth and self-perceived distress during pregnancy: associations with maternal depression and obstetric, neonatal and early childhood outcomes. Early Hum Dev. 2010;86(5):305–10.

McAllister N, Elshtewi M, Badr L, Russell I, Lindow S. Pregnancy outcomes in women with severe needle phobia. Eur J Obstet Gynecol Reprod Biol. 2012;162(2):149–52.

McAllister-Williams RH, Baldwin DS, Cantwell R, et al. British Association for Psychopharmacology consensus guidance on the use of psychotropic medication preconception, in pregnancy and postpartum 2017. J Psychopharmacol. 2017;31:519–52.

McCusker J, Boulenger JP, Boyer R, Bellavance F, Miller JM. Use of health services for anxiety disorders: a multisite study in Quebec. Can J Psychiatr. 1997;42(7):730–6.

McElhatton PR. The effects of benzodiazepine use during pregnancy and lactation. Reprod Toxicol. 1994;8(6):461–75.

Misri S, Sivertz K. Tricyclic drugs in pregnancy and lactation: a preliminary report. Int J Psychiatry Med. 1991;21(2):157–71.

Misri S, Abizadeh J, Sanders S, Swift E. Perinatal generalized anxiety disorder: assessment and treatment. J Womens Health (Larchmt). 2015;24(9):762–70.

Molenaar NM, Kamperman AM, Boyce P, et al. Guidelines on treatment of perinatal depression with antidepressants: an international review. Aust N Z J Psychiatry. 2018;52:320–7.

Myles N, Newall H, Ward H, Large M. Systematic meta-analysis of individual selective serotonin reuptake inhibitor medications and congenital malformations. Aust N Z J Psychiatry. 2013;47(11):1002–12.

Nath S, Busuulwa P, Ryan EG, Challacombe FL, Howard LM. The characteristics and prevalence of phobias in pregnancy. Midwifery. 2020;82:102590.

National Institute for Health and Care Excellence (NICE). Antenatal and postnatal mental health: Clinical management and service guidance (NICE guideline CG192); 2020.

Navarro P, García-Esteve L, Ascaso C, Aguado J, Gelabert E, Martín-Santos R. Non-psychotic psychiatric disorders after childbirth: prevalence and comorbidity in a community sample. J Affect Disord. 2008;109(1–2):171–6.

Neuman G, Colantonio D, Delaney S, Szynkaruk M, Ito S. Bupropion and escitalopram during lactation. Ann Pharmacother. 2014;48(7):928–31.

Newport DJ, Ritchie JC, Knight BT, Glover BA, Zach EB, Stowe ZN. Venlafaxine in human breast milk and nursing infant plasma: determination of exposure. J Clin Psychiatry. 2009;70(9):1304–10.

Nishimura A, Furugen A, Umazume T, et al. Benzodiazepine concentrations in the breast milk and plasma of nursing mothers: estimation of relative infant dose. Breastfeed Med. 2021;16(5):424–31.

O'Hara MW, Wisner KL. Perinatal mental illness: definition, description and aetiology. Best Pract Res Clin Obstet Gynaecol. 2014;28(1):3–12.

Ohayon MM, Shapiro CM, Kennedy SH. Differentiating DSM-IV anxiety and depressive disorders in the general population: comorbidity and treatment consequences. Can J Psychiatr. 2000;45(2):166–72.

Orsolini L, Bellantuono C. Serotonin reuptake inhibitors and breastfeeding: a systematic review. Hum Psychopharmacol. 2015;30(1):4–20.

Ossola P, Ampollini P, Gerra ML, Tonna M, Viviani D, Marchesi C. Anxiety, depression, and cardiac outcomes after a first diagnosis of acute coronary syndrome. Health Psychol. 2018;37(12):1115–22.

Ossola P, Gerra ML, De Panfilis C, Tonna M, Viviani D, Marchesi C. Anxiety, depression, and birth outcomes in a cohort of unmedicated women. J Matern Fetal Neonatal Med. 2021;34(10):1606–12.

Patel RR, Hollins K. Clinical report: the joint obstetric and psychiatric management of phobic anxiety disorders in pregnancy. J Psychosom Obstet Gynaecol. 2015;36(1):10–4.

Patrick MJ, Tilstone WJ, Reavey P. Diazepam and breast-feeding. Lancet. 1972;1(7749):542–3.

Pleshette N, Asch S, Chase J. A study of anxiety during pregnancy, labor, the early and late puerperium. Bull N Y Acad Med. 1956;32(6):436–55.

Pogliani L, Baldelli S, Cattaneo D, et al. Selective serotonin reuptake inhibitors passage into human milk of lactating women. J Matern Fetal Neonatal Med. 2019;32:3020–5.

Rees S, Channon S, Waters CS. The impact of maternal prenatal and postnatal anxiety on children's emotional problems: a systematic review. Eur Child Adolesc Psychiatry. 2019;28(2):257–80.

Reis M, Källén B. Delivery outcome after maternal use of antidepressant drugs in pregnancy: an update using Swedish data. Psychol Med. 2010;40(10):1723–33.

Richardson JL, Martin F, Dunstan H, Greenall A, Stephens S, Yates LM, Thomas SHL. Pregnancy outcomes following maternal venlafaxine use: a prospective observational comparative cohort study. Reprod Toxicol. 2019;84:108–13.

Robertson E, Grace S, Wallington T, Stewart DE. Antenatal risk factors for postpartum depression: a synthesis of recent literature. Gen Hosp Psychiatry. 2004;26:289–95.

Ross LE, McLean LM. Anxiety disorders during pregnancy and the postpartum period: a systematic review. J Clin Psychiatry. 2006;67(8):1285–98.

Rowe H, Baker T, Hale TW. Maternal medication, drug use, and breastfeeding. Pediatr Clin N Am. 2013;60(1):275–94.

Rowe H, Baker T, Hale TW. Maternal medication, drug use, and breastfeeding. Child Adolesc Psychiatr Clin N Am. 2015;24(1):1–20.

Rubertsson C, Hellström J, Cross M, Sydsjö G. Anxiety in early pregnancy: prevalence and contributing factors. Arch Womens Ment Health. 2014;17(3):221–8.

Sachs HC. The transfer of drugs and therapeutics into human breast milk: an update on selected topics. Pediatrics. 2013;132(3):e796–809.

Saito J, Ishii M, Miura Y, et al. Brotizolam during pregnancy and lactation: Brotizolam levels in maternal serum, cord blood, breast milk, and neonatal serum. Breastfeed Med. 2021;16(7):579–82.

Sanchez SE, Puente GC, Atencio G, et al. Risk of spontaneous preterm birth in relation to maternal depressive, anxiety, and stress symptoms. J Reprod Med. 2013;58(1–2):25–33.

Schafer R, Genna CW. Physiologic breastfeeding: a contemporary approach to breastfeeding initiation. J Midwifery Womens Health. 2015;60(5):546–53.

Schoretsanitis G, Augustin M, Saßmannshausen H, Franz C, Gründer G, Paulzen M. Antidepressants in breast milk; comparative analysis of excretion ratios. Arch Womens Ment Health. 2019;22(3):383–90.

Schreier A, Wittchen HU, Höfler M, Lieb R. Anxiety disorders in mothers and their children: prospective longitudinal community study. Br J Psychiatry. 2008;192:308–9.

Serretti A, Chiesa A, Calati R, Perna G, Bellodi L, De Ronchi D. Novel antidepressants and panic disorder: evidence beyond current guidelines. Neuropsychobiology. 2011;63(1):1–7.

Shariatpanahi M, Faramarzi M, Barat S, Farghadani A, Shirafkan H. Prevalence and risk factors of prenatal anxiety disorders: a cross-sectional study. Health Sci Rep. 2023;6(8):e1491.

Smit M, Dolman KM, Honig A. Mirtazapine in pregnancy and lactation – a systematic review. Eur Neuropsychopharmacol. 2016;26(1):126–35.

Somers JM, Goldner EM, Waraich P, Hsu L. Prevalence and incidence studies of anxiety disorders: a systematic review of the literature. Can J Psychiatr. 2006;51(2):100–13.

Somerville S, Dedman K, Hagan R, Oxnam E, Wettinger M, Byrne S, Coo S, Doherty D, Page AC. The perinatal anxiety screening scale: development and preliminary validation. Arch Womens Ment Health. 2014;17:443–54.

Standley K, Soule B, Copans SA. Dimensions of prenatal anxiety and their influence on pregnancy outcome. Am J Obstet Gynecol. 1979;135(1):22–6.

Stein A, Pearson RM, Goodman SH, et al. Effects of perinatal mental disorders on the fetus and child. Lancet. 2014;384(9956):1800–19.

Sutter-Dallay AL, Giaconne-Marcesche V, Glatigny-Dallay E, Verdoux H. Women with anxiety disorders during pregnancy are at increased risk of intense postnatal depressive symptoms: a prospective survey of the MATQUID cohort. Eur Psychiatry. 2004;19(8):459–63.

Taylor D, Barnes TRE, Young AH. The Maudsley prescribing guidelines in psychiatry. 14th ed. Hoboken (NJ): Wiley-Blackwell; 2021.

Teixeira JM, Fisk NM, Glover V. Association between maternal anxiety in pregnancy and increased uterine artery resistance index: cohort based study. BMJ. 1999;318(7177):153–7.

Thorsness KR, Watson C, LaRusso EM. Perinatal anxiety: approach to diagnosis and management in the obstetric setting. Am J Obstet Gynecol. 2018;219:326–45.

Uguz F. Low-dose mirtazapine in treatment of major depression developed following severe nausea and vomiting during pregnancy. J Matern Fetal Neonatal Med. 2013;26(11):1066–8.

Uguz F. Pharmacotherapy of obsessive-compulsive disorder during pregnancy: a clinical approach. Braz J Psychiatry. 2015;37(4):334–42.

Uguz F. A pharmacological approach to panic disorder during pregnancy. J Matern Fetal Neonatal Med. 2016;29(9):1468–75.

Uguz F. Citalopram in treatment of pregnant women with panic disorder: a retrospective study. J Clin Psychopharmacol. 2020;40(6):615–7.

Uguz F. A new safety scoring system for the use of psychotropic drugs during lactation. Am J Ther. 2021;28:e118–26.

Uguz F, Sonmez EO, Sahingoz M, et al. Maternal generalized anxiety disorder during pregnancy and fetal brain development: a comparative study on cord blood brain-derived neurotrophic factor levels. J Psychosom Res. 2013;75(4):346–50.

Uguz F, Sahingoz M, Gungor B, Askin R. Low-dose imipramine for treatment of panic disorder during pregnancy: a retrospective chart review. J Clin Psychopharmacol. 2014;34(4):513–5.

Uguz F, Aydin A, Ak M, Turgut K. Low-dose imipramine for the treatment of panic disorder during postpartum period: a retrospective analysis of 6 cases. J Clin Psychopharmacol. 2016;36(3):292–3.

Uguz F, Yuksel G, Onur OS, Karsidag C, Gezginc K, Arpaci N. Neonatal outcomes in pregnant women with untreated and treated panic disorder. Compr Psychiatry. 2018;2018(87):107–11.

Uguz F, Yakut E, Aydogan S, Bayman MG, Gezginc K. The impact of maternal major depression, anxiety disorders and their comorbidities on gestational age, birth weight, preterm birth and low birth weight in newborns. J Affect Disord. 2019;259:382–5.

Umuziga MP, Adejumo O, Hynie M. A cross-sectional study of the prevalence and factors associated with symptoms of perinatal depression and anxiety in Rwanda. BMC Pregnancy Childbirth. 2020;20(1):68.

Van den Bergh BR, Marcoen A. High antenatal maternal anxiety is related to ADHD symptoms, externalizing problems, and anxiety in 8- and 9-year-olds. Child Dev. 2004;75(4):1085–97.

Van den Bergh BR, Van Calster B, Smits T, Van Huffel S, Lagae L. Antenatal maternal anxiety is related to HPA-axis dysregulation and self-reported depressive symptoms in adolescence: a prospective study on the fetal origins of depressed mood. Neuropsychopharmacology. 2008;33(3):536–45.

van der Zee-van den Berg AI, Boere-Boonekamp MM, CGM G-O, Reijneveld SA. Postpartum depression and anxiety: a community-based study on risk factors before, during and after pregnancy. J Affect Disord. 2021;286:158–65.

Veale D, Lambrou C. The psychopathology of vomit phobia. Behav Cogn Psychother. 2006;34(2):139–50.

Ware MR, DeVane CL. Imipramine treatment of panic disorder during pregnancy. J Clin Psychiatry. 1990;51(11):482–4.

Weissman AM, Levy BT, Hartz AJ, Bentler S, Donohue M, Ellingrod VL, et al. Pooled analysis of antidepressant levels in lactating mothers, breast milk, and nursing infants. Am J Psychiatry. 2004;161:1066–78.

Wenzel A, Haugen EN, Jackson LC, Robinson K. Prevalence of generalized anxiety at eight weeks postpartum. Arch Womens Ment Health. 2003;6:43–9.

Wenzel A, Haugen EN, Jackson LC, Brendle JR. Anxiety symptoms and disorders at eight weeks postpartum. J Anxiety Disord. 2005;19:295–311.

Wesson DR, Camber S, Harkey M, Smith DE. Diazepam and desmethyldiazepam in breast milk. J Psychoactive Drugs. 1985;17(1):55–6.

Wikner BN, Stiller CO, Bergman U, Asker C, Källén B. Use of benzodiazepines and benzodiazepine receptor agonists during pregnancy: neonatal outcome and congenital malformations. Pharmacoepidemiol Drug Saf. 2007;16(11):1203–10.

Williams KE, Koleva H. Identification and treatment of peripartum anxiety disorders. Obstet Gynecol Clin N Am. 2018;45(3):469–81.

Winkel S, Einsle F, Pieper L, Höfler M, Wittchen HU, Martini J. Associations of anxiety disorders, depressive disorders and body weight with hypertension during pregnancy. Arch Womens Ment Health. 2015;18(3):473–83.

Wisner KL, Sit DK, McShea MC, et al. Onset timing, thoughts of self-harm, and diagnoses in postpartum women with screen-positive depression findings. JAMA Psychiatry. 2013;70(5):490–8.

Womersley K, Ripullone K, Agius M. What are the risks associated with different selective serotonin re-uptake inhibitors (SSRIs) to treat depression and anxiety in pregnancy? An evaluation of current evidence. Psychiatr Danub. 2017;29(Suppl 3):629–44.

Wretlind M. Excretion of oxazepam in breast milk. Eur J Clin Pharmacol. 1987;33(2):209–10.

Yang L, Sun J, Nan Y, et al. Prevalence of perinatal anxiety and its determinants in mainland China: a systematic review and meta-analysis. J Affect Disord. 2023;323:193–203.

Yoshida K, Smith B, Craggs M, Kumar RC. Investigation of pharmacokinetics and of possible adverse effects in infants exposed to tricyclic antidepressants in breast milk. J Affect Disord. 1997;43(3):225–37.

Posttraumatic Stress Disorder

20

Mine Sahingoz and Serap Sari

20.1 Introduction

Posttraumatic stress disorder (PTSD) is one of the significant mental health concerns for women in the perinatal period, with prevalence estimates ranging from 0% to 35% in pregnancy (Horsch et al. 2013; Mahenge et al. 2013) and from 0% to 21% in postpartum (Schwab et al. 2012; Verreault et al. 2012). According to previous studies, the likelihood of PTSD increases during pregnancy and reaches its peak just before childbirth (Onoye et al. 2013). About one-third of women in the general population have experienced a traumatic birth, and the risk of PTSD in postpartum women is also increasing (Yildiz et al. 2017; Slade et al. 2022). It is possible that PTSD can be re-triggered by events during pregnancy and childbirth for women with a history of trauma or prior PTSD (Halvorsen et al. 2013). Several studies have identified numerous risk factors that increase the likelihood of PTSD in the perinatal period, including age, income level, history of trauma and psychological disturbances, trait anxiety, obstetric factors and complicated deliveries, and low social support (van Son et al. 2005; Cerulli et al. 2011; Grekin and O'Hara 2014; Canet-Vélez et al. 2024). Additionally, PTSD symptoms may be more severe during the peripartum period than at other life stages because the childbearing years have more potential triggers. There is strong evidence that PTSD during pregnancy is associated with poor birth outcomes, such as preterm birth (Shaw et al. 2014; Yonkers et al. 2014), and mothers with PTSD have been reported to have bonding difficulties with their babies and have more intrusive behaviors toward their babies (Davies et al. 2008; Ionio and Di 2014). Treating PTSD in the perinatal period is critical

M. Sahingoz (✉)
Meram Faculty of Medicine, Department of Psychiatry, Necmettin Erbakan University, Konya, Turkey

S. Sari
Faculty of Medicine, Department of Psychiatry, Atatürk University, Erzurum, Turkey

F. Uguz, L. Orsolini (eds.), *Perinatal Psychopharmacology*,
https://doi.org/10.1007/978-3-031-99720-4_20

because untreated PTSD may increase the risk of pregnancy complications and adverse outcomes, affect the infant's emotion regulation and development, and treatment of pregnant and lactating women with psychotropic medications also has potential risks (Bosquet Enlow et al. 2011; Garthus-Niegel et al. 2017). Unfortunately, there are currently very limited data on the treatment of PTSD in the perinatal period.

20.2 Risks of Untreated PTSD

PTSD is known to be a potentially disabling condition that can persist for decades (Kessler et al. 1995; Marmar et al. 2015). This disorder is associated with high comorbidity of psychiatric illnesses involving depression, anxiety, psychosis, personality, and substance use disorders (Galatzer-Levy et al. 2013; Gallagher and Brown 2015). It has been suggested that both PTSD and co-occurring psychological disorders increase the emergence of high-risk behaviors such as suicidal thoughts and behaviors and alcohol/substance use in general trauma literature (Yarvis and Schiess 2008). Although there is not adequate evidence, it should be considered that women with perinatal PTSD may have similar risks. Traumatic stress and PTSD during pregnancy may negatively affect birth outcomes or fetal development indirectly through risky health behaviors and poor self-care (e.g., attendance to medical care, nutrition, and sleep). Furthermore, anxiety and depression may also increase risks for preterm delivery, low birth weight, and reduced fetal growth (Morland et al. 2007). On the other hand, PTSD during pregnancy may directly predispose women to birth complications by neuroendocrine alterations, such as the dysregulation of cortisol, vasopressin, and oxytocin (Alder et al. 2007; Dunkel Schetter and Tanner 2012; Shaw et al. 2014). There are reports suggesting that posttraumatic stress is associated with preterm delivery (Shaw et al. 2014; Cook et al. 2018), decrement in infant head circumference at birth (Engel et al. 2005).

Several studies reported that maternal distress may associate with an adverse impact on maternal and child health (Alder et al. 2007; Dunkel Schetter and Tanner 2012; Ding et al. 2014; Glover 2015) and may affect child developmental outcomes and family functioning in the perinatal period (Ayers et al. 2006; Anderson and Cacola 2017). A large prospective study found that women with higher postpartum PTSD scores were significantly less likely to have breastfed their infant (Beck et al. 2011).

There is suggestive evidence that additional long-term impacts on families and infants include breastfeeding difficulties, as well as feelings of detachment with infant and mother, infant behavior, and cognitive development (Ayers et al. 2006; Creedy et al. 2000; Beck and Watson 2008). In addition, it has been suggested that untreated PTSD is associated with sexual avoidance, secondary tokophobia (fear of childbirth), disordered maternal-child bonding or overanxious/protective parenting and maternal long-term physical and emotional health issues (Nicholls and Ayers 2007; Fenech and Thomson 2014; Ionio and Di 2014; Davies et al. 2008). Given that perinatal PTSD related to high risk of pregnancy complications and adverse birth outcomes (Ayers and Ford 2014) as well as postpartum PTSD may have negative impact on women and the baby (Koen et al. 2016; Parfitt et al. 2014), it is of importance to identify and treat women with PTSD in the perinatal period.

20.3 Pharmacological Treatment

There is no distinctive guideline in the literature for the treatment of perinatal PTSD, despite evidence that PTSD occurs in a significant proportion of pregnant and in pregnant or lactating women and it is associated with poor outcomes such as preterm birth (Shaw et al. 2014; Yonkers et al. 2014). Although insufficient data, it is presumed that treatment methods known to be effective in the treatment of PTSD may also be effective in the perinatal period. Unfortunately, there is also limited data on therapeutic interventions for the PTSD non-perinatal population. The guidelines of PTSD treatment recommend that psychological treatments, especially trauma-focused psychotherapies, should be preferentially used as a routine first treatment of PTSD (Australian Centre for Posttraumatic Mental Health 2013; World Health Organization 2013). Numerous systematic reviews and meta-analyses demonstrated that the psychotherapeutic interventions, including trauma-focused cognitive behavioral therapy (CBT), exposure therapy and eye movement desensitization and reprocessing (EMDR), and debriefing and counselling, are effective on the symptoms of PTSD (Cusack et al. 2016; Chen et al. 2014; Gamble et al. 2002; Buhmann et al. 2018; Ford and Courtois 2020; Forbes et al. 2020).

Although the effectiveness of pharmacological drugs in the treatment of posttraumatic stress disorder has been discussed, they are still widely used, especially because psychological interventions cannot be found or unresponsive (Hoskins et al. 2015). It is likely that pharmacotherapies may relieve from symptoms such as sleep problems, depression, and anxiety, which are common in PTSD, rather than complete remission (Bowers and Ressler 2015).

20.3.1 General Considerations

Determining the appropriate psychiatric medications to use in the treatment of PTSD in the perinatal period is complicated by pregnancy and breastfeeding. Principally, nonpharmacological methods should be preferred firstly in the pregnant or lactating women for the treatment of PTSD. However, it is sometimes necessary to use pharmacological treatment, in patients with severe anxiety and depressive symptoms, malnutrition, or disturbance of sleep (Baldwin et al. 2014). On the other hand, trauma-focused psychotherapies can often temporarily increase symptoms. Therefore, medications that reduce PTSD symptoms can be a very useful second-line or adjunctive treatment during psychotherapy (Forbes et al. 2020; Ford and Courtois 2020). A wide range of pharmacotherapy has been tested in the treatment of PTSD, but it is unclear which pharmacological treatment should be selected among all the compounds available for perinatal PTSD. The pharmacologic treatments reported to be efficacious in the literature for the treatment of PTSD may be preferred according to their safety in pregnant or lactating women.

The primary concerns regarding the use of psychotropic medications during pregnancy and lactation include physical or neurobehavioral teratogenesis in the fetus, neonatal toxicity, and neonatal withdrawal. Before PTSD treatment is decided, it should be evaluated conditions such as severity of depression and anxiety, risk of suicide, nutrition deficiency, and sleep disturbances due to PTSD. In addition, it should be identified whether the PTSD itself or treatment of PTSD is independently associated with possible negative effects on both mother and infant as well as potential benefits of treatment. The risks and benefits of medication use during pregnancy or breastfeeding should be weighed individually. Finally, clinicians should inform both mother and father about the possible risks of treated or untreated PTSD. Parents and physicians must decide together for the regimen of treatment.

Psychotropic medicines should be selected with respect to evidence for both efficacy and safety in the perinatal period. If possible, psychotropics should be used at the lowest doses and shortly and avoided use of combination of medications. Due to the pharmacokinetic changes in pregnancy, clinicians should closely monitor patients, especially during the third trimester and the antepartum period, to maintain a therapeutic blood level and to avoid toxicity.

20.3.2 First-Line Pharmacotherapy of PTSD

Most guidelines agree that serotonin reuptake inhibitor antidepressants (SSRIs) are the drugs of first choice, being backed by a large body of evidence from randomized controlled trials (RCTs) (Davidson 2016; Jeffreys et al. 2012; Watts et al. 2013). SSRIs often produce modest results despite having currently the most evidence of efficacy on PTSD treatment (Ipser and Stein 2012). The use of selective norepinephrine-serotonin reuptake inhibitors (SNRIs), particularly venlafaxine, is also supported by clinical guidelines (National Academies Press 2014).

There are only two medications approved for the treatment of PTSD by the U.S. Food and Drug Administration (FDA), sertraline and paroxetine. All other medications for PTSD are considered off-label use. Paroxetine, sertraline, and fluoxetine were found to be superior to placebo in treating PTSD (Martenyi et al. 2002; Martenyi and Soldatenkova 2006; Davidson et al. 2005). Furthermore, there is evidence that fluoxetine, paroxetine, and venlafaxine are statistically significantly superior to placebo in the treatment of PTSD, while sertraline is ineffective or less effective (Hoskins et al. 2015; Buhmann and Andersen 2017). A large multinational RCT found venlafaxine was effective for PTSD re-experiencing and avoidance/numbing clusters, but not for hyperarousal (Davidson et al. 2006). Although venlafaxine demonstrated a large initial effect, this decreased over time (Lee et al. 2016). Other SSRIs, such as citalopram and fluvoxamine, currently have far less evidence for their effectiveness in PTSD (Shalev et al. 2012; Escalona et al. 2002). Fluvoxamine showed improvement in subjective sleep quality and PTSD symptoms in a few studies (Neylan et al. 2001).

To date, SSRIs are the most studied medications in pregnancy and lactation among available psychotropic drugs (McAllister-Williams et al. 2017). Paroxetine has stronger support for the efficacy in the treatment of non-perinatal PTSD than sertraline (Ipser and Stein 2012). However, paroxetine and fluoxetine are not recommended during pregnancy due to evidence suggesting increased risk of fetal defects (Jain and Lacy 2005; Womersley et al. 2017). The literature shows that paroxetine and fluoxetine have the strongest association with congenital malformations and negative birth outcomes while the associations between sertraline and citalopram with negative outcomes remain weaker. Citalopram may also be preferred in pregnant women, but it has lesser evidence than sertraline for their effectiveness in PTSD. Fluvoxamine is not recommended during pregnancy because of limited data on both its safety in the fetus and efficacy in PTSD treatment (Larsen et al. 2015). Limited data on venlafaxine show that use of venlafaxine during pregnancy does not increase the teratogenic risk (Einarson et al. 2001; Einarson et al. 2009). Considering sertraline is supported by a large body of data for the treatment of PTSD and has the largest safety data on its use in pregnancy, it is recommended to choose sertraline from the class of SSRIs as the first-line medicine for the treatment of PTSD in pregnant women. (Womersley et al. 2017; Thomson and Sharma 2021). However, in cases where a patient has previously responded to an alternative first-line drug, it may be preferred to this medication during pregnancy also.

Several studies on antidepressants and breastfeeding indicated that paroxetine and sertraline produce lower infant plasma levels than other antidepressants while citalopram and especially fluoxetine produce the highest plasma levels in infants. Therefore, sertraline and paroxetine should be preferred as first-line drugs during the lactation period (Womersley et al. 2017; Ram and Gandotra 2015; Larsen et al. 2015). Among the antidepressants, sertraline seems to be the best option during the perinatal period as it can also be continued in breastfeeding. Fluoxetine and citalopram/escitalopram are not appropriate for first-line treatments of PTSD in lactation due to the high infant exposure for these drugs. Venlafaxine and fluvoxamine should not be considered as first-line therapies because of inadequate data on safety in lactation. However, other antidepressants except sertraline and paroxetine can be used in special cases such as a history of their effectivity, or if the mother has used one of these drugs during pregnancy.

20.3.3 Second-Line Pharmacotherapy of PTSD

Second-line recommended medications generally include less evidence of effectiveness on PTSD symptoms. Additionally, many of them have a greater side effect profile than SSRI or SNRI medications, for example, tricyclic antidepressants (TCAs) and monoamine oxidase inhibitors (MAOIs).

TCAs and MAOIs were the first medications tested in RCTs for treating PTSD. Despite promising results from some RCTs for TCA in PTSD, high dropout rates due to common side effects complicated the interpretation of results in these studies (Davidson et al. 1990; Reist et al. 1989; Sullivan and Neria 2009). TCAs are not generally recommended as first-line medications in guidelines for the treatment of PTSD. However, they may be considered useful as add-on therapy to another drug or psychotherapy, to enhance sleep or to resolve specific symptoms, such as dissociation, pain (Davidson 2015). A review of the literature on the safety of TCA antidepressants in pregnancy suggests that although there is a slight increase in the rates of congenital anomalies in some studies, most studies did not show any increase (Ornoy et al. 2017). However, a meta-analysis has shown that exposure to TCAs during late gestation was associated with poor neonatal adaptation (Gentile 2010). The use of TCAs (except doxepin) appears to be a relatively safe option during breastfeeding (Eberhard-Gran et al. 2006), but there is a case of amitriptyline presenting with severe sedation and poor nutrition in the breastfed baby (Uguz 2017). When the limited data on both efficacy in the treatment of PTSD and safety for the maternal use of TCAs in gestation and lactation are considered, their use during the perinatal period is restricted.

Phenelzine provided mixed evidence for its efficacy in the treatment of PTSD (Shestatzky et al. 1988; Kosten et al. 1991); nevertheless, brofaromine failed to produce efficacy on PTSD symptoms in two placebo-controlled trials (Katz et al. 1994; Baker et al. 1995). For MAOIs, the necessity of a low tyramine diet to avoid hypertensive crisis and their contraindication in combination with other antidepressants and sympathomimetics means this class also has limited use (Sullivan and Neria 2009). There is also a very limited amount of data on the safety of MAOIs during both pregnancy and breastfeeding (Kennedy et al. 2017; Bauer et al. 2017). It is recommended to avoid these medications due to dietary and medication restrictions, along with the potential to cause hypertensive crises in the perinatal period (Lusskin et al. 2018).

Nefazodone has been shown to significantly improve most PTSD symptoms, including intrusive thoughts, avoidant behaviors, emotional numbing, nightmares, sleep, depression, and anger, but unadvisable because of the risk of hepatotoxicity in pregnant or lactating women (Lee et al. 2016; Detweiler et al. 2016). Trazodone is one of the most prescribed medications in the treatment of PTSD patients with insomnia or nightmares. There have been no RCTs to demonstrate its efficacy for sleep disturbances related to PTSD despite it has beneficial effects on sleep habits (Warner et al. 2001; Detweiler et al. 2016). Limited available data of trazodone in the perinatal period suggest that it is safe to use both during pregnancy due to the low risk of malformation and during breastfeeding due to a low relative infant dose (Smit et al. 2016; Kristensen et al. 2007; Klier et al. 2007). Mirtazapine was reported to improve PTSD symptoms and associated anxiety as well as useful in reducing the frequency and intensity of nightmares (Davidson et al. 2005; Detweiler et al. 2016). However, it should be noted that the data on mirtazapine support its use as an augmenting agent in addition to another medication, most commonly sertraline, rather than as a monotherapy in improving PTSD symptoms (Schneier et al. 2015; Thomson and Sharma 2021). Most of the data show that mirtazapine does not increase the risk of malformation in pregnancy and is also relatively reliable in lactation (Einarson et al. 2003; Smit et al. 2016). Therefore, mirtazapine and trazodone may be used in pregnant or breastfeeding women with PTSD for the treatment of sleep disturbances.

Atypical antipsychotics have also been used for PTSD if the treatment use of SSRIs does not show efficacy. The relatively large body of evidence of pharmacological treatment for PTSD indicates that atypical antipsychotics may be effective in PTSD with promising initial findings (Ipser and Stein 2012; Ahearn et al. 2011). Although many studies were performed on the use of antipsychotics as augmentation agents, there is less evidence on these medications as monotherapy in PTSD treatment (Carey et al. 2012; Berger et al. 2009). While there are some studies recommending antipsychotics to treat co-morbid psychotic symptoms/disorders or co-morbid bipolar disorder in PTSD patients (Hamner et al. 1999; Hamner et al. 2003a), others reported that second-generation antipsychotics (SGAs) were used primarily to target refractory insomnia/sleep disturbances in patients with PTSD (Hermes et al. 2014). Many reviews and meta-analyses to date have found that risperidone and olanzapine generally have greater evidence of effectiveness than quetiapine or aripiprazole in the treatment of non-perinatal PTSD (Koek et al. 2016).

For risperidone, there are positive results in the reduction of several PTSD symptom clusters such as re-experiencing and hyperarousal subscale scores with adjunctive risperidone for antidepressant-resistant PTSD (Reich et al. 2004). Some placebo-controlled studies of risperidone monotherapy indicated that it may be utilized as an effective in the management of PTSD (Padala et al. 2006); in contrast, others did not (Rothbaum et al. 2008).

As both monotherapy and augmentation with SSRIs in PTSD patients, the use of olanzapine is supported by evidence on symptom improvement in placebo-controlled trials (Stein et al. 2002; Carey et al. 2012). In addition, olanzapine has also been shown to have positive effects in improving sleep problems (Carey et al. 2012). However, in a controlled study of olanzapine monotherapy in PTSD, the clinical response to olanzapine ($n = 10$) was inadequate (Butterfield et al. 2001). There is limited data in the literature for the use of quetiapine in PTSD, but quetiapine is one of the most prescribed anti-nightmare medications in PTSD (Detweiler et al. 2016). Especially, for the sleep disturbances related to PTSD, quetiapine was found to be beneficial in some but not all trials (Sokolski et al. 2003; Hamner et al. 2003b). A recent systematic review suggests that aripiprazole as monotherapy or adjunct therapy for PTSD appears to improve symptoms associated with PTSD, such as anxiety, avoidance, hyperarousal, re-experiencing symptoms, and quality and length of sleep (Britnell et al. 2017). A small placebo-controlled study hypothesized significantly lower PTSD and depressive symptoms in the ziprasidone versus placebo group, but researchers terminated the study because intolerable adverse effects occurred in a significant proportion of patients receiving ziprasidone (Kellner et al. 2010).

There are very little data for the second-generation antipsychotic drugs, with respect to teratogenic or toxic effects on the fetus. A recent review reported that a slight increase in the rate of congenital anomalies following prenatal risperidone was observed in some smaller studies (Ornoy et al. 2017). A few studies have suggested that these agents may increase the risk of hyperglycemia in pregnant women as well as the rate of poor neonatal adaptation (Gentile 2004). However, most available studies on the safety of the second-generation antipsychotics in pregnancy and lactation demonstrated that they did not increase the risk of overall deformity (McKenna et al. 2005; Ornoy et al. 2017). Given the amount of clinical data on the safety in the perinatal period and efficacy in PTSD treatment of the second-generation antipsychotics, it is recommended to use risperidone and olanzapine during pregnancy, and olanzapine and quetiapine during lactation. There are controversial results on the efficacy of augmentation of antipsychotics with SSRIs in non-perinatal PTSD (Stein et al. 2002; Hamner et al. 2003b; Britnell et al. 2017). Moreover, antipsychotic augmentation may lead to higher adverse effects than monotherapy on the fetus or breastfed infant. As such, these treatments should be considered when women have failed to respond to monotherapies or have a comorbid condition such as bipolar disorder; and they should be used at as low doses as possible.

There are various recommendations among the guidelines and treatment algorithms for antiadrenergic agents in PTSD treatment (Koek et al. 2016). Several RCTs of prazosin observed that it had beneficial effects on nightmares and insomnia related to PTSD (Taylor et al. 2008), but results have been mixed regarding its efficacy for the full PTSD syndrome (Raskind et al. 2007). Some reports recommend prazosin as the first-line pharmacotherapy in PTSD patients with sleep disturbances before SSRIs (Bajor et al. 2011), while Ipser and Stein (2012) recommended it for sleep and nightmares unresponsive to SSRIs. In contrast with prazosin, there have been inadequate evidence on sleep disturbances or PTSD symptoms for both guanfacine and clonidine (Neylan et al. 2006; Alao et al. 2012). Although available limited data on the use of prazosin in pregnancy do not support an association between prazosin and congenital defects, the use of prazosin is not recommended during pregnancy and breastfeeding due to insufficient data on prazosin safety (Lubbe and Hodge 1981).

Most of the studies of propranolol have been examined in the prevention of post-traumatic symptoms and it has been found that beneficial in reducing the development of PTSD after trauma by some investigators (Pitman et al. 2002) although not others (Hoge et al. 2012). Additionally, Brunet et al. (2014) found that propranolol administration during an exposure session reduced physiological hyperarousal during later re-exposure. Propranolol has been extensively used to treat a variety of conditions such as hypertension and pheochromocytoma in the mother, and tachyarrhythmias in both the mother and fetus during pregnancy, and no teratogenicity associated with this agent has been documented (Ferrero et al. 2004). However, since adverse fetal effects have occasionally been noted, it is only recommended for use in pregnant women with PTSD when the benefit outweighs the risk (Meidahl Petersen et al. 2012). Despite no adverse effects in the breastfed infant have been reported and propranolol levels in breast milk are low, it is recommended that monitoring the signs of beta blockade of the infant and planning the feeding at least 3 hours after administration of maternal propranolol (Taylor and Turner 1981; Thorley and McAinsh 1983).

To date, there is little evidence to support the use of antiepileptics in the treatment of PTSD. Bajor et al. (2011) found evidence effectiveness of lamotrigine or topiramate on re-experiencing symptoms, lamotrigine on avoidance/numbing symptoms, and levetiracetam on global symptoms in patients with PTSD. Several reports recommended topiramate for PTSD symptoms including nightmares (Watts et al. 2013; Detweiler et al. 2016), while others did not (Hoskins et al. 2015). In addition, numerous systematic reviews indicated that antiepileptics failed to achieve significance for treating PTSD symptoms (Lee et al. 2016).

Exposure to antiepileptics, including valproic acid and carbamazepine, during pregnancy is known to be associated with an increased risk of major congenital malformations (Ornoy et al. 2017). Similarly, current evidence suggests topiramate may be teratogenic and may also lead to an increase in the rate of developmental problems (Hernandez-Diaz et al. 2018; Alsaad et al. 2015). Infants who were breastfed by mothers treated with topiramate were found to have very low serum levels and no side effects (Gentile 2009). Lamotrigine has a good safety profile compared with other antiepileptics and most studies found no increase in the rate of major congenital anomalies (Cunnington et al. 2011). On the other hand, it should not be forgotten that data about neurodevelopmental outcomes are rather limited. Lamotrigine is considered moderately safe during breastfeeding (Davanzo et al. 2013). Given both the inconclusive evidence on the efficacy of antiepileptics in the treatment of PTSD and concerns about their effects on the infant, antiepileptics are not recommended for use in pregnant or lactating women with PTSD.

Numerous systematic reviews indicated that benzodiazepines have no benefit in PTSD, despite they historically one of the medications most prescribed in patients with PTSD (Katzman et al. 2014; Hoskins et al. 2015; Jeffreys et al. 2012). However, eszopiclone, a hypnotic drug, was found useful in only one study (Pollack et al. 2011). According to several guidelines, benzodiazepines are contraindicated for patients with disinhibition and addiction problems (Jeffreys et al. 2012; Foa et al. 2008).

Recent reviews suggest that NMDA receptor modulators may have potential for benefit in treating PTSD by playing a role on the glutamatergic receptor subtype NMDA in fear extinction and reconsolidation (Kerbage and Richa 2015; Bernardy and Friedman 2015). However, there have been limited clinical data.

20.3.4 Prevention of PTSD After Trauma

It is estimated that up to 80% of the whole people will experience at least one potentially traumatic event (de Vries and Olff 2009; Frans et al. 2005). Fortunately, PTSD or other psychopathology does not develop in many people. Therefore, it is hypothesized that posttraumatic stress symptoms may be prevented in individuals exposed to trauma (Birur et al. 2017; Horn et al. 2016; Qi et al. 2016). There are many approaches to PTSD prevention, the most common of which is psychotherapy. The findings of systematic reviews and controlled trials suggest that trauma-focused CBT is potentially beneficial in preventing chronic posttraumatic symptoms, when provided within 6 months of the incident (Roberts et al. 2009). Also, few evidence indicate that the use of pharmacological interventions immediately after exposure to trauma may reduce the risk of developing of PTSD (Nash and Watson 2012). Several medications such as propranolol, glucocorticoids, opioids, antidepressants, neuroleptics, and salbutamol have been tested in the early aftermath of trauma with an attempt to prevent PTSD (Birur et al. 2017; Horn et al. 2016; Qi et al. 2016; Nash and Watson 2012).

A placebo-controlled randomized study found that acute administration of propranolol (160 mg/day) was superior to placebo in reducing subsequent posttraumatic symptoms and physiological hyper-activity to reminders of trauma, but did not reduce the emergence of posttraumatic stress disorder at 1 month (Pitman et al. 2002). A naturalistic study shows that acute administration of propranolol (120 mg/day) prevented the emergence of PTSD at 2 months (Vaiva et al. 2003), but not all evidence is consistent (Nugent et al. 2010; Stein et al. 2007). Based on scientific evidence on effectivity of propranolol for preventing traumatic symptoms in non-perinatal patients, propranolol can be given in pregnant and lactating women at low doses and for short periods after exposure to trauma.

Findings from controlled trials of glucocorticoids such as hydrocortisone (Delahanty et al. 2013; Schelling et al. 2001) are promising and support suggestions that cortisol administration after trauma may be a useful approach in preventing PTSD (Schelling et al. 1999). But this strategy does not appropriate during pregnancy and lactation due to cortisol may disrupt the hypothalamic–pituitary–adrenal axis.

While benzodiazepines are widely used in acute trauma settings, the rationale for their use in treating trauma has been undermined by the negative findings of a non-randomized controlled trial of clonazepam or alprazolam (Gelpin et al. 1996). Early administration of temazepam following life-threatening incidents resulted in a larger proportion of participants developing PTSD in a small randomized, placebo-controlled trial (Mellman et al. 2002). There is evidence for the efficacy for sertraline in preventing posttraumatic symptoms (Stoddard Jr et al. 2011), but not for gabapentin (Stein et al. 2007) or escitalopram (Shalev et al. 2012). A small number of randomized double-blind placebo-controlled relapse prevention studies find evidence for the efficacy of longer-term treatment, for fluoxetine (Martenyi et al. 2002) and sertraline (Davidson et al. 2005).

20.4 Conclusion

Management of women with PTSD during perinatal period is important given that they are not only at higher risk of pregnancy complications and adverse perinatal outcomes (Ayers and Ford 2014) but also postpartum PTSD which may have negative impact on women and the baby (Koen et al. 2016; Parfitt et al. 2014). Nevertheless, there are no published guidelines regarding the clinical approach to women with PTSD during the perinatal period. Especially, pregnant women determined to be in risk groups should be monitored closely and necessary support

Table 20.1 Expert recommendations based on scientific evidence and clinical experience

There are risks of untreated PTSD as well as the medications on the fetus or infants
Before PTSD treatment is decided, it should be evaluated conditions such as severity of depression and anxiety, risk of suicide, nutrition deficiency, and sleep disturbances due to PTSD
Clinicians and patients are concerned about the possible risks associated with PTSD and the medications
The treatment should be individualized
Both the patients and the exposed fetus or infant should be closely monitored
Monotherapy and lowest therapeutic doses are preferred
The first-line medications recommended for treating PTSD are sertraline, paroxetine, venlafaxine, and fluoxetine
According to their safety, sertraline may be preferred during pregnancy and sertraline and paroxetine may preferred during lactation
Trazodone, mirtazapine, followed by, and olanzapine are the most useful and reliable medications for sleep disturbances such as nightmares and insomnia in perinatal PTSD
Risperidone, olanzapine lesser to quetiapine and ziprasidone are the most preferable antipsychotic drugs for augmentation treatment in PTSD
In cases where the first-line medications cannot be used such as in comorbid bipolar disorder or ineffective, it is recommended to use risperidone and olanzapine during pregnancy, and olanzapine and quetiapine during lactation
Propranolol can be given to pregnant and lactating women at low doses and for short periods within 48 hours after exposure to trauma
Benzodiazepines should be avoided in the treatment of PTSD

PTSD posttraumatic stress disorder

should be provided. Clinicians should carefully consider the anticipated benefits and risks of pharmacological treatment of PTSD in pregnant or lactating women, including the potential risks of harm to a developing child; therefore, treatment should be individualized (Table 20.1).

References

Ahearn EP, Juergens T, Cordes T, Becker T, Krahn D. A review of atypical antipsychotic medications for posttraumatic stress disorder. Int Clin Psychopharmacol. 2011;26:193–200.

Alao A, Selvarajah J, Razi S. The use of clonidine in the treatment of nightmares among patients with co-morbid PTSD and traumatic brain injury. Int J Psychiatry Med. 2012;44:165–9.

Alder J, Fink N, Bitzer J, Hösli I, Holzgreve W. Depression and anxiety during pregnancy: a risk factor for obstetric, fetal and neonatal outcome? A critical review of the literature. J Matern Fetal Neonatal Med. 2007;20:189–209.

Alsaad AM, Chaudhry SA, Koren G. First trimester exposure to topiramate and the risk of oral clefts in the offspring: a systematic review and meta-analysis. Reprod Toxicol. 2015;53:45–50.

Anderson C, Cacola P. Implications of preterm birth for maternal mental health and infant development. Am J Matern Child Nurs. 2017;42:108–14.

Australian Centre for Posttraumatic Mental Health. The Australian guidelines for the treatment of acute stress disorder and posttraumatic stress disorder. Melborne: Australian Centre for Posttraumatic Mental Health (ACPMH); 2013.

Ayers S, Ford E. Post-traumatic stress during pregnancy and the postpartum period. In: Wenzel A, editor. Oxford handbook of perinatal psychology. Oxford: Oxford University Press; 2014.

Ayers S, Eagle A, Waring H. The effects of childbirth-related post-traumatic stress disorder on women and their relationships: a qualitative study. Psychol Health Med. 2006;11:389–98.

Bajor LA, Ticlea AN, Osser DN. The psychopharmacology algorithm project at the Harvard south shore program: an update on posttraumatic stress disorder. Harv Rev Psychiatry. 2011;19:240–58.

Baker DG, Diamond BI, Gillette G, Hamner M, Katzelnick D, Keller T, Mellman TA, Pontius E, Rosenthal M, Tucker P, et al. A double-blind, randomized, placebo-controlled, multi-center study of brofaromine in the treatment of post-traumatic stress disorder. Psychopharmacology. 1995;122:386–9.

Baldwin DS, Anderson IM, Nutt DJ, Allgulander C, Bandelow B, den Boer JA, Christmas DM, Davies S, Fineberg N, Lidbetter N, Malizia A, McCrone P, Nabarro D, O'Neill C, Scott J, van der Wee N, Wittchen HU. Evidence-based pharmacological treatment of anxiety disorders, post-traumatic stress disorder and obsessive-compulsive disorder: a revision of the 2005 guidelines from the British Association for Psychopharmacology. J Psychopharmacol. 2014;28:403–39.

Bauer RL, Orfei J, Wichman CL. Use of transdermal selegiline in pregnancy and lactation: a case report. Psychosomatics. 2017;58:450–2.

Beck CT, Watson S. Impact of birth trauma on breast-feeding: a tale of two pathways. Nurs Res. 2008;57:228–36.

Beck CT, Gable RK, Sakala C, Declercq ER. Posttraumatic stress disorder in new mothers: results from a two-stage U.S. National Survey. Birth. 2011;38:216–27.

Berger W, Mendlowicz MV, Marques-Portella C, Kinrys G, Fontenelle LF, Marmar CR, Figueira I. Pharmacologic alternatives to antidepressants in posttraumatic stress disorder: a systematic review. Prog Neuro-Psychopharmacol Biol Psychiatry. 2009;33:169–80.

Bernardy NC, Friedman MJ. Psychopharmacological strategies in the management of posttraumatic stress disorder (PTSD): what have we learned? Curr Psychiatry Rep. 2015;17:564.

Birur B, Moore NC, Davis LL. An evidence-based review of early intervention and prevention of posttraumatic stress disorder. Community Ment Health J. 2017;53:183–201.

Bosquet Enlow M, Kitts RL, Blood E, Bizarro A, Hofmeister M, Wright RJ. Maternal posttraumatic stress symptoms and infant emotional reactivity and emotion regulation. Infant Behav Dev. 2011;34:487–503.

Bowers ME, Ressler KJ. An overview of translationally informed treatments for posttraumatic stress disorder: animal models of pavlovian fear conditioning to human clinical trials. Biol Psychiatry. 2015;78:15–27.

Britnell SR, Jackson AD, Brown JN, Capehart BP. Aripiprazole for post-traumatic stress disorder: a systematic review. Clin Neuropharmacol. 2017;40:273–8.

Brunet A, Thomas É, Saumier D, Ashbaugh AR, Azzoug A, Pitman RK, Orr SP, Tremblay J. Trauma reactivation plus propranolol is associated with durably low physiological responding during subsequent script-driven traumatic imagery. Can J Psychiatr. 2014;59:228–32.

Buhmann CB, Andersen HS. Diagnosing and treating post-traumatic stress disorder. Ugeskr Laeger. 2017;179(24)

Buhmann CB, Nordentoft M, Ekstroem M, Carlsson J, Mortensen EL. Long-term treatment effect of trauma-affected refugees with flexible cognitive behavioral therapy and antidepressants. Psychiatry Res. 2018;264:217–23.

Butterfield MI, Becker ME, Connor KM, Sutherland S, Churchill LE, Davidson JR. Olanzapine in the treatment of post-traumatic stress disorder: a pilot study. Int Clin Psychopharmacol. 2001;16:197–203.

Canet-Vélez O, Besa ME, Sanromà-Ortíz M, et al. Incidence of perinatal post-traumatic stress disorder in Catalonia: an observational study of protective and risk factors. Healthcare (Basel). 2024;12(8):826.

Carey P, Suliman S, Ganesan K, Seedat S, Stein DJ. Olanzapine monotherapy in posttraumatic stress disorder: efficacy in a randomized, double-blind, placebo-controlled study. Hum Psychopharmacol. 2012;27:386–91.

Cerulli C, Talbot NL, Tang W, Chaudron LH. Co-occurring intimate partner violence and mental health diagnoses in perinatal women. J Women's Health. 2011;20:1797–803.

Chen YR, Hung KW, Tsai JC, Chu H, Chung MH, Chen SR, Liao YM, Ou KL, Chang YC, Chou KR. Efficacy of eye-movement desensitization and reprocessing for patients with posttraumatic-stress disorder: a meta-analysis of randomized controlled trials. PLoS One. 2014;9:103676.

Cook N, Ayers S, Horsch A. Maternal posttraumatic stress disorder during the perinatal period and child outcomes: A systematic review. J Affect Disord. 2018;225:18–31.

Creedy DK, Shochet IM, Horsfall J. Childbirth and the development of acute trauma symptoms: incidence and contributing factors. Birth. 2000;27:104–11.

Cunnington MC, Weil JG, Messenheimer JA, Ferber S, Yerby M, Tennis P. Final results from 18 years of the international lamotrigine pregnancy registry. Neurology. 2011;76:1817–23.

Cusack K, Jonas DE, Forneris CA, Wines C, Sonis J, Middleton JC, Feltner C, Brownley KA, Olmsted KR, Greenblatt A, Weil A, Gaynes BN. Psychological treatments for adults with posttraumatic stress disorder: a systematic review and meta-analysis. Clin Psychol Rev. 2016;43:128–41.

Davanzo R, Dal Bo S, Bua J, Copertino M, Zanelli E, Matarazzo L. Antiepileptic drugs and breast-feeding. Ital J Pediatr. 2013;39:50.

Davidson J. Vintage treatments for PTSD: a reconsideration of tricyclic drugs. J Psychopharmacol. 2015;29(3):264–9.

Davidson J. Pharmacotherapy of post-traumatic stress disorder: going beyond the guidelines. Br J Psych Open. 2016;2:16–8.

Davidson J, Kudler H, Smith R, Mahorney SL, Lipper S, Hammett E, Saunders WB, Cavenar JO Jr. Treatment of posttraumatic stress disorder with amitriptyline and placebo. Arch Gen Psychiatry. 1990;47:259–66.

Davidson JR, Bernik M, Connor KM, Friedman MJ, Jobson KO, Kim Y, Lecrubier Y, Ma H, Njenga F, Stein DJ. A new treatment algorithm for posttraumatic stress disorder. Psychiatr Ann. 2005;35:887–98.

Davidson J, Baldwin D, Stein DJ, Kuper E, Benattia I, Ahmed S, Pedersen R, Musgnung J. Treatment of posttraumatic stress disorder with venlafaxine extended release: a 6-month randomized controlled trial. Arch Gen Psychiatry. 2006;63:1158–65.

Davies J, Slade P, Wright I, Stewart P. Posttraumatic stress symptoms following childbirth and mothers' perceptions of their infants. Infant Ment Health J. 2008;29:537–54.

de Vries GJ, Olff M. The lifetime prevalence of traumatic events and posttraumatic stress disorder in The Netherlands. J Trauma Stress. 2009;22:259–67.

Delahanty DL, Gabert-Quillen C, Ostrowski SA, Nugent NR, Fischer B, Morris A, Pitman RK, Bon J, Fallon W. The efficacy of initial hydrocortisone administration at preventing posttraumatic distress in adult trauma patients: a randomized trial. CNS Spectr. 2013;18:103–11.

Detweiler MB, Pagadala B, Candelario J, Boyle JS, Detweiler JG, Lutgens BW. Treatment of post-traumatic stress disorder nightmares at a veterans affairs medical center. J Clin Med. 2016;5(12):pii: E117.

Ding XX, Wu YL, Xu SJ, Zhu RP, Jia XM, Zhang SF, Huang K, Zhu P, Hao JH, Tao FB. Maternal anxiety during pregnancy and adverse birth outcomes: a systematic review and meta-analysis of prospective cohort studies. J Affect Disord. 2014;159:103–10.

Dunkel Schetter C, Tanner L. Anxiety, depression and stress in pregnancy: implications for mothers, children, research, and practice. Curr Opin Psychiatry. 2012;25:141–8.

Eberhard-Gran M, Eskild A, Opjordsmoen S. Use of psychotropic medications in treating mood disorders during lactation: practical recommendations. CNS Drugs. 2006;20:187–98.

Einarson A, Fatoye B, Sarkar M, Lavigne SV, Brochu J, Chambers C, Mastroiacovo P, Addis A, Matsui D, Schuler L, Einarson TR, Koren G. Pregnancy outcome following gestational exposure to venlafaxine: a multicenter prospective controlled study. Am J Psychiatry. 2001;158:1728–30.

Einarson A, Bonari L, Voyer-Lavigne S, Addis A, Matsui D, Johnson Y, Koren G. A multicentre prospective controlled study to determine the safety of trazodone and nefazodone use during pregnancy. Can J Psychiatr. 2003;48:48106–10.

Einarson A, Choi J, Einarson TR, Koren G. Incidence of major malformations in infants following antidepressant exposure in pregnancy: results of a large prospective cohort study. Can J Psychiatr. 2009;54:242–6.

Engel SM, Berkowitz GS, Wolff MS, Yehuda R. Psychological trauma associated with the world trade center attacks and its effect on pregnancy outcome. Paediatr Perinat Epidemiol. 2005;19:334–41.

Escalona R, Canive JM, Calais LA, Davidson JR. Fluvoxamine treatment in veterans with combat-related post-traumatic stress disorder. Depress Anxiety. 2002;15:29–33.

Fenech G, Thomson G. Tormented by ghosts from their past': a meta-synthesis to explore the psychosocial implications of a traumatic birth on maternal well-being. Midwifery. 2014;30(2):185–93.

Ferrero S, Colombo BM, Ragni N. Maternal arrhythmias during pregnancy. Arch Gynecol Obstet. 2004;269:244–53.

Foa EB, Keane TM, Friedman MJ, Cohen JA. Effective treatments for PTSD: practice guidelines from the International Society for Traumatic Stress Studies. 2nd ed. New York: Guilford; 2008.

Forbes D, Bisson JI, Monson CM, Berliner L. Effective treatments for PTSD: practice guidelines from the International Society for Traumatic Stress Studies. 3rd ed. Guilford Press; 2020.

Ford JD, Courtois CA. Treating complex traumatic stress disorders in adults: scientific foundations and therapeutic models. Guilford Publications; 2020.

Frans O, Rimmö PA, Aberg L, Fredrikson M. Trauma exposure and post-traumatic stress disorder in the general population. Acta Psychiatr Scand. 2005;111:291–9.

Galatzer-Levy IR, Nickerson A, Litz BT, Marmar CR. Patterns of lifetime PTSD comorbidity: a latent class analysis. Depress Anxiety. 2013;30:489–96.

Gallagher MW, Brown TA. Bayesian analysis of current and lifetime comorbidity rates of mood and anxiety disorders in individuals with posttraumatic stress disorder. J Psychopathol Behav Assess. 2015;37:60–6.

Gamble JA, Creedy DK, Webster J, Moyle W. A review of the literature on debriefing or non-directive counselling to prevent postpartum emotional distress. Midwifery. 2002;18:72–9.

Garthus-Niegel S, Ayers S, Martini J, von Soest T, Eberhard-Gran M. The impact of postpartum post-traumatic stress disorder symptoms on child development: a population-based, 2-year follow-up study. Psychol Med. 2017;47:161–70.

Gelpin E, Bonne O, Peri T, Brandes D, Shalev AY. Treatment of recent trauma survivors with benzodiazepines: a prospective study. J Clin Psychiatry. 1996;57:390–4.

Gentile S. Clinical utilization of atypical antipsychotics in pregnancy and lactation. Ann Pharmacother. 2004;38:1265–71.

Gentile S. Topiramate in pregnancy and breastfeeding. Clin Drug Investig. 2009;29:139–41.

Gentile S. On categorizing gestational, birth, and neonatal complications following late pregnancy exposure to antidepressants: the prenatal antidepressant exposure syndrome. CNS Spectr. 2010;15:167–85.

Glover V. Prenatal stress and its effects on the fetus and the child: possible underlying biological mechanisms. Adv Neurobiol. 2015;10:269–83.

Grekin R, O'Hara MW. Prevalence and risk factors of postpartum posttraumatic stress disorder: a meta-analysis. Clin Psychol Rev. 2014;34:389–401.

Halvorsen L, Nerum H, Oian P, Sørlie T. Giving birth with rape in one's past: a qualitative study. Birth. 2013;40:182–91.

Hamner MB, Frueh BC, Ulmer HG, Arana GW. Psychotic features and illness severity in combat veterans with chronic posttraumatic stress disorder. Biol Psychiatry. 1999;45:846–52.
Hamner MB, Faldowski RA, Ulmer HG, Frueh BC, Huber MG, Arana GW. Adjunctive risperidonee treatment in post-traumatic stress disorder: a preliminary controlled trial of effects on comorbid psychotic symptoms. Int Clin Psychopharmacol. 2003a;18:1–8.
Hamner MB, Deitsch SE, Brodrick PS, Ulmer HG, Lorberbaum JP. Quetiapine treatment in patients with posttraumatic stress disorder: an open trial of adjunctive therapy. J Clin Psychopharmacol. 2003b;23:15–20.
Hermes E, Sernyak M, Rosenheck R. The use of second-generation antipsychotics for posttraumatic stress disorder in a US Veterans Health Administration MedicalCenter. Epidemiol Psychiatr Sci. 2014;23(3):281–8.
Hernandez-Diaz S, Huybrechts KF, Desai RJ, Cohen JM, Mogun H, Pennell PB, Bateman BT, Patorno E. Topiramate use early in pregnancy and the risk of oral clefts: a pregnancy cohort study. Neurology. 2018;90:342–51.
Hoge EA, Worthington JJ, Nagurney JT, Chang Y, Kay EB, Feterowski CM, Katzman AR, Goetz JM, Rosasco ML, Lasko NB, Zusman RM, Pollack MH, Orr SP, Pitman RK. Effect of acute post trauma propranolol on PTSD outcome and physiological responses during script-driven imagery. CNS Neurosci Ther. 2012;18:21–7.
Horn SR, Charney DS, Feder A. Understanding resilience: new approaches for preventing and treating PTSD. Exp Neurol. 2016;284(Pt B):119–32.
Horsch A, Brooks C, Fletcher H. Maternal coping, appraisals and adjustment following diagnosis of fetal anomaly. Prenat Diagn. 2013;33:1137–45.
Hoskins M, Pearce J, Bethell A, Dankova L, Barbui C, Tol WA, van Ommeren M, de Jong J, Seedat S, Chen H, Bisson JI. Pharmacotherapy for post-traumatic stress disorder: systematic review and meta-analysis. Br J Psychiatry. 2015;206:93–100.
Ionio C, Di Blasio P. Post-traumatic stress symptoms after childbirth and early mother–child interactions: an exploratory study. J Reprod Infant Psychol. 2014;32:163–81.
Ipser JC, Stein DJ. Evidence-based pharmacotherapy of post-traumatic stress disorder (PTSD). Int J Neuropsychopharmacol. 2012;15:825–40.
Jain AE, Lacy T. Psychotropic drugs in pregnancy and lactation. J Psychiatr Pract. 2005;11:177–91.
Jeffreys M, Capehart B, Friedman MJ. Pharmacotherapy for posttraumatic stress disorder: review with clinical applications. J Rehabil Res Dev. 2012;49:703–15.
Katz RJ, Lott MH, Arbus P, Crocq L, Herlobsen P, Lingjaerde O, Lopez G, Loughrey GC, MacFarlane DJ, McIvor R, et al. Pharmacotherapy of post-traumatic stress disorder with a novel psychotropic. Anxiety. 1994;1:169–74.
Katzman MA, Bleau P, Blier P, Chokka P, Kjernisted K, Van Ameringen M, et al. Canadian clinical practice guidelines for the management of anxiety, posttraumatic stress and obsessive-compulsive disorders. BMC Psychiatry. 2014;14(Suppl 1):S1.
Kellner M, Muhtz C, Wiedemann K. Primary add-on of ziprasidone in sertraline treatment of posttraumatic stress disorder: lessons from a stopped trial? J Clin Psychopharmacol. 2010;30:471–3.
Kennedy D, Webster WS, Hill M, Ritchie HE. Abnormal pregnancy outcome associated with high-dose maternal tranylcypromine therapy: case report and literature review. Reprod Toxicol. 2017;69:146–9.
Kerbage H, Richa S. Non-antidepressant long-term treatment in post-traumatic stress disorder (PTSD). Curr Clin Pharmacol. 2015;10:116–25.
Kessler RC, Sonnega A, Bromet E, Hughes M, Nelson CB. Posttraumatic stress disorder in the National Comorbidity Survey. Arch Gen Psychiatry. 1995;52:1048–60.
Klier CM, Mossaheb N, Lee A, Zernig G. Mirtazapine and breastfeeding: maternal and infant plasma levels. Am J Psychiatry. 2007;164:348–9.
Koek RJ, Schwartz HN, Scully S, Langevin JP, Spangler S, Korotinsky A, Jou K, Leuchter A. Treatment-refractory posttraumatic stress disorder (TRPTSD): a review and framework for the future. Prog Neuro-Psychopharmacol Biol Psychiatry. 2016;70:170–218.

Koen N, Brittain K, Donald KA, Barnett W, Koopowitz S, Maré K, Zar HJ, Stein DJ. Psychological trauma and posttraumatic stress disorder: risk factors and associations with birth outcomes in the Drakenstein child health study. Eur J Psychotraumatol. 2016;7:28720.

Kosten TR, Frank JB, Dan E, McDougle CJ, Giller EL Jr. Pharmacotherapy for posttraumatic stress disorder using phenelzine or imipramine. J Nerv Ment Dis. 1991;179:366–70.

Kristensen JH, Ilett KF, Rampono J, Kohan R, Hackett LP. Transfer of the antidepressant mirtazapine into breast milk. Br J Clin Pharmacol. 2007;63:322–7.

Larsen ER, Damkier P, Pedersen LH, Fenger-Gron J, Mikkelsen RL, Nielsen RE, Linde VJ, Knudsen HE, Skaarup L. Use of psychotropic drugs during pregnancy and breast-feeding. Acta Psychiatr Scand. 2015;445:1–28.

Lee DJ, Schnitzlein CW, Wolf JP, Vythilingam M, Rasmusson AM, Hoge CW. Psychotherapy versus pharmacotherapy for posttraumatic stress disorder: systemic review and meta-analyses to determine first-line treatments. Depress Anxiety. 2016;33:792–806.

Lubbe WF, Hodge JV. Combined alpha- and beta-adrenoceptor antagonism withprazosin and oxprenolol in control of severe hypertension in pregnancy. N Z Med J. 1981;94(691):169–72.

Lusskin SI, Khan SJ, Ernst C, Habib S, Fersh ME, Albertini ES. Pharmacotherapy for perinatal depression. Clin Obstet Gynecol. 2018;61:544.

Mahenge B, Likindikoki S, Stöckl H, Mbwambo J. Intimate partner violence during pregnancy and associated mental health symptoms among pregnant women in Tanzania: a cross-sectional study. BJOG. 2013;120:940–6.

Marmar CR, Schlenger W, Henn-Haase C, Qian M, Purchia E, Li M, Corry N, Williams CS, Ho CL, Horesh D, Karstoft KI, Shalev A, Kulka RA. Course of posttraumatic stress disorder 40 years after the Vietnam war: findings from the National Vietnam Veterans Longitudinal Study. JAMA Psychiatry. 2015;72:875–81.

Martenyi F, Soldatenkova V. Fluoxetine in the acute treatment and relapse prevention of combat-related post-traumatic stress disorder: analysis of the veteran group of a placebo-controlled, randomized clinical trial. Eur Neuropsychopharmacol. 2006;16:340–9.

Martenyi F, Brown EB, Zhang H, Koke SC, Prakash A. Fluoxetine v. placebo in prevention of relapse in post-traumatic stress disorder. Br J Psychiatry. 2002;181:315–20.

McAllister-Williams RH, Baldwin DS, Cantwell R, Easter A, Gilvarry E, Glover V, Green L, Gregoire A, Howard LM, Jones I, Khalifeh H, Lingford-Hughes A, McDonald E, Micali N, Pariante CM, Peters L, Roberts A, Smith NC, Taylor D, Wieck A, Yates LM, Young AH. British Association for Psychopharmacology consensus guidance on the use of psychotropic medication preconception, in pregnancy and postpartum 2017, vol. 31. J Psychopharmacol; 2017. p. 519–52.

McKenna K, Koren G, Tetelbaum M, Wilton L, Shakir S, Diav-Citrin O, Levinson A, Zipursky RB, Einarson A. Pregnancy outcome of women using atypical antipsychotic drugs: a prospective comparative study. J Clin Psychiatry. 2005;66:444–9.

Meidahl Petersen K, Jimenez-Solem E, Andersen JT, Petersen M, Brødbæk K, Køber L, Torp-Pedersen C, Poulsen HE. β-Blocker treatment during pregnancy and adverse pregnancy outcomes: a nationwide population-based cohort study. BMJ Open. 2012;2(4):e001185.

Mellman TA, Bustamante V, David D, Fins AI. Hypnotic medication in the aftermath of trauma. J Clin Psychiatry. 2002;63:1183–4.

Morland L, Goebert D, Onoye J, Frattarelli L, Derauf C, Herbst M, Matsu C, Friedman M. Posttraumatic stress disorder and pregnancy health: preliminary update and implications. Psychosomatics. 2007;48:304–8.

Nash WP, Watson PJ. Review of VA/DOD clinical practice guideline on management of acute stress and interventions to prevent posttraumatic stress disorder. J Rehabil Res Dev. 2012;49:637–48.

National Academies Press. Treatment for posttraumatic stress disorder in military and veteran populations: final assessment. Washington: National Academies Press (US); 2014.

Neylan TC, Metzler TJ, Schoenfeld FB, Weiss DS, Lenoci M, Best SR, Lipsey TL, Marmar CR. Fluvoxamine and sleep disturbances in posttraumatic stress disorder. J Trauma Stress. 2001;14:461–7.

Neylan TC, Lenoci M, Samuelson KW, Metzler TJ, Henn-Haase C, Hierholzer RW, Lindley SE, Otte C, Schoenfeld FB, Yesavage JA, Marmar CR. No improvement of posttraumatic stress disorder symptoms with guanfacine treatment. Am J Psychiatry. 2006;163:2186–8.

Nicholls K, Ayers S. Childbirth-related post-traumatic stress disorder in couples: a qualitative study. Br J Health Psychol. 2007;12(Pt 4):491–509.

Nugent NR, Christopher NC, Crow JP, Browne L, Ostrowski S, Delahanty DL. The efficacy of early propranolol administration at reducing PTSD symptoms in pediatric injury patients: a pilot study. J Trauma Stress. 2010;23:282–7.

Onoye JM, Shafer LA, Goebert DA, Morland LA, Matsu CR, Hamagami F. Changes in PTSD symptomatology and mental health during pregnancy and postpartum. Arch Womens Ment Health. 2013;16(6):453–63.

Ornoy A, Weinstein-Fudim L, Ergaz Z. Antidepressants, antipsychotics, and mood stabilizers in pregnancy: what do we know and how should we treat pregnant women with depression. Birth Defects Res. 2017;109:933–56.

Padala PR, Madison J, Monnahan M, Marcil W, Price P, Ramaswamy S, Din AU, Wilson DR, Petty F. Risperidonee monotherapy for post-traumatic stress disorder related to sexual assault and domestic abuse in women. Int Clin Psychopharmacol. 2006;21(5):275–80.

Parfitt Y, Pike A, Ayers S. Infant developmental outcomes: a family systems perspective. Infant Child Dev. 2014;23:353–73.

Pitman RK, Sanders KM, Zusman RM, Healy AR, Cheema F, Lasko NB, Cahill L, Orr SP. Pilot study of secondary prevention of posttraumatic stress disorder with propranolol. Biol Psychiatry. 2002;51:189–92.

Pollack MH, Hoge EA, Worthington JJ, Moshier SJ, Wechsler RS, Brandes M, Simon NM. Eszopiclone for the treatment of posttraumatic stress disorder and associated insomnia: a randomized, double-blind, placebo-controlled trial. J Clin Psychiatry. 2011;72:892–7.

Qi W, Gevonden M, Shalev A. Prevention of post-traumatic stress disorder after trauma: current evidence and future directions. Curr Psychiatry Rep. 2016;18(2):20.

Ram D, Gandotra S. Antidepressants, anxiolytics, and hypnotics in pregnancy and lactation. Indian J Psychiatry. 2015;57(Suppl 2):354–71.

Raskind MA, Peskind ER, Hoff DJ, Hart KL, Holmes HA, Warren D, Shofer J, O'Connell J, Taylor F, Gross C, Rohde K, McFall ME. A parallel group placebo-controlled study of prazosin for trauma nightmares and sleep disturbance in combat veterans with post-traumatic stress disorder. Biol Psychiatry. 2007;61:928–34.

Reich DB, Winternitz S, Hennen J, Watts T, Stanculescu C. A preliminary study of risperidonee in the treatment of posttraumatic stress disorder related to childhood abuse in women. J Clin Psychiatry. 2004;65:1601–6.

Reist C, Kauffmann CD, Haler RJ, Sangdahl C, DeMet EM, Chicz-DeMet A, Nelson JN. A controlled trial of desipramine in 18 men with posttraumatic stress disorder. Am J Psychiatry. 1989;146:513–6.

Roberts NP, Kitchiner NJ, Kenardy J, Bisson JI. Systematic review and meta-analysis of multiple-session early interventions following traumatic events. Am J Psychiatry. 2009;166:293–301.

Rothbaum BO, Killeen TK, Davidson JR, Brady KT, Connor KM, Heekin MH. Placebo-controlled trial of risperidonee augmentation for selective serotonin reuptake inhibitor-resistant civilian posttraumatic stress disorder. J Clin Psychiatry. 2008;69:520–5.

Schelling G, Stoll C, Kapfhammer HP, Rothenhäusler HB, Krauseneck T, Durst K, Haller M, Briegel J. The effect of stress doses of hydrocortisone during septic shock on posttraumatic stress disorder and health-related quality of life in survivors. Crit Care Med. 1999;27:2678–83.

Schelling G, Briegel J, Roozendaal B, Stoll C, Rothenhäusler HB, Kapfhammer HP. The effect of stress doses of hydrocortisone during septic shock on posttraumatic stress disorder in survivors. Biol Psychiatry. 2001;50:978–85.

Schneier FR, et al. Combined mirtazapine and SSRI treatment of PTSD: a placebo-controlled trial. Depress Anxiety. 2015;32(8):570–9.

Schwab W, Marth C, Bergant AM. Post-traumatic stress disorder postpartum: the impact of birth on the prevalence of post-traumatic stress disorder (PTSD) in multiparous women. Geburtshilfe Frauenheilkd. 2012;72(1):56–63.

Shalev AY, Ankri Y, Israeli-Shalev Y, Peleg T, Adessky R, Freedman S. Prevention of posttraumatic stress disorder by early treatment: results from the Jerusalem trauma outreach and prevention study. Arch Gen Psychiatry. 2012;69:166–76.

Shaw JG, Asch SM, Kimerling R, Frayne SM, Shaw KA, Phibbs CS. Posttraumatic stress disorder and risk of spontaneous preterm birth. Obstet Gynecol. 2014;124:1111–9.

Shestatzky M, Greenberg D, Lerer B. A controlled trial of phenelzine in posttraumatic stress disorder. Psychiatry Res. 1988;24(2):149–55.

Slade P, Murphy A, Hayden E. Identifying post-traumatic stress disorder after childbirth. BMJ. 2022;377:e067659.

Smit M, Dolman KM, Honig A. Mirtazapine in pregnancy and lactation – a systematic review. Eur Neuropsychopharmacol. 2016;26:126–35.

Sokolski KN, Denson TF, Lee RT, Reist C. Quetiapine for treatment of refractory symptoms of combat-related post-traumatic stress disorder. Mil Med. 2003;168:486–9.

Stein MB, Kline NA, Matloff JL. Adjunctive olanzapine for SSRI-resistant combat-related PTSD: a double-blind, placebo-controlled study. Am J Psychiatry. 2002;159:1777–9.

Stein MB, Kerridge C, Dimsdale JE, Hoyt DB. Pharmacotherapy to prevent PTSD: results from a randomized controlled proof-of-concept trial in physically injured patients. J Trauma Stress. 2007;20:923–32.

Stoddard FJ Jr, Luthra R, Sorrentino EA, Saxe GN, Drake J, Chang Y, Levine JB, Chedekel DS, Sheridan RL. A randomized controlled trial of sertraline to prevent posttraumatic stress disorder in burned children. J Child Adolesc Psychopharmacol. 2011;21:469–77.

Sullivan GM, Neria Y. Pharmacotherapy in post-traumatic stress disorder: evidence from randomized controlled trials. Curr Opin Investig Drugs. 2009;10:35–45.

Taylor EA, Turner P. Anti-hypertensive therapy with propranolol during pregnancy and lactation. Postgrad Med J. 1981;57(669):427–30.

Taylor FB, Martin P, Thompson C, Williams J, Mellman TA, Gross C, Peskind ER, Raskind MA. Prazosin effects on objective sleep measures and clinical symptoms in civilian trauma posttraumatic stress disorder: a placebo-controlled study. Biol Psychiatry. 2008;63:629–32.

Thomson M, Sharma V. Pharmacotherapeutic considerations for the treatment of posttraumatic stress disorder during and after pregnancy. Expert Opin Pharmacother. 2021;22(6):705–14.

Thorley KJ, McAinsh J. Levels of the beta-blockers atenolol and propranolol in the breast milk of women treated for hypertension in pregnancy. Biopharm Drug Dispos. 1983;4:299–301.

Uguz F. Poor feeding and severe sedation in a newborn nursed by a mother on a low dose of amitriptyline. Breastfeed Med. 2017;12:67–8.

Vaiva G, Ducrocq F, Jezequel K, Averland B, Lestavel P, Brunet A, Marmar CR. Immediate treatment with propranolol decreases posttraumatic stress disorder two months after trauma. Biol Psychiatry. 2003;54:947–9.

van Son M, Verkerk G, van der Hart O, Komproe I, Pop V. Prenatal depression, mode of delivery and perinatal dissociation as predictors of postpartum posttraumatic stress: an empirical study. Clin Psychol Psychother. 2005;12:297–312.

Verreault N, Da Costa D, Marchand A, Ireland K, Banack H, Dritsa M, Khalifé S. PTSD following childbirth: a prospective study of incidence and risk factors in Canadian women. J Psychosom Res. 2012;73:257–63.

Warner MD, Dorn MR, Peabody CA. Survey on the usefulness of trazodone in patients with PTSD with insomnia or nightmares. Pharmacopsychiatry. 2001;34:128–31.

Watts BV, Schnurr PP, Mayo L, Young-Xu Y, Weeks WB, Friedman MJ. Meta-analysis of the efficacy of treatments for posttraumatic stress disorder. J Clin Psychiatry. 2013;74:541–50.

Womersley K, Ripullone K, Agius M. What are the risks associated with different selective serotonin re-uptake inhibitors (SSRIs) to treat depression and anxiety in pregnancy? An evaluation of current evidence. Psychiatr Danub. 2017;29(Suppl 3):629–44.

World Health Organization. Guidelines for the management of conditions specifically related to stress. Geneva: WHO Press; 2013.

Yarvis JS, Schiess L. Subthreshold posttraumatic stress disorder (PTSD) as a predictor of depression, alcohol use, and health problems in veterans. J Workplace Behav Health. 2008;23:395–424.

Yildiz PD, Ayers S, Phillips L. The prevalence of posttraumatic stress disorder in pregnancy and after birth: a systematic review and meta-analysis. J Affect Disord. 2017;208:634–45.

Yonkers KA, Smith MV, Forray A, Epperson CN, Costello D, Lin H, Belanger K. Pregnant women with posttraumatic stress disorder and risk of preterm birth. JAMA Psychiatry. 2014;71:897–904.

RETRACTED CHAPTER: Alcohol Use Disorders

21

Laura Orsolini, Rosa Volgare, Giulia Francesconi, Giovanni Martinotti, and Umberto Volpe

21.1 Introduction

Alcohol consumption among women of childbearing age is increasing globally (WHO 2018). The COVID-19 pandemic has indeed worsened alcohol consumption worldwide (Rehm et al. 2020). About 10% of women declared to regularly drink alcohol during pregnancy, with some variability across worldwide countries (WHO 2018). Certain groups, such as women with substance use disorders (SUD), low socioeconomic status or coming from marginalized communities/cultural minorities, seemed to be more at risk to develop AUD during the perinatal period (Popova et al. 2017; Dozet et al. 2023).

In general, as stated by the guidelines proposed by the Australian Government Department of Health (2018), clinicians should always advise all women who are pregnant or planning a pregnancy that not drinking is the safest option as maternal alcohol consumption may adversely affect the developing fetus (NHMRC 2009). Although no conclusive evidence shows that low levels of prenatal alcohol exposure cause fetal harm, periodic binge drinking or regular heavy drinking (i.e., drinking on average 70 grams alcohol weekly) during pregnancy can lead to serious adverse outcomes (Woodruff and Roberts 2019). In fact, alcohol intake during pregnancy is associated with an increased risk of miscarriage, preterm birth, stillbirth and sudden infant death syndrome (SIDS) as well as it may determine the onset of a range of lifelong behavioural, intellectual and physical disabilities (i.e., 'fetal alcohol spectrum disorders' [FASDs]) (CDC 2024). To date, literature supports that there is no

The original version of this chapter was retracted: The retraction note to this chapter is available at https://doi.org/10.1007/978-3-031-99720-4_25

L. Orsolini (✉) · R. Volgare · G. Francesconi · U. Volpe
Unit of Clinical Psychiatry, Department of Experimental and Clinical Medicine (DIMSC), Polytechnic University of Marche, Ancona, Italy
e-mail: l.orsolini@staff.univpm.it

G. Martinotti
University "G. D'Annunzio" di Chieti-Pescara, Chieti, Italy

F. Uguz, L. Orsolini (eds.), *Perinatal Psychopharmacology*,
https://doi.org/10.1007/978-3-031-99720-4_21

safe time for alcohol use during pregnancy nor there is no known safe amount of alcohol use during pregnancy (CDC 2024).

However, despite some strong evidence that alcohol intake could determine often unpredictable and serious irreversible detrimental consequences on maternal and fetal outcomes both throughout the pregnancy and postpartum periods, few research information and well-designed clinical studies provided clear flowchart and treatment management strategies to support the use of specific pharmacological interventions for AUD during pregnancy and breastfeeding. Similarly, few studies addressed how to manage alcohol detoxification programs among pregnant and breastfeeding women, as well as the use of benzodiazepines (BZDs) in pregnant women is still controversial in many studies. Coherently, many policies have been developed addressing alcohol use in pregnancy (Drabble et al. 2014). Among these policies there are supportive initiatives which include measures giving pregnant women priority access to alcohol treatment or mandating point-of-sale signage warning of the risks of drinking during pregnancy; and punitive initiatives which include measures requiring mandatory reporting of patients who abuse alcohol during pregnancy to Child Protective Services or allowing civil commitment of alcohol-abusing pregnant women to involuntary treatment or protective custody of the state (Roberts et al. 2017).

The present chapter will provide an overview about the epidemiology of AUDs in pregnancy and breastfeeding, the associated risks about the development of major and minor malformations and perinatal complications, with a particular focus on the foetal alcohol spectrum disorder (FASD) and foetal alcohol syndrome (FAS), and, finally, will provide some clinical guidelines for the management (pharmacological and not-pharmacological) of AUD both in pregnancy and postpartum period (Table 21.1).

21.2 Epidemiology

According to the National Survey on Drug Use and Health (NSDUH 2022), around 8.5% of pregnant women in the United States consumed at least one alcoholic drink in the previous 30 days, 5.3% drank five or more drinks (aka '*binge drinking*') during one episode in the previous 30 days and 1.7% had five or more drinks on the same occasion five or more times (aka '*heavy drinking*') in the last 30 days. However, overall pregnant women have been reported to on average consume less alcohol, compared to non-pregnant women (8.5% vs 55.1% drank at least once in the last 30 days; 5.3% vs 27.0% reported binge drinking; 1.7% vs 5.7% reported heavy drinking) (NSDUH 2022). In fact, some studies also documented that around 85% of women who regularly intake alcohol, when they become pregnant, usually decide to discontinue alcohol consumption, mainly due to the fear of causing detrimental fetal consequences (Alvik et al. 2006). However, the epidemiological trend seemed to document a progressive increase of pregnancy alcohol use and binge drinking rates in recent years. In fact, between 2018 and 2020, about one in seven pregnant women reported drinking alcohol in the past 30 days, with 40% of them

Table 21.1 Expert recommendations based on scientific evidence and clinical experience

Clinicians should advise women who intend to plan a pregnancy to discontinue alcohol consumption, as there is a good quality evidence that drinking excessive amounts of alcohol during pregnancy may damage foetal development
Clinicians and researchers do not still know the minimum or threshold level at which alcohol begins to pose a significant threat to pregnancy, hence, it is preferred not using alcohol at all
Clinicians should know that alcohol is a teratogen agent, therefore, it should be avoided during pregnancy, especially during the first trimester
The likelihood of developing foetal malformations increases with increased volume and frequency of alcohol consumption during the first trimester, hence, it is preferred not having binge or heavy drinking during this period
During antenatal visits, it is important to collect a complete medical history (paying particular attention to indicators of possible AUD such as hepatitis, experiences of sexual and/or physical abuse, presence of psychiatric comorbidities, recognizing that some pregnant women may hesitate to disclose substance use due to fear of repercussions, involvement with social services, losing custody of children or judgmental treatment
A screening assessment for alcohol consumption, specifically designed for pregnant and/or nursing women, may help clinicians to adopt preventive tools, provide advice to stop alcohol consumption, and therapeutic strategies for the management of AUD
Laboratory testing can aid in measuring prenatal alcohol exposure
After identifying pregnant and/or nursing women at risk of AUD, clinicians should suggest involving a drug and/or alcohol specialist in counselling and care
AUD during pregnancy may contribute to an increased risk of congenital malformations or later intellectual disability
AUD during pregnancy may contribute to the onset of FASD
The optimal management approach for pregnant women with AUD involves a combination of pharmacological treatment, specialist consultation, and psychosocial interventions
Pregnant women should be given priority access to withdrawal management and treatment
Research on the safety of alcohol pharmacotherapies during pregnancy is limited. In the United States, the Food and Drug Administration (FDA) has approved only three medications for the treatment of AUD: Naltrexone, disulfiram, and acamprosate
Psychosocial interventions appear to reduce the frequency of alcohol use especially with interventions that combine parenting skills with a substance use component. Peer support groups seem to be very helpful too
Special attention should be paid to the postnatal period where the risk of relapse is very high

engaging in binge drinking (Gosdin et al. 2022). In particular, pregnant women who experienced frequent mental distress (i.e., 14 or more days of poor mental health in the past 30 days) and those women who did not have a usual healthcare provider were more likely to report alcohol intake (Gosdin et al. 2022).

21.3 Risk of Congenital Major Malformations and Perinatal Complications

The French paediatrician Paul Lemoine firstly identified alcohol as a teratogenic agent in 1967, by describing 127 cases of a similar pattern of abnormalities in those children exposed to a 'chronic alcoholism' of their mothers (Lemoine et al. 1968;

Lemoine 2012). Subsequently, Jones and Smith clearly described this specific spectrum of dysmorphologies associated with AUD during pregnancy and firstly introduced the associated terminology '*Fetal Alcohol Syndrome*' (FAS) (Jones et al. 1973). FAS is a clinically complex congenital disorder of the fetus determined by the mother's consumption of alcohol during pregnancy (Seo et al. 2021). Indeed, it has been demonstrated that alcohol consumption occurring also from around 3–4 months before conception and throughout the pregnancy can affect fetal development. The prevalence of FAS in the general population is 14.6 per 10,000 people. In addition, it has been estimated that one out of 67 pregnant women who consumed alcohol will have a child developing a FAS, resulting in approximately 119,000 babies born with FAS each year worldwide (Popova et al. 2017). The FAS is characterized by craniofacial, limb, and cardiovascular defects associated with prenatal-onset growth deficiency and development delay (Jones et al. 1973; Seo et al. 2021).

Indeed, another not-full FAS condition was also identified and described within the terminology of '*foetal alcohol spectrum disorders*' (FASD). FASD is represented by a pattern of dysmorphologies comprising all not-fully FAS clinical presentations. FASD is an umbrella term describing the range of developmental deviations, such as craniofacial mal-development or neurodevelopmental abnormalities that can occur in an individual whose mother consumed alcohol during pregnancy (Hoyme et al. 2016). FASD may include a low birth weight, preterm birth, small for gestational age, spontaneous abortions, behavioural problems, developmental delay, cognitive deficits, related to dose-response pattern to alcohol use during pregnancy (Blume 1985; Streissguth et al. 1989; Sood et al. 2001; O'Callaghan et al. 2007; Sayal et al. 2007; Patra et al. 2011).

Overall, the extent of developmental abnormalities seemed to depend on the prenatal alcohol amount, pattern of consumption, and timing throughout pregnancy. No level of alcohol consumption is safe during pregnancy. Binge drinking in the first 6 weeks of pregnancy and chronic alcohol consumption throughout pregnancy, which is often associated with poor maternal nutrition and reduced BMI, have been reported to be associated with the highest incidence of FASD (Grzywacz et al. 2023). However, many etiopathogenetic determinants, including genetic, epigenetic, and social environmental factors, may also influence the development and manifestations of FASD and associated disabilities (Murawski et al. 2015). Approximately 30–40% of children with significant prenatal alcohol exposure meet the criteria for FASD (Grzywacz et al. 2023). Most children affected with FASD may experience difficulties in daily life, e.g., deficit in motor control, eyesight, hearing, attention, concentration and impulse control (Riley et al. 2011). Furthermore, it has been documented the association between FASD and the development of autism spectrum disorder (ASD), attention-deficit-hyperactivity disorder (ADHD), and intellectual disability in newborns exposed to antenatal maternal alcohol consumption (Popova et al. 2016).

FASD is a broad diagnosis which includes four distinct diagnostic categories: (a) classical FAS; (b) fetal partial alcohol syndrome (PFAS); (c) alcohol-related neurodevelopmental disorder (ARND); and (d) alcohol-related birth defects (ARBD)

(Hoyme et al. 2016). FAS refers to those babies who fulfil all complete/classical criteria and comprise facial dysmorphologies, growth inhibition and dysfunction of the central nervous system (Hoyme et al. 2016). Children with FAS display central nervous system abnormalities (i.e., microcephaly, tremors, hyperactivity, lack of motor skills, attention deficit, learning disabilities, intellectual or cognitive deficits, and seizures), a pre and/or postnatal growth disturbance and characteristic facial abnormalities (i.e., hort eyelid slits, epicantal folds, flat midface, hypoplastic philtrum, and a thin upper vermilion border) (Hoyme et al. 2016). Diagnosis is often overlooked, misdiagnosed, or delayed, with an average delay of about 48.3 months after birth, which prevents affected children from receiving necessary services promptly. To diagnose FAS, physicians must collect a detailed history related to prenatal alcohol exposure. Significant exposure is defined as at least one of the following:

- 6+ drinks per week for 2+ weeks during pregnancy
- 3+ drinks per occasion on 2+ occasions during pregnancy
- Alcohol-related social or legal issues during pregnancy.
- Documented intoxication via blood, breath, or urine tests.
- Positive alcohol biomarkers (e.g., fatty acid ethyl esters, phosphatidylethanol) in maternal or fetal samples.
- Increased prenatal risk from alcohol use identified by a validated screening tool.

If there was no history of prenatal alcohol use in the 3 months before recognizing pregnancy or at the time of a positive test, FAS can be excluded (Hoyme et al. 2016). A summary of the FAS diagnostic process has been provided in Table 21.2. Updated diagnostic criteria for the diagnosis of fetal alcohol spectrum disorders are reported in Table 21.3.

21.4 Prenatal Alcohol Exposure and Children's Outcomes

Several studies documented an increased risk of unfavourable outcomes in children of mothers with heavy prenatal alcohol consumption. These include a range of behavioural problems, developmental challenges, as well as more severe outcomes such as intellectual disability, cerebral palsy, preterm birth, low birth weight, stillbirth, sudden infant death syndrome (SIDS), and infant mortality (Mattson et al. 2013; Flak et al. 2014; Hutchinson et al. 2014). These outcomes are attributed to both the biological effects of prenatal alcohol exposure and social/environmental factors including increased risk of parental mental health problems, other substance use, economic disadvantage, family instability, poor parenting skills and social isolation (O'Leary et al. 2020).

Prenatal alcohol exposure (PAE) has been associated with several neurodevelopmental deficits, including attention difficulties, learning delays, poor memory and impaired social skills. Children prenatally exposed to alcohol may face behavioural problems, poor academic performance, and interactions with the justice system.

Table 21.2 Criteria for FAS and partial FAS

1. Evidence of prenatal or postnatal growth impairment, in at least 1 of the following (FAS only):	Birth weight or birth length at or below the tenth percentile for gestational age Height or weight at or below the tenth percentile for age Disproportionately low weight-to-height ratio at or below the tenth percentile
2. Simultaneous presentation of the following facial anomalies at any age (FAS all 3, partial FAS any 2):	Short palpebral fissure length (2 or more SDs below the mean) Smooth or flattened philtrum (rank 4 or 5 on the lip-philtrum guide) Thin upper lip (rank 4 or 5 on the lip-philtrum guide)
3. Evidence of impairment in 3 or more of the following CNS domains (FAS, partial FAS, and ARND):	Hard and soft neurologic signs Brain structure Cognition (IQ) Communication Academic achievement vi. Memory Executive functioning and abstract reasoning Attention deficit/hyperactivity Adaptive behaviour Social skills Social communication
4. Confirmed maternal alcohol exposure (partial FAS)[a]	

SD standard deviation, *CNS* central nervous system, *IQ* intelligence quotient
[a]FAS can be diagnosed without this if (1) to (3) are all present

ADHD is a neurodevelopmental disorder and is the most frequently diagnosed cognitive and behavioural disorder among school-age children, with an estimated worldwide prevalence of 7.2% for children and adolescents and 2.5% for adults (Chaulagain et al. 2023). The aetiology of the disorder remains unclear, despite several genetic and environmental factors having been proposed to increase susceptibility to the disorder, one of which is PAE (Banerjee et al. 2007; Wetherill et al. 2018; Gibson and Porter 2022). This could be related to an altered brain development, which appears to be negatively affected by prenatal exposure to alcohol, with PEA being associated with reduced brain volume and subsequent attention difficulties and impulsivity (Lebel et al. 2011; Paolozza et al. 2014). Studies in animal models also indicated that even low levels of prenatal alcohol exposure can negatively affect neurodevelopment. For instance, reduced brain volume and response inhibition deficits have been documented in individuals with PAE, highlighting its long-lasting impact on cognitive and behavioural functioning (Sood et al. 2001). However, data from the current published literature appeared contradictory, with some studies indicating that prenatal alcohol consumption—whether light, moderate, or heavy—is not associated with an increased risk of ADHD in offspring (Mitchell and Sevigny-Resetco 2020).

The effect of PAE also seemed to depend on a set of genetic factors. A recent study by Miyake et al. (2024) aimed at investigating the role of polymorphisms of

Table 21.3 Updated Institute of Medicine (IOM) diagnostic criteria for the diagnosis of fetal alcohol spectrum disorders

FAS	With or without documented prenatal alcohol exposure Requires all the following features: A characteristic pattern of facial anomalies, including at least 2 among the following: (1) short palpebral fissures; (2) thin vermilion border of the upper lip; (3) smooth philtrum Prenatal and/or postnatal growth deficiency Deficient brain growth, abnormal morphogenesis or abnormal neurophysiology, including at least 1 of the following head circumference ≤10th percentile; (1) structural brain anomalies; (2) recurrent nonfebrile seizures (other causes of seizures having been ruled out) Neurobehavioural impairment
PFAS	With or without documented prenatal alcohol exposure Requires all the following features: A characteristic pattern of facial anomalies, including at least 2 among the following: (1) short palpebral fissures; (2) thin vermilion border of the upper lip; (3) smooth philtrum Neurobehavioural impairment
ARND	This diagnosis cannot be made before the age of three Requires all the following features: Documented prenatal alcohol exposure Neurobehavioural impairment
ARBD	Requires all the following features: Documented prenatal alcohol exposure One or more specific major malformations due to prenatal alcohol exposure: (1) cardiac (atrial septal defects, aberrant great vessels, ventricular septal defects, conotruncal heart defects); (2) skeletal (radioulnar synostosis, vertebral segmentation defects, large joint contractures, scoliosis); (3) renal (aplastic/hypoplastic/dysplastic kidneys, 'horseshoe' kidneys/ureteral duplications); (4) eyes (strabismus, ptosis, retinal vascular anomalies, optic nerve hypoplasia); (5) ears (conductive hearing loss, neurosensory hearing loss)

FAS fetal alcohol syndrome, *PFAS* partial fetal alcohol syndrome, *ARND* alcohol-related neurodevelopmental disorder, *ARBD* alcohol-related birth defect

the ADH1B and ALDH2 genes, both demonstrated to be involved in alcohol metabolism, in maternal alcohol consumption during pregnancy and their association with the risk of developmental delays in offspring in a Japanese population. Analysis of maternal polymorphisms of the ALDH2 gene showed that alcohol consumption by mothers with wild-type genotype specifically increased the risk of communication delays. In contrast, mothers with the heterozygous genotype were associated with an increased risk of developmental delays (Miyake et al. 2024). While the influence of the polymorphism of the ADH1B gene on developmental outcomes could not be clearly determined (Miyake et al. 2024).

PAE has also been reported to be associated with the increased probability of alcohol and substance use in adolescents, but its specific impact is difficult to determine because of concomitant risk factors, including parental substance use, home environment, access to substances and genetics (Jacobson et al. 1998). The impact of PAE seems to depend on drinking patterns, with binge drinking causing the most harm (Duko et al. 2020, 2022). Streissguth's Seattle 500 study showed that PAE is more predictive of adolescent alcohol use at age 14 than family history of alcohol problems (Baer et al. 1998, 2003). The Mater University study of Pregnancy showed that maternal consumption of more than 3 drinks is more predictive of alcohol use at age 14 (Alati et al. 2008). In contrast, according to another study, strong PAE in the first trimester predicted higher alcohol consumption in offspring at 16 and 22 years of age, regardless of childhood behavioural problems or family history of alcohol use (Goldschmidt et al. 2019). In a study conducted by Dodge et al. (2023), PAE has been reported to significantly impact on the amount of alcohol consumed per occasion and on tolerance, rather than on the frequency of consumption, much more likely due to an increased sensitivity to the rewarding effects of alcohol.

21.5 Alcohol Intake During Breastfeeding and Children's Outcomes

There is limited research available on the alcohol use during lactation. It is known that alcohol passes rapidly to breast milk, where it is found in a similar concentration to maternal blood (CDC 2024). It has been documented that alcohol intake during breastfeeding may have a negative impact on infant brain development, being also associated with the development of detrimental cognitive and academic outcomes (Haastrup et al. 2020). Alcohol use during lactation has also been associated with an increased prevalence of ADHD and altered infant sleep patterns (Haastrup et al. 2020; Gibson and Porter 2020). However, the literature reports conflicting data with some studies, such as that carried out by Gibson and colleagues showing no correlation between maternal alcohol consumption during breastfeeding and the risk of ADHD or ASD (Gibson and Porter 2022). Alcohol intake while breastfeeding may still be harmful to children or disrupt the lactation process when consumed during breastfeeding. For this reason, the safest choice for breastfeeding women seems to be abstaining from alcohol consumption (Gibson and Porter 2018, 2020, 2022).

21.6 Screening Tools for AUD During Pregnancy

An increased predisposition to the development of AUD has been observed during the reproductive age, especially in the presence of comorbid psychiatric or neurodevelopmental disorders (e.g., ADHD) (Luderer et al. 2021). Most women who use alcohol more commonly reduce their consumption during pregnancy. Generally, women avoid initiating the use of potentially harmful substances once they become aware of their pregnancy. Those capable of quitting independently typically manage to do so (Prince et al. 2023). Approximately half of pregnant women report drinking shortly before pregnancy, with more than 10% who display a binge drinking pattern that is also being associated with a higher risk of subsequent alcohol consumption during pregnancy (Naimi et al. 2003; Kitsantas et al. 2014).

Hence, a careful and prompt identification of AUD and/or risky alcohol intake could help clinicians to provide an appropriate and timely support before/during/after pregnancy which has been suggested to be crucial for maternal and neonatal health (McGovern et al. 2021; Prince et al. 2023). A thorough medical history and physical examination often reveal an alcohol use. However, many women do not disclose sensitive information about their alcohol intake, so doctors must rely on other methods to identify those women at-risk to be diagnosed with AUD. Ideally, all pregnant women should be screened and those who test positive should be treated, with access to effective interventions if indicated, as part of comprehensive antenatal care in collaboration with pregnant women (ACOG 2018; Prince et al. 2023).

Regarding the clinical assessment, clinicians currently have several validated screening tools for AUD such as the CAGE (Cut down, Annoyed, Guilty, Eye-opener) (Ewing 1984), the Alcohol Use Disorders Identification Test (AUDIT-C) (Saunders et al. 1993), the Michigan Alcoholism Screening Test (MAST) (Selzer 1971), the Tolerance, Worried, Eye-opener, Amnesia, K/Cut down attempts (TWEAK) (Russel et al. 1994) and the Tolerance, Annoyance, Cut down attempts, Eye opener (T-ACE-R3) (Chang et al. 1998). However, several of these screening tools have not been specifically developed and/or validated for the pregnant population (such as the CAGE and MAST tools), either they have been designed to accurately identify alcohol use patterns in male samples, by particularly focusing on alcohol dependence. Hence, they may be less effective in identifying problem drinking amongst women, especially among pregnant and/or nursing women. Therefore, positive cut-off scores for these AUD screening tools need to be set differently for women than for men. In fact, women usually experience higher blood alcohol levels at identical exposures (doses) and women are more susceptible to irreversible and severe alcohol-dependent organ damages, compared to the male counterpart (Urbano-Marquez et al. 1995; Graham et al. 1998; Jones et al. 2013). So far, only T-ACE, TWEAK, AUDIT-C, 4P's Plus and the 1-Question Screen have been validated for AUD screening in pregnant women. In particular, T-ACE, AUDIT-C, and TWEAK questionnaires are considered the most promising screening tools for detecting at-risk alcohol drinking in pregnant women (WHO 2014; Montag 2016; Poole et al. 2019; Chang 2020; Dozet et al. 2023). However, a positivity to the screening tools, it appears to not be enough to take a diagnosis, being needed to be accompanied by a structured and complete clinical interview about the frequency of alcohol intake and current alcohol pattern. Finally, laboratory-based screening tools could be useful to measure prenatal alcohol exposure through ethanol biomarkers, such as fatty acid ethyl esters, found in blood, maternal and neonatal hair, placenta, cord blood, and meconium (Prince et al. 2023).

21.7 Pharmacological Management of Alcohol Use Disorders During the Perinatal Period

The optimal management strategy for pregnant women with AUD includes pharmacological treatment, consultation with a multidisciplinary team comprising several specialists, and psychosocial interventions. A psychoeducational approach (also preventive) addressed to at-risk pregnant women, those not still pregnant women who intend to start a pregnancy and those displaying risky factors associated with a higher probability to develop an AUD and/or a risky alcohol intake should be the first therapy target strategy. The first recommendation should include educating about the consequences of alcohol intake during pregnancy for both the mother and the fetus in the short- as well as in the long-term (US Preventive Services Task Force 2018). The second recommendation should provide advice to refer to the speciality treatment service, incentivize access and ask for professional help for the management of alcohol intake and act by using a harm reduction strategy (US Preventive Services Task Force 2018). Motivational interviewing and brief interventions are more effective than judgmental or punitive approaches in encouraging positive behavioural change (Prince et al. 2023). Patient education, counselling, and monitoring do not end with childbirth, as women with AUD are at the highest risk of developing a postpartum relapse and must be educated about the dangers of resuming substance use after childbirth. They need to be closely monitored, particularly during the first postpartum year. Psychosocial interventions appear to reduce the frequency of alcohol intake by parents. Integrated interventions that combine parenting skills with an alcohol use component seem to be the most promising, although it appears that mothers may benefit less from these interventions than fathers (McGovern et al. 2021). Peer support groups seem to be very helpful (Forray et al. 2015; Morton Ninomiya et al. 2023).

Overall, there is limited evidence regarding the potential risks associated to pharmacological treatment prescribed by clinicians to those at-risk and/or those pregnant women affected by AUD (Briggs and Freeman 2015). The highest risk could be much more likely during an explosion to pharmacotherapy during the first trimester of pregnancy (Mitchell et al. 2011). The American Psychiatric Association (Reus et al. 2018) recommends that for pregnant or nursing women with AUD, pharmacological treatments should not be prescribed, except for managing an acute alcohol withdrawal through BZDs or for managing a dual disorder (i.e., a concomitant psychiatric disorder) (ACOG 2018).

Regarding the pharmacotherapy for AUD, there are a number of approved medications used for the treatment of AUD including naltrexone, disulfiram, acamprosate, nalmefene, and baclofen, as well as repurposed topiramate and gabapentin (Burnette et al. 2022). However, the use of these medications in pregnancy is typically not recommended due to the unknown fetal risks and the lack of evidence regarding the long-term safety and efficacy. Indeed, there is also a lack of agreement between health organization guidelines for the pharmacological management of AUD in pregnancy. Some guidelines suggest that relapse prevention medications should not be initiated in pregnant women, due to the low level of evidence

(Lingford-Hughes et al. 2012; Rolland et al. 2016; Reus et al. 2018; Thibaut et al. 2019). Some guidelines also recommend to consider the management on a case-by-case basis (Lingford-Hughes et al. 2012; Rolland et al. 2016; Reus et al. 2018), particularly in those women on alcohol pharmacotherapy prior to conceiving. Overall, data coming from animal studies do not recommend the use of disulfiram due to the lack of supporting studies, while a moderate risk is associated with the use of naltrexone and a high risk with acamprosate, a possible risk for use of gabapentin and topiramate (Briggs and Freeman 2015). Regarding breastfeeding, even though limited data is available, there may be potential for toxicity with disulfiram, naltrexone and topiramate (Briggs and Freeman 2015), whereas acamprosate and gabapentin are noted to be 'probably compatible' with breastfeeding (Briggs and Freeman 2015).

21.7.1 Naltrexone Use

Naltrexone is a mu opioid receptor antagonist that has been shown to decrease the risk of heavy drinking to 83% of the risk in placebo groups and decrease drinking days by about 4% (Rösner et al. 2010). Naltrexone is available in both oral and long-acting injectable formulations. However, there are no published studies on the safety or efficacy of either formulation of naltrexone for use in AUD in pregnant women. Naltrexone is classified as a category C medication by the Food and Drug Administration (FDA), meaning that animal studies have shown adverse effects on the fetus, but there are no adequate studies on reproductive effects and safety in human pregnancy (Zagon et al. 1998). In fact, a small number of clinical studies has examined the safety of naltrexone in pregnancy, by indeed investigating the treatment of pregnant women with opioid use disorders and not AUD (Hulse and O'Neil 2002; Hulse et al. 2001, 2004; Kelty and Hulse 2017a, b, c; Towers et al. 2020). A retrospective cohort study of birth outcomes in neonates exposed to naltrexone in utero reported that naltrexone-exposed neonates were generally not significantly different to buprenorphine-exposed neonates ($n = 124$), but significantly lower rates of neonatal abstinence syndrome (7.5 vs. 41.8%) and shorter hospital length of stay (5.5 vs. 8.0 days) in naltrexone-exposed neonates. Compared with the control group of neonates ($n = 569$), naltrexone-exposed neonates were not significantly different in terms of overall rates of congenital anomalies, stillbirths and neonatal mortality. However, naltrexone-exposed neonates were significantly smaller (3137.1 vs. 33[illegible]3.0 g), spent more time in hospital following birth (5.5 vs. 4.3 days) and had higher rates of NAS (7.5 vs. 0.2%) (Kelty and Hulse 2017a, b, c). Despite concerns about higher rates of some pregnancy complications, the general consensus is that naltrexone is the safest option than alcohol use during pregnancy. Based on the currently available data, and the known teratogenic effects of alcohol exposure, naltrexone would likely be the first to be considered in the treatment of AUD in pregnancy.

21.7.2 Disulfiram Use

Disulfiram (an aldehyde dehydrogenase inhibitor that results in a severe reaction when alcohol is consumed concurrently with it, resulting in a strong deterrent effect) is also a category C medication. There are no clinical studies on disulfiram exposure in pregnancy. This is probably due to research conducted between the 1970s and 1980s (Nora et al. 1977; Gardner and Clarkson 1981; Dehaene et al. 1984) that demonstrated an association between disulfiram use in pregnancy and an elevated risk of adverse neonatal health outcomes, including congenital anomalies, miscarriages and stillbirths, probably due to the mechanism of action (Briggs et al. 2017). There is some evidence, albeit inconsistent, that exposure to disulfiram in the first trimester may increase the risk of fetal malformations (Nora et al. 1977; Helmbrecht and Hoskins 1993; Reitnauer et al. 1997). Furthermore, the intensity of the disulfiram-alcohol reaction, which can involve severe acute autonomic instability, including hypertension, can also be considered a risk to the pregnant woman and her fetus, although there have been no studies specifically assessing the magnitude of this specific risk. While the only three preclinical studies on disulfiram exposure during pregnancy present conflicting findings (Harding and Edwards 1993; Johnson et al. 2007; Teng et al. 2023). Therefore, although there was an absence of safety data on the use of disulfiram in pregnancy, it is thought to be harmful and should not be used. In particular, limited data documented that disulfiram acts as a copper chelating agent, lowering blood and tissue copper levels which can harm the pregnancy and the exposed neonate causing early embryonic death, congenital anomalies and impaired cognitive and behavioural function. Moreover, combination of disulfiram and alcohol causes severe autonomic instability including dizziness, tachycardia, and so forth which are risk factors for pregnant women and their developing fetus.

21.7.3 Acamprosate Use

Acamprosate, which is believed to exert its action through modulation of glutamate neurotransmission thereby reducing post-acute withdrawal symptoms and consequently helping to maintain sobriety, is also a category C medication (Rösner et al. 2010). Animal data suggest possible teratogenic effects of acamprosate, but there are no human trial data to support this evidence. Overall, animal studies indicate that prenatal exposure to acamprosate was not associated with adverse maternal or neonatal health outcomes, nor with neurodevelopmental or behavioural impairments (Kelty et al. 2019). The same study did not report any stillbirths or neonatal deaths, and there was no difference in rates of low birth weight, preterm birth or congenital abnormalities between acamprosate-treated pregnant women versus those not exposed (Kelty et al. 2019). However, the effects of acamprosate on short-term memory remain unclear. A study by Quintrell et al. (2023) suggested a potential neuroprotective action exerted by acamprosate against damage caused by alcohol exposure in utero. Therefore, as very minimal research has been conducted on the safety of acamprosate in pregnancy, preliminary evidence has suggested little cause for concern. In the few studies carried out, there were no adverse effects associated with prenatal exposure to acamprosate. However, further research is needed to draw definitive conclusions about considering acamprosate as a first-line pharmacotherapeutical approach for the treatment of AUD in pregnancy.

21.7.4 Nalmefene Use

Nalmefene is produced in tablet form and approved by the European Medical Agency (EMA) in 2013 for the treatment of AUD (EMA 2022). The oral formulation has not still approved by the FDA in the USA and is therefore unavailable. No human or preclinical/animal studies investigating the safety of nalmefene in pregnancy.

21.7.5 Baclofen Use

Baclofen could be typically used in the treatment of AUD as off-label medication, except for the more recent approval in France (Rolland et al. 2020). Few animal studies investigating the use of baclofen in pregnancy reported a risk of neural tube defects (Briner 1996, 2001). Clinical studies on the safety of baclofen in pregnancy are limited and do not allow to draw definitive conclusions.

21.7.6 Other Medications

Regarding other commonly prescribed medications for the treatment of AUD, topiramate was extensively investigated even though studies so far available did not investigate its safety and use in AUD in pregnancy. Among children exposed to prenatal topiramate has been documented the occurrence of an increased risk for congenital anomalies (such as oral clefts, hypospadias), perinatal complications (i.e., ischemic placental disease, preeclampsia, placental abruption, small for gestational age, or preterm birth), increased risk of poor neurodevelopmental outcomes and intellectual disabilities including ASD, ADHD, learning disabilities. Furthermore, topiramate can induce weight loss during pregnancy which may mediate the medication's impact on fetal growth. Although gabapentin was not found to be associated with an increased risk of major congenital anomalies, several studies documented an increased risk of preterm birth, small size for gestational age and neonatal intensive care unit (NICU) access. Therefore, several concerns regarding the use of topiramate and gabapentin in pregnancy have been identified and overall it is not recommended to prescribe them to pregnant women.

Finally, the use of benzodiazepines during pregnancy could be necessary in the management of alcohol withdrawal syndrome (AWS) in those pregnant women who abruptly stopped alcohol consumption during the perinatal period. AWS is a common medical condition with varying presentation from mild hangover to life-threatening seizures, and delirium tremens (Amato et al. 2011). The impact of AWS during the prenatal and postpartum periods remains largely unexplored (Bhat and Hadley 2015; McDonald et al. 2018). At-risk pregnant women require diligent monitoring, preventive strategies and specialized care to mitigate effects due to AWS in pregnancy. The first recommendation should provide early and routine screening for alcohol use in pregnancy to identify high-risk women before the onset of severe AWS. The second step should include to offer timely and effective treatment to manage AWS and mitigate associated risks. Ongoing monitoring of both maternal health and fetal development is crucial to detect complications early, allowing for interventions that can prevent more severe outcomes for both mother and child, including benzodiazepine therapy (Meng et al. 2024).

21.8 Conclusions

Overall, alcohol is a known teratogen, and its use during pregnancy results in a set of severe and complicated detrimental physical, psychological, and cognitive outcomes. In fact, alcohol intake during pregnancy is associated with an increased risk of miscarriage, preterm birth, stillbirth and sudden infant death syndrome (SIDS) as well as it may determine the onset of a range of lifelong behavioural, intellectual and physical disabilities (i.e., 'fetal alcohol spectrum disorders' [FASDs]) (CDC 2024). To date, literature supports that there is no safe time for alcohol use during pregnancy nor there is no known safe amount of alcohol use during pregnancy (CDC 2024).

A multi-step preventive and treatment approach could be effective in managing and in improving harm reduction strategies among pregnant and/or breastfeeding women with AUD. A first step should be an educational and informational approach, including preventive interventions addressed to general population and all pregnant women (Primary prevention). A second step should include a screening approach in order to identify at-risk women before the conception among those who desire to plan a pregnancy, in order to provide all detailed information and preventive strategies to manage the potential occurrence and maintenance of an AUD and/or alcohol intake during pregnancy. A third step should include to promptly identify and screen all pregnant women at-risk for alcohol intake. All conditions associated with any amount of alcohol intake during pregnancy and/or lactation periods should be considered potentially risky for the development of AUD and for the occurrence of detrimental maternal, fetal and newborns' detrimental outcomes. Alcohol should be recommended to be discontinued at any dosage and/or alcohol pattern intake at all.

Regarding the pharmacological management of AUD in pregnancy and breastfeeding, there are not conclusive and reassuring clinical guidelines. A nonpharmacological approach should be always associated and prioritized over the pharmacological approach, except for the management of AWS during pregnancy. All psychosocial interventions addressed to alcohol harm reduction, counselling and motivational approach to discontinue alcohol intake and a psychotherapeutic approach should be preferred. Based on the currently available data, and the known teratogenic effects of alcohol exposure, naltrexone would likely be the first medication to be considered in the treatment of AUD in pregnancy. Other approved and/or not-officially approved medications should not be recommended due to limited data on their safety and efficacy in pregnancy for the fetus. Regarding breastfeeding and use of pharmacological drugs for AUD also require an individualized discussion with the woman and the infant's paediatrician in balancing the benefits of breastfeeding and potential harms of exposure to medication in breastmilk.

References

ACOG. American Congress of Obstetricians and Gynecologists (ACOG). Alcohol and pregnancy, 2018.

Alati R, Clavarino A, Najman JM, O'Callaghan M, Bor W, Mamun AA, Williams GM. The developmental origin of adolescent alcohol use: findings from the mater university study of pregnancy and its outcomes. Drug Alcohol Depend. 2008;98(1–2):136–43. https://doi.org/10.1016/j.drugalcdep.2008.05.011. Epub 2008 Jul 17

Alvik A, Heyerdahl S, Haldorsen T, Lindemann R. Alcohol use before and during pregnancy: a population-based study. Acta Obstet Gynecol. 2006;85:1292–8.

Amato L, Minozzi S, Davoli M. Efficacy and safety of pharmacological interventions for the treatment of the alcohol withdrawal syndrome. Cochrane Database Syst Rev. 2011;2011:Cd008537.

Baer JS, Barr HM, Bookstein FL, Sampson PD, Streissguth AP. Prenatal alcohol exposure and family history of alcoholism in the etiology of adolescent alcohol problems. J Stud Alcohol. 1998;59(5):533–43. https://doi.org/10.15288/jsa.1998.59.533.

Baer JS, Sampson PD, Barr HM, Connor PD, Streissguth AP. A 21-year longitudinal analysis of the effects of prenatal alcohol exposure on young adult drinking. Arch Gen Psychiatry. 2003;60(4):377–85. https://doi.org/10.1001/archpsyc.60.4.377.

Banerjee TD, Middleton F, Faraone SV. Environmental risk factors for attention-deficit hyperactivity disorder. Acta Paediatr. 2007;96(9):1269–74. https://doi.org/10.1111/j.1651-2227.2007.00430.x.

Bhat A, Hadley A. The management of alcohol withdrawal in pregnancy – case report, literature review and preliminary recommendations. Gen Hosp Psychiatry. 2015;37:273.

Blume SB. Is social drinking during pregnancy harmless? There is reason to think not. Adv Alcohol Subst Abuse. 1985;5(1–2):209.

Briggs GF, Freeman RK. Drugs in pregnancy and lactation: a reference guide to fetal and neonatal risk. Philadelphia: Wolters Kluwer/Lippincott Williams & Wilkins Health; 2015.

Briggs GF, Towers RK, Craig V, Forinash AB. Drugs in pregnancy and lactation: a reference guide to fetal and neonatal risk. Lippincott Williams & Wilkins; 2017.

Briner W. Muscimol- and baclofen-induced spina bifida in the rat. Med Sci Res. 1996;24(9):639–40.

Briner W. The effect of GABA receptor ligands in experimental spina bifida occulta. BMC Pharmacol. 2001;1:2. https://doi.org/10.1186/1471-2210-1-2.

Burnette EM, Nieto SJ, Grodin EN, Meredith LR, Hurley B, Miotto K, Gillis AJ, Ray LA. Novel agents for the pharmacological treatment of alcohol use disorder. Drugs. 2022;82(3):251–74. https://doi.org/10.1007/s40265-021-01670-3.

CDC. US Centers for Disease Control and Prevention. Data and Statistics on Alcohol and Pregnancy; 2024. Avaible at https://www.cdc.gov/alcohol-pregnancy/data-research/facts-stats/index.html

Chang G. Maternal substance use: consequences, identification, and interventions. Alcohol Res. 2020;40(2):06.

Chang G, Wilkins-Haug L, Berman S, Goetz MA, Behr H, Hiley A. Alcohol use and pregnancy: improving identification. Obstet Gynecol. 1998;91:892–8.

Chaulagain A, Lyhmann I, Halmøy A, Widding-Havneraas T, Nyttingnes O, Bjelland I, Mykletun A. A systematic meta-review of systematic reviews on attention deficit hyperactivity disorder. Eur Psychiatry. 2023;66(1):e90. Published 2023 Nov 17. https://doi.org/10.1192/j.eurpsy.2023.2451.

Dehaene P, Titran M, Dubois D. Syndrome de Pierre Robin et malformations cardiaques chez un nouveau-né. Rôle du disulfirame pendant la grossesse? [Pierre Robin syndrome and heart malformations in a newborn infant. The role of disulfiram during pregnancy?]. Presse Med. 1984;13(22):1394–5. French

Department of Health. Clinical practice guidelines: pregnancy care. Short form guideline. Canberra: Australian Government Department of Health; 2018.

Dodge NC, Jacobson JL, Lundahl LH, Jacobson SW. Prenatal alcohol exposure and attention-deficit/hyperactivity disorder independently predict greater substance use in young adulthood. Alcohol Clin Exp Res (Hoboken). 2023;47(6):1143–55. https://doi.org/10.1111/acer.15076.

Dozet D, Burd L, Popova S. Screening for alcohol use in pregnancy: a review of current practices and perspectives. Int J Ment Health Addict. 2023;21(2):1220–39. https://doi.org/10.1007/s11469-021-00655-3.

Drabble L, Thomas S, O'Connor L, Roberts SC. State responses to alcohol use and pregnancy: findings from the alcohol policy information system (APIS). J Soc Work Pract Addict. 2014;14(2):191–206. https://doi.org/10.1080/1533256X.2014.900409.

Duko B, Pereira G, Betts K, Tait RJ, Newnham J, Alati R. Associations of prenatal alcohol exposure and offspring harmful alcohol use: findings from the Raine study. Drug Alcohol Depend. 2020;217:108305. https://doi.org/10.1016/j.drugalcdep.2020.108305. Epub 2020 Sep 20

Duko B, Pereira G, Tait RJ, Betts K, Newnham J, Alati R. Prenatal alcohol and tobacco exposures and the risk of cannabis use in offspring: findings from a population-based cohort study. Neurotoxicol Teratol. 2022;90:107064. https://doi.org/10.1016/j.ntt.2022.107064. Epub 2022 Jan 7

European Medicines Agency. Selincro nalmefene. 2022. Available from: https://www.ema.europa.eu/en/medicines/human/EPAR/selincro. Accessed 22 Jan 2025.

Ewing JA. Detecting alcoholism: the CAGE questionnaire. JAMA. 1984;252:1905–7.

Flak AL, Su S, Bertrand J, Denny CH, Kesmodel US, Cogswell ME. The association of mild, moderate, and binge prenatal alcohol exposure and child neuropsychological outcomes: a meta-analysis. Alcohol Clin Exp Res. 2014;38(1):214–26. https://doi.org/10.1111/acer.12214.

Forray A, Merry B, Lin H, Ruger JP, Yonkers KA. Perinatal substance use: a prospective evaluation of abstinence and relapse. Drug Alcohol Depend. 2015;150:147–55. https://doi.org/10.1016/j.drugalcdep.2015.02.027.

Gardner RJ, Clarkson JE. A malformed child whose previously alcoholic mother had taken disulfiram. N Z Med J. 1981;93(680):184–6.

Gibson L, Porter M. Drinking or smoking while breastfeeding and later cognition in children. Pediatrics. 2018;142(2):e20174266. https://doi.org/10.1542/peds.2017-4266.

Gibson L, Porter M. Drinking or smoking while breastfeeding and later academic outcomes in children. Nutrients. 2020;12(3):829. https://doi.org/10.3390/nu12030829.

Gibson L, Porter M. Alcohol and tobacco use while breastfeeding and risk of autism spectrum disorder or attention deficit/hyperactivity disorder. J Autism Dev Disord. 2022;52(3):1223–34. https://doi.org/10.1007/s10803-021-05027-3.

Goldschmidt L, Richardson GA, De Genna NM, Cornelius MD, Day NL. Prenatal alcohol exposure and offspring alcohol use and misuse at 22 years of age: a prospective longitudinal study. Neurotoxicol Teratol. 2019;71:1–5. https://doi.org/10.1016/j.ntt.2018.11.001.

Gosdin LK, Deputy NP, Kim SY, Dang EP, Denny CH. Alcohol consumption and binge drinking during pregnancy among adults aged 18-49 years – United States, 2018-2020. MMWR Morb Mortal Wkly Rep. 2022;71(4):156. https://doi.org/10.15585/mmwr.mm7104a4.

Graham K, Wilsnack R, Dawson D, Vogeltanz N. Should alcohol consumption measures be adjusted for gender differences? Addiction. 1998;93:1137–47.

Grzywacz E, Brzuchalski B, Śmiarowska M, Malinowski D, Machoy-Mokrzyńska A, Białecka MA. Significance of selected environmental and biological factors on the risk of FASD in women who drink alcohol during pregnancy. J Clin Med. 2023;12(19):6185. https://doi.org/10.3390/jcm12196185.

Haastrup MB, Pottegard A, Damkier P. Alcohol and breastfeeding. In: Basic & clinical pharmacology & toxicology; 2020.

Harding AJ, Edwards MJ. Retardation of prenatal brain growth of Guinea pigs by disulfiram. Congenit Anom. 1993;33(3):197–202. https://doi.org/10.1111/j.1741-4520.1993.tb00526.x.

Helmbrecht GD, Hoskins IA. First trimester disulfiram exposure: report of two cases. Am J Perinatol. 1993;10(1):5–7.

Hoyme HE, Kalberg WO, Elliott AJ, Blankenship J, Buckley D, Marais AS, Manning MA, Robinson LK, Adam MP, Abdul-Rahman O, Jewett T, Coles CD, Chambers C, Jones KL, Adnams CM, Shah PE, Riley EP, Charness ME, Warren KR, May PA. Updated clinical guidelines for diagnosing fetal alcohol spectrum disorders. Pediatrics. 2016;138:e20154256.

Hulse G, O'Neil GK. Using naltrexone implants in the management of the pregnant heroin user. Aust N Z J Obstet Gynaecol. 2002;42(5):569–73. https://doi.org/10.1111/j.0004-8666.2002.548_14.x.

Hulse GK, O'Neill G, Pereira C, et al. Obstetric and neonatal outcomes associated with maternal naltrexone exposure. Aust N Z J Obstet Gynaecol. 2001;41(4):424–8. https://doi.org/10.1111/j.1479-828X.2001.tb01322.x.

Hulse GK, O'Neil G, Arnold-Reed D. Methadone maintenance vs. implantable naltrexone treatment in the pregnant heroin user. IntJ Gynecol Obstet. 2004;85(2):170–1. https://doi.org/10.1016/j.ijgo.2003.10.001.

Hutchinson D, Mattick R, Braunstein D et al. The impact of alcohol use disorders on family life: a review of the empirical literature. Report No.: NDARC Technical Report No. 325. Sydney, Australia: University of New South Wales; 2004.

Jacobson JL, Jacobson SW, Sokol RJ, Ager JW Jr. Relation of maternal age and pattern of pregnancy drinking to functionally significant cognitive deficit in infancy. Alcohol Clin Exp Res. 1998 Apr;22(2):345–51. https://doi.org/10.1111/j.1530-0277.1998.tb03659.x.

Johnson CS, Zucker RM, Hunter ES, et al. Perturbation of retinoic acid (RA)-mediated limb development suggests a role for diminished RA signaling in the teratogenesis of ethanol. Birth Defects Res Part A Clin Mol Teratol. 2007;79(9):631–41. https://doi.org/10.1002/bdra.20385.

Jones KL, Smith DW, Ulleland CN, Streissguth AP. Pattern of malformation in offspring of chronic alcohol mothers. Lancet. 1973;301(7815):1267–71.

Jones TB, Bailey BA, Sokol RJ. Alcohol use in pregnancy: insights in screening and intervention for the clinician. Clin Obstet Gynecol. 2013;56(1):114–23.

Kelty E, Hulse G. A retrospective cohort study of obstetric outcomes in opioid-dependent women treated with implant naltrexone, oral methadone or sublingual buprenorphine, and non-dependent controls. Drugs. 2017a;77(11):1199–210. https://doi.org/10.1007/s40265-017-0762-9.

Kelty E, Hulse G. A retrospective cohort study of birth outcomes in neonates exposed to naltrexone in utero: a comparison with methadone-, buprenorphine-and non-opioid-exposed neonates. Drugs. 2017b;77(11):1211–9. https://doi.org/10.1007/s40265-017-0763-8.

Kelty E, Hulse G. A retrospective cohort study of the health of children prenatally exposed to methadone, buprenorphine or naltrexone compared with non-exposed control children. Am J Addict. 2017c;26(8):845–51. https://doi.org/10.1111/ajad.12642.

Kelty E, Tran D, Lavin T, Preen DB, Hulse G, Havard A. Prevalence and safety of acamprosate use in pregnant alcohol-dependent women in New South Wales, Australia. Addiction. 2019;114(2):206–15. https://doi.org/10.1111/add.14429.

Kitsantas P, Gaffney KF, Wu H, Kastello JC. Determinants of alcohol cessation, reduction and no reduction during pregnancy. Arch Gynecol Obstet. 2014;289(4):771–9. https://doi.org/10.1007/s00404-013-3056-9. Epub 2013 Oct 23

Lebel C, Roussotte F, Sowell ER. Imaging the impact of prenatal alcohol exposure on the structure of the developing human brain. Neuropsychol Rev. 2011;21(2):102–18. https://doi.org/10.1007/s11065-011-9163-0.

Lemoine P. The history of alcoholic fetopathies. J Popul Ther Clin Pharmacol. 2012;19(2):224–6.

Lemoine P, Harousseau H, Borteyru JP, Menuet JC. Children of alcoholic parents-observed anomalies: discussion of 127 cases. Ouest Med. 1968;8:476–82.

Lingford-Hughes AR, Welch S, Peters L, Nutt DJ. British Association for Psychopharmacology, expert reviewers group. BAP updated guidelines: evidence-based guidelines for the pharmacological management of substance abuse, harmful use, addiction and comorbidity: recommendations from BAP. J Psychopharmacol. 2012;26(7):899–952. https://doi.org/10.1177/0269881112444324.

Luderer M, Ramos Quiroga JA, Faraone SV, Zhang James Y, Reif A. Alcohol use disorders and ADHD. Neurosci Biobehav Rev. 2021;128:648–60. https://doi.org/10.1016/j.neubiorev.2021.07.010.

Mattson SN, Roesch SC, Glass L, et al. Further development of a neurobehavioral profile of fetal alcohol spectrum disorders. Alcohol Clin Exp Res. 2013;37(3):517–28. https://doi.org/10.1111/j.1530-0277.2012.01952.x.

McDonald PLL, Jia L, Vipler S. Alcohol withdrawal management and relapse prevention in pregnancy. Can J Addict. 2018;9:32–41.

McGovern R, Newham JJ, Addison MT, Hickman M, Kaner EF. Effectiveness of psychosocial interventions for reducing parental substance misuse. Cochrane Database Syst Rev. 2021;3(3):CD012823.

Meng LC, Lin CW, Chuang HM, Chen LK, Hsiao FY. Benzodiazepine use during pregnancy and risk of miscarriage. JAMA Psychiatry. 2024;81(4):366–73. https://doi.org/10.1001/jamapsychiatry.2023.4912.

Mitchell SH, Sevigny-Resetco D. Effort-related decision-making in ADHD. J Psychiatr Brain Sci. 2020;5:e200027. https://doi.org/10.20900/jpbs.20200027.

Mitchell AA, Gilboa SM, Werler MM, et al. National Birth Defects Prevention Study: medication use during pregnancy, with particular focus on prescription drugs: 1976–2008. Am J Obstet Gynecol. 2011;205(1):51.e1–8.

Miyake K, Otawa S, Kushima M, Yui H, Shinohara R, Horiuchi S, Akiyama Y, Ooka T, Kojima R, Yokomichi H, Yamagata Z. Maternal alcohol consumption during pregnancy and child development: role of ADH1B and ALDH2 gene polymorphisms-the Yamanashi adjunct study of the Japan environment and children's study. Alcohol Clin Exp Res (Hoboken). 2024;49:117.

Montag AC. Fetal alcohol spectrum disorders: identifying at-risk mothers. International. J Women's Health. 2016;8:311–23.

Morton Ninomiya ME, Almomani Y, Dunbar Winsor K, et al. Supporting pregnant and parenting women who use alcohol during pregnancy: a scoping review of trauma-informed approaches. Womens Health (Lond). 2023;19:17455057221148304. https://doi.org/10.1177/17455057221148304.

Murawski NJ, Moore EM, Thomas JD, Riley EP. Advances in diagnosis and treatment of fetal alcohol spectrum disorders: from animal models to human studies. Alcohol Res. 2015;37(1):97–108.

Naimi TS, Lipscomb LE, Brewer RD, Gilbert BC. Binge drinking in the preconception period and the risk of unintended pregnancy: implications for women and their children. Pediatrics. 2003;111(5 Pt 2):1136–41.

NHMRC. Australian guidelines to reduce health risks from drinking alcohol. Canberra: National Health and Medical Research Council; 2009.

Nora H, Nora J, Blu J. Limb reduction anomalies in infants born to disulfiram-treated alcohol mothers. Lancet. 1977;3:664–9.

NSDUH. Substance Abuse and Mental Health Services Administradion (SAMHSA). 2022 National Survey on Drug Use and Health (NSDUH); 2022. Avaible at https://www.samhsa.gov/data/release/2022-national-survey-drug-use-and-health-nsduh-releases

O'Callaghan FV, O'Callaghan M, Najman JM, Williams GM, Bor W. Prenatal alcohol exposure and attention, learning and intellectual ability at 14 years: a prospective longitudinal study. Early Hum Dev. 2007;83(2):115–23.

O'Leary C, Lawrence D, Hafekost K, Zubrick SR, Bower C. Maternal alcohol-use disorder and child outcomes. Pediatrics. 2020;145(3):e20191574. https://doi.org/10.1542/peds.2019-1574.

Paolozza A, Rasmussen C, Pei J, Hanlon-Dearman A, Nikkel SM, Andrew G, McFarlane A, Samdup D, Reynolds JN. Deficits in response inhibition correlate with oculomotor control in children with fetal alcohol spectrum disorder and prenatal alcohol exposure. Behav Brain Res. 2014;259:97–105. https://doi.org/10.1016/j.bbr.2013.10.040.

Patra J, Bakker R, Irving H, Jaddoe VWV, Malini S, Rehm J. Dose-response relationship between alcohol consumption before and during pregnancy and the risks of low birth weight, preterm birth and small-size-for-gestational age (SGA)- a systematic review and meta-analysis. BJOG. 2011;118(12):1411–21.

Poole N, Schmidt RA, Bocking A, Bergeron J, Fortier I. The potential for fetal alcohol spectrum disorder prevention of a harmonized approach to data collection about alcohol use in pregnancy cohort studies. Int J Environ Res Public Health. 2019;16(11):2019. https://doi.org/10.3390/ijerph16112019.

Popova S, Lange S, Shield K, Mihic A, Chudley AE, Mukherjee RAS, Bekmuradov D, Rehm J. Comorbidity of fetal alcohol spectrum disorder: a systematic review and meta-analysis. Lancet. 2016;387:978–87.

Popova S, Lange S, Probst C, Gmel G, Rehm J. Estimation of national, regional, and global prevalence of alcohol use during pregnancy and fetal alcohol syndrome: a systematic review and meta-analysis. Lancet Glob Health. 2017;5(3):e290–9. https://doi.org/10.1016/S2214-109X(17)30021-9.

Prince MK, Daley SF, Ayers D. Substance use in pregnancy. 2023. In: StatPearls [Internet]. Treasure Island (FL): StatPearls Publishing; 2025.

Quintrell E, Wyrwoll C, Rosenow T, Larcombe A, Kelty E. The effects of acamprosate on maternal and neonatal outcomes in a mouse model of alcohol use disorders. Physiol Behav. 2023;259:114037. https://doi.org/10.1016/j.physbeh.2022.114037.

Rehm J, Kilian C, Ferreira-Borges C, Jernigan D, Monteiro M, Parry CDH, Sanchez ZM, Manthey J. Alcohol use in times of the COVID 19: implications for monitoring and policy. Drug Alcohol Rev. 2020;39(4):301–4. https://doi.org/10.1111/dar.13074.

Reitnauer PJ, Callanan NP, Farber RA, Aylsworth AS. Prenatal exposure to disulfiram implicated in the cause of malformations in discordant monozygotic twins. Teratology. 1997;56(6):358–62.

Reus VI, Fochtmann LJ, Bukstein O, Eyler AE, Hilty DM, Horvitz-Lennon M, Mahoney J, Pasic J, Weaver M, Wills CD, McIntyre J, Kidd J, Yager J, Hong SH. The American Psychiatric Association practice guideline for the pharmacological treatment of patients with alcohol use disorder. Am J Psychiatry. 2018;175(1):86–90. https://doi.org/10.1176/appi.ajp.2017.1750101.

Riley EP, Infante MA, Warren KR. Fetal alcohol spectrum disorders: an overview. Neuropsychol Rev. 2011;21(2):73–8.

Roberts SCM, Thomas S, Treffers R, Drabble L. Forty years of state alcohol and pregnancy policies in the USA: best practices for public health or efforts to restrict women's reproductive rights? Alcohol Alcohol. 2017;52(6):715–21. https://doi.org/10.1093/alcalc/agx047.

Rolland B, Paille F, Gillet C, Rigaud A, Moirand R, Dano C, Dematteis M, Mann K, Aubin HJ. Pharmacotherapy for alcohol dependence: the 2015 recommendations of the French alcohol society, issued in partnership with the European Federation of Addiction Societies. CNS Neurosci Ther. 2016;22(1):25–37. https://doi.org/10.1111/cns.12489.

Rolland B, Simon N, Franchitto N, Aubin HJ. France grants an approval to baclofen for alcohol dependence. Alcohol Alcohol. 2020;55(1):44–5. https://doi.org/10.1093/alcalc/agz082.

Rösner S, Hackl-Herrwerth A, Leucht S, Vecchi S, Srisurapanont M, Soyka M. Opioid antagonists for alcohol dependence. Cochrane Database Syst Rev. 2010;8(12):CD001867.

Russel M, Martier SS, Sokol RJ, Mudar P, Bottoms S, Jacobson S, Jacobson J. Screening for pregnancy risk-drinking. Alcohol Clin Exp Res. 1994;18(5):1156–61.

Saunders JB, Aasland OG, Babor TF, de la Fuente JR, Grant M. Development of the alcohol use disorders identification test (AUDIT): WHO collaborative project on early detection of persons with harmful alcohol consumption-II. Addiction. 1993;88:791–804.

Sayal K, Heron J, Golding J, Emond A. Prenatal alcohol exposure and gender differences in childhood mental health problems: a longitudinal population-base study. Pediatrics. 2007;119(2):e426–34.

Selzer ML. The Michigan alcoholism screening test: the quest for a new diagnostic instrument. Am J Psychiatry. 1971;127(12):89–94.

Seo BA, Kim SG, Huh SY, Lee DH, An SH, Lee SY, Lee DH, An HS, Lee SY, Kim HK, Choi JM. Changes of drinking behavior in Korean pregnant women for the last 20 year. J Public Health (Oxf). 2021;43(4):e632–6. https://doi.org/10.1093/pubmed/fdaa143.

Sood B, Delaney-Black V, Covington C, Nordstrom-Klee B, Ager J, Templin T, Janisse J, Martier S, Sokol RJ. Prenatal alcohol exposure and childhood behavior at age 6 to 7 years: I. Dose-response effect. Pediatrics. 2001;108(2):e34.

Streissguth AP, Sampson PD, Barr HM. Neurobehavioral dose-response effects of prenatal alcohol exposure in humans from infancy to adulthood. Ann N Y Acad Sci. 1989;562:145–58.

Teng M, Luo Y, Wang C, et al. Effect of disulfiram on the reproductive capacity of female mice. Int J Mol Sci. 2023;24(3):2371. https://doi.org/10.3390/ijms24032371.

Thibaut F, Chagraoui A, Buckley L, Gressier F, Labad J, Lamy S, Potenza MN, Rondon M, Riecher-Rössler A, Soyka M, Yonkers K. WFSBP * and IAWMH ** guidelines for the treatment of alcohol use disorders in pregnant women. World J Biol Psychiatry. 2019;20(1):17–50. https://doi.org/10.1080/15622975.2018.1510185.

Towers CV, Katz E, Weitz B, et al. Use of naltrexone in treating opioid use disorder in pregnancy. Am J Obstet Gynecol. 2020;222(1):83.e1–8. https://doi.org/10.1016/j.ajog.2019.07.037.

Urbano-Marquez A, Estruch R, Fernandez-Sola J. The greater risk of alcoholic cardiomyopathy and myopathy in women compared with men. JAMA. 1995;274:149–54.

US Preventive Services Task Force, et al. Screening and behavioral counseling interventions to reduce unhealthy alcohol use in adolescents and adults: US preventive services task force recommendation statement. JAMA. 2018;320(18):1899–909. https://doi.org/10.1001/jama.2018.16789.

Wetherill L, Foroud T, Goodlett C. Meta-analyses of externalizing disorders: genetics or prenatal alcohol exposure? Alcohol Clin Exp Res. 2018;42(1):162–72. https://doi.org/10.1111/acer.13535.

WHO. Guidelines for the identification and management of substance use and substance use disorders in pregnancy. World Health Organization, 2014. Available at https://www.who.int/publications/i/item/9789241548731

WHO. Global status report on alcohol and health. World Health Organization, 2018. Available at https://www.who.int/publications/i/item/9789241565639

Woodruff K, Roberts SCM. "Alcohol during pregnancy? Nobody does that anymore": state legislators' use of evidence in making policy on alcohol use in pregnancy. J Stud Alcohol Drugs. 2019;80(3):380–8. https://doi.org/10.15288/jsad.2019.80.380.

Zagon IS, Tobias SW, Hytrek SD, McLaughlin PJ. Opioid receptor blockade throughout prenatal life confers long-term insensitivity to morphine and alters mu opioid receptors. Pharmacol Biochem Behav. 1998;59:201–7.

22 Substance Use Disorders

Laura Orsolini, Giulia Francesconi, Rosa Volgare, Fabrizio Schifano, and Umberto Volpe

22.1 Introduction

Epidemiological studies report that substance use disorders (SUDs) are a growing public and health concern, broadly spanning into all stages of life. The Diagnostic and Statistical Manual of Mental Disorders in its fifth edition, revised (DSM-5-TR) defines SUD as a cluster of cognitive, behavioural and physiological symptoms indicating that the individual persists in using the substance despite significant substance-related issues (APA 2022). According to the 2020 National Survey of Substance Abuse and Mental Health Services Administration (SAMHSA), SUD during pregnancy is dramatically increasing among women of childbearing age, having been reported use of an illicit drug, tobacco or alcohol in the past month in some 8–11% of pregnant women (SAMHSA 2020). In the USA, 15.4% of women reported to use illicit drugs, being younger women (aged 18–29) those with the highest risk (Pacho et al. 2023). Among women, substances are more commonly misused and/or abused for weight control, pain management, and as a self-medication strategy for managing mental health issues (Pacho et al. 2023; Pentecost et al. 2021). Substance use during pregnancy affects 15% of newborns, causing serious maternal and neonatal health risks like miscarriage, birth defects, and withdrawal symptoms in infants (Pacho et al. 2023; Pentecost et al. 2021). Overall, perinatal substance use was reported to be less prevalent among women in later trimesters, with lower odds of past-month substance use observed in the second

L. Orsolini (✉) · G. Francesconi · R. Volgare · U. Volpe
Unit of Clinical Psychiatry, Department of Experimental and Clinical Medicine (DIMSC), Polytechnic University of Marche, Ancona, Italy
e-mail: l.orsolini@staff.univpm.it

F. Schifano
Psychopharmacology, Drug Misuse and Novel Psychoactive Substances Research Unit, School of Life and Medical Sciences, Hatfield, UK

F. Uguz, L. Orsolini (eds.), *Perinatal Psychopharmacology*,
https://doi.org/10.1007/978-3-031-99720-4_22

trimester across tobacco and marijuana (Odds Ratios [ORs] = 0.29–0.47), when compared to first trimester of pregnancy (Peltier et al. 2022). A similar lower rate was observed in the third trimester compared to the first trimester, across tobacco and marijuana use, as well as cocaine, prescription pain medication and tranquilizer use (ORs = 0.02–0.42). Conversely, polysubstance use was lower among women in their second and third trimesters compared to their first trimester (ORs = 0.09–0.46) (Peltier et al. 2022).

However, despite the relatively significant prevalence of SUD in women of reproductive age, there are still limited data to draw definitive conclusions on the impact of SUDs on pregnancy, foetal and postpartum outcomes, including insights on the short- and long-term impact of a foetal and/or neonatal exposure to substances of abuse. Furthermore, the situation could be complicated by the type of the clinical population under investigation, as pregnant women may present with a comorbidity of a pre-existing and/or a subclinical psychiatric condition, reported in up to 60–72% of cases among SUD individuals; this could act as a confounding variable when interpreting clinical data on pregnancy and foetal outcomes (SAMHSA 2020). In addition, a comorbid psychiatric condition has been associated with a high risk for polysubstance consumption (Kandel et al. 2001). On the other hand, SUDs could be a direct or indirect consequence of a previous and/or a current history of a physical/sexual abuse, as a sort of coping strategy to manage negative affective situations or to normalize dysregulated emotional states. The abovementioned concurrent conditions could also determine detrimental foetal and/or neonatal outcomes, by acting as confounder determinants as well. Beyond the concurrent mental conditions, in the management of a pregnant/puerperal woman clinicians should also evaluate the potential psychological consequences for the newborn in being exposed to a nursing SUD woman (e.g., poor parenting, failure to thrive, child neglect, child abuse, abandonment and so forth).

22.2 Tobacco, Caffeine and Tea Intake During the Perinatal Period

A global estimate reported that up to 30–53% of women who are daily smokers continue with their nicotine intake during their pregnancy (Lange et al. 2018; Puga et al. 2024). Tobacco exposure has been reported to be highly prevalent particularly during the first trimester of pregnancy (e.g., at around 22.9%), followed by the third (15.3%) and the second (14.3%) trimester (National Survey on Drug Use and Health 2007). Moreover, despite many women quitting tobacco consumption once pregnant, a substantial number tend to restart their habit post-delivery (Bushi et al. 2024). Smoking rates among SUD women in the perinatal period are influenced and perpetuated by a set of psychosocial challenges such as stigma, concurrent mental conditions, traumatic history, intimate partner violence and child protection issues (Jackson et al. 2022). Tobacco smoking may negatively impact on pregnancy outcomes. Yuan et al. (2021) identified tobacco among those risk factors implicated in early pregnancy termination, in being associated with dysfunctional placental development, placental abruption (Odds Ratio [OR] = 1.80) and placenta praevia (OR = 1.42). Tobacco smoking has been associated with higher rates of stillbirth (50%), neonatal death (22%), and perinatal death (33%) (Yuan et al. 2021). In particular, tobacco exposure has been supposed to determine epigenetic changes that affect gene expression and contribute to offspring health issues (Gould et al. 2020). Tobacco exposure during intrauterine life appears to double the risk of intrauterine growth issues, low birth weight, as well as increasing the risk of both spina bifida (OR = 1.55) and cleft lip/palate syndrome (OR = 1.36), up to 10–30% (Gould et al. 2020; Bushi et al. 2024). Maternal smoking during pregnancy has been associated with abnormal development of the central nervous system (Honein et al. 2001) and behavioural problems in the offspring (Haustein 1999; Wakschlag et al. 2002). Evidence-based management strategies of tobacco cessation treatments in pregnancy include nicotine replacement therapy (NRT), contingency management (CM), and behavioural counselling, despite limited evidence of their effectiveness in the perinatal period (Jackson et al. 2022). A recent systematic review identified 3 studies using CM, 5 studies investigating behavioural counselling and one offering NRT, with most of these studies however being methodologically weak or of low quality. Furthermore, some studies reported a growth in e-cigarette usage among expecting mothers, with around 7% of pregnant women who turn to e-cigarettes during their pregnancy, and a significant 45% of them who believe that e-cigarette could represent a safer alternative than traditional cigarettes and that could aid in either quitting or reducing their smoking habits during pregnancy (Kapaya et al. 2019; Siu et al. 2015). A recent meta-analysis indicated an overall prevalence of 4.6% for dual users of tobacco smoking and e-cigarette use in pregnant women, with subgroup analyses showing a prevalence of 4.9% for the USA and 8.1% for the UK (Bushi et al. 2024). However, although e-cigarettes do not contain tobacco, the vapour inhaled by the user often contains nicotine and is therefore considered a tobacco product by some organizations, including the U.S. Food and Drug Administration (FDA) (Havard et al. 2022) and hence not considered safe to use during pregnancy (U.S. Centers for Disease Control and Prevention 2010). In fact, studies reported that offspring born to mothers exposed to e-cigarettes might face a range of neonatal adverse effects, including neurodevelopmental challenges, compromised lung growth, elevated inflammatory markers and oxidative stress, as well as reductions in crown-rump length and overall foetal weight (Bushi et al. 2024).

Caffeine has been reported to be consumed by around 75–93% of pregnant women (Frary et al. 2005; Kaiser and Allen 2008). Caffeine is a central nervous system stimulant that can also cross the placenta during pregnancy. During pregnancy, caffeine clearance substantially decreases by potentially increasing its effect in the pregnant woman and her foetus. Observational studies suggested that excessive caffeine intake can be associated with growth restriction, low birth weight, preterm birth, miscarriage or stillbirth, and childhood obesity (Greenwood et al. 2014; Wikoff et al. 2017; Arabzadeh et al. 2024). Moreover, caffeine during pregnancy has been associated with an increase in heart rate and blood pressure for the mother (Arafa et al. 2024). In fact, caffeine exerts its effects by antagonizing adenosine receptors in the central nervous system and peripheral tissues, resulting in increased blood pressure (Ribeiro and Sebastião 2010). In addition, caffeine stimulates the release of catecholamines (e.g., noradrenaline, adrenaline) from the adrenal glands, leading to increased heart rate and cardiac output and peripheral vasoconstriction. Other issues associated with caffeine intake may include the stimulation of renin release from the kidneys through the release of angiotensin II, a potent vasoconstrictor which stimulates the release of aldosterone, leading to sodium and water retention, further contributing to increased blood pressure (Tanuma et al. 2003). Another caffeine effect involves the impairment of insulin sensitivity and glucose metabolism, both representing risk factors for hypertension and cardiovascular disease (Sakr et al. 2023). A recent meta-analysis and systematic review by Chen et al. (2022) observed that caffeine exposure during pregnancy was not significantly associated with the risk of gestational hypertension or pre-eclampsia, suggesting that more prospective and long-term studies should be implemented to draw up definitive conclusions. Santana et al. (2024) concluded in their systematic review that the evidence so far published is insufficient to confirm with certainty that prenatal caffeine exposure may lead to neurobehavioural disorders in the newborns. In conclusion, evidence supports the recommendation of a caffeine consumption up to 300 mg daily in healthy pregnant women as an intake that is generally not associated with adverse reproductive and developmental effects (Chen et al. 2022; Wikoff et al. 2017).

Furthermore, tea and other consumed beverages which could contain bioactive compounds including caffeine, catechins and polyphenols have been investigated in their potential detrimental impact on gestational, foetal and neonatal outcomes (Arafa et al. 2024). The highest frequencies of antenatal tea drinking were associated with increased ORs of hypertensive disorders of pregnancy (OR = 1.16) (Arafa et al. 2024). Therefore, it could be prudent for pregnant women to minimize tea consumption as well. However, well-designed prospective cohort studies are needed to establish causality and explore potential dose-response relationships between tea consumption during pregnancy and gestational and/or foetal and/or neonatal outcomes.

22.3 Cannabis and Cannabimimetics Use During the Perinatal Period

Cannabis sativa L. (aka *Canapa, Indian Canapa, Marijuana, Mary Jane, Hashish, pot, herb, Maria, Hagga, Puf, Maconha*, etc.) is a commonly used drug during pregnancy, with its use having increased among pregnant women in recent years (Young-Wolff et al. 2017, 2019). Epidemiological evidence shows that cannabis use during the gestational period is quite common, ranging from 3% to 16% worldwide reaching higher levels in some demographic subgroups (Angeliki Gerede et al. 2024). Marijuana has antiemetic properties, and prenatal cannabis use is most prevalent in the first trimester of pregnancy for managing nausea and vomiting in pregnancy and hyperemesis syndrome (Ainiti et al. 2023). In addition, marijuana use can be reported among pregnant women to self-manage other pregnancy-related symptoms, including anxiety, depression, pain or for recreational purposes (Young-Wolff et al. 2019; Brown et al. 2019). Cannabis passes placental transfer to the foetus (Pertwee 2010) and its levels can be detected in the cord (Hanuš 2007) with levels which are proportionately smaller than those of the mother (Hanuš 2007). In urine samples of neonates, significant levels of cannabis have been detected (Al-Hayani et al. 2001). The potentially adverse effects of marijuana use during pregnancy are aggravated by the consumption of high potency marijuana (i.e., marijuana consisting of high Δ9-THC content of 9% or higher), with the risk of an increased effect in developing central nervous system anomalies of embryo/foetus (Psychoyos and Vinod 2013).

In utero exposure to cannabis has also been associated with increased neonatal care requirements and risk for miscarriage (Gurm et al. 2021). Furthermore, cognitive, motor and social dysfunctions as well as neurobehavioural complications have been described in the offspring following maternal exposure to cannabis during pregnancy (Orsolini et al. 2017). Indeed, prenatal cannabis exposure has been linked to a wide range of effects in offspring, including:

1. *Cognitive impairments*: Studies showed that cannabis exposure during pregnancy negatively impacts foetal neurodevelopment reducing performance in cognitive domains such as verbal language, memory and visual function (Gurm et al. 2021; Ramon Portillo et al. 2024). Cannabidiol (CBD) can disrupt tryptophan metabolism in the human placenta, altering the balance of serotonin and kynurenine (KYN) pathways thus possibly increasing the risk of cognitive impairments in newborns and small-for-gestational-age births (Ramon Portillo et al. 2024). Prenatal cannabis exposure has been linked to changes in the development of fronto-limbic white matter, particularly the fornix, a critical pathway for emotional learning and memory (Evanski et al. 2023). These deficits may be persistent thus extending into childhood, adolescence, and even adulthood (Murnan et al. 2021).
2. *Neuro-behavioural effects*: Prenatal cannabis exposure is associated with increased impulsivity, hyperactivity, and emotional dysregulation in children (Odom et al. 2020). THC, CBD, and their combination can produce sex-specific behavioural changes during adolescence, such as altered impulsivity, anxiety, memory, and sensory gating (DeVuono et al. 2024).
3. *Psychiatric illnesses*: Children exposed to cannabis during intrauterine life show a higher likelihood of developing ADHD symptoms/disorders, psychotic-like experiences and autism spectrum disorder (Tadesse et al. 2024; Paul et al. 2021).
4. *Physical abnormalities:* Perinatal cannabis exposure is associated with gastroschisis, particularly in mothers aged over 34, although further research is required to determine causality and age-related variations (Delker et al. 2024).

Studies observed that the above-mentioned risks are dose- and time-dependent, with increased levels of prenatal cannabis exposure associated with higher risks to induce detrimental obstetrical, foetal and neonatal effects (Klebanoff et al. 2021). According to a recent systematic review and meta-analysis, among all associations documented so far in the published literature between cannabis exposure and a specific set of gestational, foetal and neonatal outcomes, only two outcomes presented convincing evidence of in utero cannabinoids exposure harmful effects, i.e., low birth weight (OR = 1.43) and small for gestational age (OR = 1.61) with Class I evidence (Solmi et al. 2008). Conversely, preterm delivery (OR = 1.32) and neonatal intensive care unit admission (OR = 1.41) displayed Class III evidence following in utero cannabis exposure (Solmi et al. 2008). Current literature conducted on humans still lacks solid association data which limits them to draw definitive conclusions, due to potential concomitant confounding variables such as polysubstance use and lifestyle issues. However, due to significant concerns regarding impaired neurodevelopment, as well as maternal and foetal exposure to the adverse effects of marijuana consumption, pregnant women or those contemplating pregnancy should be encouraged to discontinue cannabis and cannabis-like products. Before pregnancy and in early pregnancy, clinicians should always be asked to all women about their current and/or recent/past use of marijuana, investigating motivations and counsel women about concerns regarding potential adverse health effects during the perinatal period. There is insufficient data to evaluate the effects of marijuana use on infants during breastfeeding, hence, marijuana consumption also during breastfeeding should be discouraged (ACOG 2017; National Council of State Boards of Nursing 2018). Furthermore, clinicians should be discouraged from prescribing or recommending the use of marijuana for medical purposes during the period before pregnancy and during pregnancy and lactation. Further high-quality studies regarding the effects of marijuana and other cannabis-containing products on pregnancy and breastfeeding are needed, including indications about the exposure and prescription to medical cannabis during pregnancy and postpartum period.

The use of cannabidiol (CBD) is becoming increasingly popular and is being marketed for various mental conditions. Non-approved Food and Drug Administration (FDA) commercial CBD products are available over-the-counter but may significantly differ in composition from those used in clinical studies for medical use. CBD is one of many chemical compounds, together with Δ9-THC, found in the cannabis plant. The FDA has approved one cannabis-derived (CBD) drug product (Epidiolex) for the treatment of two forms of severe epilepsy and three THC-related drug products for the treatment of nausea and vomiting caused by cancer chemotherapy or weight loss/poor appetite in patients affected with AIDS. These medications are only available with a prescription from a licensed healthcare provider. There is no data on CBD exposure during pregnancy and breastfeeding; hence, CBD use should be avoided in these populations. FDA did not approve the use of CBD products for managing nausea and vomiting or 'gravidarum hyperemesis', hence, CBD should not be prescribed or recommended to pregnant women (ACOG 2017; FDA 2019).

The current urging increase in the dissemination and consumption of pseudo-cannabis-like products, such as synthetic cannabimimetics, 'Spice' drugs, Synthetic Cannabinoids (SCBs) pose a further public and clinical concern (for a comprehensive review, see Orsolini et al. 2017). Blends falling under the brand 'Spice' are composed of herbals mixed/sprayed with cannabimimetics, with some of them possessing extremely high potency levels compared to traditional cannabis. The use of SCBs has become more popular due to their increased availability and the fact that they are undetectable in routine drug screenings. However, SCBs are more toxic and harmful compared to natural Δ9-tetrahydrocannabinol (Δ9-THC) due to differences in activity, chemical structure, and concentration in commercial products (Schifano et al. 2015). Research conducted by a Texas-based international team revealed a significant decrease in foetal brain vessel diameter and area density, indicating that acute prenatal SCB exposure causes significant brain vasoconstriction during critical brain development stages (Raghunathan et al. 2019). However, adverse effects due to perinatal SCB exposure are still unknown, as analytical data are scarce (Carlier et al. 2020). Hence, due to limited data, clinicians should recommend caution and suggest to avoid SCB consumption during pregnancy and postpartum period to all women in their reproductive age.

22.4 Stimulant Use During the Perinatal Period

Stimulant drugs, including cocaine, ecstasy, methamphetamines and prescription stimulants, represent the second most widely used and abused class of substances, with a lifetime prevalence among adults of around 30% (EMCDDA 2024). Psychostimulants ('uppers') refer to any drug able to increase activity of the central nervous system or those with sympathomimetic properties. Psychostimulants are prescribed also for medical purposes, including mood disorders, impulse control disorders such as Attention Deficit and Hyperactivity Disorder (ADHD), sleep disorders and obesity (Schifano et al. 2015). Stimulants are usually misused and/or abused due to their recreational euphoric and disinhibiting effect as well as for their performance-enhancing purposes (Schifano et al. 2016). Women appeared to be disproportionately vulnerable to developing stimulant misuse and abuse due to factors related to hormonal profiles and reinforcement of gender constructs, as well as in progressing to an addiction faster than men (Roth et al. 2004; Miller et al. 2015). Epidemiological data reported a stimulant use among pregnant women in a consistent increasing trend over the last decade (Smid et al. 2019).

In the late 1980s and early 1990s, cocaine dependence was labelled an epidemic by the US government, with 30% of young adult women reporting recent use (SAMHSA 2007). Cocaine use during pregnancy received considerable media attention, when photographers documented the first newborns exposed to crack/cocaine in utero (the '*crack babies*' phenomenon; Chavkin 2001). Cocaine use is associated in around 10% with women in their reproductive age, who also use opioids for non-medical purposes (Jarlenski et al. 2017). In 2015, cocaine represented the second most common illicit substance used by pregnant women, with 3.4% of pregnant women having used cocaine in the past month (Smid et al. 2019). Sociodemographic associated risk factors are older age, African-American ethnicity and low socioeconomic status (Day et al. 1993). Moreover, cocaine represents the leading cause of ante-partum hospitalizations for substance use among pregnant women (Cox et al. 2008). Cocaine acts on the central nervous system primarily by the inhibition of dopaminergic reuptake, and through the activation of noradrenergic and serotoninergic sites in the basal forebrain and cerebral cortex (Malanga and Kosofsky 1999). In preclinical studies, exposure to cocaine during gestation has been shown to affect brain function, particularly the dopaminergic systems, causing anatomical, physiological, and behavioural changes. However, human studies often reported only mild alterations in attention, language, and memory influenced by environmental factors such as socioeconomic status and other drug use (Betancourt et al. 2011). Neurotoxic effects of in utero cocaine exposure can manifest in foetal and long-term growth outcomes, as well as structural abnormalities, determining an impaired neurodevelopment. Maternal complications following in utero cocaine exposure include cardiovascular complications (e.g., hypertension, myocardial infarction, ischaemia), renal failure, hepatic rupture, cerebral haemorrhage/ischaemia/infarction and maternal death (Smid et al. 2019). Evidence supports that cardiovascular complications are not dose-dependent, by underlining that also small doses may lead to cardiac morbidity and mortality in healthy pregnant women. Moreover, clinicians should also consider that pregnancy may increase cardiovascular toxicity due to an increased cardiac muscle's sensitivity to cocaine through an increased progesterone concentration (Plessinger and Woods Jr. 1991). Cocaine toxicity may cause severe hypertension, hyperreflexia, oedema, seizures and proteinuria in pregnant women (Smid et al. 2019). A systematic review and meta-analysis conducted by Gouin et al. (2011) on 31 studies reported an increased risk for preterm delivery, low birth weight, small for gestational age infants, earlier gestational age at delivery and reduced birth weight. Postpartum psychological distress experienced by mothers with prenatal cocaine exposure was greater compared to mothers not using cocaine (Smid et al. 2019). The long-term effects on child growth and development are uncertain, though some research indicates slower growth in children up to age 10. Cocaine exposure is linked to neurodevelopmental issues like cognitive impairments, behavioural problems (e.g., ADHD), and language delays. However, sociodemographic and environmental factors may contribute as much, or more, to these outcomes. Protective factors, such as family support and better socioeconomic status, can help mitigate the negative effects of prenatal cocaine exposure (Cressman et al. 2014). Higher rates of psychopathological symptoms (e.g., depression, anxiety, psychosis and paranoia) amongst cocaine-using women were reported by Singer et al. (2000) which were associated with higher levels of reduced head circumference and birthweight. A dose-response correlation between a prenatal cocaine exposure and a lower height and weight-for-height z scores at 6 years was reported by Minnes et al. (2005). Several large longitudinal prospective cohort studies reported stable negative effects on language skills in cocaine-exposed infants and children up to 7 years of age, beyond the effect of the home environment or other confounding factors (Singer et al. 2001; Morrow et al. 2003; Bandstra et al. 2004). Other studies on language development showed mixed findings. In fact, whilst gestational cocaine exposure may not cause the severe deficits once feared, it may still result in subtle cognitive impairments that could affect academic and work performance later in life. Since brain maturation continues into adulthood, the full impact may only become evident in adolescence or adulthood, making further research necessary to understand its long-term effects (Betancourt et al. 2011). The extent of these negative consequences depends on the dosage, timing, and duration of a mother's cocaine use, and therefore on how long the baby was exposed to the drug (American Addiction Centre 2024).

Methamphetamine ([2S]-N-methyl-1-phenyl-propan-2-amine; aka 'meth', 'ice', 'crystal meth', 'crank') is the methylated derivative of dextroamphetamine, its use had significantly increased over the past two decades. Between 2010 and 2014, the rate of methamphetamine-related overdoses doubled. In 2015, 1.7 million people (0.6% of the population) used methamphetamine in the past year, with over half (52.7%) having used it in the past month (Smid et al. 2019). Ecstasy (MDMA, i.e., 3,4-methylenedioxy-N-methylamphetamine; aka 'molly') is an amphetamine-type substance commonly consumed by younger populations, including women of reproductive age (Center for Behavioral Health Statistics and Quality. Results from the 2015 National Survey on Drug Use and Health: Detailed Tables. Substance Abuse and Mental Health Services Administration 2016). Although MDMA and methamphetamines are the most commonly abused drugs in party/rave settings, it has been supposed that such parties would be less likely joined by women once pregnant. Conversely, one would argue that it would be more likely to be exposed to unwanted pregnancy in those women with risky behaviour due to MDMA-related disinhibiting and pro-social effect. The DAISY (*Drugs and Infancy*) study documented a trend in both MDMA and methamphetamine use particularly in the first trimester of pregnancy among those women who declared a pre-conception use (respectively, in 35% and 9% of cases); conversely, the persistence of this consumption declined throughout the pregnancy, with only 4% who confirmed its use also in the second and third trimester (Moore et al. 2009). The DAISY study observed as well that those pregnant women who declared a stimulant intake during the first trimester usually also took concomitantly cannabis, tobacco and alcohol, with one third of them having persisted in cannabis intake throughout the pregnancy period (Moore et al. 2009).

Methamphetamine is a central nervous system stimulant which acts by increasing presynaptic release of dopamine, serotonin and norepinephrine. Methamphetamine use determines intense euphoria and increased levels of energy. It can be snorted, smoked, used rectally and injected. It can be manufactured from commonly available items such as over-the-counter cough syrups and decongestants. Methamphetamine intake has been associated with an increased risk of developing myocardial infarction, hypertension, cardiomyopathy and stroke, as well as increased risk of infection including HIV and HCV and severe dental disease (Miller et al. 2009). Pregnant women using methamphetamine are typically younger (under 24), unemployed, and more likely to have psychiatric disorders, live in poverty, and have a lower perceived quality of life. They also face higher risks of legal issues and are more likely to have family and friends who use substances (Smid et al. 2019). Methamphetamine exposure during the pregnancy has been associated with adverse perinatal outcomes including stillbirth, small for gestational age, preterm delivery, caesarean delivery, and maternal intensive care unit admission, despite most studies not having controlled the effect of potential confounding factors (e.g., maternal co-morbidities, tobacco smoking, other drugs, contaminants in non-pharmaceutical preparations and poverty; Smid et al. 2019). A comprehensive meta-analysis, including eight studies, found that methamphetamine use during pregnancy was associated with earlier gestational age at delivery, low birthweight and small head circumference (Kalaitzopoulos et al. 2018). Congenital malformations reported following in utero methamphetamine use included cardiac malformations, gastroschisis, limb reduction, biliary atresia and neural tube defects, despite prospective studies having failed to confirm a causal association, except for cleft palate (Smid et al. 2019). Newborns exposed to methamphetamine during pregnancy reported jitteriness, drowsiness and respiratory distress at a level in need of monitoring within intensive neonatal care units (Oro and Dixon 1987; Smith et al. 2003). An analysis of neurobehavior at birth revealed that methamphetamine-exposed infants demonstrated poor movement quality and high levels of physiological stress (Smith et al. 2003; LaGasse et al. 2012). Moreover, infants with a history of heavy methamphetamine exposure showed lower arousal and reduced excitability levels compared to non-exposed infants (Wouldes et al. 2023). Furthermore, although methamphetamine is neurotoxic, studies investigating the effect of methamphetamine exposure during pregnancy on the foetal brain are mostly pre-clinical and overall suggesting a gestational age-dependent effect with exposure in early to mid-trimester; there are concerns relating to the long-lasting effects on the serotonergic development of the foetal brain (Won et al. 2001, 2002). Prenatal methamphetamine exposure negatively affects brain development, particularly during early to mid-trimester, leading to long-lasting neurotoxic effects. Studies show smaller brain volumes and altered metabolism in methamphetamine-exposed children, but results are influenced by concurrent alcohol and tobacco use (Jablonski et al. 2016; Chang et al. 2004). Similarly, long-term studies of children exposed to methamphetamine are limited. The Infant Development, Environment and Lifestyle study (IDEAL) followed 412 maternal-child pairs (204 methamphetamine exposed vs 208 unexposed pairs) from the U.S.A. and New Zealand, from delivery throughout childhood; they reported increased likelihood of admission to the neonatal intensive care unit, decreased arousal and increased physiological stress among exposed neonates at 1 month (Kiblawi et al. 2014). Heavy (e.g., more than 3 days a week) prenatal methamphetamine exposure was associated with anxiety, depression and attention problems by age 3- and 5-years-old after controlling for other substances and caregiver/environmental risk factors (Derauf et al. 2012; LaGasse et al. 2012). Conversely, children exposed to methamphetamine at age 7 displayed poorer cognitive functioning compared to unexposed (Diaz et al. 2014).

MDMA is a powerful monoaminergic agonist which inhibits the reuptake and promotes the release of serotonin and, to a lesser extent, of dopamine. A chronic maternal MDMA intake may impair memory functioning, frontal executive processing, problem solving, decision making and social and emotional intelligence; these issues may be the result of altered parental style, newborn/child-focused attention, communication and attachment style, and cognitive impairment (Rodgers 2000; Rodgers et al. 2003; Fisk et al. 2005; Rendell et al. 2007). Pregnant women who use MDMA during pregnancy are more likely to suffer negative consequences, including work- and social-related impairment (Singer et al. 2012). There is limited data on foetuses and infants of women exposed to MDMA during pregnancy. Most data come from animal studies which documented an increased mortality, retinal eye defects, cleft palate, rib malformations, decreased physical growth and delayed motor development. There are only isolated reports of cardiac defects, cleft lip and biliary atresia after amphetamine in utero exposure in human infants, a reduced growth and increased foetal distress (Eriksson et al. 1978, 1981; Billing et al. 1980; Dixon and Bejar 1989; Catanzarite and Stein 1995; Plessinger 1998). Using MDMA during pregnancy can harm both the mother and the baby. In a single-centre study, pregnant women using methamphetamine were more likely to experience pre-term delivery, caesarean section and maternal ICU admission. However, the study did not consider other factors such as smoking, other drug use, or socioeconomic status (Good et al. 2010). Pregnant women who use MDMA are more likely to display higher rates of unplanned pregnancies, therapeutic abortions, binge drinking, smoking and using other drugs. The drug can also negatively affect the mother's health, causing stress, high body temperature, appetite loss, sadness and sleep disturbances (American Addiction Center 2024). Babies exposed to ecstasy in utero may face increased risks of congenital defects (cleft palate, gastroschisis, biliary atresia, and neural tube defects), cardiovascular (cardiac defects) and musculoskeletal issues (limb reduction), low birth weight, smaller head circumference at birth, motor delays, and developmental problems (Landry 2002). However, prospective studies have not consistently found such associations, except for cleft palate. Infants exposed to methamphetamines may experience amphetamine withdrawal syndrome with symptoms like jitteriness, drowsiness, and respiratory distress, though only a few need a pharmacological treatment (Smid et al. 2019). MDMA exposure in the first trimester can lead to long-term memory and learning issues in children.

22.5 Opioids/Opiates in the Perinatal Period

A large cohort study involving pregnant women who use prescription opioids reported a 30–60% increase in the risk of neonatal drug withdrawal associated with co-exposure to other psychotropic drugs compared with opioids alone (Huybrechts et al. 2017). A chronic untreated addiction to heroin in pregnancy has been associated with lack of prenatal care, increased risk of foetal growth restriction, abruptio placentae, foetal death, preterm labour, and intrauterine passage of meconium (CSAT 2005). Babies born from heroin-dependent mothers often present with a neonatal abstinence syndrome, which manifests as restlessness, yawning, acute crying, tremors, watery stools, hypertonia, seizures and vomiting. There is also a risk of sudden unexplained death in infancy (Dryden et al. 2009; Wachman et al. 2011; Hwang et al. 2016; Huybrechts et al. 2017; Flannagan et al. 2020; Varney et al. 2024). According to some studies, naloxone, a specific opioid antagonist, could be used to treat infants with cardiorespiratory or neurological depression due to intrauterine opioid exposure. However, current evidence from randomized controlled trials is insufficient to determine whether naloxone provides significant benefits given some concerns about its safety (Moe-Byrne et al. 2018). Moreover, rates of unwanted pregnancy among women using opioids are remarkably high, with unwanted pregnancies reported in 85% of women using opioids during pregnancy, compared to 45% of the general population (Auerbach et al. 2021). Furthermore, an untreated opioid use disorder has been associated with engagement in high-risk activities, such as prostitution, trading sex for drugs, and criminal activities. Long-term outcomes of infants with in utero opioid exposure have been evaluated in several observational studies, reporting no significant differences in cognitive development between children up to 5 years of age exposed to methadone in utero and control groups matched for age, race and socioeconomic status, although scores were often lower in both groups compared with general population (Kaltenbach and Finnegan 1984).

The safety of opioids during early pregnancy has been evaluated in several observational studies. Earlier reports have not shown an increased risk of birth defects after prenatal exposure to oxycodone, meperidine and propoxyphene (Bracken and Holford 1981; Jick et al. 1981). An association between first-trimester use of codeine and congenital abnormalities has been reported in some studies (Zierler and Rothman 1985; Broussard et al. 2011) but not in others (Shaw et al. 1992; Nezvalova-Henriksen et al. 2011). An observational study found a possible association between use of opioids during the first trimester and neural tube defects (Yazdy et al. 2013; Wang et al. 2022). Some studies have also identified a link between prenatal opioid exposure and birth defects, albeit rare, such as congenital heart defects, cleft palate and clubfoot (Yazdy et al. 2013; Källén et al. 2013; Lind et al. 2017; Wang et al. 2022). Developmental delays in children exposed to opioids are possible compared to their non-exposed peers (Welton et al. 2019).

In contrast, recent studies have shown that tapering the dosage, or carrying out an opioid detoxification, does not increase the risk of adverse pregnancy outcomes, resulting in neither an increased foetal risk associated with detoxification nor an increased risk of preterm delivery (Towers et al. 2020). Comparing detoxification treatment with opioid substitution therapy (ORT) shows an increased risk of relapse with detoxification treatment compared to ORT; however, detoxification does not alter the risk of stillbirth, preterm birth (PTB) nor neonatal abstinence syndrome (NAS) (Wang et al. 2019). Methadone is commonly used as an opioid agonist medication, providing stability of opioid levels, preventing withdrawal cycles, and improving engagement with obstetric care. However, its use is limited by stringent observation protocols and the risk of overdose. Children born to mothers who were prescribed with methadone during pregnancy have a high risk for behavioural problems, poor motor performance, poor fine motor coordination, short attention span, and low cognitive performance. Nystagmus and strabismus are more frequent in methadone-exposed children than in non-methadone-exposed peers (Monnelly et al. 2019). Another alternative to methadone is buprenorphine. As a partial opioid receptor agonist, it has a limiting effect on respiratory depression, reducing the risk of harm in the event of an overdose. It also offers a more favourable neonatal opioid withdrawal profile than methadone and has been associated with more positive neonatal outcomes than methadone. These include better levels of birth weight, longer body length at birth, and reduced risk of prematurity (Kinsella et al. 2022). Pregnant women receiving treatment for opioid use disorder with the buprenorphine-naloxone combination have comparable pregnancy outcomes to those undergoing treatment with other forms of opioid agonist medication-assisted therapy (Link et al. 2020; Ordean and Tubman-Broeren 2023).

Fentanyl, a highly potent synthetic opioid commonly used in patients undergoing general anaesthesia, including women undergoing various surgical procedures during pregnancy and for epidural analgesia during labour, rapidly transfers to the placenta and foetal brain, with detectable accumulation in these tissues (British Columbia Centre on Substance Use 2018; Alipio et al. 2021). Studies in animals suggest prenatal fentanyl exposure may lead to increased newborn mortality, withdrawal symptoms, ADHD, autism-like traits and schizophrenia. These findings highlight the complex risks of opioid exposure during pregnancy, particularly with potent opioids like fentanyl (Wouldes et al. 2023).

22.6 Pharmacological Management of Substance Use Disorders During the Perinatal Period

In general, substance-dependent pregnant women should be optimally treated with a multi-disciplinary and multi-professional approach with treatment being tailored individually to the kind of substance dependence (Woolf et al. 2003; Metz et al. 2012; WHO 2014) (Table 22.1).

There are no officially approved pharmacological treatments for the management of a cannabis use disorder in pregnancy. No medication is approved specifically for the treatment of cannabis intoxication. Pregnant women could usually manifest mild cannabis withdrawal symptoms including sleep disturbances, irritability, loss of appetite, restlessness, nausea and cramps which could be managed by prescribing symptomatic pharmacotherapy (Rayburn and Bogenschutz 2004; CAMH 2012). Evidence advice for all pregnant women is to discontinue cannabis use, although for some women this may not be possible without professional support. Pharmacological interventions for cannabis withdrawal have been explored, though studies often have small sample sizes (Connor et al. 2022). Some trials using standardized withdrawal scoring systems reported better symptom relief with medications compared to placebo. Effective treatments include dronabinol (Levin et al. 2011), quetiapine (Mariani et al. 2021), nabiximols (Trigo et al. 2016), gabapentin (Mason et al. 2012), and oral THC (Budney et al. 2007), which reduced withdrawal symptoms and cravings in cannabis-dependent individuals. To date, dronabinol has been the medication most investigated. Dronabinol has been assigned by the Food and Drug Administration (FDA) to pregnancy category C, i.e., animal studies have revealed evidence of decreased maternal weight gain and decreased number of offspring, increased foetal mortality, and early foetal resorptions. Exposure to dronabinol during pregnancy and lactation in mice caused anxiety-like and depressive behaviours, cognitive impairments, and disruptions in the reward system, with increased motivation for alcohol consumption in offspring. These effects, linked to

Table 22.1 Practical recommendations based on scientific evidence and clinical experience (based on WHO, 2014)

Recommendation(s)
All pregnant women or those planning a pregnancy should be regularly screened for tobacco, caffeine, prescription medications, illicit drugs and legal highs, and engaged in discussion about the risks of SUDs during pregnancy and how to reduce them
Healthcare providers should ask pregnant women about tobacco, caffeine, prescription medications, illicit drugs and legal highs use (past and current) early in pregnancy and at every antenatal visits, as some women could disclose sensitive information and substance-related data, only once trust is established with their clinician
A comprehensive clinical assessment should include: 1. Complete drug history (name of drug, amount, frequency, duration, route of administration, last use, etc.) 2. Clinical and therapeutical staging of SUD 3. Concomitant medical infective, chronic conditions 4. Concomitant medications 5. Psychiatric history 6. Social history (family, custody status, housing condition, legal status, financial status, nutrition, child protection agency involvement, child safety concerns) 7. Investigating about feelings, impressions/ideas, functioning, expectations about pregnancy and drug use
Drug toxicology testing is not recommended for universal screening. Whereas there is a clinical indication, healthcare professionals should ask for a drug screening test just during the first prenatal assessment and, in case of positivity, it should be proposed periodically throughout pregnancy and postpartum (Suspected cases should include women concerned about providing a sample or reluctant to do so. In these cases, healthcare providers should build a trust alliance with the woman and try to collect her informed consent) The urine drug screening testing is appropriate for routine clinical use due to low costs
Before any maternal drug screening and confirmatory tests, informed consent must be obtained from the woman before maternal drug toxicology and documented in the medical record. In case of maternal refusal, clinicians must document the refusal in the medical record and testing should not be performed. It should be recommended, particularly in complex cases, to provide an informative and motivational session to the woman together with her partner/husband/caregiver/family member
Neonatal toxicology testing may be performed without consent of the parent(s) if the person requesting this testing has a legislative right to make decisions for the infant to be tested. Parent(s) should be informed that the neonate is being tested
Healthcare providers should apply a flexible and non-judgemental approach when caring for a woman with substance use problems. A trusting, collaborative and empowering relationship could improve treatment adherence and follow-up clinical monitoring
Healthcare providers should be skilled in providing a "brief individual therapeutic intervention" (5–30 min) comprising a motivational approach to implement harm reduction strategies and a psychoeducational approach to reduce/limit substance use during pregnancy, with follow-up and potential referral to treatment if necessary

(continued)

Table 22.1 (continued)

Recommendation(s)
Healthcare providers should be aware about high concurrent prevalence of trauma (i.e., sexual and physical abuse) history among SUD women. Therefore, clinicians should be adequately skilled in a trauma-informed practice (e.g., trauma awareness, safety and trustworthiness, choice, collaboration and connection; strengths-based approaches and skill building)
Pregnant women dependent on alcohol or drugs should be advised to cease the use and referred to detox services if needed. Withdrawal from opioids may require treatment. Methadone or buprenorphine can be used for opioid dependence
Opiate-dependent women should be informed that neonates exposed to opiates, prescription opioids, methadone, or buprenorphine during pregnancy are monitored closely for symptoms and signs of neonatal withdrawal (neonatal abstinence syndrome)
Hospitals providing obstetric care should develop a protocol for identification, assessment, monitoring and management of neonates exposed to substances of abuse during pregnancy
The withdrawal syndrome from other substances, such as psychostimulants, has not been deemed sufficient to warrant the use of psychotropic medication
Combining psychosocial support (cognitive-behavioural therapy and motivational enhancement) with pharmacotherapy is recommended as it has been shown to be superior to pharmacotherapy alone
Treatment should provide interventions also addressed to the mother-infant dyad (e.g., assessing motivation and exploring ideas for change; developing a holistic treatment plan, not only medical but also social; promoting strategies for managing stress; considering nutritional asset, housing and security needs, etc.)
Whereas available, harm reduction strategies should be implemented to reduce substance-related consequences, including HIV and hepatitis C infection, overdose death, and improve neonatal outcomes (i.e., fewer preterm births, higher birth weights, etc.)
Antenatal planning for intrapartum and postpartum analgesia may be offered for all women in consultation with appropriate healthcare providers

neurodevelopment-related gene and protein changes, were sex-dependent (Navarro et al. 2024). Cognitive-behavioural therapy, motivational enhancement and contingency management therapies have been demonstrated to be effective for reducing cannabis use in women, even though they have not been specifically studied amongst pregnant women. Studies on interventions for substance use during pregnancy found that both electronic screening with brief intervention and tailored text messaging were feasible and acceptable. For treating cannabis use disorder, psychotherapeutic approaches, including cognitive-behavioural therapy, motivational enhancement therapy, and abstinence-based incentives, remain the most effective, as no pharmacological treatments have proven to be clinically effective (Ondersma et al. 2012; Hayer et al. 2023).

Regarding cocaine use disorder, evidence recommends psychosocial and psychotherapeutic interventions, including cognitive-behavioural therapies (CBT), community reinforcement approach, seeking safety, motivational interviewing, rather than psychopharmacotherapy (SAMHSA 2010). In fact, there is currently no approved pharmacological treatment for cocaine dependence. Some researchers proposed disulfiram, a medication approved to treat alcohol use disorder, which indeed is contraindicated during pregnancy (Traccis et al. 2024). For the management of other stimulant use disorders, evidence recommends psychosocial and psychotherapeutic interventions, particularly addressing drug-using behaviours and lifestyles which could negatively affect the baby's needs (McCarthy et al. 2009). As there are currently no replacement therapies for amphetamine dependence, the pregnant amphetamine user must be encouraged to moderate and cease drug use, but this may be an unrealistic expectation. A priority in prenatal care for the known amphetamine user is to ensure that she has adequate shelter and nutrition, that co-existing psychiatric morbidities are optimally treated, and that she is encouraged to attend regular antenatal care (Good et al. 2010). While there are currently no medical treatments specifically for ecstasy addiction, behavioural therapy may be beneficial (Savard et al. 2024).

The first-line treatment for opioid-dependent pregnant women is opioid maintenance therapy (OMT) with methadone or alternatively buprenorphine (Winklbaur-Hausknost et al. 2013). It has been well-documented and demonstrated that OMT may outweigh any neonatal risks associated with opioid agonists (British Columbia Centre on Substance Use 2018). OMT may eliminate or substantially reduce non-medical opioid use and associated health risks, leading to improved neonatal outcomes in comparison to untreated opioid use disorder and/or rapid withdrawal management (WHO 2009; Minozzi et al. 2013). Treatment with methadone improves outcomes compared to heroin but it may negatively impact the pregnancy outcomes (Zelson et al. 1973; Finnegan 1978; Olofsson et al. 1983a, b). Methadone crosses the placenta, impacting foetal motor activity, breathing, heart rate and neurodevelopment. Infants exposed to methadone are at higher risk of preterm birth and, if born at term, are smaller for gestational age (i.e., they display low weight, low height, and reduced head circumference) than those exposed to non-opioid drugs. Additionally, methadone-exposed infants face an increased risk of sudden unexpected death in infancy, strabismus, nystagmus and hyaline membrane disease compared to non-opioid-exposed infants (Jansson et al. 2005, 2009; Walhovd et al. 2012; Wouldes et al. 2020). Although methadone represents the most frequently prescribed OAT during pregnancy, growing scientific evidence levels support the equal efficacy and potentially superior safety of buprenorphine and buprenorphine/naloxone for the treatment of opioid use disorder in pregnancy (Jones et al. 2008, 2010; Minozzi et al. 2013; Noormohammadi et al. 2016; Zedler et al. 2016). However, the benefits may also be linked to social or psychological factors (Piske et al. 2021; Kinsella et al. 2022; Suarez et al. 2022; Wouldes et al. 2023). Buprenorphine combined with naloxone is typically used to treat opioid use disorders outside of pregnancy, but during pregnancy buprenorphine alone is preferred due to limited safety data on the combination. However, the few studies conducted show that pregnant women treated with buprenorphine-naloxone generally have similar pregnancy outcomes to those receiving other opioid agonist therapies (Link et al. 2020; Mullins et al. 2020). However, unless clinically indicated, transitioning between methadone, buprenorphine/naloxone and slow-release oral morphine is not advisable for pregnant women stable on one of these agents during pregnancy and postpartum period, as reducing and titrating medication dosage during transition may determine a re-emergence of withdrawal symptoms and increase the risk of relapse (British Columbia Centre on Substance Use 2018). The continuity of care and adequate suppression of withdrawal symptoms during pregnancy represent the most important factors associated with improved maternal and neonatal outcomes (Wright et al. 2016; American Society of Addiction Medicine 2017).

22.7 Conclusions

Although obtaining clear and accurate prevalence data on SUDs in pregnancy remains extremely complex primarily due to the stigma and prejudice against pregnant women who use substances, it is widely recognized that SUDs in pregnancy and perinatal period should be early identified; carefully managed; and properly treated in order to protect and adequately treat the dyad mother-foetus/newborn. All substances largely and variably pass across the placenta during pregnancy, by affecting both gestational and neonatal outcomes. Thus, the foetus may be exposed to substances of abuse and their potential complications during pregnancy. Risks associated with the exposure comprise a set of variable outcomes depending on the type of substance taken by the mother, the timing of the intake, the pattern of substance use, and so forth. Most commonly reported detrimental outcomes include organ minor and/or major malformations (teratogenicity), obstetrical complications (i.e., preterm delivery, low birth rate, delivery complications, low Apgar score), perinatal complications (i.e., neonatal toxicity which includes behavioural symptoms appearing immediately after birth such as jitteriness) and long-term postnatal behavioural and mental consequences (e.g., behavioural teratogenicity).

References

Ainiti DF, Lykeridou A, Nanou C, Deltsidou A. Cannabis use during pregnancy and its effect on the fetus, newborn and later childhood: a systematic review. Eur J Midwifery. 2023;7:19. https://doi.org/10.18332/ejm/168727.

Al-Hayani A, Wease KN, Ross RA, Pertwee RG, Davies SN. The endogenous cannabinoid anandamide activates vanilloid receptors in the rat hippocampal slice. Neuropharmacology. 2001;41(8):1000–5.

Alipio JB, Haga C, Fox ME, Arakawa K, Balaji R, Cramer N, Lobo MK, Keller A. Perinatal fentanyl exposure leads to long-lasting impairments in somatosensory circuit function and behavior. J Neurosci. 2021;41(15):3400–17. https://doi.org/10.1523/JNEUROSCI.2470-20.2020.

American College of Obstetricians and Gynecologists. ACOG Committee opinion no. 722: marijuana use during pregnancy and lactation. Obstet Gynecol. 2017;130:e205.

American Psychiatric Association. Diagnostic and statistical manual of mental disorders: diagnostic and statistical manual of mental disorders. 5th ed. Arlington: American Psychiatric Association; 2022.

American Society of Addiction Medicine. Substance Use, Misuse, and Use Disorders During and Following Pregnancy, with an Emphasis on Opioids. January 18, 2017. Available from: http://www.asam.org/advocacy/and-a-policy-statement/view-policy-statement/public-policy-statements/2017/01/19/substance-use-misuse-and-use-disorders-during-and-following-pregnancy-with-an-emphasis-on-opioids

Arabzadeh H, Doosti-Irani A, Kamkari S, Farhadian M, Elyasi E, Mohammadi Y. The maternal factors associated with infant low birth weight: an umbrella review. BMC Pregnancy Childbirth. 2024;24(1):316. https://doi.org/10.1186/s12884-024-06487-y.

Arafa A, Sheerah HA, Alzaydan OK, Sabr Y. The association between antenatal tea drinking and hypertensive disorders of pregnancy: a systematic review and meta-analysis. Epidemiologia. 2024;5(2):200–10. https://doi.org/10.3390/epidemiologia5020014.

Auerbach SL, Agbemenu K, Ely GE, Lorenz R. A review of unintended pregnancy in opioid-using women: implications for nursing. J Addict Nurs. 2021;32(2):107–14. https://doi.org/10.1097/JAN.0000000000000396.

Bandstra ES, Vogel AL, Morrow CE, Xue L, Anthony JC. Severity of prenatal cocaine exposure and child language functioning through age seven years: a longitudinal latent growth curve analysis. Substance Use Misuse. 2004;39:25–59.

Betancourt LM, Yang W, Brodsky NL, Gallagher PR, Malmud EK, Giannetta JM, Farah MJ, Hurt H. Adolescents with and without gestational cocaine exposure: longitudinal analysis of inhibitory control, memory and receptive language. Neurotoxicol Teratol. 2011;33(1):36–46. https://doi.org/10.1016/j.ntt.2010.08.004.

Billing L, Eriksson M, Larsson G, Zetterström R. Amphetamine addiction and pregnancy. III. One year follow-up of the children. Psychosocial and pediatric aspects. Acta Paediatr Scand. 1980;69:675–80.

Bracken MB, Holford TR. Exposure to prescribed drugs in pregnancy and association with congenital malformations. Obstet Gynecol. 1981;58:336–44.

British Columbia Centre on Substance Use. B.C. Ministry of Health, B.C. Ministry of Mental Health and Addictions, & Perinatal Services BC. A Guideline for the Clinical Management of Opioid Use Disorder – Pregnancy Supplement. Published June 1, 2018. Available at: http://www.bccsu.ca/care-guid-ance-publications/

Broussard CS, Rasmussen SA, Reefhuis J, Friedman JM, Jann MW, Riehle-Colarusso T, et al. Maternal treatment with opioid analgesics and risk for birth defects. National Birth Defects Prevention Study. Am J Obstet Gynecol. 2011;204(314):e1–11.

Brown JD, Winterstein AG. Potential adverse drug events and drug-drug interactions with medical and consumer Cannabidiol (CBD) use. J Clin Med. 2019;8(7):989. https://doi.org/10.3390/jcm8070989.

Budney AJ, Vandrey RG, Hughes JR, Moore BA, Bahrenburg B. Oral delta-9-tetrahydrocannabinol suppresses cannabis withdrawal symptoms. Drug Alcohol Depend. 2007;86(1):22–9. https://doi.org/10.1016/j.drugalcdep.2006.04.014.

Bushi G, Khatib MN, Balaraman AK, Ballal S, Bansal P, Tomar BS, Ashraf A, Kumar MR, Sinha A, Rawat P, Gaidhane AM, Sah S, Syed R, Sharma G, Mehta RAGMT, Chilakam N, Pandey S, Brar M, Shabil M. Prevalence of dual use of combustible tobacco and E-cigarettes among pregnant smokers: a systematic review and meta-analysis. BMC Public Health. 2024;24(1):3200. https://doi.org/10.1186/s12889-024-20746-9.

CAMH. The Centre for Addiction and Mental Health; 2012. Available at: http://knowledgex.camh.net/primary_ care/guidelines_materials/pregnancy_lactation/pages/ per_cannabis.aspx. Accessed August 25, 2018.

Carlier J, Huestis MA, Zaami S, Pichini S, Busardò FP. Monitoring perinatal exposure to cannabis and synthetic cannabinoids. Ther Drug Monit. 2020;42(2):194204. https://doi.org/10.1097/FTD.0000000000000667.

Catanzarite VA, Stein DA. 'Crystal' and pregnancy – methamphetamine-associated maternal deaths. West J Med. 1995;162:454–7.

Chang L, Smith LM, LoPresti C, Yonekura ML, Kuo J, Walot I, Ernst T. Smaller subcortical volumes and cognitive deficits in children with prenatal methamphetamine exposure. Psychiatry Res. 2004;132(2):95–106. https://doi.org/10.1016/j.pscychresns.2004.06.004.

Chavkin W. Cocaine and pregnancy – time to look at the evidence. JAMA. 2001;285(12):1626–8.

Chen B, Zhang M, He Y, Si Y, Shi Y, Jiang K, Shen J, Hong J, Ni S. The association between caffeine exposure during pregnancy and risk of gestational hypertension/preeclampsia: a meta-analysis and systematical review. J Obstet Gynaecol Res. 2022;48(12):3045–55. https://doi.org/10.1111/jog.15445.

Connor JP, Stjepanović D, Budney AJ, Le Foll B, Hall WD. Clinical management of cannabis withdrawal. Addiction. 2022;117(7):2075–95. https://doi.org/10.1111/add.15743.

Cox S, Posner SF, Kourtis AP, Jamieson DJ. Hospitalizations with amphetamine abuse among pregnant women. Obstet Gynecol. 2008;111(2):341–7.

Cressman AM, Natekar A, Kim E, Koren G, Bozzo P. Cocaine abuse during pregnancy. Journal of obstetrics and gynaecology Canada: JOGC = Journal d'obstetrique et gynecologie du Canada: JOGC. 2014;36(7):628–31. https://doi.org/10.1016/S1701-2163(15)30543-0.

CSAT (Center for Substance Abuse Treatment). Medication-assisted treatment for opioid addiction during pregnancy. In: Medication-assisted treatment for opioid addiction in opioid treatment programs. Treatment Improvement Protocol (TIP) Series, No. 43. Rockville (MD): Substance Abuse and Mental Health Services Administration; 2005: 211–24.

Day NL, Cottreau CM, Richardson GA. The epidemiology of alcohol, marijuana, and cocaine use among women of childbearing age and pregnant women. Clin Obstet Gynecol. 1993;36(2):232–45.

Delker E, Baer RJ, Kelly AE, Chambers C, Bandoli G. Prenatal cannabis use disorder and gastroschisis in California, 2007-19. Int J Epidemiol. 2024;53(2):dyae042. https://doi.org/10.1093/ije/dyae042.

Derauf C, LaGasse LL, Smith LM, et al. Prenatal methamphetamine exposure and inhibitory control among young school-age children. J Pediatr. 2012;161(3):452–9.

DeVuono MV, Nashed MG, Sarikahya MH, Kocsis A, Lee K, Vanin SR, Hudson R, Lonnee EP, Rushlow WJ, Hardy DB, Laviolette SR. Prenatal tetrahydrocannabinol and cannabidiol exposure produce sex-specific pathophysiological phenotypes in the adolescent prefrontal cortex and hippocampus. Neurobiol Dis. 2024;199:106588. https://doi.org/10.1016/j.nbd.2024.106588.

Diaz SD, Smith LM, LaGasse LL, et al. Effects of prenatal methamphetamine exposure on behavioral and cognitive findings at 7.5 years of age. J Pediatr. 2014;164(6):1333–8.

Dixon SD, Bejar R. Echoencephalographic findings in neonates associated with maternal cocaine and methamphetamine use: incidence and clinical correlates. J Pediatr. 1989;115:770–8.

Dryden C, Young D, Hepburn M, Mactier H. Maternal methadone use in pregnancy: factors associated with the development of neonatal abstinence syndrome and implications for healthcare resources. BJOG. 2009;116(5):665–71.

EMCDDA. European Monitoring Centre for Drugs and Drug Addiction. 2024.

Eriksson M, Larsson G, Winbladh B, Zetterström R. The influence of amphetamine addiction onpregnancy and the newborn infant. Acta Paediatr Scand. 1978;67:95–9.

Eriksson M, Larsson G, Zetterström R. Amphetamine addiction and pregnancy. II. Pregnancy, delivery, and the neonatal period. Socio-medical aspects. Acta Obstet Gynecol Scand. 1981;60:253–9.

Evanski JM, Zundel CG, Baglot SL, Desai S, Gowatch LC, Ely SL, Sadik N, Lundahl LH, Hill MN, Marusak HA. The first hit to the endocannabinoid system? Associations between prenatal cannabis exposure and Frontolimbic white matter pathways in children. Biol Psychiatry Glob Open Sci. 2023;4(1):11–8. https://doi.org/10.1016/j.bpsgos.2023.09.005.

FDA. United States Department of Health and Human Services, U.S. Food and Drug Administration. (2019). FDA regulation of cannabis and cannabis-derived products: Questions and answers. Retrieved from https://www.fda.gov/news-events/public-healthfocus/fda-regulation-cannabis-and-cannabis-derivedproducts-questions-and-answers#cosmetics

Finnegan LP. Management of pregnant drug-dependent women. Ann New York Acad Sci. 1978;311:135–46. https://doi.org/10.1111/j.1749-6632.1978.tb16770.x.

Fisk JE, Montgomery C, Wareing M, Murphy PN. Reasoning deficits in ecstasy (MDMA) polydrug users. Psychopharmacology. 2005;181:550–9.

Flannagan KS, Sjaarda LA, Mumford SL, Schisterman EF. Prescription opioid use among populations of reproductive age: effects on fertility, pregnancy loss, and pregnancy complications. Epidemiol Rev. 2020;42(1):117–33. https://doi.org/10.1093/epirev/mxaa007.

Frary CD, Johnson RK, Wang MQ. Food sources and intakes of caffeine in the diets of persons in the United States. J Am Diet Assoc. 2005;105(1):110–3. https://doi.org/10.1016/j.jada.2004.10.027.

Gerede A, Stavros S, Chatzakis C, Vavoulidis E, Papasozomenou P, Domali E, Nikolettos K, Oikonomou E, Potiris A, Tsikouras P, Nikolettos N. Cannabis use during pregnancy: an update. Medicina (Kaunas, Lithuania). 2024;60(10):1691. https://doi.org/10.3390/medicina60101691.

Good MM, Solt I, Acuna JG, Rotmensch S, Kim MJ. Methamphetamine use during pregnancy: maternal and neonatal implications. Obstet Gynecol. 2010;116(2 Pt 1):330–4.

Gouin K, Murphy K, Shah PS. Effects of cocaine use during pregnancy on low birthweight and preterm birth: systematic review and metaanalyses. Am J Obstet Gynecol. 2011;204(4):340.

Gould GS, Havard A, Lim LL. The Psanz Smoking In Pregnancy Expert Group, & Kumar, R. Exposure to Tobacco, Environmental Tobacco Smoke and Nicotine in Pregnancy: A Pragmatic Overview of Reviews of Maternal and Child Outcomes, Effectiveness of Interventions and Barriers and Facilitators to Quitting. Int J Environ Res Public Health. 2020;17(6):2034. https://doi.org/10.3390/ijerph17062034.

Greenwood DC, Thatcher NJ, Ye J, Garrard L, Keogh G, King LG, Cade JE. Caffeine intake during pregnancy and adverse birth outcomes: a systematic review and dose-response meta-analysis. Eur J Epidemiol. 2014;29(10):725–34. https://doi.org/10.1007/s10654-014-9944-x.

Gurm H, Hirota JA, Raha S. Cannabinoid signalling in immune-reproductive crosstalk during human pregnancy. Biomedicine. 2021;9(3):267. https://doi.org/10.3390/biomedicines9030267.

Hanuš LO. Discovery and isolation of anandamide and other endocannabinoids. Chem Biodivers. 2007;4(8):1828–41.

Haustein K. Cigarette smoking, nicotine and pregnancy. Int J Clin Pharmacol Ther. 1999;37:417–27.

Havard A, Chandran JJ, Oei JL. Tobacco use during pregnancy. Addiction. 2022;117(6):1801–10. https://doi.org/10.1111/add.15792.

Hayer S, Mandelbaum AD, Watch L, Ryan KS, Hedges MA, Manuzak JA, Easley CA 4th, Schust DJ, Lo JO. Cannabis and pregnancy: a review. Obstet Gynecol Surv. 2023;78(7):411–28. https://doi.org/10.1097/OGX.0000000000001159.

Honein MA, Paulozzi LJ, Watkins ML. Maternal smoking and birth defects: validity of birth certificate data for effect estimation. Public Health Rep. 2001;116:327–55.

Huybrechts KF, Bateman BT, Desai RJ, Hernandez-Diaz S, Rough K, Mogun H, Kerzner LS, Davis JM, Stover M, Bartels D, Cottral J, Patorno E. Risk of neonatal drug withdrawal after intrauterine co-exposure to opioids and psychotropic medications: cohort study. BMJ. 2017:358. https://doi.org/10.1136/bmj.j3326.

Hwang CS, Kang EM, Kornegay CJ, et al. Trends in the concomitant prescribing of opioids and benzodiazepines, 2002-2014. Am J Prev Med. 2016;51(2):151–60.

Jablonski SA, Williams MT, Vorhees CV. Mechanisms involved in the neurotoxic and cognitive effects of developmental methamphetamine exposure. Birth Defects Res C Embryo Today Reviews. 2016;108(2):131–41. https://doi.org/10.1002/bdrc.21130.

Jackson MA, Baker AL, Gould GS, Brown AL, Dunlop AJ, McCarter K. Smoking cessation interventions for pregnant women attending treatment for substance use disorders: a systematic review. Addiction. 2022;117(4):847–60. https://doi.org/10.1111/add.15663.

Jansson LM, Dipietro J, Elko A. Fetal response to maternal methadone administration. Am J Obstet Gynecol. 2005;193(3 Pt 1):611–7. https://doi.org/10.1016/j.ajog.2005.02.075.

Jansson LM, Dipietro JA, Velez M, Elko A, Knauer H, Kivlighan KT. Maternal methadone dosing schedule and fetal neurobehaviour. The journal of maternal-fetal & neonatal medicine : the official journal of the European Association of Perinatal Medicine, the Federation of Asia and Oceania Perinatal Societies, the International Society of Perinatal Obstetricians. 2009;22(1):29–35. https://doi.org/10.1080/14767050802452291.

Jarlenski M, Barry CL, Gollust S, Graves AJ, Kennedy-Hendricks A, Kozhimannil K. Polysubstance use among US women of reproductive age who use opioids for nonmedical reasons. Am J Public Health. 2017;107(8):1308–10.

Jick H, Holmes LB, Hunter JR, Madsen S, Stergachis A. First-trimester drug use and congenital disorders. JAMA. 1981;246:343–6.

Jones HE, Martin PR, Heil SH, Kaltenbach K, Selby P, Coyle MG, Stine SM, O'Grady KE, Arria AM, Fischer G. Treatment of opioid dependent pregnant women: clinical and research issues. J Subst Abus Treat. 2008;35(3):245–59.

Jones HE, Kaltenbach K, Heil SH, Stine SM, Coyle MG, Arria AM, O'Grady KE, Selby P, Martin PR, Fisher G. Neonatal abstinence syndrome after methadone or buprenorphine exposure. N Engl J Med. 2010;363(24):2320–31.

Kaiser L, Allen LH, American Dietetic Association. Position of the American dietetic association: nutrition and lifestyle for a healthy pregnancy outcome. J Am Diet Assoc. 2008;108(3):553–61. https://doi.org/10.1016/j.jada.2008.01.030.

Kalaitzopoulos DR, Chatzistergiou K, Amylidi AL, Kokkinidis DG, Goulis DG. Effect of methamphetamine hydrochloride on pregnancy outcome: a systematic review and meta-analysis. J Addict Med. 2018;12(3):220–6.

Källén B, Borg N, Reis M. The use of central nervous system active drugs during pregnancy. Pharmaceuticals (Basel, Switzerland). 2013;6(10):1221–86. https://doi.org/10.3390/ph6101221.

Kaltenbach K, Finnegan LP. Developmental outcome of children born to methadone maintained women: a review of longitudinal studies. Neurobehav Toxicol Teratol. 1984;6:271–5.

Kandel DB, Huang FY, Davies M. Comorbidity between patterns of substance use dependence and psychiatric syndromes. Drug Alcohol Depend. 2001;64(2):233–41.

Kapaya M, D'Angelo DV, Tong VT, England L, Ruffo N, Cox S, Warner L, Bombard J, Guthrie T, Lampkins A, King BA. Use of electronic vapor products before, during, and after pregnancy among women with a recent live birth – Oklahoma and Texas, 2015. Morb Mortal Wkly Rep. 2019;68(8):189.

Kiblawi ZN, Smith LM, Diaz SD, et al. Prenatal methamphetamine exposure and neonatal and infant neurobehavioral outcome: results from the IDEAL study. Subst Abus. 2014;35(1):68–73.

Kinsella M, Halliday LOE, Shaw M, Capel Y, Nelson SM, Kearns RJ. Buprenorphine compared with methadone in pregnancy: a systematic review and meta-analysis. Subst Use Misuse. 2022;57(9):1400–16. https://doi.org/10.1080/10826084.2022.2083174.

Klebanoff MA, Wilkins DG, Keim SA. Marijuana use during pregnancy and preterm birth: a prospective cohort study. Am J Perinatol. 2021;38(S 01):e146–54. https://doi.org/10.1055/s-0040-1708802.

LaGasse LL, Derauf C, Smith LM, et al. Prenatal methamphetamine exposure and childhood behavior problems at 3 and 5 years of age. Pediatrics. 2012;129:2011–209.

Landry MJ. MDMA: a review of epidemiological data. J Psychoactive Drugs. 2002;34(2):163–9.

Lange S, Probst C, Rehm J, Popova S. National, regional, and global prevalence of smoking during pregnancy in the general population: a systematic review and meta-analysis. Lancet Global Health. 2018;6(7):e769.

Levin FR, Mariani JJ, Brooks DJ, Pavlicova M, Cheng W, Nunes EV. Dronabinol for the treatment of cannabis dependence: a randomized, double-blind, placebo-controlled trial. Drug Alcohol Depend. 2011;116(1–3):142–50. https://doi.org/10.1016/j.drugalcdep.2010.12.010.

Lind JN, Interrante JD, Ailes EC, Gilboa SM, Khan S, Frey MT, Dawson AL, Honein MA, Dowling NF, Razzaghi H, Creanga AA, Broussard CS. Maternal use of opioids during pregnancy and congenital malformations: a systematic review. Pediatrics. 2017;139(6):e20164131. https://doi.org/10.1542/peds.2016-4131.

Link HM, Jones H, Miller L, Kaltenbach K, Seligman N. Buprenorphine-naloxone use in pregnancy: a systematic review and metaanalysis. Am J Obstet Gynecol MFM. 2020;2(3):100179. https://doi.org/10.1016/j.ajogmf.2020.100179.

Malanga CJ, Kosofsky BE. Mechanisms of action of drugs of abuse on the developing foetal brain. ClinPerinatol. 1999;26:17–37.

Mariani JJ, Pavlicova M, Jean Choi C, Basaraba C, Carpenter KM, Mahony AL, Brooks DJ, Bisaga A, Naqvi N, Nunes EV, Levin FR. Quetiapine treatment for cannabis use disorder. Drug Alcohol Depend. 2021;218:108366. https://doi.org/10.1016/j.drugalcdep.2020.108366.

Mason BJ, Crean R, Goodell V, Light JM, Quello S, Shadan F, Buffkins K, Kyle M, Adusumalli M, Begovic A, Rao S. A proof-of-concept randomized controlled study of gabapentin: effects on cannabis use, withdrawal and executive function deficits in cannabis-dependent adults. Neuropsychopharmacology : official publication of the American College of Neuropsychopharmacology. 2012;37(7):1689–98. https://doi.org/10.1038/npp.2012.14.

McCarthy S, Cranswick N, Potts L, Taylor E, Wong IC. Mortality associated with attention-deficit hyperactivity disorder (ADHD) drug treatment: a retrospective cohort study of children, adolescents and young adults using the general practice research database. Drug Saf. 2009;32(11):1089–96.

Metz V, Köchl B, Fischer G. Should pregnant women with substance use disorders be managed differently? Neuropsychiatry (London). 2012;2(1):29–41.

Miller CL, Kerr T, Fischer B, Zhang R, Wood E. Methamphetamine injection independently predicts hepatitis C infection among street-involved youth in a Canadian setting. J Adolesc Health. 2009;44(3):302–4.

Miller J, Carbone-Lopez K, Gunderman MV. Gendered narratives of self, addiction, and recovery among women methamphetamine users. In: Narrative criminology: understanding stories of crime; 2015. p. 69–95.

Minnes S, Singer LT, Arendt R, Satayathum S. Effects of prenatal cocaine/polydrug use on maternal–infant feeding interactions during the first year of life. Dev Behav Pediatr. 2005;26:194–200.

Minozzi S, Amato L, Bellisario C, Ferri M, Davoli M. Maintenance agonist treatments for opiate-dependent pregnant women. Cochrane Database Syst Rev. 2013;12:Cd006318.

Moe-Byrne T, Brown JVE, McGuire W. Naloxone for opioid-exposed newborn infants. Cochrane Database Syst Rev. 2018;10(10):CD003483. https://doi.org/10.1002/14651858.CD003483.pub3.

Monnelly VJ, Hamilton R, Chappell FM, Mactier H, Boardman JP. Childhood neurodevelopment after prescription of maintenance methadone for opioid dependency in pregnancy: a systematic review and meta-analysis. Dev Med Child Neurol. 2019;61(7):750–60. https://doi.org/10.1111/dmcn.14117.

Moore DG, Turner JD, Parrott AC, Goodwin JE, Fulton SE, Min MO, Fox HC, Braddick FM, Axelsson EL, Lynch S, Ribeiro H, Frostick CJ, Singer LT. During pregnancy, recreational drug-using women stop taking ecstasy (3,4-methylenedioxy-N-methylamphetamine) and reduce alcohol consumption but continue to smoke tobacco and cannabis initial findings from the development and infancy study. J Psychopharmacol. 2009;24:1403. https://doi.org/10.1177/0269881109348165.

Morrow CE, Bandstra ES, Anthony JC, Ofir AY, Xue L, Reyes MB. Influence of prenatal cocaine exposure on early language development: longitudinal findings from four months to three years of age. J Dev Behav Pediatr. 2003;24:39–50.

Mullins N, Galvin SL, Ramage M, Gannon M, Lorenz K, Sager B, Coulson CC. Buprenorphine and naloxone versus buprenorphine for opioid use disorder in pregnancy: a cohort study. J Addict Med. 2020;14(3):185–92. https://doi.org/10.1097/ADM.0000000000000562.

Murnan AW, Keim SA, Yeates KO, Boone KM, Sheppard KW, Klebanoff MA. Behavioral and cognitive differences in early childhood related to prenatal marijuana exposure. J Appl Dev Psychol. 2021;77:101348. https://doi.org/10.1016/j.appdev.2021.101348.

National Council of State Boards of Nursing. The NCSBN national nursing guidelines for medical marijuana. J Nurs Regul. 2018;9(Suppl. 2):S1–S60.

National Survey on Drug Use and Health. United States Department of Health and Human Services. Substance Abuse and Mental Health Services Administration. Office of Applied Studies. National Survey on Drug Use and Health, 2007. Ann Arbor, MI: Inter-university Consortium for Political and Social Research [distributor], 2015-11-23. https://doi.org/10.3886/ICPSR23782.v5.

Navarro D, Gasparyan A, Navarrete F, Manzanares J. Fetal cannabinoid syndrome: Behavioral and brain alterations of the offspring exposed to Dronabinol during gestation and lactation. Int J Mol Sci. 2024;25(13):7453. https://doi.org/10.3390/ijms25137453.

Nezvalova-Henriksen K, Spigset O, Nordeng H. Effects of codeine on pregnancy outcome: results from a large population-based cohort study. Eur J Clin Pharmacol. 2011;67:1253–61.

Noormohammadi A, Forinash A, Yancey A, Crannage E, Campbell K, Shyken J. Buprenorphine versus methadone for opioid dependence in pregnancy. Ann Pharmacother. 2016;50(8):666–72.

Olofsson M, Buckley W, Andersen GE, Friis-Hansen B. Investigation of 89 children born by drug-dependent mothers. I Neonatal course. Acta Paediatr Scand. 1983a;72(3):403–6. https://doi.org/10.1111/j.1651-2227.1983.tb09736.x.

Olofsson M, Buckley W, Andersen GE, Friis-Hansen B. Investigation of 89 children born by drugdependent mothers. II. Follow-up 1-10 years after birth. Acta Paediatr Scand. 1983b;72(3):407–10. https://doi.org/10.1111/j.1651-2227.1983.tb09737.x.

Ondersma SJ, Svikis DS, LeBreton JM, Streiner DL, Grekin ER, Lam PK, Connors-Burge V. Development and preliminary validation of an indirect screener for drug use in the perinatal period. Addiction. 2012;107(12):2099–106. https://doi.org/10.1111/j.1360-0443.2012.03982.x.

Ordean A, Tubman-Broeren M. Safety and efficacy of buprenorphine-naloxone in pregnancy: a systematic review of the literature. Pathophysiology. 2023;30(1):27–36. https://doi.org/10.3390/pathophysiology30010004.

Oro AS, Dixon SD. Perinatal cocaine and methamphetamine exposure: maternal and neonatal correlates. J Pediatr. 1987;111(4):571–8.

Orsolini L, Papanti D, Corkery J, De Luca MA, Cadoni C, Di Chiara G, Schifano F. Is there a teratogenicity risk associated with cannabis and synthetic Cannabimimetics' ('spice') intake? CNS Neurol Disord Drug Targets. 2017;16(5):585–91. https://doi.org/10.2174/1871527316666170413101257.

Pacho M, Aymerich C, Pedruzo B, Salazar de Pablo G, Sesma E, Bordenave M, Dieguez R, Lopez-Zorroza I, Herrero J, Laborda M, Fernandez-Rivas A, Garcia-Rizo C, Gonzalez-Torres MA, Catalan A. Substance use during pregnancy and risk of postpartum depression: a systematic review and metaanalysis. Front Psych. 2023;14:1264998. https://doi.org/10.3389/fpsyt.2023.1264998.

Paul SE, Hatoum AS, Fine JD, Johnson EC, Hansen I, Karcher NR, Moreau AL, Qu Y, Carter EB, Rogers CE, Agrawal A, Barch DM, Bogdan R. Associations between prenatal cannabis exposure and childhood outcomes: results from the ABCD study. JAMA Psychiatry. 2021;78(1):64–76. https://doi.org/10.1001/jamapsychiatry.2020.2902.

Peltier MR, Roberts W, Verplaetse TL, Burke C, Zakiniaeiz Y, Moore K, McKee SA. Licit and illicit drug use across trimesters in pregnant women endorsing past-year substance use: results from National Survey on drug use and health (2009-2019). Arch Womens Ment Health. 2022;25(4):819–27. https://doi.org/10.1007/s00737-022-01244-6.

Pentecost R, Schmidt K, Grassley JS. Health care providers' perceived barriers to screening for substance use during pregnancy. Nurs Womens Health. 2021;25(4):272–7. https://doi.org/10.1016/j.nwh.2021.05.002.

Pertwee RG. Receptors targeted by synthetic cannabinoid receptor agonists and antagonists. Curr Med Chem. 2010;17(14):1360–81.

Piske M. et al. Opioid use disorder and perinatal outcomes. Pediatrics. 2021; Kinsella M et al. Opioid substitution in pregnancy a narrative review: contemporary evidence for use of methadone and buprenorphine in pregnancy. J Subst Use. 2022

Plessinger MA. Prenatal exposure to amphetamines. Risks and adverse outcomes in pregnancy. Obstet Gynecol Clin N Am. 1998;25:119–38.

Plessinger MA, Woods JR Jr. The cardiovascular effects of cocaine use in pregnancy. Reprod Toxicol. 1991;5(2):99–113.

Portillo R, Abad C, Synova T, Kastner P, Heblik D, Kucera R, Karahoda R, Staud F. Cannabidiol disrupts tryptophan metabolism in the human term placenta. Toxicology. 2024;505:153813. https://doi.org/10.1016/j.tox.2024.153813.

Psychoyos D, Vinod KY. Marijuana, spice 'herbal high', and early neural development: implications for rescheduling and legalization. Drug Test Anal. 2013;5(1):27–45. https://doi.org/10.1002/dta.1390.

Puga TB, Dai HD, Wang Y, Theye E. Maternal tobacco use during pregnancy and child neurocognitive development. JAMA Netw Open. 2024;7(2):e2355952. https://doi.org/10.1001/jamanetworkopen.2023.55952.

Raghunathan R, Liu CH, Kouka A, Singh M, Miranda RC, Larin KV. Assessing the acute effects of prenatal synthetic cannabinoid exposure on murine fetal brain vasculature using optical coherence tomography. J Biophotonics. 2019;12(8):e201900050. https://doi.org/10.1002/jbio.201900050.

Rayburn WF, Bogenschutz MP. Pharmacotherapy for pregnant women with addictions. Am J Obstet Gynecol. 2004;191:1885–97.

Rendell PG, Gray TJ, Henry JD, Tolan A. Prospective memory impairment in "ecstasy" (MDMA) users. Psychopharmacology. 2007;194:497–504.

Ribeiro JA, Sebastião AM. Caffeine and adenosine. J Alzheimer's Dis. 2010;20(Suppl 1):S3–S15. https://doi.org/10.3233/JAD-2010-1379.

Rodgers J. Cognitive performance amongst recreational users of "ecstasy". Psychopharmacology. 2000;151:19–24.

Rodgers J, Buchanan T, Scholey AB, Heffernan TM, Ling J, Parrott AC. Patterns of drug use and the influence of gender on self-reports of memory ability in ecstasy users: a web based study. J Psychopharmacol. 2003;17:379–86.

Roth ME, Cosgrove KP, Carroll ME. Sex differences in the vulnerability to drug abuse: a review of preclinical studies. Neurosci Biobehav Rev. 2004;28(6):533–46.

Sakr HF, Sirasanagandla SR, Das S, Bima AI, Elsamanoudy AZ. Insulin resistance and hypertension: mechanisms involved and modifying factors for effective glucose control. Biomedicine. 2023;11(8):2271. https://doi.org/10.3390/biomedicines11082271.

SAMHSA: SAMHSA website. Available at http://www.samhsa.gov/index.aspx or at http://ncadistore.samhsa.gov/catalog/. Accessed May 6, 2010.

SAMHSA. Substance Abuse and Mental Health Services Administration; Rockville, MD: 2020. National Survey of Drug Use and Health (NSDUH) releases. Available at: https://www.samhsa.gov/data/release/2020-national-survey-drug-use-and-health-nsduh-release

SAMHSA OoAS. The DASIS report: cocaine route of administration trends: 1995–2005. Rockville: Substance Abuse and Mental Health Services Administration; 2007.

Santana AB, Spelta LEW, Martinez-Sobalvarro JV, Garcia RCT, Dos Reis TM, Torres LH. Prenatal caffeine consumption and neurobehavioral disorders – a systematic review. Reprod Toxicol. 2024;125:108563. https://doi.org/10.1016/j.reprotox.2024.108563.

Savard H et al. Ecstasy addiction: symptoms, effects, and rehab treatment, American addiction centers, 2024.

Schifano F, Orsolini L, Duccio Papanti G, Corkery JM. Novel psychoactive substances of interest for psychiatry. World Psychiatry. 2015;14(1):15–26. https://doi.org/10.1002/wps.20174.

Schifano F, Papanti GD, Orsolini L, Corkery JM. Novel psychoactive substances: the pharmacology of stimulants and hallucinogens. Expert Rev Clin Pharmacol. 2016;9(7):943–54. https://doi.org/10.1586/17512433.2016.1167597.

Shaw GM, Malcoe LH, Swan SH, Cummins SK, Schulman J. Congenital cardiac anomalies relative to selected maternal exposures and conditions during early pregnancy. Eur J Epidemiol. 1992;8:757–60.

Singer LT, Arendt R, Minnes S, Farkas K, Salvator A. Neurobehavioral outcomes of cocaine-exposed infants. Neurotoxicol Teratol. 2000;22:653–66.

Singer LT, Arendt RA, Minnes S, Salvator A, Siegel AC, Lewis BA. Developing language skills of cocaine-exposed infants. Pediatrics. 2001;107:1057–64.

Singer LT, Moore DG, Fulton S, et al. Neurobehavioral outcomes of infants exposed to MDMA (ecstasy) and other recreational drugs during pregnancy. Neurotoxicol Teratol. 2012;34(3):303–10.

Siu AL, et al. Behavioral and pharmacotherapy interventions for tobacco smoking cessation in adults, including pregnant women: US preventive services task force recommendation statement. Ann Intern Med. 2015;163(8):622–34.

Smid MC, Metz TD, Gordon AJ. Stimulant use in pregnancy: an under-recognized epidemic among pregnant women. Clin Obstet Gynecol. 2019;62(1):168–84. https://doi.org/10.1097/GRF.0000000000000418.

Smith L, Yonekura ML, Wallace T, Berman N, Kuo J, Berkowitz C. Effects of prenatal methamphetamine exposure on foetal growth and drug withdrawal symptoms in infants born at term. J Dev Behav Pediatr. 2003;24(1):17–23.

Solmi M, De Toffol M, Kim JY, Choi MJ, Stubbs B, Thompson T, Firth J, Miola A, Croatto G, Baggio F, Michelon S, Ballan L, Gerdle B, Monaco F, Simonato P, Scocco P, Ricca V, Castellini G, Stein MT, Drahota A, Chavira DA. Ian: a 7-year old with prenatal drug exposure and early exposure to family violence. J Dev Behav Pediatr. 2008;29:512.

Suarez EA, Huybrechts KF, Straub L, Hernández-Díaz S, Jones HE, Connery HS, Davis JM, Gray KJ, Lester B, Terplan M, Mogun H, Bateman BT. Buprenorphine versus methadone for opioid use disorder in pregnancy. N Engl J Med. 2022;387(22):2033–44. https://doi.org/10.1056/NEJMoa2203318.

Tadesse AW, Dachew BA, Ayano G, Betts K, Alati R. Prenatal cannabis use and the risk of attention deficit hyperactivity disorder and autism spectrum disorder in offspring: a systematic review and metaanalysis. J Psychiatr Res. 2024;171:142–51. https://doi.org/10.1016/j.jpsychires.2024.01.045.

Tanuma A, Saito S, Ide I, Sasahara H, Yazdani M, Gottschalk S, Nakamoto T, Abiko Y. Caffeine enhances the expression of the angiotensin II type 2 receptor mRNA in BeWo cell culture and in the rat placenta. Placenta. 2003;24(6):638–47. https://doi.org/10.1016/s0143-4004(03)00033-x.

Towers CV, Terry P, Rackley B, Hennessy M, Visconti K. Foetal outcomes with detoxification from opioid drugs during pregnancy: a systematic review. Am J Perinatol. 2020;37(7):679–88. https://doi.org/10.1055/s-0039-1688908.

Traccis F, Minozzi S, Trogu E, Vacca R, Vecchi S, Pani PP, Agabio R. Disulfiram for the treatment of cocaine dependence. Cochrane Database Syst Rev. 2024;1(1):CD007024. https://doi.org/10.1002/14651858.CD007024.pub3.

Trigo JM, Lagzdins D, Rehm J, Selby P, Gamaleddin I, Fischer B, Barnes AJ, Huestis MA, Le Foll B. Effects of fixed or self-titrated dosages of Sativex on cannabis withdrawal and cravings. Drug Alcohol Depend. 2016;161:298–306. https://doi.org/10.1016/j.drugalcdep.2016.02.020.

U.S. Centers for Disease Control and Prevention. National Center for Chronic Disease Prevention and Health Promotion; Office on Smoking and Health (U.S.). How Tobacco Smoke Causes Disease: The Biology and Behavioral Basis for Smoking-Attributable Disease: A Report of the Surgeon General. Centers for Disease Control and Prevention (US), Atlanta (GA); 2010.

Varney B, Brett J, Zoega H, Gillies MB, Powell M, Bateman BT, Shand AW, Pearson SA, Havard A. Opioid analgesic exposure during the first trimester of pregnancy and the risk of major congenital malformations in infants: a systematic review and meta-analysis†. Anaesthesia. 2024;79(9):967–77. https://doi.org/10.1111/anae.16307.

Wachman EM, Newby PK, Vreeland J, Byun J, Bonzagni A, Bauchner H, Philipp BL. The relationship between maternal opioid agonists and psychiatric medications on length of hospitalization for neonatal abstinence syndrome. J Addict Med. 2011;5(4):293–9.

Wakschlag LS, Pickett KE, Cook E Jr, Benowitz NL, Leventhal BL. Maternal smoking during pregnancy and severe antisocial behavior in offspring: a review. Am J Public Health. 2002;92:966–74.

Walhovd KB, Watts R, Amlien I, Woodward LJ. Neural tract development of infants born to methadone-maintained mothers. Pediatr Neurol. 2012;47(1):1–6. https://doi.org/10.1016/j.pediatrneurol.2012.04.008.

Wang MJ, Kuper SG, Sims B, Paddock CS, Dantzler J, Muir S, Harper LM. Opioid detoxification in pregnancy: systematic review and meta-analysis of perinatal outcomes. Am J Perinatol. 2019;36(6):581–7. https://doi.org/10.1055/s-0038-1670680.

Wang X, Wang Y, Tang B, Feng X. Opioid exposure during pregnancy and the risk of congenital malformation: a meta-analysis of cohort studies. BMC Pregnancy Childbirth. 2022;22(1):401. https://doi.org/10.1186/s12884-022-04733-9.

Welton S, Blakelock B, Madden S, Kelly L. Effects of opioid use in pregnancy on pediatric development and behaviour in children older than age 2: systematic review. Can Fam Physician. 2019;65(12):e544–51.

WHO Guidelines Approved by the Guidelines Review Committee. In: Clinical Guidelines for Withdrawal Management and Treatment of Drug Dependence in Closed Settings. Geneva: World Health Organization. Copyright (c) World Health Organization 2009; 2009.

Wikoff D, Welsh BT, Henderson R, Brorby GP, Britt J, Myers E, Goldberger J, Lieberman HR, O'Brien C, Peck J, Tenenbein M, Weaver C, Harvey S, Urban J, Doepker C. Systematic review of the potential adverse effects of caffeine consumption in healthy adults, pregnant women, adolescents, and children. Food Chem Toxicol. 2017;109(Pt 1):585–648. https://doi.org/10.1016/j.fct.2017.04.002.

Winklbaur-Hausknost B, Jagsch R, Graf-Rohrmeister K, Unger A, Baewert A, Langer M, Thau K, Fischer G. Lessons learned from a comparison of evidence-based research in pregnant opioid-dependent women. Hum Psychopharmacol. 2013;28(1):15–24. https://doi.org/10.1002/hup.2275.

Won L, Bubula N, McCoy H, Heller A. Methamphetamine concentrations in foetal and maternal brain following prenatal exposure. Neurotoxicol Teratol. 2001;23(4):349–54.

Won L, Bubula N, Heller A. Foetal exposure to methamphetamine in utero stimulates development of serotonergic neurons in three-dimensional reaggregate tissue culture. Synapse. 2002;43(2):139–44.

Woolf SH, Battista RN, Angerson GM, Logan AG, Eel W. New grades for recommendations from the Canadian task force on preventive health care. CMAJ. 2003;169:207–8.

World Health Organization. Guidelines for the identification and management of substance use and substance use disorders in pregnancy. Geneva: World Health Organization; 2014.

Wouldes TA, Woodward LJ. Neurobehavior of newborn infants exposed prenatally to methadone and identification of a neurobehavioral profile linked to poorer neurodevelopmental outcomes at age 24 months. PLoS One. 2020;15(10):e0240905. https://doi.org/10.1371/journal.pone.0240905.

Wouldes TA, Lester BM. Opioid, methamphetamine, and polysubstance use: perinatal outcomes for the mother and infant. Front Pediatr. 2023;11:1305508. https://doi.org/10.3389/fped.2023.1305508.

Wright TE, Terplan M, Ondersma SJ, Boyce C, Yonkers K, Chang G, Creanga AA. The role of screening, brief intervention, and referral to treatment in the perinatal period. Am J Obstet Gynecol. 2016;215(5):539–47.

Yazdy MM, Mitchell AA, Tinker SC, Parker SE, Werler MM. Periconceptional use of opioids and the risk of neural tube defects. Obstet Gynecol. 2013;122:838–44.

Young-Wolff KC, Tucker LY, Alexeeff S, Armstrong MA, Conway A, Weisner C, Goler N. Trends in self-reported and biochemically tested marijuana use among pregnant females in California from 2009-2016. JAMA. 2017;318(24):2490–1. https://doi.org/10.1001/jama.2017.17225.

Young-Wolff KC, Sarovar V, Tucker LY, Avalos LA, Alexeeff S, Conway A, Armstrong MA, Weisner C, Campbell CI, Goler N. Trends in marijuana use among pregnant women with and without nausea and vomiting in pregnancy, 2009–2016. Drug Alcohol Depend. 2019;196:66–70. https://doi.org/10.1016/j.drugalcdep.2018.12.009.

Yuan S, Liu J, Larsson SC. Smoking, alcohol and coffee consumption and pregnancy loss: a Mendelian randomization investigation. Fertil Steril. 2021;116(4):1061–7. https://doi.org/10.1016/j.fertnstert.2021.05.103.

Zedler BK, Mann AL, Kim MM, Amick HR, Joyce AR, Murrelle EL, Jones HE. Buprenorphine compared with methadone to treat pregnant women with opioid use disorder: a systematic review and meta-analysis of safety in the mother, fetus and child. Addiction. 2016;111(12):2115–28. https://doi.org/10.1111/add.13462.

Zelson C, Lee SJ, Casalino M. Neonatal narcotic addiction. Comparative effects of maternal intake of heroin and methadone. The New England Journal of Medicine. 1973;289(23):1216–20. https://doi.org/10.1056/NEJM197312062892303.

Zierler S, Rothman KJ. Congenital heart disease in relation to maternal use of Bendectin and other drugs in early pregnancy. N Engl J Med. 1985;313:347–52.

Pharmacological Approaches to Managing Common Sleep Disorders

23

Laura Palagini

23.1 Introduction

Women's sleep patterns during pregnancy and the postpartum period are influenced by a variety of factors, including anatomical, endocrinological, physiological, psychological, behavioral, socio-economic, and cultural elements (Pengo et al. 2018). These alterations can significantly impact sleep duration, quality, patterns, and respiratory function during sleep, thereby increasing the likelihood of sleep disturbances in pregnant women during the peripartum phase (Baglioni et al. 2020; Garbazza et al. 2020; Palagini et al. 2022). Research indicates that nearly 80% of women report experiencing sleep disruptions during this period. The most prevalent issues across all three trimesters include reduced sleep duration, diminished sleep quality, and insomnia (Baglioni et al. 2020; Palagini et al. 2022), which often persist and may worsen in the postpartum phase (Sivertsen et al. 2015). Additionally, women may experience nightmares, sleep-disordered breathing, and restless legs syndrome (Pengo et al. 2018; Garbazza et al. 2020). Accumulating evidence suggests that insomnia and sleep disruptions during pregnancy may be linked to adverse gestational and birth outcomes (Okun et al. 2011), the necessity for emergency cesarean sections (Paine et al. 2020), and the development of gestational diabetes. Notably, insomnia and poor sleep quality during the peripartum period have been identified as potential risk factors for peripartum psychopathology, including mood disorders, postpartum blues, and psychosis (Swanson et al. 2020; Palagini et al. 2023; Sharma et al. 2023; Palagini et al. 2024a, b, c). Furthermore, maternal sleep patterns during pregnancy may influence infant sleep patterns, with disrupted maternal sleep correlating with poorer infant sleep, which can subsequently affect

L. Palagini (✉)
Department of Neuroscience, Psychiatric Section, University of Pisa, Azienda Ospedaliera Universitaria Pisana (AUOP), Pisa, Italy

F. Uguz, L. Orsolini (eds.), *Perinatal Psychopharmacology*,
https://doi.org/10.1007/978-3-031-99720-4_23

maternal sleep in the postpartum period (Baglioni et al. 2020). Sleep during the perinatal period is regarded as a family concern, with potential short-term effects on the mental health of both the child and the entire family, as well as long-term implications for the child's susceptibility to mental health issues in adulthood (Baglioni et al. 2020). In this context, it is essential to evaluate and address sleep disturbances during the peripartum period. The management of these numerous conditions often necessitates the use of pharmacotherapy, which complicates the decision-making process concerning the timing and selection of treatment, as well as the most suitable approach for both the mother and her unborn child, particularly in light of drug safety and pharmacodynamic considerations. This chapter examines the physiological changes and the occurrence of sleep disorders. It will also discuss prescribing decision-making process during the peripartum with a focus on sleep disorders.

23.2 Peripartum-Related Physiological Changes and the Occurrence of Sleep Disorders

Pregnancy induces significant physiological changes that markedly impact sleep patterns. The hormonal fluctuations that occur during this period, including increased levels of various hormones, play a crucial role in altering both the circadian and homeostatic mechanisms governing sleep, thereby modifying sleep architecture. Notably, alterations in melatonin, cortisol, and gonadal steroids such as estrogen and progesterone, along with pituitary hormones like gonadotropins, prolactin, and growth hormone, can influence sleep quality. Research indicates that non-rapid eye movement (NREM) sleep is enhanced by progesterone and prolactin, while rapid eye movement (REM) sleep is diminished by progesterone and augmented by estrogens. Specifically, progesterone exerts a sleep-promoting effect on brain gamma-aminobutyric acid (GABA) receptors, leading to increased NREM sleep and potentially explaining the daytime drowsiness and fatigue often experienced during the first trimester, when progesterone levels are on the rise. Additionally, the elevated respiratory rate associated with progesterone may help prevent airway obstruction, thereby reducing the risk of sleep disorder breathing (SDB). Furthermore, progesterone's thermogenic properties raise core body temperature, and its relaxing effect on smooth muscles—including those in the gastrointestinal tract, ureters, and bladder—can disrupt sleep, resulting in more frequent awakenings and diminished sleep quality. Estrogen, which is secreted by the placenta and peaks before delivery, has stimulating effects on the nervous system and is known to reduce REM sleep. Its elevated levels during pregnancy can lead to vasodilation and nasal congestion, which may further contribute to SDB. Additionally, estrogen promotes the production of prolactin. Collectively, all these factors may contribute to the development of insomnia, SDB, and restless legs syndrome (RLS).

23.3 Most Common Sleep Disorders During Peripartum

23.3.1 Insomnia

23.3.1.1 Epidemiology and Clinical Features During the Peripartum Period

Insomnia disorder is currently recognized as a 24-h sleep-wake disorder (APA 2022), marked by symptoms that manifest both at night and during the day. This condition can be classified as episodic, lasting from 1 month to 3 months, or persistent, extending beyond 3 months; transient-episodic forms often progress to chronic insomnia. It is the most prevalent sleep disturbance, affecting nearly one-third of the general population and approximately 10% of the European population (APA 2022; Riemann et al. 2023). The frequency, severity, and pattern of insomnia symptoms may fluctuate during pregnancy, with studies indicating that it impacts over 38% of pregnant women, rising to 42.4% during the third trimester (Swanson et al. 2020; Sedov et al. 2021; Salari et al. 2021). Symptoms of insomnia tend to increase in the first 6 months following childbirth. Notably, 50% of these women continue to experience insomnia 2 years postpartum, and 15% may develop a long-term insomnia disorder (Sivertsen et al. 2015). Insomnia as a disorder may affect around 22–23% of perinatal women (Palagini et al. 2024a, b, c).

23.3.1.2 Pathophysiology

The diathesis-stress model, often referred to as the "3-P" model, serves as the most heuristic framework for understanding insomnia, particularly in the context of pregnancy and the postpartum period (Swanson et al. 2020; Palagini et al. 2021). This model delineates three categories of factors: Predisposing, Precipitating, and Perpetuating. Numerous physiological and psychosocial transformations occurring during the perinatal period significantly influence the onset and continuation of insomnia, as outlined by the diathesis-stress model of chronic insomnia, which highlights the interplay of predisposing factors, triggering events, and sustaining behaviors (Palagini et al. 2024a, b, c).

Numerous predisposing factors for insomnia arise during pregnancy. In the first trimester, hormonal changes may play a significant role in the onset of insomnia. Additional risk factors during this period include being over the age of 30, experiencing premenstrual syndrome, having no previous pregnancies, being a single mother, suffering from affective disorders prior to pregnancy, experiencing perinatal depression, and dealing with various physical symptoms. As pregnancy progresses into the second trimester, a reduction in melatonin levels, alongside hormonal changes characterized by increased estrogen, may contribute to insomnia. Physical discomforts such as snoring, heartburn, vivid dreams, and pain in the back, neck, and joints can also heighten the risk of developing insomnia. In the third trimester, hormonal influences from estrogen, cortisol, growth hormone, melatonin, and oxytocin can disrupt sleep patterns, leading to sleep fragmentation, RLS, and SDB. Physical discomfort continues to be a significant factor in the development of insomnia. Additionally, irregular uterine contractions and fetal movements toward the end of pregnancy may further exacerbate insomnia (Swanson et al. 2020; Palagini et al. 2022). Postpartum, factors contributing to insomnia include abrupt hormonal shifts, breastfeeding, cesarean delivery, sleep deprivation during labor and the peripartum period, and the irregular sleep patterns of the infant. Chronodisruption is frequently observed during the postpartum phase, which may further facilitate the onset of insomnia.

Pregnancy and childbirth, while often viewed as positive milestones, are significant life stressors that can trigger insomnia (Swanson et al. 2020). During the perinatal period, these stressors can exacerbate maladaptive cognitive and emotional regulation strategies (Swanson et al. 2020). Extensive research has established hyperarousal as a critical factor in chronic insomnia (Riemann et al. 2015; Riemann et al. 2023), characterized by heightened physiological, cognitive, and emotional arousal. This hyperarousal is believed to interact with detrimental cognitive beliefs and negative behaviors, further sustaining insomnia. The allostatic load hypothesis has been suggested in the context of pregnancy and the postpartum period. Consequently, insomnia and chronic sleep deprivation serve as both triggers and outcomes of stress, potentially leading to a state of stress overload that may result in adverse pregnancy outcomes, including peripartum psychopathology and persistent insomnia (Palagini et al. 2014, 2023, 2024a, b, c).

23.3.1.3 Insomnia Treatment in the Peripartum

Assessment and effective management are crucial in preventing potential adverse outcomes during pregnancy and the recurrence of chronic insomnia. Research indicates that a significant number of pregnant women refrain from seeking treatment for insomnia, often believing it will resolve on its own post-delivery or due to concerns regarding the impact of medication on the fetus (Bacaro et al. 2020; Baglioni et al. 2020). Consequently, it is imperative to evaluate and address sleep disturbances from the onset of pregnancy. The National Institute for Health and Clinical Excellence (NICE) guidelines on antenatal and postnatal mental health, published in 2018, advocate for psychological therapies to be prioritized as the first-line treatment for mild to moderate conditions whenever feasible. The criteria for prescribing psychotropic medications should be stringent, with such medications being considered only when psychological interventions fail to alleviate symptoms (NICE 2018). For chronic insomnia, Cognitive Behavioral Therapy for Insomnia (CBT-I) is recognized internationally as the primary treatment option (Riemann et al. 2023). CBT-I typically encompasses various behavioral strategies, including psychoeducation and sleep hygiene, relaxation techniques, stimulus control therapy, sleep restriction therapy, and cognitive strategies such as cognitive restructuring related to sleep. Within the framework of CBT-I, psychoeducation often involves imparting "sleep hygiene rules" that address health practices and environmental factors (such as light, noise, and temperature) that can either facilitate or hinder sleep. Relaxation therapy focuses on alleviating physical tension and intrusive thoughts at bedtime. Behavioral strategies include sleep restriction, which limits time spent in bed to the actual amount of sleep achieved, and stimulus control therapy, which provides behavioral guidelines to help re-establish a positive association with the bed and bedroom environment. A systematic review and meta-analysis conducted by Zheng et al. (2023) evaluated the effectiveness of CBT-I among pregnant women. This analysis encompassed eight randomized controlled trials with a total of 743 participants. The findings indicated that CBT-I led to a notable improvement in insomnia symptoms among perinatal women when compared to the control group. The National Institute for Health and Clinical Excellence (NICE) guideline on antenatal and postnatal mental health from 2018 advises that pharmacological treatment should be considered for women who do not respond to nonpharmacological therapies and exhibit severe insomnia symptoms, particularly when no alternatives are available and the benefits outweigh the risks (Kay-Stacey and Attarian 2017). The US Food and Drug Administration (FDA) has classified various medications based on their risk levels during pregnancy and lactation. However, in 2015, the FDA discontinued this classification system, replacing the ABCDX categories with the FDA Pregnancy and Lactation Labeling Rule (PLLR). This new regulation provides prescribers with essential information for informed decision-making, advocating for a shared decision-making approach when treating pregnant or lactating women. It includes three categories: (1) pregnancy, encompassing labor and delivery; (2) lactation; and (3) female individuals of reproductive potential Miller et al. (2020) proposed an algorithm for treating insomnia or other sleep conditions during pregnancy. Uguz (2021) introduced a safety scoring system for the administration of psychotropic medications during lactation, which is based on six safety parameters. The total score can range from 0 to 10, with higher scores indicating a more favorable safety profile.

Guidelines concerning the treatment of insomnia highlight various sleep-promoting agents. These include GABA modulator compounds such as benzodiazepines and related medications known as Z drugs, as well as melatonin receptor agonists like prolonged-release melatonin (2 mg) and ramelteon. Additionally, antagonists targeting the arousal-promoting system are noted, including dual orexin receptor antagonists (DORAs) such as daridorexant, suvorexant, and lemborexant. Most of sedating antidepressants with antihistaminic and anti-5HT properties, including low doses of trazodone, are considered off-label in insomnia treatment. However, other classes of medications, including various antidepressants, antihistamines, neuroleptics, and mood stabilizers, are not recommended for the treatment of insomnia (Riemann et al. 2023; Palagini et al. 2023).

Sleep-Promoting Agents in the Peripartum Period

GABA, a four-carbon non-proteinogenic amino acid, serves as the primary inhibitory neurotransmitter found in significant concentrations across various regions of the mammalian brain. GABAA receptors are distinguished by numerous allosteric binding sites, including those for benzodiazepines. Ligands that engage with these binding sites trigger a conformational alteration in GABAA receptors, thereby influencing their functionality. GABAergic neurons are crucial in modulating the sleep-wake cycle through cortico-medullary pathways. These neurons may affect both rapid eye movement (REM) and non-REM (NREM) sleep, particularly during slow wave sleep (SWS) (for an overview see Palagini and Bianchini 2022). Furthermore, the activation of GABAA receptors plays a significant role in sleep regulation, with GABAergic activity originating from the ventrolateral preoptic nucleus (VLPO) of the hypothalamus exerting inhibitory control over the ascending arousal network. This network is supported by various wake-promoting circuits, including the cholinergic basal forebrain, histaminergic tuberomammillary nucleus, serotonergic dorsal raphe, and noradrenaline-producing locus coeruleus, with orexin neurons providing excitatory projections to the thalamus and neocortex (for an overview see Palagini and Bianchini 2022). Reduced levels of GABA or dysfunctional GABAergic transmission are linked to the development and persistence of both acute and chronic insomnia and are associated with hyperarousal in insomnia cases (for an overview see Palagini et al. 2022). The GABAA receptor, a pentameric ligand-gated ion channel made up of five transmembrane glycoprotein subunits (two α, two β, and one γ), each with distinct isoforms [α1–6, β1–3, and γ1–3], binds GABA at the extracellular site. Hypnotic benzodiazepines and Z-drugs interact at the junction of the α and γ subunits of the GABAA receptor, functioning as positive allosteric modulators that facilitate a conformational change in the subunit structure. This process increases the binding site's affinity for GABA, thereby enhancing its effects (for an overview see Palagini et al. 2022). Most hypnotic benzodiazepines exhibit a high affinity for the α1, α2, α3, and α5 receptor subtypes. In contrast, Z-drugs demonstrate a comparatively lower affinity for these subunits (Palagini and Bianchini 2022). For instance, zolpidem does not bind to the α5 subunit, and its affinity for the α1 and α2, α3 GABAA receptor subtypes is approximately 10 times and 100 times lower than that of triazolam, respectively (for an overview see Palagini and Bianchini 2022). The subsequent sections will discuss commonly prescribed hypnotic benzodiazepines (such as brotizolam, temazepam, and triazolam) and Z-drugs (including zolpidem, zopiclone, eszopiclone, and zaleplon), with particular emphasis on their implications during pregnancy and the postpartum period. Estazolam, flurazepam, and lormetazepam have been recommended for the treatment of insomnia over the past years; therefore, data regarding these benzodiazepines will also be analyzed during the peripartum period (Wang et al 2022). Conversely, although lorazepam is not typically classified as a hypnotic benzodiazepine, it is often used in managing insomnia in pregnant patients (Uguz 2021). Data regarding lorazepam will be discussed elsewhere.

Hypnotic Benzodiazepines

Brotizolam

Brotizolam (8-bromo-6-(o-chlorophenyl)-1-methyl-4H triazolo[3,4-c]thieno[2,3-e]-1,4-diazepine) is classified as a thieno-triazolo diazepine derivative that interacts with α1-containing GABAA receptors. The drug has an elimination half-life that is considered “intermediate,” lasting around 5 h (for an overview see Palagini and Bianchini. 2022).

Currently, four studies involved brotizolam in pregnancy and postpartum (Table 23.1). One study was conducted in animals and showed that brotizolam does pass the placenta and the breast milk in animal (Bechtel 1983). A study was conducted with 11 women in the peripartum period, while two additional studies were presented as case reports (Nishimura et al. 2021; Saito et al. 2021; Saito et al. 2021). These studies indicated that the Relative Infant Dose (RID) was less than 10%, suggesting a relatively safe level, and the milk to plasma (M/P) ratio was below 1.

Temazepam

Temazepam, classified as a 1,4-benzodiazepine, is a hydroxylated derivative of diazepam (3-hydroxydiazepam) and exerts its effects on sleep through interaction with GABAA receptors. Its half-life ranges from approximately 5–11 h. Six studies involved the use of temazepam during the perinatal period (Table 23.1) (Kargas et al. 1985; Lebedevs et al. 1992; Cooper et al. 2001; Kelly et al. 2012; Damen et al. 2014; Ban et al. 2014). Data on pregnancy are lacking. Globally the milk to plasma (M/P) ratio was below 1. Two studies report negative outcomes: one with the interaction with diphenhydramine, the other one after using it during delivery (Kargas et al. 1985; Cooper et al. 2001). In a large cohort study, risks of system-specific major congenital anomalies were generally similar in children exposed to temazepam during the first trimester of pregnancy compared to those not exposed to such medications (Ban et al. 2014).

Triazolam

Triazolam is classified as a triazolobenzodiazepine. Its half-life is relatively brief, ranging from approximately 2–3 h, with recommended hypnotic doses between 0.125 and 0.25 mg administered at bedtime. Five studies involved triazolam in the perinatal period (Kitagawa et al. 1979; Sakai et al. 1996; Kelly et al. 2012; Noh et al. 2022; Bagger et al. 2023) (Table 23.1). Triazolam has been shown to cross the placenta in animals (Kitagawa et al. 1979) but there are no data on RID of M/P in humans. Two retrospective cohort studies showed risk for malformation after exposure during the first trimester comparable to that of non-exposed population (Noh et al. 2022; Bagger et al. 2023). Other reports are case discussions.

There are no data on other benzodiazepines sometimes prescribed for insomnia such as Flurazepam, lormetazepam, or estazolam, related to the peripartum period. Currently, there is inconclusive data on the use of hypnotic benzodiazepines in insomnia during the peripartum.

Several meta-analyses and reviews have examined the effects of these medications during the peripartum period (Chaudhry and Susser 2018; Miller et al. 2020; Grigoriadis et al. 2020; Huitfeldt et al. 2020; Uguz 2021; Wang et al. 2022; Andrade et al. 2024).

Table 23.1 Studies on pharmacological options for insomnia during the peripartuma period

Authors	Compound	Design of the study	Main results	
Hypnotic benzodiazepines				
Bechtel (1983)	Brotizolam	Safety study in animals	In animal studies brotizolam crossed the placenta, and brotizolam was found in the milk of rats as well as in that of cows	
Nishimura et al. (2021)	Brotizolam	11 pregnant women at obstetrics department The milk to plasma (M/P) ratio and relative infant dose (RID) were computed	M/P ratio for brotizolam: The value 3 days after delivery was 0.12 n/mL and 0.59 after 1 month. The RID value was 2.3% for brotizolam. No abnormalities were found in breastfeeding infants whose mothers were receiving these medications	
Saito et al. (2021)	Brotizolam	Case report oral brotizolam 0.25 mg once daily	A 28-year-old female patient with a diagnosis of bipolar II disorder was administered brotizolam during her pregnancy (from 28 to 40 weeks of gestation) and while breastfeeding, in conjunction with sertraline, alprazolam, and trazodone. There were no indications of pulmonary dysfunction or congenital anomalies. The concentrations of brotizolam in maternal serum were measured at 0.51 ng/mL and 0.22 ng/mL at 7.0 and 14.0 h post-dosing, respectively. Notably, brotizolam was absent in both cord blood and infant serum at 9.2 h following maternal administration. The concentration of brotizolam found in breast milk, collected 7.1 h after maternal dosing, was 0.12 ng/mL. The infant exhibited normal development, with no observable drug-related adverse effects noted during the 1-, 3-, and 6-month postpartum evaluations	

Saito et al. (2021)	Brotizolam	Case report oral brotizolam 0.25 mg once daily she was also in treatment with sulpiride, periciazine, alprazolam in the postpartum	A 38-year-old female patient diagnosed with dissociative disorder received treatment with brotizolam. The concentration ratios of the drug in both cord blood and maternal serum were found to be 0.33 for brotizolam. In breast milk, concentrations of brotizolam were undetectable. The newborn exhibited no congenital defects and did not show any significant withdrawal symptoms following delivery	
Kargas et al. (1985)	Temazepam	A case report of pregnant woman	Perinatal fetal mortality was related to the interaction of diphenhydramine and temazepam	
Lebedevs et al. (1992)	Temazepam	10 breastfeeding women 10–20 mg of temazepam	Mean milk to plasma (M/P) ratio 0. 18 ng/mL	
Cooper et al. (2001)	Temazepam	37 women undergoing surgical termination of pregnancy between 12 and 17 weeks. Temazepam 10 mg, approximately 1 h pre-operatively	Temazepam was identified in every fetal serum sample analyzed. The fetal to maternal (F:M) drug concentration ratio for temazepam was found to be 0.38, remaining consistent between 60 and 120 min following oral administration to the mother. Additionally, the F:M ratios exhibited variations correlated with the gestational age of the fetus, showing an increase as gestational age progressed for temazepam	
Kelly et al. (2012)	Temazepam	Retrospective study 124 women during breastfeeding Temazepam and or other benzodiazpeines	Adverse outcomes, specifically sedation was identified in only 1.6% (2 of 124) of infants and was not associated with temazepam. Mothers reporting adverse outcomes in themselves were more likely to be taking concomitantly a greater number of central nervous system depressants	

(continued)

Table 23.1 (continued)

Authors	Compound	Design of the study	Main results	
Damen et al. (2014)	Temazepam	Case report 20 mg of temazepam during delivery for therapeutic rest	A 38-week-old female neonate, delivered through a spontaneous vaginal birth facilitated by a midwife at home, was admitted to neonatal intensive care unit following an episode of apnea, bradycardia, and hypotonia 1 h after delivery. Cervical dilation was slow, prompting the midwife to administer 20 mg of temazepam to mitigate maternal fatigue during the first stage of labor. Three and a half hours post-temazepam, the mother delivered a female infant. Breastfeeding commenced immediately after birth. However, 1 h later, the infant was discovered to be nonbreathing. Initial laboratory tests indicated a venous serum lactate of 8.6 mmol/L was noted. Capillary blood gas analysis revealed a pH of 7.35, pCO_2 of 31 mmHg. Screening of urine was positive for benzodiazepines and a supratherapeutic temazepam plasma level of 145 μg/L (20–100 μg/L) was found 6 h since maternal temazepam intake. Three days later the neonate was fully recovered and could be discharged from the NICU	
Ban et al. (2014)	Temazepam	Retrospective study 379 children exposed to with temazepam during the first trimester compared with 351,785 children with no diagnosed depression/anxiety nor medication exposure	Overall major congenital anomaly prevalence was 2.9% in 379 children with temazepam. When compared with 2.7% in 351,785 children with no diagnosed depression/anxiety nor medication exposure, the adjusted odds ratio was 1.07 (0.49–2.37) for temazepam. Risks of system-specific major congenital anomaly were generally similar in children exposed and not exposed to such medications	

Kitagawa et al. (1979)	Triazolam	Safety study in animals	In animal studies triazolam crossed the placenta	
Sakai et al. (1996)	Triazolam	Case report	A female infant was delivered prematurely following the tragic suicide of her mother, who ingested a minimum of 20 triazolam tablets and subsequently hanged herself 7 h prior to the birth. The infant was born with cesarean section at 33 weeks of gestation. The infant experienced respiratory distress and required the administration of pulmonary artificial surfactant. Following extubation, she experienced apneic episodes, necessitating supplemental oxygen and aminophylline treatment. The triazolam concentration measured in the cord blood was 2.30 ng/ml. The infant was discharged from the neonatal intensive care unit at 2 months of age and demonstrated normal developmental progress by 4 months of post-conceptional age	
Kelly et al. 2012	Triazolam	Retrospective study 1 case with triazolam	Sedation was not associated with triazolam (1 case). Mothers reporting adverse outcomes in themselves were more likely to be taking concomitantly a greater number of central nervous system depressants	
Noh et al. (2022)	Triazolam	Retrospective population-based cohort study exposure to triazolam and other benzodiazepines during the first trimester 3,094,227 women	Among those exposed to triazolam, the risk for overall malformation with triazolam was 0.91 and for cardiac defect 1.12, which was comparable with non-exposed population	

(continued)

Table 23.1 (continued)

Authors	Compound	Design of the study	Main results	
Bagger et al. (2023)	Triazolam	Retrospective cohort study 800 nulliparous singleton pregnant women in the latent phase of labor presenting at the labor ward women who were treated with therapeutic rest Triazolam vs women who were not	414 women (52%) were treated with therapeutic rest. The most frequently used ($n = 206$) medication for therapeutic rest was a combination of paracetamol, triazolam, and codeine. No significant difference in neonatal admission, or neonatal resuscitation, between women treated with or without therapeutic rest	
Z-DRUGS				
Pons et al. (1989)	Zolpidem	Five lactating, healthy women were treated with a single 20 mg tablet of zolpidem 3–4 days after the delivery of a full-term baby. The drug was administered at 20.00 h, 30 min after dinner, and milk samples were collected before and 3, 13, and 16 h. venous blood 5 ml was taken before and 1.5, 3, 13, and 16 h after zolpidem administration.	The estimated apparent elimination half-life of zolpidem, derived from plasma concentrations, was found to be 2.6 h. At the 3-h mark, the quantity of zolpidem present in breast milk varied from 0.76 to 3.88 micrograms, accounting for 0.004 to 0.019% of the administered dose. No detectable levels of zolpidem (below 0.5 ng/ml) were observed in the milk during subsequent sampling intervals. The concentration ratio of zolpidem in breast milk to that in plasma at 3 h was determined to be 0.13. Furthermore, the apparent clearance of zolpidem from breast milk, calculated based on the total amount excreted in milk relative to its plasma concentration, was 1.48 ml/h. these findings indicate that the excretion of zolpidem in human milk is minimal (below 0.02%), with the majority occurring within the initial 3 h post-administration drug intake	

Cannizzaro et al. (2002)	Zolpidem	Rats prenatal exposure to zolpidem	These findings indicate a convergence on anxiety-related behaviors in the effects of prenatal exposure to diazepam and alprazolam but not of zolpidem	
Askew (2007)	Zolpidem	Case report	A 30-year-old Caucasian female with a history of zolpidem misuse experienced a spontaneous vaginal delivery at 38 weeks of gestation. The total fetal exposure to zolpidem remains uncertain; however, it is estimated to be no less than 1000 mg over a duration of at least 1 month. Typical peak plasma concentrations following a single administration of 5 mg and 10 mg of zolpidem are reported to be between 29–113 ng/ml (mean 59 ng/ml) and 58–272 ng/ml (mean 121 ng/ml), respectively. A sample of cord blood was collected for zolpidem analysis, yielding a concentration of 41 ng/ml. Notably, despite the detection of zolpidem in the cord blood, the neonate exhibited activity and alertness following a normal delivery. There were no signs of withdrawal symptoms, and both the mother and the neonate were discharged after a 48-h monitoring period. This case report illustrates that zolpidem is capable of crossing the human placenta, as evidenced by the cord blood analysis	

(continued)

Table 23.1 (continued)

Authors	Compound	Design of the study	Main results	
Juric et al. (2009)	Zolpidem	Forty-five women taking zolpidem during pregnancy were studied in comparison with non-exposed patients	The incidence of preterm delivery and low birth weight in the group exposed to zolpidem was recorded at 26.7% and 15.6%, respectively, compared to 13.3% and 4.4% in the matched control group; however, these differences were not statistically significant. The ratio of zolpidem concentrations in umbilical cord blood to maternal plasma in six pairs varied between 0.48 and 2.75. Zolpidem is capable of crossing the human placenta and is rapidly eliminated from fetal circulation. Although pregnant women with psychiatric disorders receiving zolpidem may experience less favorable obstetric outcomes, it remains uncertain whether this is attributable to the medication itself	
Wang et al. (2010)	Zolpidem	Nationwide population-based study Taiwan National Health Insurance Research Dataset (NHIRD) and birth-certificate registry. In total, the data from 2497 mothers who received zolpidem treatment during pregnancy and those from 12,485 randomly selected mothers who did not receive the drug were included in the analysis.	The findings indicate that the adjusted odds ratios (ORs) for negative pregnancy outcomes—Including low-birth-weight infants, preterm births, small-for-gestational-age infants, and cesarean sections—were significantly elevated among mothers who underwent zolpidem treatment during pregnancy when compared to the randomly selected control group (1.39 (95% confidence interval (CI) = 1.17–1.64), 1.49 (95% CI = 1.28–1.74), 1.34 (95% CI = 1.20–1.49), and 1.74 (95% CI = 1.59–1.90), respectively). In summary, the data suggest that the likelihood of experiencing adverse pregnancy outcomes is greater in women who were treated with zolpidem during their pregnancy compared to those who were not	

Wikner and Källén (2011)	Zolpidem	Swedish medical birth registry indicated that 1318 women reported the use of Z drugs during early pregnancy	The use of hypnotic benzodiazepine receptor agonists did not correlate with an elevated risk of congenital malformations. However, a statistically significant increased risk for other intestinal malformations, excluding atresias and stenosis, was identified, albeit based on a limited sample of only four infants	
Sharma et al. (2011)	Zolpidem	Case report	A case of a female patient with fetal neural tube defects has been reported, linked to her dependence on zolpidem and the consumption of high doses during the first trimester of her pregnancy	
Saito et al. (2022a, b, c, d)	Zolpidem	Case report	A woman was administered zolpidem at a dosage of 5 mg each night to aid her sleep. Breastmilk concentrations were assessed on three occasions following childbirth: On day one, 8.2 h post-dose, the concentration measured was 12.8 mcg/L; on day two, 9 h after the dose, the concentration was recorded at 6.4 mcg/L; and on day three, 2.2 h post-dose, the concentration reached 26.5 mcg/L. the authors calculated the maximum daily dose for the infant to be 4 mcg/kg, based on the measurement obtained on day three	

(continued)

Table 23.1 (continued)

Authors	Compound	Design of the study	Main results	
Saito et al. (2022a, b, c, d)	Zopidem	Three case series	Two pregnant women administered daily doses of 5 mg of zolpidem throughout their pregnancy and the postpartum period. One of the women exhibited a breastmilk concentration of zolpidem measuring 10.1 mcg/L, recorded 6.5 h following a dose on the sixth day postpartum. The second woman displayed varying milk zolpidem concentrations, with levels between 0.6 mcg/L at 18.1 h post-dose on the second day postpartum and 4.8 mcg/L at 10.1 h post-dose on the third day postpartum. Additionally, a third woman, who took a 5 mg dose as needed, showed a milk concentration of 3.4 mcg/L at 17.2 h after a dose on the first day postpartum. By the seventh day, 105 h after a dose, zolpidem was no longer detectable in the breastmilk. Three infants were breastfed by mothers who were administered zolpidem at a dosage of 5 mg daily ($n = 2$) or on an as-needed basis ($n = 1$). The breastfeeding frequency for these infants ranged from four to six times per day. Notably, all infants exhibited undetectable serum levels of zolpidem, measured at less than 0.05 mcg/L	

Saito et al. (2022a, b, c, d)	Zolpidem	Case report	A 46-year-old female patient with a diagnosis of insomnia was administered 5–10 mg/day of zolpidem during her pregnancy and lactation period, along with 8 mg/day of ramelteon while breastfeeding. She gave birth to a male infant weighing 3329 g at 38 weeks of gestation, with no congenital abnormalities detected either during the pregnancy or at birth. The infant's health was assessed as normal during the one-month postpartum follow-up. The maternal/placental ratio of zolpidem concentrations was measured at 0.1, taken 7.4 h post-maternal dosing, which aligns with findings from prior research. The estimated relative infant dose via breast milk, calculated from the peak drug concentration in breast milk at 2.2 h after maternal dosing, was found to be 2.7% for zolpidem and 0.2% for ramelteon. The concentrations of ramelteon and its metabolite (M-II) in breast milk were comparable to those in the maternal serum, although the infant's exposure to these medications through oral intake was minimal. In conclusion, ramelteon was found to be present in breast milk	
Gaillot et al. (1982)	Zopiclone	Animal studies	In nursing mothers, milk and plasma kinetics of zopiclone are similar with a milk/plasma ratio around 0.80	

(continued)

Table 23.1 (continued)

Authors	Compound	Design of the study	Main results	
Matheson et al. (1990)	Zopiclone	Cohort of 12 lactating women during the early postpartum phase after they received a single oral dose of zopiclone (7.5 mg)	The milk/plasma area under the curve ratio for zopiclone was determined to be 0.51 ± 0.09. There was notable interindividual variability in the mean milk/plasma concentration ratios of zopiclone, which ranged from 0.41 to 0.70. Furthermore, when comparing pharmacokinetic parameters in postpartum women to those previously documented in non-pregnant women, it was observed that the maximum concentration (Cmax) values were significantly elevated in the lactating mothers, with the time to reach maximum concentration (tmax) occurring later in breast milk than in maternal plasma. Assuming an average daily milk consumption of 0.15 liters per kilogram and complete absorption, the estimated dose of zopiclone received by infants through breast milk would be approximately 1.4% of the weight-adjusted dose taken by the mother	
Diav-Citrin et al. (1999)	Zopiclone	Prospective study in 40 women exposed to zopiclone	The Motherisk program, in conjunction with the Toronto teratogen information service, conducted a prospective study involving 40 women who were exposed to zopiclone during their pregnancies. The findings indicated no significant rise in the incidence of major malformations, with 0 out of 31 cases (0%) in the zopiclone group compared to 1 out of 37 cases (2.7%) in the non-teratogenic control group	

Mathieu et al. (2010)	Zopiclone		A mother who was prescribed zopiclone at a dosage of 3.75 mg four times daily for tension headaches during her pregnancy gave birth to 30-week preterm twins. The infants exhibited withdrawal symptoms within their first week of life. Starting at 2 weeks of age, they were approximately two-thirds breastfed by their mother, who maintained the same dosage of the medication. The twins showed no clinical abnormalities and were discharged from the hospital 6 weeks post-delivery.	
Wikner and Källén (2011)	Zopiclone	Swedish medical birth registry indicated that 1318 women reported the use of Z drugs during early pregnancy	The use of hypnotic benzodiazepine receptor agonists did not correlate with an elevated risk of congenital malformations	
Ban et al. (2014)	Zopiclone	Retrospective study 406 children exposed to zopiclone during the first trimester compared with 351,785 children with no diagnosed depression/anxiety nor medication use	When compared with 2.7% in 351,785 children with no diagnosed depression/anxiety nor medication use, the adjusted odds ratio was 0.96 (0.42–2.20) for zopiclone and 1.01 (0.90–1.14) for un-medicated depression/anxiety. Risks were generally similar in children exposed and not exposed to such medications	
Melatonin receptor agonists				
Schenker et al. (1998)	200 pmol/L of melatonin	Three healthy pregnant women during delivery	The equilibration of melatonin levels between the maternal and fetal compartments was achieved within 150 min	

(continued)

Table 23.1 (continued)

Authors	Compound	Design of the study	Main results	
Okatani et al. (1998)	Melatonin 3 mg immediate release	12 women who underwent spontaneous vaginal delivery without receiving melatonin, 33 women who had elective caesarean sections and were administered 3 mg of melatonin either 1, 2, 3, or 4 h prior to delivery	The findings indicated that oral administration of melatonin resulted in elevated serum melatonin levels, peaking 2 h post-administration before significantly declining over the next 2 h. The analysis revealed no significant difference in serum melatonin levels between the maternal and umbilical veins, with a strong correlation observed between the concentrations in both veins, indicating that melatonin administered to the mother is rapidly and effectively transferred to the fetal circulation	
	Melatonin immediate release	Ninety-four mothers of healthy 2 to 4-month-old infants	Exclusively breast-fed infants had a significantly lower incidence of colic attacks, lower severity of irritability attacks, and a trend for longer nocturnal sleep duration	
Miller et al. (2014)	Melatonin 8 mg daily (4 mg twice daily) from the time of recruitment until delivery	Phase I clinical trial 12 pregnant women experiencing severe early onset intrauterine restriction	The trial findings indicated that there were no adverse effects on either maternal or fetal health linked to the administration of melatonin	
Fang et al. (2016)	Melatonin 10 mg immediate release or quercetin	Randomized controlled trial 180 pregnant women 15th to the 33rd week of gestation with hyperglycemia	The study concluded that melatonin is more clinically effective than quercetin for managing hyperglycemia in pregnant women and raised no safety concerns regarding its use during pregnancy	One human volonteer

Hobson et al. (2018)	Melatonin 30 mg daily (10 mg three times a day) from the time of diagnosis until delivery	Phase I clinical trial melatonin 20 pregnant women diagnosed with early-onset preeclampsia	The findings of this trial indicated that melatonin was safe for both the mothers and their fetuses, with no reported adverse events or drug reactions among the mothers, fetuses, or neonates. However, it was noted that the neonates born to mothers receiving melatonin treatment exhibited a higher incidence of being small for gestational age compared to historical controls	
Luciani et al. (2019)	Melatonin no specified dose	Case report	An 18-month-old child with a documented history of bleeding episodes since birth. Mother taking melatonin while breastfeeding the child's mother had intermittently consumed melatonin during and after her pregnancy, although the specific dosage and frequency were not detailed. Consequently, maternal melatonin intake was halted. After a period of 3 months, platelet aggregation levels normalized, and the child experienced no further instances of bleeding	
Saito et al. (2022a, b, c, d)	Ramelteon	Case report	A 46-year-old female patient with a diagnosis of insomnia was administered 5–10 mg/day of zolpidem during her pregnancy and lactation period, along with 8 mg/day of ramelteon while breastfeeding. The estimated relative infant dose via breast milk, calculated from the peak drug concentration in breast milk at 2.2 h after maternal dosing, was found to be 2.7% for zolpidem and 0.2% for ramelteon. The concentrations of ramelteon and its metabolite (M-II) in breast milk were comparable to those in the maternal serum, although the infant's exposure to these medications through oral intake was minimal	

(continued)

Table 23.1 (continued)

Authors	Compound	Design of the study	Main results	
Dual orexin receptor antagonists (DORAs)				
Ishikawa et al. (2024a, b)	Suvorexant	2 case reports	Data from two women suggest that the levels of suvorexant present in breast milk are minimal. Both women were administered a dosage of 20 mg of suvorexant at night. They submitted milk samples "a few days" following childbirth. One woman provided a sample prior to taking the medication and another 70 min post-dose, with concentrations recorded at 1.36 and 2.85 mcg/L, respectively. The second woman submitted samples a few days and 1 month after delivery, although the exact timing of these samples was not specified, taken the day after the drug was ingested. The concentrations in these samples were 3.47 and 4.09 mcg/L, respectively. The authors calculated the relative dosages for infants to be approximately 0.17% and 0.2% for the two women, respectively	
Ishikawa et al. (2024a, b)	Lemborexant	Case report	A woman with bipolar disorder was on long-term lemborexant therapy at a dose of 5 mg every night before sleep. Milk samples were collected "a few days" after delivery at 70 and 565 min after a dose. The concentrations in breast milk were 4.69 mcg/L at 70 min and 5.12 mcg/L at 565 min after administration. The authors estimated a relative infant dose of 1.05% at 565 min after administration	

Saito et al. (2023)	Lemborexant 10 mg	Case report	A woman administered lemborexant 10 mg, brotizolam 0.25 mg, and etizolam 0.5 mg at bedtime during her pregnancy and the postpartum period. Colostrum samples were collected on days 2 and 3 postpartum, with collection times varying from 8 to 19.6 h following the medication dose. The concentrations of the substances in the milk ranged from 1.8 to 12.7 mcg/L, with the peak concentration observed in the sample taken 8 h post-dose. The estimated daily dose for the infant through breastmilk, based on the highest concentration recorded, was calculated to be 1.91 mcg/kg, resulting in a relative infant dose of 1.21%	
Rawal et al. (2024)	Lemborexant 10 mg	8 breastfeeding women	Throughout the 240-h collection period, a total of 0.0174 mg of the unchanged drug was detected in the breastmilk, with 70% of this amount being collected within the first 24 h. The researchers estimated that a fully breastfed infant would receive an average weight-adjusted relative infant dose of 1.96% of the maternal dose	
Kaufmann et al. (2024)	Daridorexant 50 mg	Single-center open-label trial, 10 women, phase I study	Blood and milk samples were collected both prior to dosing and at various intervals over a 72-h period following administration. Daridorexant was found to be rapidly absorbed into the plasma and subsequently distributed. Both daridorexant and its primary metabolites were detectable in breast milk. Over the 72-h period, the total cumulative amount of daridorexant excreted was 0.010 mg, representing 0.02% of the maternal dose. This resulted in a mean daily dose for infants of 0.009 mg/day, equating to a relative infant dose of less than 0.22% over a 24-h period. Minimal quantities of daridorexant and its metabolites were identified in the breast milk of healthy lactating women	

There exists a notable ambiguity in the literature regarding the effects of hypnotic benzodiazepines and those benzodiazepines utilized for anxiety. These two categories are often examined in a similar context (Chaudhry and Susser 2018; Miller et al. 2020; Grigoriadis et al. 2020; Huitfeldt et al. 2020; Uguz 2021; Wang et al. 2022; Andrade et al. 2024), leading to a lack of clarity concerning the specific effects of hypnotic benzodiazepines during the peripartum period.

Z-Drugs

Zolpidem

Zolpidem is an imidazopyridine compound that exhibits a preferential affinity for the α1-GABAA receptor subtype. (for an overview see Palagini et al. 2022). The bioavailability of zolpidem in humans is approximately 70%, with peak plasma concentrations reached within 1 h of administration and an elimination half-life of 1.5–2.5 h. Active metabolites are not accumulated following its degradation (for an overview see Palagini et al. 2022). Nine works involved the use of zolpidem in the peripartum period (Pons et al. 1989; Cannizzaro et al. 2002; Askew 2007; Juric et al. 2009; Wang et al. 2010; Sharma et al. 2011; Wikner and Källén 2011; Saito et al. 2022a; Saito et al. 2022b) (Table 23.1). Zolpidem has been shown to cross the placenta in humans. The ratio of zolpidem concentrations in umbilical cord blood to maternal plasma in six pairs varied between 0.48 and 2.75. The concentration of zolpidem in breast milk has been shown to be low and eliminated relatively quickly (from 0.76 to 3.88 micrograms, accounting for 0.004 to 0.019% of the administered dose). Some experts advise against the use of zolpidem while breastfeeding, mainly due to the lack of comprehensive documentation (Uguz 2021). On the other hand, American Academy of Pediatrics Committee on Drugs in 2001 (here is the citation it is in the list) recommended Zolpidem as safe for lactation (Miller et al. 2020). Some data also suggest that the likelihood of experiencing adverse pregnancy outcomes including low-birth-weight infants, preterm births, small-for-gestational-age infants, and cesarean section is greater in women who were treated with zolpidem during their pregnancy compared to those who were not. Indeed, thee data are not confirmed in other studies (Table 23.1).

Zopiclone and Eszopiclone

Zopiclone is a derivative of cyclopyrrolone believed to interact with the GABAA receptor complex. Zopiclone shows a stronger affinity for the α1 and α2 subunits compared to benzodiazepines. In contrast, eszopiclone displays high affinity and potency primarily for the α2 and α3 subunits. The elimination half-life of zopiclone ranges from 3.5 to 6.5 h (for an overview See Palagini et al. 2022). Six studies involved zopiclone during the perinatal period (Table 23.1) (Gaillot et al. 1982; Matheson et al. 1990; Diav-Citrin et al. 1999; Mathieu et al. 2010; Wikner and Källén 2011; Ban et al. 2014). In a study, the peak concentration of the drug in breast milk reached approximately 55 mcg/L approximately 2 h post-administration. The half-life of zopiclone in breast milk was found to be comparable to that in plasma, which is 5.3 h in healthy adults. Additionally, 12 nursing mothers, 2–6 days postpartum, received a single oral dose of 7.5 mg of zopiclone. The average peak concentration in breast milk was 34 mcg/L (ranging from 24 to 57 mcg/L), occurring 2.4 h (with a range of 1–6 h) after the dose. The mean half-life in breast milk was also 5.3 h (with a range of 3.5–8.6 h). The authors estimated that an exclusively breastfed infant would receive an average of 15 mcg/kg, which corresponds to 1.2–1.4% of the maternal weight-adjusted dosage of zopiclone. There are no studies about Infant Levels. Some experts advise against the use of zopiclone while breastfeeding, mainly due to the lack of comprehensive documentation (Uguz 2021). No data are available for eszopiclone during the peripartum period. Given the limited number of clinical trials examining the use of these drugs during pregnancy and breastfeeding, particularly those focused on safety and efficacy concerning sleep disorders, no definitive conclusions can be drawn from the current evidence.

Melatonin Receptor Agonists

Melatonin 2 mg Prolonged Release

Melatonin (N-acetyl-5-methoxytryptamine) is a peptide hormone produced and released by the pineal gland in the brain, entering the bloodstream directly. Its synthesis is stimulated by signals from the internal biological clock located in the suprachiasmatic nuclei (SCN) of the hypothalamus and is suppressed by light detected by the retina. Melatonin operates through various mechanisms and interacts with its specific receptors (MT1 and MT2), which belong to the G-protein-coupled receptor family (for an overview see Palagini et al. 2021; Biggio et al. 2021). The consistent daily pattern of melatonin signaling, aligned with the dark phase of the day, positions melatonin as a key internal regulator of circadian rhythms, thereby establishing its "chronobiotic action." It is noteworthy that, despite being a neurohormone, melatonin secretion does not follow the traditional negative feedback mechanism; instead, it is regulated by a unique process at the SCN level, which influences its own secretion timing. Consequently, when administered as a treatment, exogenous melatonin serves as an external regulator of circadian rhythms, capable of inducing either a phase advance or phase delay in its secretion based on the timing of administration. In summary, melatonin is a significant synchronizer of human circadian biological rhythms and functions as a principal chronobiological pacemaker (for an overview see Palagini et al. 2021). When administered exogenously, melatonin exhibits similar sleep-inducing and phase-shifting properties as endogenous melatonin. The pharmacokinetics of melatonin are influenced by the method of administration, which may include oral, immediate release (IR), prolonged release (PR), intravenous, nasal spray, anal suppository, skin patches, or cream, as well as individual absorption rates and hepatic metabolism. The only formulation approved for the treatment of insomnia is the 2 mg prolonged release melatonin formulation (Circadin® at 2 mg) for patients over 55 years of age. This formulation achieves peak plasma levels approximately 2.6 h post-ingestion, which are sustained for 3.5 h. No other melatonin formulations are recommended for the treatment of insomnia.

On the other hand, the utilization of melatonin in different doses or formulation is often used in pregnant women as oral supplementation (for an overview see Vine et al. 2022). The current review identified no clinical trials that primarily focused on the safety or efficacy of melatonin prolonged release for insomnia or other sleep disorders in pregnant individuals.

Exogenous melatonin does cross the placenta (Table 23.1) (Schenker et al. 1998). No significant difference in serum melatonin levels between the maternal and umbilical veins was found indicating that melatonin administered to the mother is rapidly and effectively transferred to the fetal circulation. Oral administration of melatonin resulted in elevated serum melatonin levels, peaking 2 h post-administration before significantly declining over the next 2 h (Okatani et al. 1998).

Three clinical trials have explored the efficacy of melatonin as an antioxidant treatment for various conditions during pregnancy (Table 23.1). Significantly elevated doses of melatonin, ranging from 8 to 30 mg per day, were administered in an immediate-release formulation. No adverse effects were observed, with the exception of one noted issue on fetal growth (Miller et al. 2014; Fang et al. 2016; Hobson et al. 2018).

Melatonin levels in breast milk exhibit a circadian rhythm, characterized by elevated concentrations at night and reduced levels during the day, as documented in various studies (for a review see Vine et al. 2022). This rhythmic pattern remains consistent throughout the different stages of breast milk maturation, although minor variations exist, particularly with milk showing higher nocturnal levels compared to colostrum. The concentration of melatonin in breast milk is approximately 35% of that found in maternal serum, and it remains stable under typical conditions. In terms of potential advantages, one study indicated that exogenous melatonin present in breast milk might correlate with a reduction in both the severity and frequency of infantile colic. On the other hand, a case study involving a breastfeeding mother who consumed exogenous melatonin suggested a possible link to non-fatal bleeding episodes in her child (Luciani et al. 2019). The current work identified a lack of clinical trials assessing the safety and efficacy of exogenous melatonin during breastfeeding, highlighting a notable gap in the existing literature (for an overview see Vine et al. 2022). Nevertheless, research involving the administration of exogenous melatonin to preterm infants has reported no adverse effects (for an overview see Vine et al. 2022). Additionally, the pharmacokinetics of melatonin in premature infants differ from those in adults, exhibiting prolonged clearance, extended half-life, and increased time to reach maximum concentration, along with a reduced volume of distribution. This underscores the importance of investigating the use of melatonin in breastfeeding mothers and its potential implications for their infants. Given the limited number of clinical trials examining melatonin use during pregnancy and breastfeeding, particularly those focused on safety and efficacy concerning sleep disorders, no definitive conclusions can be drawn from the current evidence.

Ramelteon

Ramelteon is a selective MT1 and MT2 receptor agonist with negligible affinity for other neuronal receptors including gamma-aminobutyric acid and benzodiazepine receptors. Ramelteon is currently approved in the United States and Japan for the treatment of insomnia. Ramelteon is rapidly absorbed, with a time to peak serum concentration of 0.75 h at the dose of 8 mg. Two case reports involve ramelteon in the post-partum period (Table 23.1) (Saito et al. 2022a, b, c, d; Ishikawa et al. 2024a; b), showing that it appears in the breast milk. No other works involve ramelteon in the peripartum period.

Wake-Regulating Agents in Insomnia Treatment: Implications for the Peripartum Period

Dual Receptor Orexin Antagonists (DORAs)

Orexin A and orexin B, also known as hypocretin 1 and hypocretin 2, are two neuropeptides that originate from preproorexin. Neurons that produce orexin are situated in the lateral hypothalamic area (LHA) and the posterior hypothalamus, with orexinergic fibers extending throughout the brain. The orexin 1 receptor (OX1R) is specifically activated by orexin A, while the orexin 2 receptor (OX2R) responds to both orexin A and B in a non-selective manner. The distribution of OX1R and OX2R within the brain is distinct. These neurons receive inputs from the limbic system, which may play a role in emotional arousal and fear responses. Additionally, the preoptic area, particularly the ventrolateral preoptic nucleus (VLPO), is crucial for the initiation and maintenance of non-REM sleep and receives signals from the suprachiasmatic nuclei, which serve as the central regulator of circadian rhythms based on environmental light and dark cycles. The orexinergic system plays a crucial role in regulating various functions, including sleep and arousal, behavioral and neuroendocrine responses to stress, emotional reactivity, reward-seeking behaviors, energy homeostasis, as well as learning and memory. Data such as these support the hypothesis that insomnia can be due to an inability of the brain to switch off wake-promoting systems such as the orexin system, as well as an inability to switch on sleep-promoting circuits with an instability of the flip-flop switch system (Riemann et al. 2023). In this framework, Dual Receptor Orexin Antagonists (DORAs) are a class of drugs recommended for insomnia treatment (Riemann et al. 2023; Palagini et al. 2023), Daridorexant, Lemborexant, and Suvorexant are the compounds belonging to this class.

Suvorexant

Suvorexant was approved for use in the United States in 2014, the first such orexin-based drug approved for insomnia. The recommended dose is 10 mg taken orally within 30 min of bedtime. The dose can be increased to 20 mg. Its half-life of 12 h. Currently, no data have been collected during pregnancy in humans. Two case reports indicated that it is present in the milk with dosages for infants to be approximately 0.17% and 0.2% for the two women, respectively (Ishikawa et al. 2024a, b).

Lemborexant

Lemborexant has been approved by the U.S. FDA in 2019 to treat adult patients with insomnia. Although lemborexant is a reversible competitive antagonist that binds to both OX1R and OX2R just as suvorexant does, lemborexant has a stronger inhibition effect on OX2R than QX1R. It is rapidly absorbed (peak 1–3 h), lemborexant has a half-life of 17–19 h. At present, there is a lack of data collected during pregnancy. Two different case reports have suggested that the substance is found in breast milk, with dosages for infants estimated of 1.05% or 1.21% (Saito et al. 2023; Ishikawa et al. 2024a, b). In another study with 8 lactating women the relative infant dose was of 1.96% of the maternal dose (Rawal et al. 2024).

Daridorexant

Daridorexant is a new DORA approved in USA in 2020 and in May 2022 was approved by the European Medicines Agency EMA for the treatment of insomnia. It is the first DORA available in Europe. The compound is rapidly absorbed with a time to maximum plasma concentration of 1–2 h and eliminated with a terminal half-life of approximately 8 h. Daridorexant concentrations in rat milk exceeded those in plasma by 14- to 20-fold (USFDA 2022). In a phase I study conducted in 10 lactating women, Daridorexant was found to be rapidly absorbed into the plasma and subsequently distributed. Over the 72-h period, the total cumulative amount of daridorexant excreted was 0.010 mg, representing 0.02% of the maternal dose. This resulted in a mean daily dose for infants of 0.009 mg/day, equating to a relative infant dose of less than 0.22% over a 24-h period. Minimal quantities of daridorexant and its metabolites were identified in the breast milk of healthy lactating women. (Table 23.1).

Off-Label Treatment for Insomnia Used in Pregnancy and Postpartum

Low-Sedating Antidepressants

Trazodone is an antidepressant that belongs to a group of drugs called serotonin receptor antagonists and reuptake inhibitors (SARIs). In animals at the highest dosage, trazodone was associated with a reduction in fetal viability in rats. In humans, no major congenital malformations have been reported based on a few studies (McElhatton et al. 1996; Einarson et al. 2003, 2009) also when compared to SSRI (Dao et al. 2023). Indeed in a study a recent study posed a serious concern on the effects of trazodone on the brain development of the fetus (Korade et al. 2021). The use of trazodone during lactation has been rated as possible with caution because limited data are available (Uguz 2021). Although it is not recommended for insomnia treatment, low doses are frequently used in clinical practice. One study has been conducted for insomnia treatment with trazodone in pregnancy. In a randomized controlled trial, fifty-four pregnant women experiencing insomnia were assigned at random to receive either trazodone, diphenhydramine, or a placebo. Sleep quality was evaluated through actigraphy at the beginning of the study, as well as after 2 and 6 weeks of treatment. Additionally, depressive symptoms were measured 2 and 6 weeks postpartum. After 6 weeks of treatment, both trazodone and diphenhydramine demonstrated significant improvements in sleep quality compared to the placebo group. Moreover, reductions in depressive symptoms were noted in the trazodone and diphenhydramine groups at both 2 and 6 weeks following delivery, in contrast to the placebo group. No significant differences in depressive symptoms were found between the trazodone and diphenhydramine groups (Khazaie et al. 2013). Data about bout trazodone could be promising, but they are limited.

Doxepin

Doxepin is a tricyclic antidepressant available in some countries for insomnia treatment. About doxepin, animal studies and human reports are both scarce in pregnancy and during lactation (Uguz 2021).

Antihistamines

Antihistamines are generally not advised for the treatment of insomnia (Riemann et al. 2023; Palagini et al. 2023). However, they are frequently utilized for managing insomnia during pregnancy, particularly diphenhydramine (Miller et al. 2020). Furthermore, limited research has validated their safety profiles in humans, with some studies indicating potential anomalies linked to their use in the first trimester (Kay-Stacey and Attarian 2017; Miller et al. 2020). There is a lack of data regarding the use of antihistamines during lactation. There is a randomized controlled trial with 54 pregnant women experiencing insomnia who were assigned at random to receive either trazodone, diphenhydramine, or a placebo showing reductions in depressive symptoms in the trazodone and diphenhydramine groups at both 2 and 6 weeks following delivery, in contrast to the placebo group. No significant differences in depressive symptoms were found between the trazodone and diphenhydramine groups (Khazaie et al. 2013).

23.3.2 Restless Legs Syndrome (RLS)

23.3.2.1 Epidemiology and Clinical Features in the Peripartum Period

Restless legs syndrome (RLS), also known as Willis-Ekbom disease (WED), is a prevalent sensorimotor condition marked by an overwhelming desire to move the legs, often accompanied by uncomfortable sensations. Symptoms typically manifest during periods of inactivity, are alleviated through movement, and tend to intensify in the evening hours. The diagnosis relies on the clinical criteria established by the International RLS Study Group (IRLSSG) (2003). Recent systematic reviews have indicated that the prevalence of Restless Legs Syndrome (RLS) during pregnancy varies between 11% and 34%, which is generally two to three times greater than that observed in nonpregnant women. (Chen et al. 2018). There is an increase in the prevalence of women experiencing RLS/WED during the third trimester, with many reporting a resolution of symptoms within 1 month following childbirth. The detrimental effects on sleep are frequently observed, influencing both the initiation and preservation of sleep. RLS/WED has been identified as the third most prevalent cause of insomnia in pregnant individuals. This finding is pertinent in light of recent studies indicating a correlation between sleep disorders and negative outcomes during pregnancy. In a recent review, gestational RLS heightened risks of gestational hypertension, pre-eclampsia, and peripartum depression (Steinweg et al. 2020).

23.3.2.2 Pathophysiology

Progesterone levels rise during pregnancy, reaching their highest point in the third trimester. The specific relevance of progesterone remains unclear (Prosperetti and Manconi 2015; Mendes and Silva 2022). Nonetheless, there are known interactions between progesterone and dopamine within the striatum. Additionally, thyroid hormone has been suggested to contribute to the pathophysiology of RLS during pregnancy. Iron and folate metabolism serve as essential cofactors for tyrosine hydroxylase in the synthesis of dopamine, while folate is involved in the regeneration of tetrahydrobiopterin. Consequently, a deficiency in either iron or folate may lead to a reduction in dopamine production. During pregnancy, levels of serum folate, iron, and other indicators of iron status, such as ferritin and hemoglobin, are typically lower than those observed in non-pregnant individuals. This phenomenon may be attributed to an increase in total blood volume, resulting in a dilution effect, as well as the consumption of iron and folate for fetal development. The utilization of iron and folate by the fetus begins early in pregnancy, which contributes to a rapid decrease in maternal iron stores and a decline in serum ferritin levels. Research has indicated that low serum ferritin levels prior to or during early pregnancy may serve as a predictor for the occurrence of RLS during this period. However, it is noteworthy that the symptoms of RLS tend to diminish swiftly after delivery, independent of the levels of iron and folate, as replenishing these nutrients takes a considerable amount of time (Picchietti et al. 2015; Mendes and Silva 2022).

During pregnancy, various psychological factors can intensify the symptoms of RLS, such as anxiety, stress, tension, insomnia, and increased fatigue. Additionally, conditions like neuropathy and radiculopathy may contribute to RLS symptoms. The enlarging fetus exerts mechanical pressure on the lumbosacral nerve roots, leading to the manifestation of RLS symptoms, which typically resolve after delivery. Furthermore, as pregnancy progresses, peripheral venous distension increases while peripheral vascular resistance diminishes. These changes result in leg edema and heightened pressure on the tissues surrounding the receptors of the peripheral somatosensory system, thereby amplifying their stimulation (Picchietti et al. 2015; Mendes and Silva 2022).

In a consensus (Picchietti et al. 2015), independent predictors of RLS/WED during pregnancy were calculated and included a previous diagnosis of RLS/WED in non-pregnant states, a familial history of RLS/WED, a record of RLS/WED in earlier pregnancies, and hemoglobin levels at or below 11 g/dL. Additionally, individuals with a history of RLS/WED prior to pregnancy tend to experience more severe symptoms during pregnancy compared to their pre-pregnancy state. Notably, the prevalence of RLS/WED is 1.5 to 2 times higher in women than in men.

23.4 RLS Treatment During Peripartum

A panel of specialists in the field convened in 2015 (Picchietti et al. 2015) to offer significant recommendations regarding the treatment of Restless Legs Syndrome (RLS) during pregnancy and the postpartum period. Since that time, no additional consensus or recommendations have been issued. Miller et al. revised the evidence in 2020. Nonpharmacologic interventions are recommended for RLS in pregnancy (Picchietti et al. 2015). Moderate-intensity physical activity, yoga, massage therapy, pneumatic compression devices, management of obstructive sleep apnea, and the avoidance of aggravating factors are recommended for addressing RLS/WED during pregnancy and lactation. It was advisable to minimize aggravating factors associated with RLS/WED whenever feasible including iron deficiency, Prolonged immobility, Serotonergic antidepressants, Sedating antihistamines, sleep deprivation, caffeine, alcohol, and tobacco consumption. Addressing OSA is essential, given its potential to exacerbate RLS/WED and the other adverse effects associated with untreated OSA during pregnancy. Oral iron supplementation may be appropriate for the management of RLS/WED during pregnancy and lactation when the serum ferritin level is below 75 mcg/L (Picchietti et al. 2015). Such supplements are regarded as safe for use during these periods and may offer advantages for both the mother and the infant. It is noted that maternal serum ferritin levels typically decrease to approximately 50% by mid-pregnancy, attributed to the increase in maternal red blood cell volume, as well as the development of the fetus and placental tissues. For all pregnancies, it is advisable to administer oral iron in addition to prenatal vitamins if the ferritin level falls below 30 mcg/L. Consequently, a consensus was reached that oral iron may be considered for RLS/WED during pregnancy and lactation when the serum ferritin level is under 75 mcg/L (Picchietti et al. 2015). Iron status evaluation should involve the measurement of hemoglobin, serum ferritin, total iron binding capacity, and percent iron saturation. In cases where serum ferritin levels are below 75 mcg/L, it is advisable to administer ferrous sulfate at a dosage of 65 mg of elemental iron, taken one to two times daily. Serum ferritin levels should be reassessed after a period of 6–8 weeks. Proper storage of iron is crucial, as iron overdose can be particularly dangerous, especially for young children. Intravenous (IV) iron may be considered for managing refractory Restless Legs Syndrome/Willis-Ekbom Disease during the second or third trimester of pregnancy and in the postpartum period, particularly if oral iron supplementation has proven ineffective and serum ferritin levels are below 30 mcg/L.

The available evidence does not support the recommendation of magnesium, folate, vitamin C, vitamin D, or vitamin E for the management of RLS/WED during pregnancy or lactation. Although there is substantial evidence regarding the safety of magnesium and folate in pregnant individuals, there is limited evidence to suggest that either of these nutrients is effective in treating RLS/WED, whether related to pregnancy or not.

23.4.1 Pharmacological Treatment of RLS in the Peripartum

According to Picchetti et al. (2015) pharmacological options should be taken into account for severe forms. Among pharmacological option low-dose clonazepam may be considered for managing refractory RLS/WED during the second and third trimesters of pregnancy, as well as during lactation, with a recommended dosage of

0.25 to 1 mg in the evening (Picchietti et al. 2015). It is advisable to avoid concurrent use with diphenhydramine or other anticonvulsants during pregnancy. In non-pregnant individuals, clonazepam is regarded as a secondary or adjunctive treatment for RLS/WED. It has been shown to decrease sleep arousals and may alleviate sensory symptoms associated with the condition. Although clonazepam does not seem to pose a significant teratogenic risk, a cautious approach suggests avoiding its use during the first trimester of pregnancy. Available data regarding the safety of clonazepam during pregnancy should be found in another chapter.

Dopaminergic Carbidopa/levodopa may be utilized for the management of refractory RLS during pregnancy, with a recommended dosage of 25/100 to 50/200 mg in extended-release form taken in the evening or at night (Picchietti et al. 2015). Picchetti et al. (2015) advise to avoid the combination of levodopa with benserazide. Additionally, dopaminergics are known to inhibit lactation. For non-pregnant individuals, dopaminergics are considered first-line treatments for RLS/WED. While there is comparatively less evidence supporting the efficacy of carbidopa/levodopa in relation to pramipexole, ropinirole, and rotigotine, there exists a greater body of safety data regarding carbidopa/levodopa during pregnancy. Reports indicate the use of carbidopa/levodopa in 18 cases of Parkinson's or Segawa disease and 38 cases of RLS/WED during pregnancy, with no significant evidence of major malformations or other adverse outcomes (Picchietti et al. 2015). It was recommended to limit the total daily dosage of carbidopa/levodopa to no more than 50/200 mg to mitigate the risk of augmentation and other adverse effects. Immediate-release formulations of carbidopa/levodopa may also be considered, although they have a short elimination half-life of approximately 1.5 h (Picchietti et al. 2015).

Limited data are available for pramipexole, ropinirole, and rotigotine during pregnancy. Although there is substantial literature on the safety of cabergoline and bromocriptine during the first trimester of pregnancy for hyperprolactinemia, the use of these ergots, as well as pergolide, should be avoided for RLS/WED during pregnancy because of the risk of fibrotic reactions. Dopaminergics act as prolactin inhibitors and can decrease breast milk production in a dose-dependent manner. However, if carbidopa/levodopa is administered during pregnancy, prolactin levels tend to rebound quickly.

Gabapentin, classified as an Alpha-2-delta ligand, may be considered for managing refractory RLS/WED during lactation, with a recommended dosage ranging from 300 to 900 mg in the evening or at night (Picchietti et al. 2015). Gabapentin enacarbil, gabapentin, and pregabalin are recognized as first-line treatments for chronic RLS/WED in non-pregnant individuals. However, the available safety data regarding gabapentin enacarbil and pregabalin during pregnancy is limited; it is not recommended in pregnancy. While gabapentin does transfer into breast milk, it is estimated that the infant receives only 1–4% of the maternal weight-adjusted dose, and no adverse effects have been reported in neonates (Picchietti et al. 2015). Indeed, data on gabapentin enacarbil and pregabalin during lactation are inadequate to support their recommendation (Picchietti et al. 2015).

23.5 Sleep-Disordered Breathing in Pregnancy

23.5.1 Epidemiology and Clinical Features During Peripartum

Sleep-disordered breathing (SDB) encompasses obstructive sleep apnea (OSA) and upper airway resistance syndrome (UARS). Obstructive sleep apnea (OSA) is characterized by recurrent instances of partial or complete collapse of the upper airway, which frequently leads to respiratory arousals. This disruption results in fragmented sleep and a decrease in overall sleep duration, contributing to daytime fatigue, impaired concentration, and excessive sleepiness (APA 2022). The intermittent hypoxia associated with sleep apnea triggers endothelial dysfunction, promotes inflammation, induces oxidative stress, and heightens sympathetic activity. Additionally, it causes dysregulation of the hypothalamus-pituitary-adrenal axis, which can result in various metabolic, cardiovascular, and pulmonary comorbidities.

The prevalence of OSA during the first trimester is approximately 8.4%, rising to between 15% and 19% by the third trimester (Miller et al. 2020).

Research has examined various surrogate markers of sleep-disordered breathing during pregnancy, such as snoring and UARS. The prevalence of self-reported snoring among pregnant individuals ranges from 14% to 52%. In obese pregnant women, frequent snoring, oxygen desaturation, and respiratory arousals are prevalent and tend to exacerbate in the later stages of pregnancy. SDB has emerged as a risk factor for adverse maternal–fetal outcomes in pregnancy (Miller et al. 2020).

23.5.2 Pathophysiology

As the uterus expands to accommodate the developing fetus, the diaphragm is displaced upward, resulting in a 20% decrease in functional residual capacity, which is further diminished during sleep and when in a supine position. Additionally, late pregnancy is associated with a reduction in chest wall and total respiratory compliance, which contributes to decreased maternal oxygenation and exacerbates the arterial–alveolar oxygen gradient. The interplay of estrogen, placental growth hormone, and increased blood volume during pregnancy leads to hyperemia, mucosal edema, hypersecretion, and heightened fragility of the upper airways. In the general population, nasal congestion is a known risk factor for snoring and OSA, and gestational rhinitis, which affects one in five pregnant women, can significantly impair their quality of life. Furthermore, progesterone enhances ventilatory drive and minute ventilation through its direct action on central chemoreceptors. Multiple factors may contribute to SDB in pregnancy.

23.5.3 SDB Treatment in the Peripartum

CPAP is typically well-accepted during pregnancy; however, adherence to CPAP therapy can present challenges. A review of 83 closely monitored CPAP trials involving non-pregnant individuals revealed that, on average, patients utilized CPAP therapy only 32.9% of the time. Long-term compliance rates vary between 46% and 85%. Strategies to enhance adherence encompass advancements in PAP technology, customization of mask selection based on patient preferences, educational initiatives, psychosocial support such as motivational interviewing and cognitive behavioral therapy, as well as support from peers and spouses, and the use of telemedicine. Alternative and supplementary therapies may include sleep positioning during pregnancy. Further research is necessary to evaluate the effectiveness of mandibular advancement devices, oral pressure therapy, and hypoglossal nerve stimulation (Miller et al. 2020).

23.6 Narcolepsy

Narcolepsy is a chronic neurological sleep disorder that affects approximately 0.05% of the population in the United States and 1 in every 2000 individuals worldwide. Those diagnosed with narcolepsy often suffer from significant and frequently debilitating excessive daytime sleepiness, with around 70% also experiencing cataplexy, which is characteristic of narcolepsy type 1. Current pharmacological treatments alleviate symptoms in over 90% of patients; however research focusing on pregnancy with narcolepsy remains limited (Miller et al. 2020).

The scarcity of information concerning narcolepsy in the context of pregnancy and lactation, along with the possible impacts of frequently prescribed narcolepsy medications on the developing fetus and newborn, poses significant challenges for women with narcolepsy in making family planning decisions (Barker et al. 2020). Interventions such as avoiding medications that may increase daytime drowsiness, engaging in intermittent napping, and adhering to good sleep hygiene practices can be highly beneficial (Miller et al. 2020). A global survey of sleep specialists indicated that the risks associated with narcolepsy medications during pregnancy are frequently exaggerated, leading to the discontinuation or reduction of treatment during this period (Miller et al. 2020; Barker et al. 2020). The choice to either withdraw or maintain stimulant or anticataplectic medications should be tailored to the individual, carefully considering the risks of untreated narcolepsy against the potential exposure of the fetus to these drugs (Miller et al. 2020). Pharmacological treatment may be warranted for individuals experiencing severe symptoms that could compromise maternal safety, thereby posing risks to the fetus due to potential falls or motor vehicle accidents.

A recent discovery of particular significance for individuals with narcolepsy is the identification of sodium oxybate, the primary treatment for Narcolepsy type 1, in the breast milk of lactating women who are undergoing sodium oxybate therapy. Investigation involving women with narcolepsy type 1 across pregnancies suggested that it may be possible to prevent infants from being exposed to high levels of gamma-hydroxybutyric acid (GHB) by postponing the feeding of expressed milk until the presence of exogenous GHB in the milk is no longer expected. While larger confirmatory studies are warranted, this information should be taken into account when considering treatment options for women with narcolepsy who choose to breastfeed and respond positively to sodium oxybate (Barker et al. 2020). A report detailing 150 cesarean deliveries conducted with sodium hydroxybutyrate has indicated that maternal seizures, arterial hypertension, and significant blood loss may be linked to the administration of this medication. Additionally, poor fetal condition was observed in 12% of the cases. Currently, there are no studies available that validate the safe use of this drug (Miller et al. 2020).

References

American Academy of Pediatrics Committee on Drugs. Transfer of drugs and other chemicals into human milk. Pediatrics. 2001;108(3):776–89.

American Psychiatric Association. Diagnostic and statistical manual of mental disorders, fifth edition text revised (DSM-5-TR). Arlington: American Psychiatric Publishing; 2022.

Andrade C, Varadharajan N, Bascarane S, Menon V. Gestational exposure to benzodiazepines or z-hypnotics and neurodevelopmental disorders in offspring: systematic review and meta-analysis. Acta Psychiatr Scand. 2024;150(2):65–77.

Askew JP. Zolpidem addiction in a pregnant woman with a history of second-trimester bleeding. Pharmacotherapy. 2007;27(2):306–8.

Bacaro V, Benz F, Pappaccogli A, De Bartolo P, Johann AF, Palagini L, et al. Interventions for sleep problems during pregnancy: a systematic review. Sleep Med Rev. 2020;50:101234. https://doi.org/10.1016/j.smrv.2019.101234.

Bagger NT, Milidou I, Boie S, Glavind J. Perinatal outcomes after therapeutic rest in the latent phase of labor: a cohort study. Acta Obstet Gynecol Scand. 2023;102(9):1210–8.

Baglioni C, Tang NK, Johann AF, Altena E, Bramante A, Riemann D, et al. Insomnia and poor sleep quality during peripartum: a family issue with potential long term consequences on mental health. J Matern Fetal Neonatal Med. 2020;2:1–9. https://doi.org/10.1080/14767058.2020.1854718.

Ban L, West J, Gibson JE, Fiaschi L, Sokal R, Doyle P, Hubbard R, Smeeth L, Tata LJ. First trimester exposure to anxiolytic and hypnotic drugs and the risks of major congenital anomalies: a United Kingdom population-based cohort study. PLoS One. 2014;9(6):e100996.

Barker EC, Flygare J, Paruthi S, Sharkey KM. Living with narcolepsy: current management strategies, future prospects, and overlooked real-life concerns. Nat Sci Sleep. 2020;12:453–66.

Bechtel WD. Pharmacokinetics and metabolism of brotizolam in animals. Br J Clin Pharmacol. 1983;16(Suppl 2):261S–6S.

Biggio G, Biggio F, Talani G, Mostallino MC, Aguglia A, Aguglia E, Palagini L. Melatonin: from neurobiology to treatment. Brain Sci. 2021;11(9):1121.

Cannizzaro C, Martire M, Steardo L, Cannizzaro E, Gagliano M, Mineo A, Provenzano G. Prenatal exposure to diazepam and alprazolam, but not to zolpidem, affects behavioural stress reactivity in handling-naive and handling-habituated adult male rat progeny. Brain Res. 2002;953(1–2):170–80.

Chaudhry SK, Susser LC. Considerations in treating insomnia during pregnancy: a literature review. Psychosomatics. 2018;59(4):341–8.

Chen SJ, Shi L, Bao YP, Sun YK, Lin X, Que JY, Vitiello MV, Zhou YX, Wang YQ, Lu L. Prevalence of restless legs syndrome during pregnancy: a systematic review and meta-analysis. Sleep Med Rev. 2018;40:43–54.

Cooper J, Jauniaux E, Gulbis B, Bromley L. Placental transfer of temazepam and fentanyl in early human pregnancy. Reprod Biomed Online. 2001;2(3):165–71.

Damen L, Visser DH, Sie SD, van Weissenbruch MM. Apparent life-threatening event following maternal use of temazepam during labour. Case Rep Pediatr. 2014;2014:650605.

Dao K, Shechtman S, Diav-Citrin O, George N, Richardson JL, Rollason V, Pistelli A, Eleftheriou G, Berlin M, Ekobena P, Rousson V, Addor MC, Baud D, Buclin T, Panchaud A, Winterfeld U. Reproductive safety of trazodone after maternal exposure in early pregnancy: a comparative ENTIS cohort study. J Clin Psychopharmacol. 2023;43(1):12–9.

Diav-Citrin O, Okotore B, Lucarelli K, Koren G. Pregnancy outcome following first-trimester exposure to zopiclone: a prospective controlled cohort study. Am J Perinatol. 1999;16(4):157–60.

Einarson A, Bonari L, Voyer-Lavigne S. A multicentre prospective controlled study to determine the safety of trazodone and nefazodone use during pregnancy. Can J Psychiatr. 2003;48(2):106–10. https://doi.org/10.1177/070674370304800207.

Einarson A, Choi J, Einarson TR, Koren G. Incidence of major malformations in infants following antidepressant exposure in pregnancy: results of a large prospective cohort study. Can J Psychiatr. 2009;54(4):242–6.

Fang JH, Zhang SH, Yu XM, Yang Y. Effects of quercetin and melatonin in pregnant and gestational diabetic women. Lat Am J Pharm. 2016;35:1420–5.

Gaillot J, Heusse D, Hougton GW, Marc Aurele J, Dreyfus JF. Pharmacokinetics and metabolism of zopiclone. Int Pharmacopsychiatry. 1982;17(Suppl 2):76–91.

Garbazza C, Hackethal S, Riccardi S, Cajochen C, Cicolin A, D'Agostino A, et al. Polysomnographic features of pregnancy: a systematic review. Sleep Med Rev. 2020;50:101249. https://doi.org/10.1016/j.smrv.2019.101249.

Grigoriadis S, Graves L, Peer M, Mamisashvili L, Ruthirakuhan M, Chan P, Hennawy M, Parikh S, Vigod SN, Dennis CL, Steiner M, Brown C, Cheung A, Dawson H, Rector N, Guenette M, M. Richter pregnancy and delivery outcomes following benzodiazepine exposure: a systematic review and meta-analysis can. J Psychiatry. 2020;65:821.

Hobson SR, Gurusinghe S, Lim R, Alers NO, Miller SL, Kingdom JC, et al. Melatonin improves endothelial function in vitro and prolongs pregnancy in women with early-onset preeclampsia. J Pineal Res. 2018;65:e12508. https://doi.org/10.1111/jpi.12508.

Huitfeldt A, Sundbakk LM, Skurtveit S, Handal M, Nordeng H. Associations of maternal use of benzodiazepines or benzodiazepine-like hypnotics during pregnancy with immediate pregnancy outcomes in Norway. JAMA Netw Open. 2020;3(6):e205860.

Ishikawa H, Furugen A, Nishimura A, Umazume T, Ishikawa S, Aoyagi R, Narumi K, Okamoto K, Takekuma Y, Sugawara M, Kobayashi M. Validated UPLC-MS/MS method for quantification of melatonin receptor agonists and dual orexin receptor antagonists in human plasma and breast milk: application to quantify suvorexant and lemborexant in clinical samples. J Pharm Biomed Anal. 2024a;251:116432.

Ishikawa H, Furugen A, Nishimura A, Umazume T, Ishikawa S, Aoyagi R, Narumi K, Okamoto K, Takekuma Y, Sugawara M, Kobayashi M. Validated UPLC-MS/MS method for quantification of melatonin receptor agonists and dual orexin receptor antagonists in human plasma and breast milk: application to quantify suvorexant and lemborexant in clinical samples. J Pharm Biomed Anal. 2024b;251:116432.

Juric S, Newport DJ, Ritchie JC, Galanti M, Stowe ZN. Zolpidem (Ambien) in pregnancy: placental passage and outcome. Arch Womens Ment Health. 2009;12(6):441–6.

Kargas GA, Kargas SA, Bruyere HJ Jr, Gilbert EF, Opitz JM. Perinatal mortality due to interaction of diphenhydramine and temazepam. N Engl J Med. 1985;313(22):1417–8.

Kaufmann P, Muehlan C, Anliker-Ort M, Sabattini G, Siebers N, Dingemanse JJ. Transfer of the dual orexin receptor antagonist Daridorexant into breast milk of healthy lactating women. Clin Pharmacol. 2024;64(10):1278–87.

Kay-Stacey M, Attarian HP. Managing sleep disorders during pregnancy. Gender Genome. 2017;1:34–45. https://doi.org/10.1089/gg.2016.0006.

Kelly LE, et al. Neonatal benzodiazepines exposure during breastfeeding. J Pediatr. 2012;161(3):448–51.

Khazaie H, Ghadami MR, Knight DC, Emamian F, Tahmasian M. Insomnia treatment in the third trimester of pregnancy reduces postpartum depression symptoms: a randomized clinical trial. Psychiatry Res. 2013;210(3):901–5.

Kitagawa H, Esumi Y, Kurosawa S, Sekine S, Yokoshima T. Metabolism of 8-chloro-6-(o-chlorophenyl)-1-methyl-4H-s-triazolo [4,3-alpha] [1,4] benzodiazepine, triazolam, a new central depressant. I. Absorption, distribution and excretion in rats, dogs and monkeys. Xenobiotica. 1979;9(7):415–28.

Korade Z, Allen LB, Anderson A, Tallman KA, Genaro-Mattos TC, Porter NA, Mirnics K. Trazodone effects on developing brain. Transl Psychiatry. 2021;11(1):85.

Lebedevs TH, Wojnar-Horton RE, Yapp P, Roberts MJ, Dusci LJ, Hackett LP, Ilett KF. Excretion of temazepam in breast milk. Br J Clin Pharmacol. 1992;33(2):204–6.

Luciani M, Massoud M, Foligno S, Di Felice G, Pulcinelli F, Rapini N. Melatonin antiplatelets effect through breastfeeding: a sobering case. Haemophilia. 2019;25:138–9.

Matheson I, Sande HA, Gaillot J. The excretion of zopiclone into breast milk. Br J Clin Pharmacol. 1990;30:267–71.

Mathieu O, Masson F, Thompson MA, et al. Case report: in utero exposure and safe breastfeeding in two premature twins of a chronically treated mother with high doses of zopiclone. Fundam Clin Pharmacol. 2010;24(Suppl. S1):424. https://doi.org/10.1111/j.1472-8206.2010.00819.

McElhatton PR, Garbis HM, Eléfant E. The outcome of pregnancy in 689 women exposed to therapeutic doses of antidepressants. A collaborative study of the European Network of Teratology Information Services (ENTIS). Reprod Toxicol. 1996;10(4):285–94.

Mendes A, Silva V. Possible etiologies of restless legs syndrome in pregnancy: a narrative review. Sleep Sci. 2022;15(4):471–9.

Miller SL, Yawno T, Alers NO, Castillo-Melendez M, Supramaniam VG, VanZyl N, et al. Antenatal antioxidant treatment with melatonin to decrease newborn neurodevelopmental deficits and brain injury caused by fetal growth restriction. J Pineal Res. 2014;56:283–94. https://doi.org/10.1111/jpi.12121.

Miller MA, Mehta N, Clark-Bilodeau C, Bourjeily G. Sleep pharmacotherapy for common sleep disorders in pregnancy and lactation. Chest. 2020 Jan;157(1):184–97.

National Institute for Health and Care Excellence NICE. Antenatal and postnatal mental health clinical management and service guidance updated edition; 2018.

Nishimura A, Furugen A, Umazume T, Kitamura S, Soma M, Noshiro K, Takekuma Y, Sugawara M, Iseki K, Kobayashi M. Benzodiazepine concentrations in the breast milk and plasma of nursing mothers: estimation of relative infant dose. Breastfeed Med. 2021;16(5):424–31.

Noh Y, et al. First-trimester exposure to benzodiazepines and risk of congenital malformations in offspring: a population-based cohort study in South Korea. PLoS Med. 2022;19(3):e1003945.

Okatani Y, Okamoto K, Hayashi K, Wakatsuki A, Tamura S, Sagara Y. Maternal-fetal transfer of melatonin in pregnant women near term. J Pineal Res. 1998;25:129–34. https://doi.org/10.1111/j.1600-079x.1998.tb00550.x.

Okun ML, Schetter CD, Glynn LM. Poor sleep quality is associated with preterm birth. Sleep. 2011;34(11):1493–8. https://doi.org/10.5665/sleep.1384.

Paine SJ, Signal TL, Sweeney B, Priston M, Muller D, Smith A, et al. Maternal sleep disturbances in late pregnancy and the association with emergency caesarean section: a prospective cohort study. Sleep Health. 2020;6(1):65–70. https://doi.org/10.1016/j.sleh.2019.11.004.

Palagini L, Bianchini C. Pharmacotherapeutic management of insomnia and effects on sleep processes, neural plasticity, and brain systems modulating stress: a narrative review. Front Neurosci. 2022;16:893015.

Palagini L, Gemignani A, Banti S, Manconi M, Mauri M, Riemann D. Chronic sleep loss during pregnancy as a determinant of stress: impact on pregnancy outcome. Sleep Med. 2014;15(8):853–9. https://doi.org/10.1016/j.sleep.2014.02.013.

Palagini L, Manni R, Aguglia E, Amore M, Brugnoli R, Bioulac S, Bourgin P, Micoulaud Franchi JA, Girardi P, Grassi L, Lopez R, Mencacci C, Plazzi G, Maruani J, Minervino A, Philip P, Royant Parola S, Poirot I, Nobili L, Biggio G, Schroder CM, Geoffroy PA. International expert opinions and recommendations on the use of melatonin in the treatment of insomnia and circadian sleep disturbances in adult neuropsychiatric disorders. Front Psych. 2021;12:688890.

Palagini L, Bramante A, Baglioni C, Tang N, Grassi L, Altena E, Johann AF, Geoffroy PA, Biggio G, Mencacci C, Sharma V, Riemann D. Insomnia evaluation and treatment during peripartum: a joint position paper from the European insomnia network task force "sleep and women," the Italian Marcè society and international experts task force for perinatal mental health. Arch Womens Ment Health. 2022;25(3):561–75.

Palagini L, Cipriani E, Caruso V, Sharma V, Gemignani A, Bramante A, Miniati M, Riemann D. Insomnia during the perinatal period and its association with maternal and infant psychopathology: a systematic review and meta-analysis. Curr Psychiatry Rep. 2023;25(11):617–41.

Palagini L, Cipriani E, Miniati M, Bramante A, Gemignani A, Geoffroy PA, Riemann D. Insomnia, poor sleep quality and perinatal suicidal risk: a systematic review and meta-analysis. J Sleep Res. 2024a;33(2):e14000.

Palagini L, Miniati M, Driul L, Colizzi M, Comacchio C, Gemignani A, Balestrieri M. Insomnia in pregnancy research group (IPRG). Prenatal insomnia disorder may predict concurrent and postpartum psychopathology: a longitudinal study. J Sleep Res. 2024b;33(6):e14202.

Palagini L, Manni R, Liguori C, De Gennaro L, Gemignani A, Fanfulla F, Ferri R, Nobili L, Ferini-Strambi L. Evaluation and management of insomnia in the clinical practice in Italy: a 2023 update from the Insomnia Expert Consensus Group. J Neurol. 2024c;271(4):1668–79.

Pengo MF, Won CH, Bourjeily G. Sleep in women across the life span. Chest. 2018;154(1):196–206. https://doi.org/10.1016/j.chest.2018.04.005.

Picchietti DL, Hensley JG, Bainbridge JL, Lee KA, Manconi M, McGregor JA, Silver RM, Trenkwalder C, Walters AS. International restless legs syndrome study group (IRLSSG). Consensus clinical practice guidelines for the diagnosis and treatment of restless legs syndrome/Willis-Ekbom disease during pregnancy and lactation. Sleep Med Rev. 2015;22:64–77.

Pons G, et al. Zolpidem excretion in breast milk. Eur J Clin Pharmacol. 1989;37:245–8.

Prosperetti C, Manconi M. Restless legs syndrome/willis-ekbom disease and pregnancy. Sleep Med Clin. 2015;10(3):323–9.

Rawal S, Brimhall D, Aluri J, et al. Lemborexant levels in breast milk after single doses in healthy, lactating women. Br J Clin Pharmacol. 2024;90:158–63.

Riemann D, Nissen C, Palagini L, Otte A, Perlis ML, Spiegelhalder K. The neurobiology, investigation, and treatment of chronic insomnia. Lancet Neurol. 2015;14(5):547–58. https://doi.org/10.1016/S1474-4422(15)00021-6.

Riemann D, Espie CA, Altena E, Arnardottir ES, Baglioni C, Bassetti CLA, Bastien C, Berzina N, Bjorvatn B, Dikeos D, Dolenc Groselj L, Ellis JG, Garcia-Borreguero D, Geoffroy PA, Gjerstad M, Gonçalves M, Hertenstein E, Hoedlmoser K, Hion T, Holzinger B, Janku K, Jansson-Fröjmark M, Järnefelt H, Jernelöv S, Jennum PJ, Khachatryan S, Krone L, Kyle SD, Lancee J, Leger D, Lupusor A, Marques DR, Nissen C, Palagini L, Paunio T, Perogamvros L, Pevernagie D, Schabus M, Shochat T, Szentkiralyi A, Van Someren E, van Straten A, Wichniak A, Verbraecken J, Spiegelhalder K. The European Insomnia Guideline: an update on the diagnosis and treatment of insomnia 2023. J Sleep Res. 2023;32(6):e14035. https://doi.org/10.1111/jsr.14035.

Saito J, Ishii M, Miura Y, Yakuwa N, Kawasaki H, Suzuki T, Yamatani A, Sago H, Tachibana Y, Murashima A. Brotizolam during pregnancy and lactation: brotizolam levels in maternal serum, cord blood, breast milk, and neonatal serum. Breastfeed Med. 2021;16(7):579–82. https://doi.org/10.1089/bfm.2021.0013.

Saito J, Tachibana Y, Wada YS, Yakuwa N, Kawasaki H, Suzuki T, Sago H, Yamatani A, Murashima A. Transfer of brotizolam, periciazine, and sulpiride in cord blood and breast milk, and alprazolam in breast milk: a case report. J Pharm Health Care Sci. 2022a;8(1):10.

Saito J, Tachibana Y, Sano Wada Y, et al. Presence of hypnotics in the cord blood and breast milk, with no adverse effects in the infant: a case report. Breastfeed Med. 2022b;17:349–52.

Saito J, Tachibana Y, Kawasaki H, et al. Transfer of zolpidem to cord blood and breast milk: a case series evaluating zolpidem serum levels and outcomes in birth and suckling infants. Breastfeed Med. 2022c;17:1034–8.

Saito J, Tachibana Y, Sano Wada Y, Kawasaki H, Miura Y, Oho M, Aoyagi K, Yakuwa N, Suzuki T, Yamatani A, Sago H, Murashima A. Presence of hypnotics in the cord blood and breast milk, with no adverse effects in the infant: a case report. Breastfeed Med. 2022d;17(4):349–52.

Saito J, Ishii M, Sandaiji N, et al. Lemborexant levels in maternal serum, cord blood, and breast milk during pregnancy and lactation: a case report. Psychiatry Clin Neurosci Rep. 2023;2

Sakai T, Matsuda H, Watanabe N. Triazolam (Halcion) intoxication in a neonate – a first report. Eur J Pediatr. 1996;155(12):1065–6.

Salari N, Darvishi N, Khaledi-Paveh B, Vaisi-Raygani A, Jalali R, Daneshkhah A, Bartina Y, Mohammadi M. A systematic review and meta-analysis of prevalence of insomnia in the third trimester of pregnancy. BMC Pregnancy Childbirth. 2021;21(1):284.

Schenker S, Yang Y, Perez A, Acuff RV, Papas AM, Henderson G, et al. Antioxidant transport by the human placenta. Clin Nutr. 1998;17:159–67. https://doi.org/10.1016/s0261-5614(98)80052-6.

Sedov ID, Anderson NJ, Dhillon AK, Tomfohr-Madsen LM. Insomnia symptoms during pregnancy: a meta-analysis. J Sleep Res. 2021;30(1):13207.

Sharma A, Sayeed N, Khees CR, Akhtar S. High dose zolpidem induced fetal neural tube defects. Curr Drug Saf. 2011;6(2):128–9.

Sharma V, Sharkey KM, Palagini L, Mazmanian D, Thomson M. Preventing recurrence of postpartum depression by regulating sleep. Expert Rev Neurother. 2023;23(8):1–9.

Sivertsen B, Hysing M, Dørheim SK. Eberhard-gran M trajectories of maternal sleep problems before and after childbirth: a longitudinal population-based study. BMC Pregnancy Childbirth. 2015;15:129.

Steinweg K, Nippita T, Cistulli PA, Bin YS. Maternal and neonatal outcomes associated with restless legs syndrome in pregnancy: a systematic review. Sleep Med Rev. 2020;54:101359.

Swanson LM, Kalmbach DA, Raglan GB, O'Brien LM. Perinatal insomnia and mental health: a review of recent literature. Curr Psychiatry Rep. 2020;22(12):73.

The International Restless Legs Syndrome Study Group. Validation of the international restless legs syndrome study group rating scale for restless legs syndrome. Sleep Med. 2003;4(2):121–32. https://doi.org/10.1016/s1389-9457(02)00258-7.

Uguz F. A new safety scoring system for the use of psychotropic drugs during lactation. Am J Ther. 2021;28(1):e118–26.

US Food and Drug Administration. Quviviq (Daridorexant): highlights of prescribing information. 2022. https://www.accessdata.fda.gov/drugsa. Accessed 8 No 2023.

Vine T, Brown GM, Frey BN. Melatonin use during pregnancy and lactation: a scoping review of human studies. Braz J Psychiatry. 2022;44(3):342–8.

Wang LH, Lin HC, Lin CC, Chen YH, Lin HC. Increased risk of adverse pregnancy outcomes in women receiving zolpidem during pregnancy. Clin Pharmacol Ther. 2010;88(3):369–74.

Wang X, Zhang T, Ekheden I, Chang Z, Hellner C, et al. Prenatal exposure to benzodiazepines and Z-drugs in humans and risk of adverse neurodevelopmental outcomes in offspring: a systematic review. Neurosci Biobehav Rev. 2022;137:104647.

Wikner BN, Källén B. Are hypnotic benzodiazepine receptor agonists teratogenic in humans? J Clin Psychopharmacol. 2011;31(3):356–9.

Zheng X, Zhu Z, Chen J, He J, Zhu Y, Zhang L, Qu F. Efficacy of cognitive behavioural therapy for insomnia or sleep disturbance in pregnant women: a systematic review ad meta-analysis. J Sleep Res. 2023;32(2):e13808.

[illegible]

patients who went through EMDR with tapping stimuli, the authors suggested that EMDR has desensitization effects on nausea and vomiting and on their triggers in HG cases in positive manner providing rapid recovery in the HG symptoms increasing the coping abilities of the effected women (Kavakci and Yenicesu 2014).

24.4.2 Acupuncture in HG

Because of the medical limitations in nausea and vomiting of pregnancy (NVP) and hyperemesis gravidarum HG due to pregnancy and possible fetal outcomes still mostly unclear and hard to manage as a part of study that must take place during pregnancy, the need for complementary therapies such as acupuncture is proposed to alleviate symptoms.

According to a current systematic review and meta-analysis, including twenty-four (24) randomized controlled trials involving 2390 women, acupuncture combined with western medicine is addressed to be more effective treatment for nausea and vomiting of pregnancy (NVP) than western medicine alone. PC6, ST36, and CV12 are the most commonly used acupoints (Jin et al. 2024).

24.4.3 Hypnotherapy in HG

Hypnosis or hypnotic relaxation in medical circumstances takes place more than ever in the literature because of its nature and being an option as a non-medical approach for the patients with confounding states. Especially in HG patients experiencing symptoms in the very early period of pregnancy hypnosis can be used as an only or augmenting intervention. In a review article that six studies about using hypnotherapy in HG were assessed, despite the methodology differences all reported encouraging positive outcomes (McCormack 2010).

In a Turkish study which assessed the effects of hypnosis on patients diagnosed with HG, patients were randomized to receive either conventional therapy alone ($n = 23$) or adjuvant hypnotherapy plus conventional therapy ($n = 18$). Participants in the treatment group received 2 sessions of hypnosis and were instructed in daily self-hypnosis practice. Those in the control group received treatment as usual. Results indicated that adjunctive use of hypnotherapy with patients diagnosed with HG experienced significantly reduced severity of nausea and frequency of vomiting compared to other groups of HG patients (Ozgunay et al. 2022).

24.5 Conclusion

The recent data in the literature about HG underline the multifactorial associations of etiology and pathogenesis. HG still comes out with significant burden on health care costs in all over the world. The new therapeutic options with multidisciplinary aspects and continuing updates will enlighten the problem. Social support systems

Table 24.1 Expert recommendations based on scientific evidence and clinical experience

Psychiatric examination and follow-up should be part of HG treatment
Thoughts of elective abortion or pregnancy termination should be questioned
Social support systems must be assessed
Drugs should be used for a short term, with intermittent and as low doses as possible
Also non-pharmacological interventions like EMDR, hypnotherapy, or acupuncture should be addressed as part of the solution
Possible additional pathologies must be excluded and examination including full blood and biochemical screening must be made
I.v. fluids help correct dehydration and improve symptoms whereas dextrose saline may be more effective at reducing nausea than normal saline
Primary or transient hyperparathyroidism must be assessed in women presenting with HG due to possible confounding situation

of the patient must be assessed while thoughts of elective abortion or pregnancy termination should be questioned. Psychiatric evaluation must be a basic part of the multidisciplinary aspect (Table 24.1). The HG patient must be referred to perinatal mental health specialist when needed. New studies should take place pointing not only pharmacological aspects but also non-pharmacological interventions like EMDR, hypnotherapy, and acupuncture. Women's perspectives on management and outcomes should not be ignored.

References

Aksoy H, Aksoy Ü, Karadağ Öİ, Hacimusalar Y, Açmaz G, Aykut G, Çağlı F, Yücel B, Aydın T, Babayiğit MA. Depression levels in patients with hyperemesis gravidarum: a prospective case-control study. Springerplus. 2015;4:34.

Beirne ER, Andrews LB, Murtagh LP, Browne S, Curran SB, O'Brien EC. The far-reaching burden of hyperemesis Gravidarum – an exploration of women's experiences and perceptions of healthcare support. Women Health. 2023;63(7):485–94.

Benson BC, Guinto RE, Parks JR. Primary hyperparathyroidism mimicking hyperemesis gravidarum. Hawaii J Med Public Health. 2013;72(1):11–3.

Boelig RC, Barton SJ, Saccone G, Kelly AJ, Edwards SJ, Berghella V. Interventions for treating hyperemesis gravidarum. Cochrane Database Syst Rev. 2016;2016(5):CD010607.

Erginbas Kender E, Yuksel G, Ger C, Ozer U. Eating attitudes, depression and anxiety levels of patients with hyperemesis gravidarum hospitalized in an obstetrics and gynecology clinic Düşünen Adam. J Psychiatry Neurol Sci. 2015;28:119–26.

Galvin SL, Coulson CC. Addressing cannabis consumption among patients with hyperemesis gravidarum. AJOG Glob Rep. 2023;3(2):100180.

Goodwin TM. Hyperemesis gravidarum. Obstet Gynecol Clin N Am. 2008;35:401–17.

Guttuso T Jr, Messing S, Tu X, Mullin P, Shepherd R, Strittmatter C, Saha S, Thornburg LL. Effect of gabapentin on hyperemesis gravidarum: a double-blind, randomized controlled trial. Am J Obstet Gynecol MFM. 2021;3(1):100273.

Havnen GC, Truong MB, Do MH, Heitmann K, Holst L, Nordeng H. Women's perspectives on the management and consequences of hyperemesis gravidarum – a descriptive interview study. Scand J Prim Health Care. 2019;37(1):30–40.

Hoirisch-Clapauch S, Brenner B, Nardi AE. Adverse obstetric and neonatal outcomes in women with mental disorders. Thromb Res. 2015;135(Suppl 1):S60–3.

Hussein KS. Hyperemesis Gravidarum in first-trimester pregnant Saudi women: is *helicobacter pylori* a risk factor? Front Physiol. 2020;11:575.
Jansen LAW, Koot MH, et al. The Windsor definition for hyperemesis Gravidarum: a multistakeholder international consensus definition. Eur J Obstet Gynecol Reprod Biol. 2021;266(November):15–22.
Jin B, Han Y, Jiang Y, Zhang J, Shen W, Zhang Y. Acupuncture for nausea and vomiting during pregnancy: a systematic review and meta-analysis. Complement Ther Med. 2024;85:103079.
Kavakci O, Yenicesu GI. Eye movement desensitization and reprocessing (EMDR) for hyperemesis gravidarum: a case series. Dusunen Adam J Psychiatry Neurol Sci. 2014;27(4):335–41.
Lacasse A, Rey E, Ferreira E, Morin C, Bérard A. Epidemiology of nausea and vomiting of pregnancy: prevalence, severity, determinants, and the importance of race/ethnicity. BMC Pregnancy Childbirth. 2009;9:26.
Lazarus JH. Hyperthyroidism during pregnancy: etiology, diagnosis and management. Womens Health (Lond). 2005 Jul;1(1):97–104.
London V, Grube S, Sherer DM, Abulafia O. Hyperemesis Gravidarum: a review of recent literature. Pharmacology. 2017;100(3–4):161–71.
McCormack D. Hypnosis for hyperemesis gravidarum. J Obstet Gynaecol. 2010;30:647–53.
Mitchell-Jones N, Lawson K, Bobdiwala S, Alice Farren J, Tobias A, Bourne T, Bottomley C. Association between hyperemesis gravidarum and psychological symptoms, psychosocial outcomes and infant bonding: a two-point prospective case–control multicentre survey study in an inner city setting. Br Med J Open. 2020;10(10):e039715.
O'Donnell A, McParlin C, Robson SC, Beyer F, Moloney E, Bryant A, Bradley J, Muirhead C, Nelson-Piercy C, Newbury-Birch D, Norman J, Simpson E, Swallow B, Yates L, Vale L. Treatments for hyperemesis gravidarum and nausea and vomiting in pregnancy: a systematic review and economic assessment. Health Technol Assess. 2016;20(74):1–268.
Omay O, Einarson A. Is mirtazapine an effective treatment for nausea and vomiting of pregnancy?: a case series. J Clin Psychopharmacol. 2017;37:260–1. https://doi.org/10.1097/JCP.0000000000000656.
Ozgunay SE, Dincgez B, Karasu D, Ozgen G, Taymur I, Eminoglu S, Ceylan I. Adjuvant hypnotherapy for hyperemesis Gravidarum: a randomized pilot study. Int J Clin Exp Hypn. 2022;70(3):277–85.
Shapiro F. Efficacy of the eye movement desensitization procedure in the treatment of traumatic memories. J Trauma Stress. 1989;2(2):199–223. https://doi.org/10.1002/jts.2490020207.
Soltani H, Taylor GM. Changing attitudes and perceptions to hyperemesis gravidarum. RCM Midwives. 2003;6(12):520–4.
Stoba J, Henrich W, Richter R, Sehouli J, David M. Auswirkungen einer hyperemesis gravidarum auf Schwangerschaftsverlauf und Geburtsausgang unter besonderer Berücksichtigung des Risikofaktors Migrationshintergrund [effects of hyperemesis gravidarum on the course of pregnancy and birth, with special attention to the risk factor of migration background]. Z Geburtshilfe Neonatol. 2021;225(1):39–46.
Uguz F. Low-dose mirtazapine added to selective serotonin reuptake inhibitors in pregnant women with major depression or panic disorder including symptoms of severe nausea, insomnia and decreased appetite: three cases. J Matern Fetal Neonatal Med. 2013;26:1066–8. https://doi.org/10.3109/14767058.2013.766697.
Uguz F. Low-dose mirtazapine in treatment of major depression developed following severe nausea and vomiting during pregnancy: two cases. Gen Hosp Psychiatry. 2014;36:e5–6. https://doi.org/10.1016/j.genhosppsych.2013.07.016.
Uguz F, Gezginc K, Kayhan F, Cicek E, Kantarci AH. Is hyperemesis gravidarum associated with mood, anxiety and personality disorders: a case-control study. Gen Hosp Psychiatry. 2012;34:398–402.
Yilmaz BA, Altay M, Değertekin CK, Çimen AR, Iyidir ÖT, Biri A, Yüksel O, Törüner FB, Arslan M. Hyperparathyroid crisis presenting with hyperemesis gravidarum. Arch Gynecol Obstet. 2014;290(4):811–4.